T0195190

Applied Pharmacology for Veterinary Technicians

Sixth Edition

Applied Pharmacology for Veterinary Technicians

Sixth Edition

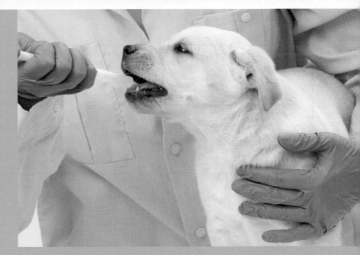

Lisa A. Martini-Johnson, DVM, CVT
Director
Veterinary Technology Program
Lehigh Carbon Community College
Schnecksville, Pennsylvania

ELSEVIER

Elsevier
1600 John F. Kennedy Blvd.
Ste 1800
Philadelphia, PA 19103-2899

APPLIED PHARMACOLOGY FOR VETERINARY TECHNICIANS,
SIXTH EDITION

ISBN: 978-0-323-68068-4

Notice

Practitioners and researchers must always rely on their own experience and knowledge in evaluating and using any information, methods, compounds or experiments described herein. Because of rapid advances in the medical sciences, in particular, independent verification of diagnoses and drug dosages should be made. To the fullest extent of the law, no responsibility is assumed by Elsevier, authors, editors or contributors for any injury and/or damage to persons or property as a matter of products liability, negligence or otherwise, or from any use or operation of any methods, products, instructions, or ideas contained in the material herein.

Previous editions copyrighted 2015, 2009, 2004, 2000, 1996

Library of Congress Control Number: 2020936210

Senior Content Strategist: Brandi Graham
Senior Content Development Specialist: Laura Klein
Publishing Services Manager: Deepthi Unni
Project Manager: Radjan Lourde Selvanadin
Design Direction: Brian Salisbury

Printed in India

Last digit is the print number: 9 8 7 6 5 4

This edition is dedicated to all veterinary technology students and graduates.

To my loving parents, Louis and Angeline, for your inspiration, support,
and encouragement. I cannot express how grateful I am for having
such wonderful parents, who taught me the value of strong principles.
I would not be where I am today without the both of you!

To my husband, Morvin, for being so incredibly supportive,
patient, and always encouraging me. You truly are my everything!

To my daughter, Mervisa, for always telling me about
my strengths I did not know I had.

In loving memory of my brother, Charles; you always
inspired me to do my very best.

PREFACE

Applied Pharmacology for Veterinary Technicians, Sixth Edition, is designed for both the graduate veterinary technician and the student. As a teaching and reference book, its purpose is to help veterinary technicians become familiar with the many veterinary pharmacologic agents and their uses, adverse side effects, and dosage forms. I believe it is very important for the veterinary technician to understand the uses of pharmacologic agents and to have the ability to provide client education under the supervision of the attending veterinarian. One of the key features of this book is that its format provides quick and easy access to important chapter content. Each chapter is introduced with learning objectives, a chapter outline, and key terms. "Technician's Notes" throughout the text provide helpful hints and emphasize important points technicians should be aware of to avoid errors and increase efficiency. The appendices provide the pharmacologic agents in alphabetical order for quick referencing. A comprehensive glossary provides the students with quick access to expand the understanding and concepts of terms used in pharmacology.

NEW TO THIS EDITION

New features have been added to the sixth edition to aid the student and veterinary technician in the study and application of pharmacology. All of the drug information throughout the book has been updated and new drugs that have entered the market since the publication of the fifth edition have been included to keep you current with the newest pharmacologic agents and their uses, adverse side effects, and dosage forms.

Additional features of this new edition include the following:

- Charts, tables, and reference boxes have been added throughout the text to reinforce the material and allow for quick access to key information. Condensed tables in Chapter 17 (Immunologic Drugs) allow the student to quickly review vaccination protocols for each species.
- A reworked structure of Chapter 3, Practical Calculations, has been expanded to better prepare students in performing drug calculations. Examples and step-by-step descriptions have been added for the different types of drug calculations.
- A large number of "Technician Notes" have been added throughout each chapter to highlight important points and concepts.
- Coverage of fluid therapy has been expanded to prepare veterinary technicians for the role they play in fluid, electrolyte, and therapeutic nutritional therapy, which can be critically important to the outcome of a case.
- A new chapter on Emergency drugs including antidotes and reversal agents.
- Numerous added sections within existing chapters.
- Case scenarios are included in each chapter to apply key concepts in a clinical situation to help reinforce learning.
- Additional review questions at the end of each chapter provides an excellent review of the chapter content, as well as a review for the Veterinary Technician National Exam (VTNE).
- This edition continues to be in color, bringing important concepts to life.
- The appendices have been updated to reflect the current pharmacologic agents and provides the student with quick referencing.

EVOLVE WEBSITE

An accompanying Evolve website is available to instructors and students using this textbook. The Evolve student resources offer the following features to reinforce textbook content and help students master key concepts:

- **Drug Administration Videos:** Twelve narrated video clips demonstrate drug administration techniques (oral, injectable, inhaled) and intravenous (IV) preparation for dogs and cats
- **Drug Calculators with Related Exercises:** Six drug calculators with accompanying word problems help students perform accurate drug calculations
- **Drug Label Image Collection:** Over 135 photos of drug labels, divided by chapters and organized alphabetically, help students become familiar with drug information and packaging encountered in practice

- **Animations:** Animations of pharmacologic processes, such as passive diffusion and receptor interaction, help students visualize and understand key concepts
- **Dosage Calculation Exercises:** Exercises reinforce calculations skills and provide valuable practice in the areas of:
  - Drug Calculation Methods
  - Oral and Enteral Medication Administration
  - Intravenous Infusion
  - Critical Care Calculations
- **Answers to Review Questions:** Answers to the chapter review questions allow students to gauge comprehension of key topics.

TEACH INSTRUCTOR RESOURCES

NEW to this edition is the Evolve TEACH Instructor Resources, which offer the following features:
- TEACH Instructor Resources
- Lesson Plans
- PowerPoint Slides
- Student Handouts
- Answer Keys
- Test Bank questions
- Image collection
- Access to student resources

The goal of this book is to focus on key topics and combine the comprehensiveness of a veterinary pharmacology textbook with the coverage of pharmacologic fundamentals needed by veterinary technicians. No longer will veterinary technician educators have to draw from two sources for this type of coverage; the new TEACH instructor resources will also assist in classroom planning, organization, and preparation. The scope and organization of the information in this book will make it a useful reference for the practicing veterinary technician as well.

Lisa A. Martini-Johnson, DVM, CVT

ACKNOWLEDGMENTS

I would like to acknowledge and thank the editors and staff at Elsevier including Brandi Graham and Laura Klein for their support, guidance, and patience throughout the writing and editing stages of this new edition. Your professional support and reminders kept the project on track. I would also like to thank Radjan Lourde Selvanadin, the project manager, for providing me direction and support through the final stages of the new edition.

I would like to express my sincere appreciation to Tara J. Fetzer, DVM, DACVECC, who was not only one of my graduates but continued her education and earned her Doctorate in Veterinary Medicine. She is also a Diplomate of ACVECC. Dr. Fetzer developed an emergency triage flow chart for the new emergency drug chapter and contributed case scenarios throughout some of the chapters.

I particularly would like to thank my veterinary technician students, past and present, for sharing their thoughts, making suggestions, and giving me valuable feedback in providing new ideas for the sixth edition. I would like to thank and acknowledge the previous two authors, Boyce P. Wanamaker, DVM and Kathy Lockett Massey, LVMT for sharing their expertise of pharmacologic concepts and valuable content of previous editions.

Lastly, I would like to recognize veterinary technicians for their commitment to the profession and their desire for knowledge while promoting competent care and humane treatment of animals. Continue to inspire those around you and make decisions that define the level of integrity for the profession as a whole.

TABLE OF CONTENTS

General Pharmacology

OBJECTIVES

After studying this chapter, you should be able to
1. Define terms related to general pharmacology.
2. List common sources of drugs used in veterinary medicine.
3. Outline the basic principles of pharmacotherapeutics.
4. Define the difference between prescription (legend) and over-the-counter drugs.
5. Describe the events that occur after a drug is administered to a patient.
6. List and describe the routes used for administration of drugs and why the bioavailability differs among the various routes.
7. Discuss drug distribution, define *biotransformation,* and list common chemical reactions involved in the process of biotransformation.
8. List the routes of drug excretion.
9. Discuss in basic terms the mechanisms by which drugs produce their effects in the body.
10. Discuss the mechanisms of clinically important drug interactions.
11. Discuss the different names that a particular drug is given.
12. List the items that should be included on a drug label.
13. List the steps and discuss the processes involved in gaining approval for a new drug.
14. List the government agencies involved in the regulation of animal health products.
15. Describe reasons for dispensing rather than prescribing drugs in veterinary medicine.
16. Discuss the primary methods of drug marketing.
17. List acceptable methods of drug disposal.

OUTLINE

KEY TERMS

Adverse drug event
Adverse drug reaction
Agonist
Antagonist
Bioavailability
Compounding
Drug
Efficacy
Extralabel use
First-pass effect
Half-life
Legend

Loading dose
Manufacturing
Metabolism (biotransformation)
Over-the-counter drugs
Parenteral
Partition coefficient
Prescription (legend) drug
Regimen
Residue
Therapeutic index
Veterinarian–client–patient relationship
Withdrawal time

INTRODUCTION

Veterinary technicians are an essential component of the efficient health care delivery team in veterinary medicine. One of the important tasks that veterinary technicians carry out is administration of **drugs** to animals on the order of a veterinarian. It is mandatory that technicians have a thorough knowledge of the types and actions of drugs used in veterinary medicine because this task may have serious consequences in terms of the outcome of a case. Technicians should have an understanding of the reasons for using drugs, called *indications*, and the reasons for not using drugs, called *contraindications* (pharmacotherapeutics). They also should know what happens to drugs once they enter the body (pharmacokinetics), how drugs exert their effects (pharmacodynamics), and how adverse drug reactions manifest themselves (toxicity). Because veterinarians dispense a large number of drugs, technicians also must be well versed in the components of a valid **veterinarian–client–patient relationship (VCPR)**, the importance of proper labeling of dispensed products, and methods of client education on the proper use of products to avoid toxic effects or residue. Finally, technicians should have a basic understanding of the laws that apply to drug use in veterinary medicine and the concept of the marketing of veterinary drugs. In short, veterinary technicians must have a working knowledge of the science of veterinary pharmacology.

TECHNICIAN NOTES

- A valid VCPR must exist for a veterinarian to prescribe medication.

BOX 1.1 Case Scenario

An owner was out of town with her dog, Mia, and noticed that there was only one more tablet of phenobarbital left which was prescribed by her veterinarian for seizures. The owner went to a local veterinary hospital with Mia to obtain a refill of phenobarbital and gave the receptionist the prescription bottle. The receptionist stated that they would not be able to refill her prescription and that she would need to speak with the veterinarian. The attending vet spoke with the owner about the need to contact her primary vet, who prescribed the medication, in order to discuss Mia's condition and medical history and the dose of the drug. The primary vet stated that, 3 months ago, Mia was seen for her yearly wellness visit, she was up-to-date on her vaccines and a blood profile was performed in which her liver values were within normal limits and her phenobarbital levels were in the therapeutic range. The owner signed a consent form that the primary vet faxed to the hospital so Mia's medical records could be faxed over. The attending veterinarian reviewed the medical records and performed a physical examination on Mia and made a clinical judgement to continue the dose of phenobarbital for her seizures and gave her 30 tablets of phenobarbital. In this case, a valid VCPR exists as the attending veterinarian obtained a history, performed a physical exam and reviewed Mia's prior medical records. The veterinarian gave her his business card and told her if she has any questions or concerns to give him a call.

DRUG SOURCES

Traditional sources of drugs are plants (botanical) and minerals. Plants have long been a source of drugs. The active components of plants that are useful as drugs include alkaloids, glycosides, gums,

TABLE 1.1   Inactive Ingredients.

Inactive Ingredient	Function	Examples
Binder	Holds tablet together	Cellulose, lactose, methylcellulose, sorbitol, starch, xylitol, and others
Coating	Protects tablet from breaking, absorbing moisture, and early disintegration	Beeswax, carob extract, methylcellulose, cellulose acetate, acrylic resin, and others
Coloring agents	Provide color and enhance appearance	Yellow No. 5, annatto, caramel color, titanium oxide, FD&C Blue No. 1, FD&C Red No. 3, and others
Disintegrants	Expand when exposed to liquid, allowing tablets and capsules to dissolve and disperse their active ingredients	Cellulose products, crospovidone, sodium starch glycolate, and starch
Emulsifiers	Allow fat-soluble and water-soluble agents to mix so they do not separate	Stearic acid, xanthan gum, lethicin, and vegetable oils
Fillers/diluents	Increase bulk or volume	Calcium carbonate, calcium sulfate, cellulose lactose, mannitol, sorbitol, starch, sucrose, and vegetable oils
Flavor agents	Create a desired taste or mask an undesirable taste	Beeswax, carob extract, glyceryl triacetate, and natural orange
Flow agents	Prevent powders from sticking together	Calcium stearate, glyceryl triacetate, polyethylene glycol, silica, sodium benzoate, and talc
Humectants	Hold moisture in a product	Glycerin, glycerol, glycerol triacetate, and sorbitol
Preservatives	Prevent degradation and extend the shelf life of a product	Citric acid, glycerol, potassium benzoate, sodium benzoate, and others
Sweetening agents	Improve taste	Aspartate, fructose, glycerin, sorbitol, sucrose, and xylitol
Thickening agents	Increase the viscosity of a product	Methylcellulose, povidone, sorbitol, and others

Adapted from ConsumerLab.com: Review article: Inactive ingredients in supplements (website). https://www.consumerlab.com/reviews/Inactive_Ingredients_in_Supplements/inactiveingredients. Accessed July 30, 2013.

resins, and oils. The names of alkaloids usually end in -ine, and the names of glycosides end in -in (Williams & Baer, 1990). Examples of alkaloids include atropine, caffeine, and nicotine. Digoxin and digitoxin are examples of glycosides. Bacteria and molds (e.g., *Penicillium*) produce many of the antibiotics (penicillin) and anthelmintics (ivermectin) in use today. Animals once were important as a source of hormones such as insulin and as a source of anticoagulants such as heparin. Today, most hormones are synthesized in a laboratory. Mineral sources of drugs include electrolytes (sodium, potassium, and chloride), iron, selenium, and others. Laboratories are one of the most important sources of currently used drugs because chemists are finding methods of reproducing drugs previously obtained through plant and animal sources. Advances in recombinant deoxyribonucleic

acid (DNA) technology have made it possible for animal and human products (e.g., insulin) in bacteria to be produced in large quantities.

INACTIVE INGREDIENTS

Veterinary pharmaceutic products and supplements may contain substances in addition to active ingredients. Inactive ingredients are classified as binders, coatings, coloring agents, disintegrants, emulsifiers, fillers, flavorings, flow agents, humectants, preservatives, sweeteners, and thickeners (Table 1.1).

PHARMACOTHERAPEUTICS

Veterinarians are challenged by the task of assessing a patient to determine a diagnosis and arrive at a plan of treatment. If the plan of treatment includes the use of drugs, the veterinarian must choose an appropriate drug and a drug regimen. The drug is selected through the use of one or more broadly defined methods called *diagnostic, empirical,* or *symptomatic.* The diagnostic method involves assessment of a patient, including a history, physical examination, laboratory tests, and other diagnostic procedures, to arrive at a specific diagnosis. Once the diagnosis has been determined, the causative microorganism or altered physiologic state is revealed to allow selection of the appropriate drug. The empirical method calls on the use of practical experience and common sense when the drug choice is made. In other instances, drugs are chosen to treat the symptoms or signs of a disease if a specific diagnosis cannot be determined. In veterinary medicine, the comparative cost of a drug also may be an important consideration in selection of an appropriate drug. Once the drug to be used in treatment has been decided, the next step for the veterinarian is to design the plan for administering the drug. This plan, called a **regimen**, includes details about the following:

- The route of administration.
- The total amount to be given (dose).
- How often the drug is to be given (frequency).
- How long the drug will be given (duration).

Every drug has the potential to cause harmful effects if it is given to the wrong patient or according to the wrong regimen. Some medications have greater potential than others for producing harmful outcomes. According to the U.S. Food and Drug Administration (FDA), when a drug has potential toxic effects or must be administered in a way that requires the services of trained personnel, that drug cannot be approved for animal use except when given under the supervision of a veterinarian. In such a case, the drug is classified as a **prescription drug** and must be labeled with the following statement: "Caution: Federal law restricts the use of this drug to use by or on the order of a licensed veterinarian." This statement sometimes is referred to as the *legend*, and the drug is called a *legend (prescription) drug*. Labels that state "For veterinary use only" or "Sold to veterinarians only" do not designate prescription drugs. Technicians should be aware that prescription drugs often have been approved by the FDA for use in specific species or for particular diseases or conditions. Veterinarians have some discretion to use a drug in ways not indicated by the label, if they take responsibility for the outcome of use. Use of a drug in a way not specified by the label is called **extralabel use**.

Federal law and sound medical practices dictate that prescription drugs should not be dispensed indiscriminately. Before prescription drugs are issued or extralabel use is undertaken, a valid VCPR must exist. For this relationship to occur, several conditions must be met. These include but are not limited to the following:

- The veterinarian has assumed responsibility for making clinical judgments about the health of the animal(s) and the need for treatment, and the client has agreed to follow the veterinarian's instructions.
- The veterinarian has sufficient knowledge of the animal(s) to issue a diagnosis. The veterinarian must have seen the animal recently and must be acquainted with its husbandry.
- The veterinarian must be available for follow-up evaluation of the patient.

Drugs that do not have enough potential to be toxic or that do not require administration in special ways do not require the supervision of a veterinarian for administration. These drugs are called *over-the-counter drugs* because they may be purchased without a prescription; these drugs contain ingredients that are very safe or have low concentrations of an active ingredient. Drugs that have the potential for abuse or dependence have been classified as *controlled substances.* Careful records of the inventory and use of these drugs must be maintained, and some of them must be kept in a locked storage area.

When a drug and its regimen have been selected, veterinary technicians often are directed through verbal or written orders to administer the drug. Technicians have several important responsibilities in carrying out these orders:

1. Ensuring that the correct drug is being administered
2. Administering the drug by the correct route and at the correct time
3. Carefully observing the animal's response to the drug
4. Questioning any medication orders that are not clear
5. Creating and affixing labels to medication containers accurately
6. Explaining administration instructions to clients
7. Recording appropriate information in the medical record

Technicians should be aware that even when the correct drug is administered in a correct manner, an unexpected adverse reaction might occur in a patient. All adverse events or reactions should be reported immediately to the veterinarian.

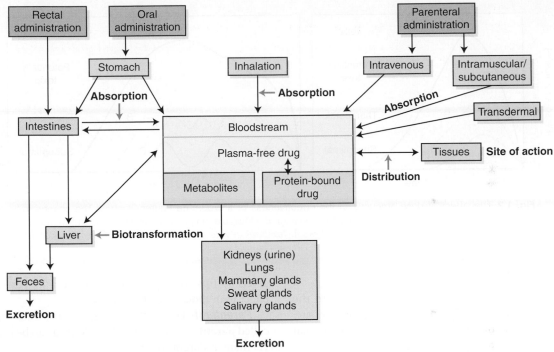

Fig. 1.1 Diagram of the possible sequence of events that a drug may follow in an animal's body.

PHARMACOKINETICS

Pharmacokinetics is the complex sequence of events that occurs after a drug is administered to a patient (Fig. 1.1). Once a drug has been given, it is available for absorption into the bloodstream and delivery to the site where it will exert its action. After a drug is absorbed, it is distributed to various fluids and tissues in the body. It is not enough, however, for the drug simply to reach the desired area. It also must accumulate in that fluid or tissue at the required concentration to be effective. Because the body immediately begins to break down and excrete the drug, the amount available to the target tissue becomes less and less over time. The veterinarian then must administer the drug repeatedly and at fixed time intervals to maintain the drug at the site of action in the desired concentration. Some drugs are administered at a high dose (**loading dose**) until an appropriate blood level is reached to establish therapeutic concentrations. Then the dose is reduced to an amount that replaces the amount lost through elimination. Doses of other drugs are at the replacement level throughout the regimen. The point at which drug accumulation equals drug elimination is

called the *steady state* or *distribution equilibrium*. This equilibrium represents the state where the amount of drug leaving the plasma for tissue equals the amount of drug leaving the tissue for the plasma. Underdosing leads to less-than-effective levels in tissue, and overdosing may result in toxic levels (Fig. 1.2). Drug levels can be measured in blood, urine, cerebrospinal fluid, and other appropriate body fluids to help a veterinarian determine whether an appropriate level has been achieved. This procedure, which is called *therapeutic drug monitoring*, is being used increasingly in veterinary practice. Nonsteroidal antiinflammatory drugs (NSAIDs), cardiac drugs, anticonvulsants, and thyroid drugs are commonly monitored.

The primary factors that influence blood concentration levels of a drug and a patient's response to it include the following:
- Rate of drug absorption
- Amount of drug absorbed
- Distribution of the drug throughout the body
- Drug metabolism or biotransformation
- Rate and route of excretion

These factors are explored after the drug administration routes have been discussed.

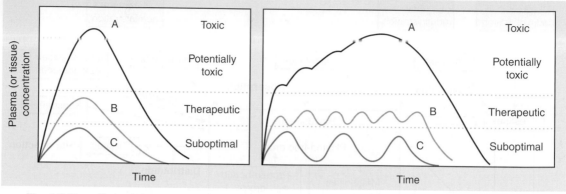

Fig. 1.2 The effect of dose amounts on the effectiveness of a drug. The figures illustrate the change in plasma drug concentration. **A.** Toxic range (overdosing). **B.** Desirable range, or **C.** Suboptimal or subtherapeutic range (underdosing). (From Jenkins, W. L. [1983]. *Textbook of veterinary internal medicine, diseases of the dog and cat.* St. Louis: WB Saunders.)

Routes of Administration

A drug is of no use unless it can be delivered to the patient in an appropriate form at an appropriate site. The way in which a drug is administered to an animal patient is influenced by several factors:

- Available pharmaceutic form of the drug
- Physical or chemical properties (irritation) of the drug
- How quickly onset of action should occur
- Use of restraint or behavioral characteristics of the patient
- Nature of the condition being treated

The routes of administration of drugs to animal patients are as follows.

Oral. In veterinary medicine, drugs commonly are administered through the oral route. Medications given by this route may be placed directly in the mouth or may be given via a tube passed through the nasal passages (nasogastric tube) or through the mouth (orogastric tube). The mucosa of the digestive tract is a large absorptive surface area with a rich blood supply. Drugs given by this route, however, are not absorbed as quickly as drugs administered by injection, and their effects are subject to species (e.g., ruminants vs. animals with a simple stomach) and individual differences. Many factors may influence the absorption of drugs from the digestive tract, including the pH of the drug, its solubility (fat vs. water), the size and shape of the molecule, the presence or absence of food in the digestive tract, the degree of gastrointestinal (GI) motility, and the presence and nature of disease processes. *This route is not suitable for animals that are vomiting or have diarrhea.* Drugs

given by this route generally produce a longer lasting effect than those given by injection.

Parenteral. Drugs that are given by injection are called **parenteral** drugs (Fig. 1.3). A drug can be injected via many different routes:

- Intravenous (IV)
- Intramuscular (IM)
- Subcutaneous (SC)
- Intradermal (ID)
- Intraperitoneal (IP)
- Intraarterial (IA)
- Intraarticular
- Intracardiac
- Intramedullary
- Epidural/subdural

Drugs given by the *intravenous route* produce the most rapid onset of action, accompanied by the shortest duration. As soon as the drug enters systemic circulation it reaches its peak plasma concentration. Medications that are irritating to tissue generally are given by this route because of the diluting effect of blood. Intravenous medications should be administered slowly to lessen the possibility of a toxic or allergic reaction. Unless a product is specifically labeled for IV use, it should never be given by this route. Oil-based drugs and those with suspended particles (i.e., those that look cloudy or thick) generally should not be given intravenously because of the possibility of an embolism. Special care should be taken to ensure that irritating drugs are injected into the vein and not around it, to avoid causing phlebitis.

The *intramuscular route* of administration produces a slower onset of action than the IV route but usually

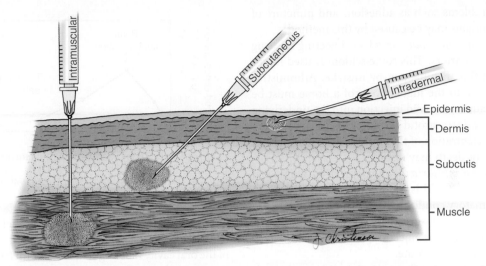

Fig. 1.3 Common parenteral routes of administration. (From Christenson, D. E. [2009]. *Veterinary medical terminology* [2nd ed.]. St. Louis: Saunders/Elsevier.)

provides a longer duration of action. The onset of action by this route can be relatively fast with a water-based form (aqueous) and is slower with other diluents (vehicles) such as oil or with other forms such as microfine crystals. When an injectable drug is placed in a substance that delays its absorption, this may be referred to as a *depot* preparation. Altering the molecule of the drug itself can influence its onset or duration of action. Onset of action usually is inversely related to duration of action. Irritating drugs should not be given by the IM route, and back pressure always should be applied to the syringe plunger before IM administration of a drug to ensure that the injection is not directed into a blood vessel.

The *subcutaneous route* produces a slower onset of action but a slightly longer duration than the intramuscular route. The absorption rate is slower as the drug must diffuse through the SC tissue to reach the capillaries and then be absorbed into systemic circulation. Irritating or hyperosmotic solutions (i.e., those with a greater number of suspended particles than are found in body fluid) should not be given by this route (see Chapter 15).

Quantities of medications that are appropriate for the species or individual being treated should be used to prevent possible dissection of the skin from underlying tissue, which could lead to death or loss (sloughing) of surface skin.

The *intradermal route* involves injecting a drug into the skin. This route is used in veterinary medicine primarily for testing for tuberculosis and allergies.

BOX 1.2   Case Scenario

The veterinarian asks you to administer two different drugs to "Sasha," a 4-year-old female spayed Golden Retriever, that is hospitalized. Drug X must be administered IV and Drug Y must be administered SC. The veterinarian selected these routes of administration based on how quickly the drug needs to take effect within the patient (onset of action), the duration of effect, and the form or concentration available.

Before administering Drug X the label of the drug bottle is checked to ensure the drug is labeled for IV administration. Drug X is administered directly into the cephalic vein slowly. Giving this drug IV produces a rapid onset of action and reaches its peak plasma concentration immediately as there is no absorption phase due to being administered directly into the bloodstream. The duration of effect is short in comparison to other routes of administration.

Drug Y is administered subcutaneously. Giving this drug SC produces a slower onset of action as it must diffuse through the subcutaneous tissue to reach the capillaries, and then be absorbed into systemic circulation.

Routes of administration greatly affect bioavailability by varying the number of barriers a drug must cross before reaching systemic circulation (Bardal, 2010).

The *intraperitoneal route* is used to deliver drugs into the abdominal cavity. The onset and duration of action of drugs given by this route are variable. This route is used to administer fluids, blood, and other medications when normal routes are not available or are not practical. Problems such as adhesions and puncture of abdominal organs may be caused by this method.

The *intraarterial route* involves injecting a drug directly into an artery. This route seldom is used intentionally, but this may happen by mistake. Administration of drugs into the jugular vein of a horse must be done with caution to avoid injection into the underlying carotid artery. Intracarotid injection results in delivery of a high concentration of the drug directly to the brain, and seizures or death may result.

Through the *intraarticular route*, a drug is injected directly into a joint. This method is used primarily to treat inflammatory conditions of the joint. Extreme care must be exercised to ensure that sterile technique is used when an intraarticular injection is given. Technicians usually do not use this route.

The *intracardiac route* is used to inject drugs through the chest wall directly into the chambers of the heart. This provides immediate access to the bloodstream and ensures that the drug is delivered quickly to all tissue in the body. This method is often used in cases of cardiopulmonary resuscitation and in euthanasia.

The *intramedullary route* is another route that is seldom used in veterinary medicine. It involves injection of the substance directly into the bone marrow. The bones used most often are the femur and the humerus. The intramedullary route usually is used to provide blood or fluids to animals with very small or damaged veins or for treatment of animals with very low blood pressure.

When spinal anesthesia is provided, drugs may be injected into the *epidural or subdural space*. The epidural space is outside the dura mater (meninges) but inside the spinal canal. The subdural space is inside the dura mater. Injection of drugs into the subdural space (cerebrospinal fluid) is also called the *intrathecal route*. A veterinarian usually carries out these methods of drug delivery.

Inhalation. Medications may be delivered to a patient in inspired air by converting a liquid form into a gaseous form through the use of a vaporizer or nebulizer. Examples of drugs that may be given by this route include anesthetics, antibiotics, bronchodilators, and mucolytics.

Topical. Drugs that are administered topically are placed on the skin or on mucous membranes. Drugs generally are absorbed more slowly through the skin than through other body membranes. The rate of absorption may be increased or absorption facilitated by placement

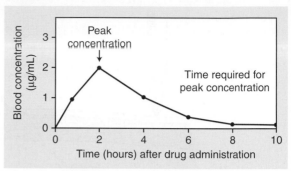

Fig. 1.4 The blood level of a drug varies with the passage of time.

of the drug in a vehicle such as dimethyl sulfoxide (DMSO). Medication also may be applied to the mucosa of the oral cavity (sublingual), the rectum (suppositories), the uterus, the vagina, the mammary glands, the eyes, and the ears. In horses, caustic materials may be applied topically to inhibit the growth of exuberant granulation tissue (proud flesh).

Transdermal drug administration is a form of topical administration that involves the use of a patch applied to the skin to deliver a drug through intact skin directly into the blood. This method is used most commonly to administer an analgesic in a slow, continuous manner or to administer compounded drugs to animals when oral administration may be difficult (e.g., cats).

Drug Absorption

Before drugs can reach their site of action, they must pass across a series of cellular membranes that make up the absorptive surfaces of the sites of administration. The degree to which a drug is absorbed and reaches the systemic circulation is called *bioavailability*.

The **manufacturing** process can have a significant effect on the physical and chemical characteristics of drug molecules that influence their bioavailability. The generic equivalent form of a drug may differ somewhat from a trademark form in overall efficacy because of manufacturing differences. Bioavailability often is demonstrated with the use of a blood level curve (Fig. 1.4). Factors that may affect the absorption process include the following:

- Mechanism of absorption
- pH and ionization status of the drug
- Absorptive surface area
- Blood supply to the area
- Solubility of the drug

- Dosage form
- Status of the GI tract (motility, permeability, and thickness of the mucosal epithelium)
- Interaction with other medications

Drugs pass across cellular membranes through three common methods. Passive absorption (transport) occurs by simple diffusion of a drug molecule from an area of high concentration of drug on one side of the membrane to an area of lower concentration on the other side. This method requires no expenditure of energy by the cell. The drug may pass through small pores in the cell membrane or may dissolve into the cell membrane on one side, pass through the membrane, and exit on the other side. For example, a disintegrated tablet or capsule results in a high concentration of drug in the GI tract. This concentration then passes through the cellular membranes of intestinal villi and adjacent capillaries, and the drug then appears in lesser concentration in the bloodstream. Alternatively, a drug may cross a membrane passively with the help of a carrier.

Drug transporters also play a major role in drug absorption. The best described transporter is the P-glycoprotein (P-gp). P-gp is produced at the direction of the MDR1 (ABCB1) gene. It uses adenosine triphosphate (ATP) as an energy source to pump drugs from cells. It is found in most mammalian tissue and appears to act in a protective manner. It is useful in intestinal, renal, placental, liver, and brain tissue, where it helps to pump transported drugs out of the body or away from protected sites. The protection is achieved by pumping the drugs into the intestine, bile, or urine for elimination or away from the fetus or brain (Boothe, 2012).

Some small drug molecules such as electrolytes may simply move with fluid through pores in cell membranes. Active transport of drugs across cell membranes moves molecules from an area of lower concentration to an area of higher concentration and requires that the cell use energy. This is the usual mechanism for the absorption of sodium, potassium, and other electrolytes. In pinocytosis, a third method of passive transport, cells engulf drug molecules by invaginating their cell membrane to form a vesicle that then breaks off from the membrane in the interior of the cell. The method of absorption that occurs in a particular situation depends on whether the drug is fat soluble or water soluble, the size and shape of the drug molecule, and the degree of ionization of the drug.

Many drugs can pass through a cell membrane only if they are nonionized (i.e., not positively or negatively charged). Most drugs exist in the body in a state that consists of both ionized and nonionized forms. The pH of a drug and the pH of the area in which the drug is located can determine the degree to which a drug becomes ionized and thus is absorbed. Weakly acidic drugs in an acidic environment do not ionize readily and therefore are absorbed well. The absorption of basic drugs is more favorable in an alkaline environment. If a drug is placed in an environment in which it readily ionizes, such as a mildly acidic drug in an alkaline environment or a mildly alkaline drug in an acidic environment, it does not diffuse and may become trapped in that environment.

As the absorptive surface of the area of drug placement increases, so does the rate of absorption. One of the largest absorptive surfaces in the body is found in the small intestine because the efficient design of the villi maximizes the surface area.

At any site of drug administration, as the blood supply to an area increases, so does the rate of absorption of the drug. Drugs are absorbed from an intramuscular site at a faster rate than from a subcutaneous site because of the proportionately greater blood supply to the muscle. Initiating the fight-or-flight response increases blood flow to the muscle but decreases blood flow to the intestines. Heat and massage also increase blood flow to an area. Poor circulation, which may occur during shock or cardiac failure, decreases blood flow, as does cooling or elevation of a body part. These factors then can positively or negatively influence drug absorption.

Another important factor that determines the rate at which drugs pass across cell membranes is the solubility of the drug. The lipid (fat) solubility of a drug tends to be directly proportional to the degree of drug nonionization. As was stated previously, the nonionized form is the one that usually is absorbed. The degree of lipid solubility of a drug often is expressed as its lipid **partition coefficient**. A high lipid partition coefficient indicates enhanced drug absorption.

Drug absorption rates often depend on the formulation of the drug. Various inert ingredients, such as carriers (vehicles), binding agents, and coatings, are used to prepare dosage forms. These substances have major effects on the rate at which formulations dissolve. *Depot* and *spansule* are terms that are associated with prolonged- or sustained-release formulations in veterinary medicine. Subcutaneous implants that contain growth stimulants that break down slowly and release their products over prolonged periods are used in some situations.

When drugs are given orally, the condition of the GI tract can have a major influence on the rate and extent of drug absorption. Factors such as degree of intestinal motility, emptying time of the stomach, irritation or inflammation of the mucosa (e.g., gastritis, enteritis), damage to or loss of villi (e.g., viral diseases), composition and amount of food material, and changes in intestinal microorganisms can affect the rate and extent of absorbance of medications. Another consideration regarding drugs that are absorbed from the GI tract is the **first-pass effect**. This refers to the fact that substances are absorbed from the GI tract into the portal venous system, which delivers the drug to the liver before it enters the general circulation. In some instances, a drug then is metabolized in the liver to altered forms; this process may make the drug inactive or less active.

The process of combining some drugs with other drugs or with certain foods can negatively affect drug absorption. The availability of tetracycline is reduced if it is administered with milk or milk products. Antacids may reduce the absorption of phenylbutazone or iron products. Technicians always should consult appropriate references about potential interactions before administering new drugs.

Drug Distribution

Drug distribution is the process by which a drug is carried from its site of absorption to its site of action. Drugs move from the absorption site into the plasma of the bloodstream, from the plasma into the interstitial fluid that surrounds cells, and from the interstitial fluid into the cells, where they combine with cellular receptors to create an action. Equilibrium soon is established between these three compartments while the drug moves from the blood into the tissue and then from the tissue back into the blood (Fig. 1.5). How well a drug is distributed throughout the body depends on several factors.

The rate of movement of drug molecules from one of the previously listed compartments to the other is proportional to the differences between the amounts of drug in all areas. The difference between the amounts of drug in two compartments is called the *concentration gradient,* and as the gradient increases (difference), so

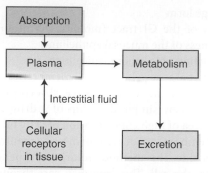

Fig. 1.5 Drug distribution establishes an equilibrium between the amount of drug at the site of absorption, the amount in the plasma, and the amount at the cellular receptor sites.

does the tendency of the drug to move from the area of higher concentration to the area of lower concentration.

A drug within the plasma comes into contact with various proteins (e.g., albumin) and binds with them or remains free. When a drug is bound to a protein, it becomes inactive and is unavailable for binding with cell receptors or for metabolism. A bound drug may be regarded as a temporary storage site of a drug because a bound drug eventually frees itself from the protein. Low levels of plasma proteins may occur in malnutrition or in certain diseases, and plasma binding may be reduced.

Drugs that are highly lipid soluble tend to move readily from the plasma into the interstitial fluid. Drugs in the nonionized form follow a similar pattern. Once a drug is present in a tissue, it may become bound or stored there. Tissues such as fat, liver, kidney, and bone may act as storage sites for drugs such as barbiturates, inhalation anesthetics, and others. When a drug moves from the storage tissue back into the blood and additional doses are given, an exaggerated or prolonged effect may result because of the additive effects.

Barriers that exist in particular tissues tend to retard the movement of all or certain classes of drugs into them. The exact nature of these barriers has not been well explained in the literature although the P-gp transporter may play an important role. The placenta acts as a barrier to some drugs that could be toxic to a fetus and permits the passage of others. Anesthetics that do not excessively depress a fetus must be chosen when a cesarean section is performed. The so-called blood–brain barrier is generally minimally permeable to all drugs, although it becomes relatively permeable to many antibiotics on inflammation. A defect in the P-gp drug transporter in the blood–brain barrier has been identified in individuals of several dog breeds, including collies, Old English sheepdogs, Australian shepherds, Shetland sheepdogs, and English shepherds and can result in potential toxicity to drugs like ivermectin. The eye also has a barrier that impedes some drugs from diffusing into its tissue.

Disease processes can interfere with drug distribution. Antibiotics usually do not diffuse well into abscesses or exudates. Heart failure and shock can reduce normal blood flow to tissue and thus impede drug distribution. Kidney failure (uremia) can alter the plasma binding of some drugs such as furosemide and phenylbutazone. Liver failure can cause a reduction in the amount of protein (albumin) available for protein binding.

Some clinicians believe that reptiles have a renal–portal system that can distribute potentially toxic levels of a drug to the kidney if the drug is injected into the posterior one third of the body.

Biotransformation/Metabolism

Biotransformation, or metabolism, is the body's ability to change a drug chemically from the form in which it was administered into a form that can be eliminated from the body. Most biotransformation occurs in the liver because of the action of microsomal enzymes called *cytochrome P450 enzymes* found in liver cells. These enzymes induce chemical reactions that change the drug chemically to allow elimination in the urine or bile. Once a drug has been biotransformed, it is called a *metabolite*. Metabolites are usually inactive, but in some cases, may have similar, less, or more activity. Some biotransformation does occur in other tissues such as the kidney, lung, and nervous system.

The following four chemical reactions are induced by microsomal enzymes in the liver to biotransform drugs:
1. Oxidation—loss of electrons
2. Reduction—gain of electrons
3. Hydrolysis—splitting of the drug molecule and addition of a water molecule to each of the split portions
4. Conjugation—the addition of glucuronic acid or similar compounds to the drug molecule; when these compounds are attached to a drug molecule, the drug becomes much more water soluble

Biotransformation reactions involving oxidation, reduction, or hydrolysis are called phase I reactions, while reactions involving conjugation are called phase II reactions. Drugs may be processed through both phases or only phase II. As a rule, phase I reactions make drugs more water soluble and because of this more susceptible to phase II metabolism. Phase II reactions generally make the drugs water soluble enough for elimination by the kidneys (Boothe, 2012).

Many factors, including species, age, nutritional status, tissue storage, and health status, can alter drug metabolism. Cats have limited ability to metabolize aspirin, narcotics, phenols, and barbiturates because of their reduced ability to form glucuronic acid. Young animals usually have poor ability to biotransform drugs because their liver enzyme systems are not fully developed until around 3 months of age. Old animals have a decreased capacity to biotransform because their ability to synthesize needed liver enzymes may be impaired. Malnourished animals have fewer protein raw materials available for use in manufacturing enzymes for biotransformation, and animals with liver disease are not able to process the raw materials available for enzyme production. Drugs present in storage compartments such as fat or plasma proteins are not available to be metabolized.

TECHNICIAN NOTES

- Most biotransformation or metabolism of a drug occurs in the liver.

Drug Excretion

Most drugs are metabolized by the liver and then are eliminated from the body by the kidneys via the urine. They can be excreted, however, by the liver (bile), mammary glands, lungs, intestinal tract, sweat glands, salivary glands, and skin. An understanding of the route of excretion of drugs is very important because alterations or diseases of a particular organ can cause a reduced capacity to excrete the drug, and toxic accumulation may result. For example, the anesthetic agent ketamine can cause serious central nervous system (CNS) depression in cats with urinary obstruction because the kidneys excrete this drug.

Kidneys excrete drugs by two principal mechanisms. The first method is called *glomerular filtration*. A glomerulus and its corresponding tubule make up the individual functional unit of the kidney, called a *nephron*. A glomerulus acts like a sieve to filter drug molecules (metabolites) from the blood into the glomerular filtrate, which is then eliminated as urine (Fig. 1.6). The second mechanism that kidneys use to excrete drugs is called *tubular secretion*. Kidney tubule cells secrete metabolites from the capillaries surrounding the tubule and into the glomerular filtrate, which becomes urine as

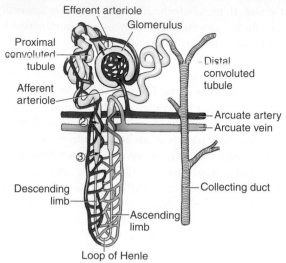

Fig. 1.6 The kidneys eliminate or conserve drug metabolites by glomerular filtration *(1)*, tubular reabsorption *(2)*, and tubular secretion *(3)*.

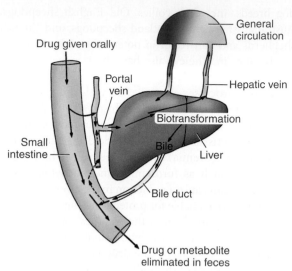

Fig. 1.7 Drugs or their metabolites in the intestine may be eliminated in the feces or absorbed/reabsorbed for a pass through the liver.

it exits the kidneys. In some instances, drug molecules may be reabsorbed from the glomerular filtrate back into the blood through *tubular reabsorption.*

It is important that the nephrons (glomerulus and corresponding tubule) are healthy and that they have an adequate blood supply, so they can do an effective job of excreting metabolites. The lower urinary tract (bladder and urethra) also must be functioning normally, so filtered or secreted metabolites can be eliminated. If any part of this system from the glomerulus to the urethra is compromised or diseased, toxic levels of a drug may accumulate.

The liver excretes drugs by first incorporating them into bile, which is eliminated into the small intestine. In the small intestine, the drug then may become a part of the feces and be eliminated from the body, or it may be reabsorbed into the bloodstream (Fig. 1.7).

Some drugs or their metabolites may pass directly from the blood and into the milk via the mammary glands. This is an important consideration because of the potential effects of the drug on nursing offspring or on people who drink the milk. Quantities of drug that remain in animal products when they are consumed are called *residues.* Residues found in milk, eggs, or meat products are potentially dangerous to people for the following reasons:

- People may be allergic to the drug.
- Prolonged exposure to antibiotic residues can result in resistant strains of bacteria.
- Residue of some drugs may cause cancer in humans.

Drugs that convert readily between a liquid and a gaseous state (gas anesthetics) may be eliminated from the blood via the lungs. These gas molecules move from the blood into the alveoli of the lungs to be eliminated in expired air.

Drugs that are given orally and are not absorbed readily from the intestinal tract may pass through the tract and be eliminated through feces. As was mentioned previously, some drugs are excreted through the bile into the intestinal tract, and a few may be actively secreted across the intestinal mucosa into the intestine for elimination.

Some drugs are eliminated through sweat and saliva, although these routes usually are not clinically important. The rate of drug loss from the body can be estimated by calculating the drug's **half-life**. The half-life is the time required for the amount of drug present in the body to be reduced by one half (Fig. 1.8).

PHARMACODYNAMICS

Pharmacodynamics is the study of the mechanisms by which drugs produce physiologic changes in the body. Drugs may enhance or depress the physiologic activity of a cell or a tissue. Drug molecules combine with components of the cell membrane or with internal components of the cell to cause alterations in cell function. The way in which drugs combine with structures (receptors)

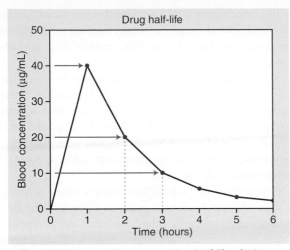

Fig. 1.8 This graph illustrates a drug half-life of 1 hour.

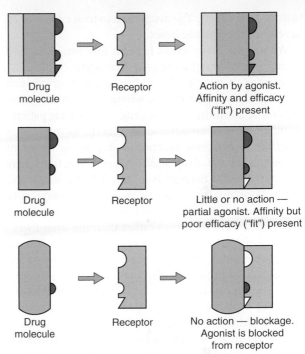

Fig. 1.9 Drug molecules must combine with specific cellular receptors to exert their effects.

on or in a cell can be compared with a lock-and-key model. The geometric match of a drug molecule and a cellular receptor must be exact for the appropriate action to occur (Fig. 1.9). The tendency of a drug to combine with a receptor is called *affinity,* and the degree to which the drug binds with its receptor helps to determine drug efficacy. A drug with a high level of affinity and efficacy causes a specific action and is an **agonist**. A drug with less affinity and efficacy is a partial agonist. A drug that blocks another drug from combining with a receptor is an **antagonist**. The combining of a drug with its receptor causes a particular drug action, and this interaction produces a particular drug effect. Examples of drug effects include stimulation, depression, irritation, and cell death. Sometimes, a drug replaces a substance that is missing or is in short supply in the body.

 TECHNICIAN NOTES

- An agonist is a drug that activates certain receptors and causes a specific action to occur.
- An antagonist is a drug that blocks another drug from combining with a receptor and prevents a specific action from occurring.

A dose–response curve displays the relationship between the dose of a drug and the body's response. The dose–response curve shows that as a dose increases, an increase in response occurs until a maximum response or plateau is achieved. *No drug produces a single effect.* Low doses of a narcotic may be used to treat patients with diarrhea. Higher doses may be used for pain relief, and even higher doses may depress the respiratory system. The *potency* of a drug is described as the amount of a drug needed to produce a desired response and is represented by a position along the dose–response curve.

The **efficacy** of a drug represents the degree to which a drug produces its desired response in a patient. Once the efficacy level of a drug has been reached, increasing the dose does not improve the effect.

The *therapeutic index* is the relationship between a drug's ability to achieve the desired effect and its tendency to produce toxic effects. The therapeutic index, which is expressed as the ratio between the LD_{50} and the ED_{50}, quantitates the drug's margin of safety. The LD_{50} is the dose of a drug that is lethal to 50% of the animals in a dose-related trial. The ED_{50} is the dose of a drug that produces the desired effect in 50% of the animals in a dose-related trial. The index is calculated as follows: therapeutic index = LD_{50}/ED_{50}.

The larger the number that is produced by dividing the LD_{50} by the ED_{50}, the greater the level of safety. Drugs with a narrow margin of safety (low therapeutic index) must be administered with caution to prevent toxic or fatal effects. The drugs used to treat cancer often have a low therapeutic index.

An **adverse drug event** is harm to a patient caused by administration of a drug for therapeutic or diagnostic reasons. It may be due to a medication error such as using the wrong drug, the wrong dose, or the wrong interval or administering the drug to the wrong patient. Another cause of an adverse event is the **adverse drug reaction**. An adverse reaction is due to the inherent properties of the drug itself. Adverse reactions may range from mild dermatitis to anaphylactic shock and death. Poor quality or purity of the drug may cause an adverse reaction. Some patients may react to carriers or binders of the drugs rather than the drug themselves. Aminoglycosides can cause harm to the kidney or eighth cranial nerve and impair hearing. Drugs can cause changes in the skin that make it more sensitive to light. This type of reaction is called *photosensitivity*.

Other types of adverse responses include abortion, liver or kidney damage, infertility, vomiting or diarrhea, and cancer. An unusual or unexpected reaction is called an *idiosyncratic drug reaction*. All adverse reactions should be reported to the drug manufacturer or the FDA. If the report is made to the drug company, the company is obligated to report the incident to the FDA.

DRUG INTERACTIONS

An altered pharmacologic response to a drug that is caused by the presence of a second drug is called a *drug interaction*. The normal response to the drug may be increased or decreased as a consequence of this interaction. The interaction may be beneficial or harmful to the patient.

Drug interactions can be classified as pharmacokinetic, pharmacodynamic, or pharmaceutic. A pharmacokinetic interaction is one in which plasma or tissue levels of a drug are altered by the presence of another. This alteration may be due to changes in absorption, distribution, metabolism, or excretion of the other drug. Metoclopramide hastens gastric emptying and promotes the delivery of a drug to the small intestine for absorption. When calcium and tetracycline are administered at the same time orally, calcium binds the tetracycline and the complex is not absorbed. Displacement of albumin-bound drugs by other drugs with a greater binding affinity may result in an increase in the free drug, leading to an increased response. Many drugs are metabolized by the cytochrome P-450 enzyme system found in the liver, and several drugs can alter (increase or decrease) the activity of the P-450 system, causing drug interactions.

A pharmacodynamic interaction is one in which the action or effect of one drug is altered by another. These reactions occur at the site of drug action. These actions may be antagonistic (reversal of an alpha agonist with yohimbine), additive (CNS depression with combinations of preanesthetics), or synergistic (sulfonamide-trimethoprim combinations).

A pharmaceutic interaction occurs when physical or chemical reactions take place as a result of mixing of drugs in a syringe or other container. Amphotericin B may form a precipitate when mixed with electrolyte solutions other than 5% dextrose. Diazepam may precipitate if mixed with certain drugs. Furosemide may be chemically inactivated if mixed with an acid medium (Boothe, 2012).

Drug interactions are described as involving an object drug (the one being acted on) and a precipitant drug (the one that influences the other; Mealey, 2002). Table 1.2 lists selected drug combinations that may have undesirable consequences.

 TECHNICIAN NOTES

- It generally is recommended that mixing of drugs in the same syringe or fluid administration system should be avoided unless the drugs are known to be compatible.
- When two drugs metabolized by the liver are given, one should anticipate a drug interaction.
- Concurrent use of drugs from the "behavior modifying" category can cause serious problems such as serotonin syndrome or hypertensive reactions.

DRUG NAMES

When a company completes the exhaustive research and development necessary to gain FDA approval to market a drug, it names this drug and has exclusive rights to the drug for the duration of the patent. During this time, no other company can manufacture the drug. This allows the original manufacturer time to recoup the cost of research and development and to earn a profit. On expiration of the patent, other companies may produce the drug. When other companies manufacture this previously developed product it is called a generic equivalent.

TABLE 1.2 Drug Combinations That May Have Undesirable Consequences.

Precipitant Drug	Object Drug	Consequences
Antacids	Tetracycline	Reduced absorption of tetracycline
Ketoconazole	Digoxin, cyclosporine, tricyclic antidepressants	Decreased metabolism of object drugs, except digoxin which is unchanged Increased absorption of digoxin
Sucralfate	Fluoroquinolones	Reduced absorption of quinolones
Fluoroquinolones	Theophylline	Decreased metabolism of theophylline
Omeprazole	Ketoconazole/itraconazole	Decreased oral absorption of object drugs
Phenobarbital	Theophylline, doxycycline, beta blockers	Increased metabolism of object drugs (cytochrome P-450 induction)
Cimetidine	Diazepam and theophylline	Decreased metabolism of object drugs (cytochrome P-450 inhibition)
MAO Inhibitors	Amitraz, selective serotonin reuptake inhibitors, tricyclic antidepressants, other MAOs	Dangerous accumulation of biogenic amines leading to serotonin syndrome or hypertensive state
Tetracyclines	Penicillins	Tetracyclines slow bacterial growth and inhibit penicillins that are most effective against rapidly growing bacteria

MAO, Monoamine oxidase.

During the course of its testing, development, and marketing, a drug may be assigned several different names. These multiple names can be a source of confusion. For practical purposes, drugs are given the following types of names:

- *Chemical*—the name that describes the molecular structure of a drug. These names are scientifically very accurate, but they are complex and impractical for use in clinical settings.
- *Code or laboratory*—the name given to a drug by the research and development investigators. It is used for communication between research teams and consists of abbreviations and code numbers.
- *Compendial*—the name listed in the *United States Pharmacopoeia (USP)*. The *USP* is the legally accepted compendium that lists drugs and standards for their quality and purity.
- *Official*—usually the same as the compendial or generic name.
- *Proprietary or trade*—the name chosen by the manufacturing company. When it is registered, it is the exclusive property of the company. A name that is short and can be easily recalled is usually selected for the proprietary name. Federal copyright and trademark laws protect this name. On drug container labels, in package inserts, and in drug references, the proprietary name can be distinguished by a superscript R with a circle around it after the name.
- *Generic*—the common name chosen by the company. It is not the exclusive right of the company. It may be the same as the official or compendial name. These are drugs with patents that have expired, or they were never patented.

Table 1.3 provides chemical, generic, and proprietary names of three common drugs.

In textbooks and other scholarly works, generic names begin with a lowercase letter, and proprietary names begin with a capital letter. This practice is followed throughout this text (e.g., ketamine [Ketaset]).

DRUG LABELS

The Center for Veterinary Medicine (CVM) of the FDA requires that drug container labels list the following items (Webb & Aeschbacher, 1993):

- Drug names (both generic and trade names)
- Drug concentration and quantity
- Name and address of the manufacturer
- Controlled substance status (if applicable)
- Manufacturer's control or lot number
- Drug's expiration date

It is required that the label also list instructions for use of the drug and warnings of possible adverse effects of the drug. Many manufacturers list this added information in an insert because the label on the container usually has limited space. An insert is a small folder that is placed inside the box with the drug container or is provided as a tear-off portion of the label.

The trade name usually is placed first on a drug label and is scripted in bold letters (Fig. 1.10). The generic name typically follows the trade name in smaller print. The label must display the concentration (strength) of a drug and the total quantity in the container. Drug strength often is expressed as milligrams or units per dosage unit (e.g., mg/mL or mg/capsule). Some drugs are sold in different concentrations with similar labels, resulting in underdosing or overdosing. When the same drug is marketed in different strengths with similar labels, some companies use different sizes of bottles for the different strengths and display the concentrations in bold print. Atropine and xylazine are examples of drugs that are marketed in different concentrations for large and small animals.

TABLE 1.3 Drug Chemical, Generic, and Trade Names.

Chemical Name	Generic Name	Trade Name
22,23-Dihydroavermectin B1a	Ivermectin	Heartguard
22,23-Dihydroavermectin B1b		Ivomec
		Eqvalan
dl 2-(o-chlorophenyl)-2-(methylamino) cyclohexanone hydrochloride	Ketamine hydrochloride	Ketaset
		Ketaject
		Vetalar
D(-)-α-amino-p-hydroxybenzyl-penicillin trihydrate	Amoxicillin	Amoxil
		Amoxi-Tabs
		Trimox

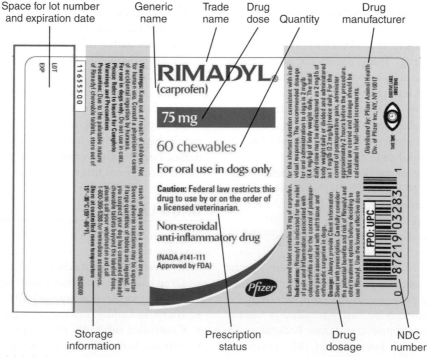

Fig. 1.10 A label showing the components of a drug as required by the U.S. Food and Drug Administration. (Courtesy Zoetic, Inc., Exton, PA.)

The label must include the name and address of the manufacturer of the drug. This is important so that one can know whom to contact if adverse drug reactions occur or if other problems with the drug arise.

Drugs that have potential for abuse by humans are controlled under the Comprehensive Drug Abuse Prevention and Control Act of 1970. The Drug Enforcement Administration places drugs into categories or schedules according to their potential for abuse and requires that the label of a container for a controlled substance be identified with a capital C, followed by a Roman numeral that identifies which of the five categories is appropriate. This labeling must be placed on the upper right side of the container label.

Drug labels must list an expiration date for the product. This is to ensure that dispensed drugs have the intended safety and efficacy. Drugs are tested during development to determine the effective shelf life and proper storage conditions. Some drugs must be stored in refrigeration, and others must be stored in light-resistant (amber) containers to ensure that the shelf life is not shortened. *Storage instructions on the label should be followed carefully so as not to invalidate the expiration date.*

All drugs must have a lot or batch number on the label. The purpose of the lot number is to allow the manufacturer to know the exact time and date of production of the product and the quality and quantity of the ingredients. The lot number is determined by the manufacturer and may consist of numbers or numbers and letters.

Another feature that is often found on a drug label but that is not required by the FDA is the national drug code (NDC) number. The NDC is a 10-digit number that identifies the manufacturer or distributor, the drug formulation, and the package size.

Drugs intended for animals that may later be consumed by humans must have the appropriate withdrawal time listed on the insert or label.

DEVELOPMENT AND APPROVAL OF NEW DRUGS

The federal government requires that, before any new animal health product can be marketed, its safety and efficacy must be proved through rigorous testing. This testing requires the expenditure of much time and money. It has been estimated that, on average, it takes 10 years or more at a cost of millions of dollars to the manufacturer to place a new drug on the market. The steps in this process are outlined in Fig. 1.11.

The development of new animal health products begins in the research and development department of the manufacturing company. The company wants to ensure that the drug not only is safe and effective for animals but also is safe for the environment and for the people who will consume products from animals treated with the drug. The company wants to be certain that a market is available for the product, that it will be produced at a cost that is reasonable for consumers, and that the product will be profitable for the company.

Regulatory Agencies

The three agencies of the U.S. government that regulate animal health products are the FDA, the Environmental Protection Agency (EPA), and the U.S. Department of Agriculture (USDA). The FDA regulates the development and approval of animal drugs and feed additives through its CVM. The EPA regulates the development and approval of animal topical pesticides, and the USDA regulates the development and approval of biologics (vaccines, serums, antitoxins, and similar products).

The Food Animal Residue Avoidance Databank

The Food Animal Residue Avoidance Databank (FARAD), a project sponsored by the USDA Extension Service, serves as a repository of **residue** avoidance information and educational materials. The FARAD provides expert advice concerning the avoidance of drug residues in an effort to achieve its goal of producing "safe foods of animal origin." The FARAD produces a compendium of FDA-approved drugs and provides information about withholding times for milk and preslaughter **withdrawal times** for meat. The information in this compendium is available online (www.farad.org), and direct telephone access is provided for situations in which online information is not sufficient.

Steps in the Development of a New Drug
Preliminary Trials

When a new drug or product shows the potential for development by a company, it is first subjected to a series of preliminary trials. The company wants to know whether the product will actually perform as expected, whether it has potentially harmful adverse effects, and whether it will be profitable to market. If these concerns are satisfactorily answered, testing begins. First, the product is tested in a laboratory on simple organisms such as bacteria, yeasts, or molds. Computer models may be used to simulate animal models at this time.

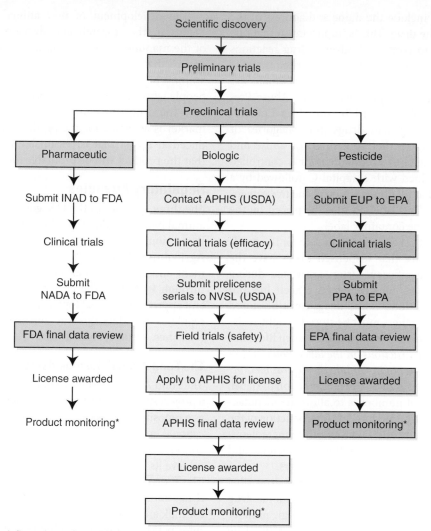

Fig. 1.11 A flow chart of the animal health product approval process. *Throughout its market life, a product is monitored by the manufacturer and the appropriate government agency to ensure its continued safety. *APHIS,* Animal and Plant Health Inspection Service; *EPA,* Environmental Protection Agency; *EUP,* Experimental Use Permit; *FDA,* U.S. Food and Drug Administration; *INAD,* Investigational New Animal Drug; *NADA,* New Animal Drug Application; *NVSL,* National Veterinary Services Laboratory; *PPA,* Pesticide Permit Application; *USDA,* U.S. Department of Agriculture. (From Etchison, K. [1993]. The path to approval: How research discoveries become federally licensed products. *Top Vet Med 4*:13.)

Preclinical (Animal Safety) Trials

If preliminary trial findings prove satisfactory, the next step involves preclinical trials. These trials usually are carried out with the use of laboratory animals to gather information about appropriate doses of the drug. A few target (intended species) animals also may be used. If the results of the preclinical trials are satisfactory, the company then notifies the appropriate government agency that a new drug is under investigation. It does this by filing

an Investigational New Animal Drug (INAD) application with the FDA. If the product is a pesticide, the company files for an Experimental Use Permit (EUP) from the EPA. If a biologic is involved, the company contacts the Animal and Plant Health Inspection Service of the USDA.

Clinical Trials

By this time, the manufacturer has compiled enough information to decide whether the product should be tested in the target species. These tests must prove that the drug is safe and effective. Potential toxic and adverse effects must be identified. Tissue residue and withdrawal time information must be accumulated if the product will be used in food-producing animals. Possible toxic effects on pregnant animals are explored, along with information about the potential for birth defects (teratogenesis). Shelf life studies also must be conducted to establish expiration date data. Results of these studies are validated through the use of statistical analysis.

Submission of a New Animal Drug Application

If the manufacturing company decides to market the drug, it then must file with the FDA a New Animal Drug Application (NADA). Procedures for pesticides and biologics are similar.

Final Review by the Food and Drug Administration

Volumes of research are submitted to the FDA, EPA, or USDA for review. Approval and a license for manufacture are granted if the appropriate agency validates the information.

Product Monitoring

As long as a product is marketed, it is monitored constantly by the company and the government to ensure its continuing safety and efficacy.

The Green Book

The Green Book is a list of all animal drug products that have been approved by the FDA for safety and effectiveness. This list was first published in 1989 as a cooperative, nonprofit effort between the USDA and Virginia Polytechnic Institute and State University. It is funded through an interagency agreement between the USDA and the FDA. Monthly updates are made to the list, and the entire list is published each January. *The Green Book* is available electronically at the FDA-CVM Web site (http://www.fda.gov/AnimalVeterinary/Products/ApprovedAnimalDrugProducts/default.htm).

FEDERAL LAWS RELATED TO DRUG DEVELOPMENT AND USE

In 1906, Congress passed the first legislation designed to regulate the manufacture, use, and sale of drugs. Table 1.4 provides a list of the major acts of legislation related to drug development and use and briefly describes the significance of each.

The Animal Medicinal Drug Use Clarification Act

In 1994, Congress passed the Animal Medicinal Drug Use Clarification Act (AMDUCA). This legislation made extralabel use of approved veterinary drugs legal under specific well-defined conditions. This act came about because of the lobbying efforts of the American Veterinary Medical Association (AVMA) and other groups in response to the FDA, which had tightened its policies on extralabel use of veterinary drugs. Previously, veterinarians had been permitted to use any drug as long as it could be legally obtained, was used according to sound professional practice, and left no residue in food products. However, public concerns over food safety issues related to residues of substances such as diethylstilbestrol, chloramphenicol, and antibiotics caused the FDA to issue compliance policy guidelines (CPGs) that made extralabel use illegal. Even though the FDA would not routinely prosecute veterinarians for extralabel use after issuance of the CPGs, practitioners nonetheless were placed in the position of breaking federal law to meet their obligations to animals and their owners. The AMDUCA allows veterinarians to legally select the most efficacious drugs for their patients. The AVMA issued an *AMDUCA Guidance Brochure* in 1998. This brochure outlines requirements of the act and provides an algorithm that can be used to determine when extralabel use is appropriate.

A section of the AMDUCA states that the FDA may prohibit or restrict extralabel use in animals if the agency finds that such use presents a risk to the public health. The following drugs and substances are prohibited or restricted for extralabel use in all food-producing animals.

Prohibited
- Chloramphenicol—Antibiotic
- Clenbuterol—Bronchodilator
- Diethylstilbestrol or DES—estrogen hormone
- Fluoroquinolone-class antibiotics
- Glycopeptides—all agents including vancomycin
- Nitroimidazoles—all agents, including dimetridazole, ipronidazole, metronidazole and others
- Medicated feeds
- Nitrofurans—all agents, including furazolidone, nitrofurazone, and others

Restricted
- Antiviral agents
- Cephalosporin-class antibiotics except cephapirin (cattle, chickens, pigs, and turkeys)

TABLE 1.4   **Federal Laws Regulating the Use of Pharmaceutics.**

Date	Legislation	Summary
1058	Food additives amendment	Regulation of substances added to food for human consumption. Delaney clause specifies that no additive that causes cancer in humans or animals may be used
1962	Kefauver-Harris amendment	Provided for safety and effectiveness of drugs by strict control of manufacturing for new animal drugs
1968	Animal drug amendment	Provided regulations for new animal drugs
1970	Comprehensive drug abuse and control act	Placed controlled substances into schedules according to their potential for abuse. Called for registration of veterinarians
1988	Generic animal drug and patent term restoration act	Allowed companies to produce and sell generic versions of animal drugs approved after October 1962 without duplicating original research
1994	Animal medicinal drug use clarification act (AMDUCA)	Allows veterinarians under specific conditions to prescribe veterinary drugs in an off-label manner. It also allows human drugs to be used in animals under certain conditions
1996	Animal drug availability act	Created a new category of drugs, Animal Feed Drugs. Allows animal drugs to be added to animal feeds under the direction of a veterinarian. Supports flexible labeling of dosages on some products
2003	Animal drug user fee act	Allows the FDA to collect fees from sponsoring companies for the review of certain animal drug applications
2004	Minor use and minor species health act	Allows FDA-approved drugs to be used for treating minor species and for uncommon uses in major species
2008	Animal generic drug user fee	Allows FDA to collect fees from sponsoring companies to study means of expediting the animal generic drug review process

FDA, U.S. Food and Drug Administration.

- Phenylbutazone (all female dairy cattle 20 months of age or older)
- Sulfonamide-class antibiotics (lactating dairy cattle)
- Indexed drugs (legally marketed unapproved drugs)

Compounding of Veterinary Drugs

FDA-approved drugs are labeled for specific therapeutic uses in defined species. It is not always possible to use an approved drug for every clinical situation because veterinarians must treat a variety of animal species that may vary greatly in size; therefore, veterinarians may have to dilute or combine (compound) existing medications. Compounding is defined by the Federal Food, Drug, and Cosmetic Act (FFDCA) as any manipulation of a drug by combining, mixing, or altering ingredients to create a different dosage form other than what is approved by the FDA to accommodate a specific patient's needs. For example, it may be in the best interest of a horse to combine more than one drug in a single syringe to minimize the number of injections. It also may be essential to dilute

an injectable agent to obtain an appropriate concentration for a bird or mouse or to prepare an antidote (e.g., sodium sulfate) that is not commercially available. None of these activities would be permitted under a strict interpretation of FDA regulations, which traditionally have not distinguished the act of diluting or combining drugs from the act of manufacturing. Any alteration of a drug by a veterinarian or their employees that changes the concentration of the active ingredient, the preservatives, or the vehicles results in a new animal drug that is subject to the FDA approval process (Davidson, 1997). Compounded drugs are not FDA approved. This means that the FDA does not verify the safety, effectiveness, and quality of compounded drugs. In food animal medicine, compounding laws were developed to safeguard the public by preventing drug residues in meat, egg, and milk products. In small animal medicine compounding from FDA approved drug products is allowed as long as it complies with the FDA's Extra-label Drug Use (ELDU); Federal Food, Drug, and Cosmetic Act (FFDCA); and the Animal Medicinal

Drug Use Clarification Act (AMDUCA) rules as well as state regulations. The following conditions for which compounding is permitted include but may not be limited to (1) a valid VCPR must exist; (2) identification of a legitimate veterinary medical need; (3) the need for an appropriate regimen for a particular species, size, gender, or medical condition; (4) lack of an approved animal or human drug that when used as labeled is clinically ineffective; (5) the compounded drug is made only from an FDA approved veterinary or human drug; (6) the compounded drug must be safe and effective; (7) if used in food producing animals withdrawal times must be established; and (8) all compounded drugs are appropriately labeled (FDA and AVMA websites).

 TECHNICIAN NOTES

- Compounding preparations can provide effective therapeutic flexibility in treating medical conditions if done correctly.
- Examples of compounded drugs include crushing tablets for an oral suspension, mixing two injectable drugs, or adding flavoring to a drug.

The Veterinary Feed Directive

Congress established the Veterinary Feed Directive (VFD) as part of the Animal Drug Availability Act of 1996. The VFD established a new category of drugs "as an alternative to prescription status" for certain antimicrobial animal feed additives. Before this directive, all commercially available animal drugs for use in medicated feeds were available on an over-the-counter basis. The VFD therefore provides the FDA CVM greater control over the use of some new animal feed additives. The use of VFD drugs requires a valid VCPR and the issuance of a VFD form by a veterinarian. The animal producer must secure the VFD form from the veterinarian and must present it to a feed mill to receive the medicated feed. The FDA has on its website "Blue Bird" labels to guide feed mills when labeling feeds treated with medication premixes. These labels ensure the safe and appropriate use of these feeds.

The Minor Use and Minor Species Animal Health Act

There is a shortage in the United States of approved animal drugs intended for use in less common animal

species or those with less common conditions. The drugs that do exist may not be used legally in the animals that need the treatment. The Minor Use and Minor Species (MUMS) Animal Health Act of 2004 is intended as a mechanism to provide FDA-authorized drugs for those less common species and indications, similar to the human Orphan Drug Act of 1983. The Minor Use and Minor Species Animal Health Act specifically defines the provision of labeled drugs for minor species, including sheep, goats, game birds, emus, ranched deer, alpacas, llamas, deer, elk, rabbits, guinea pigs, pet birds, reptiles, ornamental and other fish, shellfish, wildlife, and zoo and aquarium animals. The MUMS Animal Health Act is also designed to provide major species (e.g., cats, dogs, horses, cattle, swine, turkeys, chickens) with needed drugs for uncommon indications (minor uses).

DISPENSING VERSUS PRESCRIBING DRUGS

Although most physicians prescribe drugs, most veterinarians prescribe and dispense them. The primary reason why veterinarians maintain a pharmacy in their hospitals is that drug sales represent an important source of income. Food animal practitioners in particular use profit from drug sales to supplement their income because it may be difficult for them to charge sufficiently for their time. Another reason why veterinarians dispense drugs from their hospitals is that human pharmacies usually do not stock veterinary drugs. A few drugs are available only from human pharmacies, and others are used so infrequently that veterinarians find it more practical and economical to write a prescription for them.

MARKETING OF DRUGS

Pharmaceutic products are purchased by veterinarians from various sources. Some products are purchased directly from the manufacturer by telephone or by mail; others are obtained from sales representatives (detail persons) who call on veterinary clinics. Distributors (wholesalers) are companies that buy products from many different manufacturers and then resell the products to veterinarians through sales representatives or by phone. Generic drug companies sell generic products under their own label, usually by mail order.

Most of the pharmaceutic manufacturers are large companies that have separate divisions. One division sells products to veterinarians only, and the other sells over the counter products. It should be noted that the statement "sold to graduate veterinarians only" on a drug label does not mean that the product is a prescription drug. It only indicates a sales policy of the company. In a few instances, the same product is sold under different labels to veterinarians only and to over-the-counter markets. Some feed stores and cooperatives are able to sell over-the-counter products (similar to products sold by veterinarians) to consumers at prices lower than veterinarians can charge because of the quantity purchasing power of the stores. This can be a source of tension between veterinarians and retail markets.

In recent years, Internet pharmacies have emerged on the marketing scene. Many clients attempt to use these resources because of the reduced cost of some products. The primary concern in the veterinary community is that some Internet pharmacies are supplying prescription drugs to consumers without the authorization of a veterinarian with a VCPR. The prescription may be issued by an out-of-state veterinarian who responds to client questionnaire information rather than through actual patient and client contact. Solving these problems may be difficult because the FDA regulates the drug products themselves, not the practice of the pharmacy. The board of pharmacy in the individual states where the Internet pharmacy is located and registered regulates the practice of pharmacy. The board of pharmacy in states where consumers are given prescriptions enforces requirements for out-of-state pharmacies. A program called "Vet-VIPPS" may be used to help validate the legitimacy of online pharmacies. Vet-VIPPS is a voluntary certification program that was created by the National Association of Boards of Pharmacy (www.nabp.net). The Vet-VIPPS seal of approval validates that the online pharmacy is appropriately licensed and is conducting business legitimately. A related issue is the sale of "ethical products" by these Internet companies. These are products for which the manufacturer has voluntarily limited their sale to veterinarians as a marketing decision. Some flea and tick control products are ethical products registered with the EPA or the FDA in the over-the-counter category. Improper sale of these ethical products may then be an ethical rather than a legal issue. Another controversial issue involving Internet pharmacies is the alleged use of imported drugs that have not been approved by the FDA.

DISPOSAL OF UNWANTED DRUGS

Improper disposal of unused drugs can be a potential risk to people, animals, and the environment. When unwanted drugs are placed in the trash without placement in a secure container, accidental poisonings of people or animals are possible. Several studies have found pharmaceuticals in drinking water, lakes, and rivers. The AVMA recommends six basic practices for the disposal of unwanted pharmaceuticals to avoid potential risks of improper disposal of these products (Anonymous, 2012):

1. Incinerate unwanted drugs when possible. The drugs should be placed in leak-proof, tamper-resistant packing to prevent diversion. An absorbent such as kitty litter should be added to liquids. Liquids in syringes should be evacuated in an absorbent material and the material placed in a leak-proof container for disposal. Drugs in a labeled container should have all personal information blacked out; however the drug information should be visible. The drugs should be placed in a leak-proof, tamper resistant container. The containers with the drugs scheduled for disposal should be marked "For Incineration Only" and stored in a locked container until time for disposal. State and federal guidelines should be followed when incinerating unwanted pharmaceuticals.

2. Unused drugs should be sent to the landfill when incineration is not possible. Drugs should be prepared for sending to the landfill in a similar manner to those being incinerated. The containers should be marked for landfill disposal and kept locked until the time of disposal.

3. Never flush unwanted pharmaceuticals down the toilet or drain. Drugs flushed down the toilet or drain may show up in the water supply and may be a cause of potential danger to consumers similar to those caused by drug residues in animal products. Antibiotic resistance, allergic responses, and poisonings are some of the potential consequences.

4. Maintain close inventory control. Keeping a close watch over practice inventories can reduce the amount of expired and unused drugs. Prescriptions may be written for infrequently used drugs to prevent in-house expiration. Drugs nearing their expiration date should be returned to the distributor when feasible.

5. Always follow federal and state guidelines. While reverse distributors may be used to dispose of controlled substances held by veterinary clinics (Appendix F), the AVMA recommends that law enforcement agencies be used by clients for the disposal of unwanted controlled substances prescribed for their pets.
6. Educate clients on proper disposal.

REVIEW QUESTIONS

1. Define the following terms:
   a. Agonist
   b. Contraindication
   c. Efficacy
   d. Over-the-counter drug
   e. Prescription drug
   f. Receptor
   g. Therapeutic index
   h. Withdrawal time
   i. Veterinarian–client–patient relationship
2. List four sources of drugs used in veterinary medicine.
3. What are four components of a drug regimen?
4. Discuss the conditions that must be met before a valid veterinarian–client–patient relationship can be shown to exist.
5. Describe the difference between a prescription (legend) drug and an over-the-counter drug.
6. Discuss the responsibilities of a veterinary technician in the administration of drug orders.
7. Describe the sequence of events that a drug undergoes from administration to excretion.
8. List 11 possible routes for administering a drug to a patient, and discuss the advantages and/or disadvantages of each.
9. List some of the factors that influence drug absorption.
10. Drugs usually produce their effects by combining with specific cellular _____.

11. What are six items that must be included on a drug label?
12. What are three government agencies that regulate the development, approval, and use of animal health products?
13. Why do many veterinary clinics dispense rather than prescribe most of the drugs that they use?
14. Describe the marketing of animal health products.
15. What is the purpose of FARAD?
16. Extralabel veterinary drug use was made legal (under prescribed circumstances) by what act of Congress?
17. Define compounding.
18. What are the potential dangers of residues in animal products?
19. List three classes of drug interactions.
   a. _____
   b. _____
   c. _____
20. Drug interaction can be anticipated when two drugs are given that are both metabolized by the _____.
21. Define "ethical product."
22. Once a drug has been biotransformed, it is called a _____.
23. An(a) _____ is a reason to use a drug.
   a. contraindication
   b. indication
24. List the six practices recommended by the AVMA for the safe disposal of unwanted drugs.
25. The _____ of a drug represents the degree to which a drug produces its desired response in a patient.
   a. pharmacodynamics
   b. pharmacokinetics
   c. efficacy
   d. metabolism

REFERENCES

American Veterinary Medical Association. *Disposal of controlled substances* (website). https://www.avma.org/Advocacy/National/Federal/Pages/Disposal-of-Controlled-Substances.aspx. Accessed January 31, 2012.

American Veterinary Medical Association. *Compounding* (website). https://www.avma.org/KB/resources/reference/pages/compounding.aspx. Accessed April 6, 2019.

American Veterinary Medical Association. *ELDU and AMDUCA* (website). https://www.avma.org/KB/Resources/FAQs/Pages/ELDU-and-AMDUCA-FAQs.aspx. Accessed April 4, 2019.

Anonymous. (2012). Partnership to promote proper vet drug disposal. *Journal of the American Veterinary Medical Association, 116,* 240.

Bardal, S., Waechter, J., and Martin, D. Applied Pharmacology. 2010. Elsevier Health Sciences.

Boothe, D. M. (2012). Principles of drug therapy. In D. M. Boothe (Ed.), *Small animal clinical pharmacology* (2nd ed.). Philadelphia: WB Saunders.

Davidson, G. (1997). Pharmacy update: New FDA policy gives clear guidance for compounding. *Veterinary Technician, 18*(3), 195–201.

FDA. *Drugs prohibited from extra-label uses in animals* (website). https://www.fda.gov/AnimalVeterinary/ResourcesforYou/ucm380135.htm#. Accessed April 6, 2019.

FDA. *Compounding and the FDA* (website). https://www.fda.gov/drugs/guidancecomplianceregulatoryinformation/pharmacycompounding/ucm339764.htm. Accessed April 6, 2019.

Mealey, K. L. (2002). Clinically significant drug interactions. *Compend Contin Educ Proc Pract Vet, 24*(1), 10–22.

Webb, A. I., & Aeschbacher, G. (1993). Animal drug container labels: A guide to the reader. *Journal of the American Veterinary Medical Association, 202,* 1591–1599.

Williams, B. R., & Baer, C. (1990). Introduction to pharmacology. In B. R. Williams, & C. Baer (Eds.), *Essentials of clinical pharmacology in nursing.* Springhouse, PA: Springhouse Corp.

Routes and Techniques of Drug Administration

OBJECTIVES

After studying this chapter, you should be able to

1. Discuss the many types of available drug forms.
2. Discuss drug preservatives and solvents.
3. List and explain the six rights of administering medication.
4. Explain the techniques available for administering medications, the routes commonly used, and how the treatment should be documented. In addition, name available types of syringes and needles, describe their common uses, and correctly read doses in a syringe.
5. Describe what is involved in preparing a prescription and explain how the prescription is posted to the medical record.
6. Describe proper labeling of dispensed medications.
7. Discuss some of the U.S. Drug Enforcement Administration (DEA) requirements for the use of controlled substances in a veterinary practice to include storage, logging, and dispensing.

OUTLINE

KEY TERMS

Cerumen
Controlled or scheduled drugs
Counterirritant
Cream
Elixir
Emulsion
Enteric coating

Intravenous bolus
Intravenous infusion
Liniment
Ointment
Parenteral administration
Speculum
Suspension

INTRODUCTION

In a busy veterinary practice, a veterinary technician often administers treatments ordered by the veterinarian. Proper administration techniques should be used along with accurate documentation on the medical record. Additionally, a veterinary technician must be knowledgeable about dosage forms, syringe construction, and hatch marks and must be able to draw correct amounts of medication within a syringe, know the six rights of drug administration, be capable of administering medication by all available routes, be knowledgeable in the area of client education regarding drugs, and know how to properly handle controlled substances. Proper documentation of administered treatments is of utmost importance and ensures that the same treatment is not repeated by other veterinary personnel. Knowledge of adverse reactions that animals may have to particular medications is also crucial. The veterinary technician is the veterinarian's most important employee in a busy practice. Through observation of the patient during treatments, the technician is able to provide the veterinarian with information regarding the patient's response. The doctor, thus informed, can easily reach decisions regarding adjustment of the treatment regimen. The technician who recognizes the importance of administering proper treatment to the patient and who uses observation skills in assessing patient response to that treatment is an invaluable asset to the practice.

DOSAGE FORMS

Pharmaceutic companies manufacture drugs in various forms. Some drugs are available in a variety of forms; others may be available for administration in only one form. Most pharmaceutic companies endeavor to provide comfort to the patient and ensure ease of administration when formulating their drugs. Some common drug preparations may be administered orally, parenterally, intrarectally, or topically or through inhalation. The most common type of preparation is an oral medication. Oral preparations are usually easy to administer, have extended expiration dates, and are manufactured uniformly with respect to the content of the drug.

Tablets are the most commonly used oral form (Fig. 2.1). A tablet may be scored or unscored. A scored tablet

---

BOX 2.1 Case Scenario

The veterinarian just finished his appointment with Mrs. Smith and her cat, Rebel, and asks you to prepare medications that Rebel needs to take orally and would like you to discuss with Mrs. Smith the proper way to give the medications, by mouth, at home. The veterinarian tells you that Rebel is a smart cat and will not be fooled by giving the medication in food. He is prescribing a tablet that is to be given, by mouth, once daily for 14 days.

You meet with Mrs. Smith and show her the medications that you prepared for Rebel and discuss that they are to be given, by mouth, once a day for 14 days and that she needs to be sure to give the medication each day until they are finished. Mrs. Smith explains that she has a pilling device that was given to her quite a few years ago but needs a refresher on how to use it.

You demonstrate how to place the tablet in the soft nozzle at the end of the pilling device and how to push on the plunger to allow the pill to be released. Mrs. Smith feels comfortable doing that and demonstrates her technique. You then explain that gentle, safe restraint of Rebel is important, and it helps if you have two people—one person to give the tablet and one to hold the cat. Rebel can be on your lap, table, or the floor; anywhere he feels comfortable. You demonstrate how to gently grasp the cat's head from above with one hand, by placing your thumb on one side of the upper jaw and your fingers on the other side; the pilling device is in the other hand. Then you show her how to tilt the cat's head back so that her nose points toward the ceiling and the jaw should drop open slightly. You explain that she will need to quickly place the pilling device into the back of the cat's mouth (at the base of the tongue), depress the plunger, and close the cat's mouth and hold it closed while allowing the head to return to a normal position. You discuss how important it is for her to gently stroke the cat's neck or blow lightly on its nose to encourage swallowing and when the cat licks its nose with its tongue it will have swallowed the pill.

Mrs. Smith feels confident and demonstrates pilling Rebel in front of you with success.

You tell Mrs. Smith that it would be a good idea after pilling Rebel to give him some positive reinforcement like petting or brushing him or even giving a treat.

You end the conversation letting her know to contact the hospital if she has any problems or cannot manage giving the medication and they will discuss another option with the veterinarian.

This illustrates knowledge in the area of client education and ensures that the client feels comfortable medicating Rebel.

has indentions that have been made into its surface, allowing it to be broken into halves or quarters. Therefore, a scored tablet provides a way of administering a smaller dose to the patient. A tablet that is unscored may be cut into a smaller size with the use of a pill cutter device. However, scored tablets break more readily and are less likely to fragment. Some tablets have an **enteric coating** (acid resistant coating) to prevent them from dissolving in acid environments such as the stomach and are activated only when they pass through an alkaline environment such as the small intestine. Capsules are containers that house medication. The capsule itself may be made of gelatin and glycerin. The contents of a capsule may be in powder or liquid form. Capsules may be advantageous to use because they allow a patient to be treated without an unpalatable taste coming into contact with the oral mucosa. Unfortunately, capsules cannot be broken down the way a scored tablet can to provide a smaller dose. Boluses are large rectangular tablets that may be scored or unscored. Boluses are used in the treatment of large animals (e.g., cattle, horses, sheep). Boluses usually are administered to bovines with the aid of a special instrument called a *balling gun*.

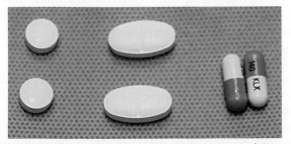

Fig. 2.1 Tablets and capsules are the most common forms of oral medications.

Liquid preparations for oral administration may be purchased in several different forms (e.g., mixtures, emulsions, syrups, or elixirs). Mixtures consist of aqueous solutions (i.e., water) and suspensions for oral administration. A **suspension** usually separates after long periods of shelf life and must be shaken well before it is used so that a uniform dose is provided. Syrups contain the drug and a flavoring in a concentrated solution of sugar water or other aqueous liquid. In veterinary medicine, an antibiotic (e.g., doxycycline) may be mixed with a liquid vitamin (e.g., Lixotinic) to ensure a more palatable taste for the patient. **Elixirs** usually consist of a hydroalcoholic liquid that contains sweeteners, flavoring, and a medicinal agent. **Emulsions** consist of oily substances dispersed in an aqueous medium with an additive that stabilizes the mixture. All liquid oral medications should be administered slowly to allow the patient to swallow before more liquid is given. Rapid administration of oral medication can result in aspiration into the lungs, thereby causing pulmonary problems.

> ### TECHNICIAN NOTES
>
> Rapid administration of oral medication can cause the liquid to be aspirated into the lungs, thereby causing pulmonary problems.

Two forms of parenteral injection that are available are injections and implants. Injections are available as single-dose vials, multidose vials, ampules, or large-volume bottles that may be used to administer intravenous (IV) infusions (Fig. 2.2). A vial is a bottle that is sealed with a rubber diaphragm. A vial may contain a single dose or multiple doses. A single-dose vial must be

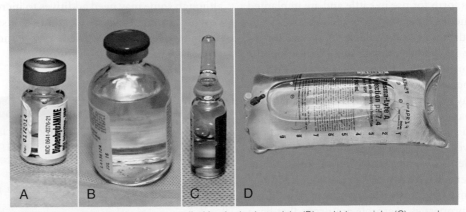

Fig. 2.2 (A) Parenteral medications are supplied in single-dose vials, (B) multidose vials, (C) ampules, and (D) large-volume bottles or bags used for intravenous administration.

discarded after one use (dose). Multidose vials usually contain preservatives that enable them to have a longer shelf life; thus they may be used for more than one dose. Ampules contain a single dose of medication in a small glass container with a thin neck, which is usually scored so that it can be snapped off easily. Some drugs may be unstable in solution and may require reconstitution with sterile water or another diluent; these may be used immediately for injection (Procedure 2.1).

TECHNICIAN NOTES

It is a good idea to place a paper towel over the neck of an ampule before breaking it, to protect the fingers from glass cuts.

Syringes and needles are used for parenteral administration of drugs (Box 2.2). This equipment must be sterile. Drugs should never be stored in syringes for a long time before administration occurs because some drugs may be absorbed into the plastic makeup of the syringe, resulting in an inadequate dose or inactivation of vaccines.

TECHNICIAN NOTES

All used needles should be discarded properly into a sharps container.

Implants are very hard sterile pellets that contain a chemical or a hormonal agent. Implants are inserted subcutaneously and are absorbed by the body over an extended time. Growth hormones are commonly manufactured in this form for use in cattle and are implanted in the subcutaneous dorsal aspect of the ear.

Topical medications are available in several forms. Liniments are medicinal preparations for use on the skin as a counterirritant or to relieve pain. Lotions are liquid suspensions or solutions with soothing substances that may be applied to the skin. An ointment is a semisolid preparation of oil and water, plus a medicinal agent. The water in an ointment evaporates after application and leaves the drug behind on the skin's surface. Dusting powders (e.g., flea powder) are mixtures of drugs in powder form for topical application. Additionally, powders may have adsorbent (cornstarch) or lubricant (talcum) properties. Aerosols are drugs that have been incorporated into a suitable solvent and packaged under pressure with a propellant. Dusting powders and aerosols are common forms for some topical insecticides and wound dressings.

Microencapsulation is a drug form that stabilizes substances commonly considered unstable. Microencapsulation also may be used for drugs intended to be released slowly over a period of time (e.g., moxidectin [ProHeart injection]). When the drug's active ingredients are microencapsulated, a protective environment is formed against harmful substances and the stability of the product is improved. Microencapsulation completely masks the flavor of a drug and allows oral treatments to be administered with greater ease because the patient is unable to taste or smell the ingredients.

DRUG PRESERVATIVES AND SOLVENTS

In addition to the active ingredient, many drugs contain organic or inorganic agents as additives or pharmaceutic aids. These inactive (or inert) ingredients facilitate tablet administration, improve solubility, or increase stability. Although the quantity of inert ingredients is usually small, these ingredients can cause adverse effects, or a patient may be sensitive or may smell the ingredients.

Parenterally administered drugs often contain chemical preservatives that are used to prevent destruction and loss of potency through oxidation or hydrolysis. The amount of preservative in the formulation of parenterally administered drugs is an optimal concentration, and the reconstituted medication should be used immediately to prevent the possibility of fungal or bacterial growth. Dilution of the drug reduces the effectiveness of the preservatives. Most drugs are water soluble, although some may need additives to increase solubility. Glycols are one example of additives used to increase solubility. Generally, propylene glycol and polyethylene glycols are preferred.

TECHNICIAN NOTES

Some vaccines may contain antibiotic preservatives. Care should be taken by personnel during reconstitution of these vaccines because liquid that escapes from the rubber seal of the vial could be sprayed inadvertently into an allergic person's eye (e.g., those persons with hypersensitivity to penicillin).

Materials Needed

Syringe of adequate size for the amount of diluent with a needle attached

70% isopropyl alcohol

Cotton swab

Invert the diluent vial and withdraw the desired amount of diluent.

3. Inject the diluent into the medication vial and withdraw the syringe and needle. Shake the vial to mix well (Fig. 2.3C).

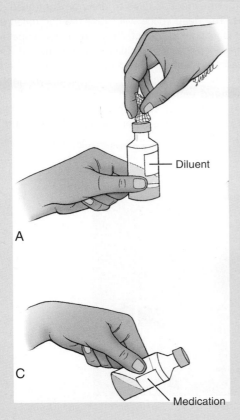

A

C

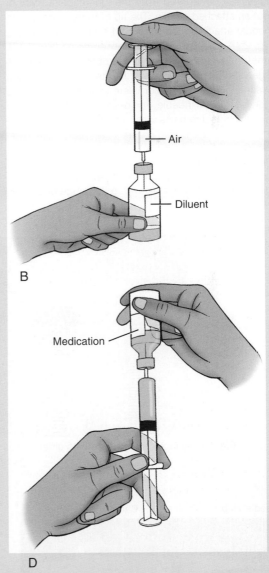

B

D

Fig. 2.3

Procedure

1. Clean the rubber diaphragm of the medication vial and the diluent vial with an alcohol swab (Fig. 2.3A).
2. Remove the needle cap and pull back on the plunger to fill the barrel with air equal to the desired amount of diluent. Inject the air into the vial of diluent to create positive pressure and to ease withdrawal (Fig. 2.3B).
3.

4. Positive pressure may be created in the freshly mixed medication vial before the desired amount of medication has been withdrawn. Once the medication has been withdrawn (Fig. 2.3D), label the syringe, and administer the drug to the patient. After withdrawing the patient's medication, dispose of the vial, or store it according to the label.

BOX 2.2   Syringes and Needles

Syringes

Syringes are available in various sizes and styles. The most commonly used sizes are 3, 6, 12, 20, 35, and 60 mL. Syringes may be ordered from the manufacturer with or without an attached needle. The tip of the syringe, where the needle attaches, can be one of four types: Luer-Lok tip (Fig. 2.4A), slip tip (Fig. 2.4B), eccentric tip (Fig. 2.4C), or catheter tip (Fig. 2.4D). Each type of tip has its own advantages and disadvantages and is often chosen because of personal preference. A complete syringe consists of a plunger, barrel, hub, needle, and dead space (Fig. 2.5). The area in which fluid remains when the plunger is completely depressed is called *dead space*.

Tuberculin Syringe

A tuberculin syringe (Fig. 2.6) holds up to 1 mL of medication. It usually is available with a 25-gauge or smaller attached needle. This syringe is commonly used for injections of less than 1 mL. Some tuberculin syringes have a dead space. Although the patient receives the proper amount of medicine, some liquid remains in this dead space, thus wasting the drug and costing the practice money. This is also important to remember when a tuberculin syringe is used to draw up controlled substances. The dead space will cause the controlled substance log book to reflect more controlled substance used than was actually administered from the vial. Thus, the dead space should be considered when amounts used are documented. Some tuberculin syringes are manufactured with low dead space or no dead space at all. In the case of syringes with no dead space, the needle screws into the tuberculin syringe instead of attaching to the tip.

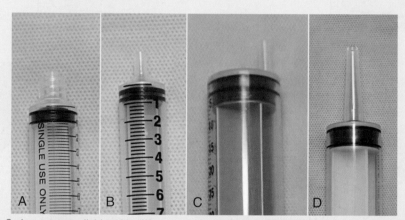

Fig. 2.4 Syringes are available with different tips, such as (A) Luer-Lok, (B) slip, (C) eccentric, and (D) catheter.

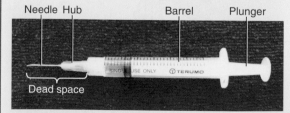

Fig. 2.5 The parts of a needle and syringe. (From Sirois, M. [2013]. *Elsevier's veterinary assisting textbook*. St. Louis: Elsevier.)

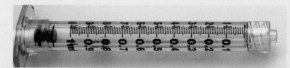

Fig. 2.6 A tuberculin syringe. (From Mulholland, J. [2011]. *The nurse, the math, the meds*. St. Louis: Elsevier.)

BOX 2.2 Syringes and Needles—Cont'd

Multidose Syringe

A multidose syringe (Fig. 2.7) is commonly used for large animals in cases when several animals require the same injection. It allows the user to set the dose and to give repeated injections until the barrel is empty of medication. This type of syringe may be disassembled and disinfected for reuse.

Insulin Syringe

An insulin syringe (Fig. 2.8) usually is supplied with a 25-gauge needle, and differing from other syringes, it has no dead space. The syringe is divided into units in-stead of milliliters and should be used only for insulin injection.

Fig. 2.9 illustrates the importance of being familiar with the different types of syringes and the units of measurement found on each. This is necessary to ensure that one can draw up an accurate amount of medication.

Needles

Needles are available in various sizes and styles, but all needles have the following three parts: hub, shaft, and bevel (Fig. 2.10). Needle sizes vary by gauge and by length (Table 2.1 and Fig. 2.11). The gauge refers to the inside diameter of the shaft; the larger the gauge number, the smaller the diameter. The length of the needle is measured from the tip of the hub to the end of the shaft.

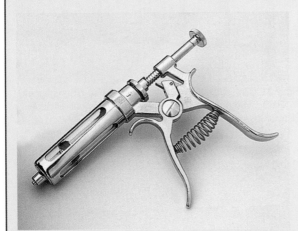

Fig. 2.7 A multidose syringe. (Courtesy Jorgensen Laboratories, Inc., Loveland, CO. In Sonsthagen, T. [2019]. *Veterinary instruments and equipment*. St. Louis: Elsevier.)

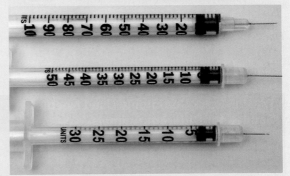

Fig. 2.8 Insulin syringes. (From Mulholland, J. [2011]. *The nurse, the math, the meds*. St. Louis: Elsevier.)

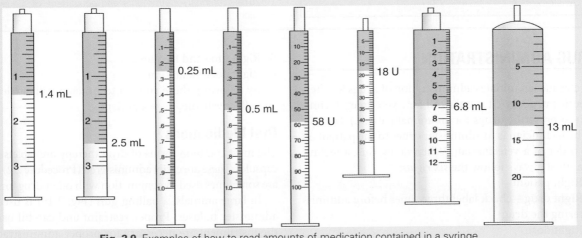

Fig. 2.9 Examples of how to read amounts of medication contained in a syringe.

Continued

BOX 2.2   Syringes and Needles—Cont'd

Lengths longer than 1 inch usually are used in large animals and occasionally for biopsy. The bevel is the angle of the opening at the needle tip. It is often helpful when venipuncture is performed to have the beveled side of the needle facing up before the needle is inserted into the patient.

Bleeding needles (Fig. 2.12) may be up to 3 inches long, are large gauge (14 to 16 gauge), and usually are used for obtaining blood from cattle and swine. These needles are made of stainless steel and are reusable after proper cleaning and disinfecting.

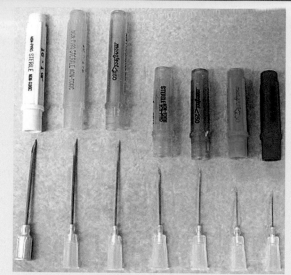

Fig. 2.11 Disposable hypodermic needles. (From Sonsthagen, T. [2019]. *Veterinary instruments and equipment.* St. Louis: Elsevier.)

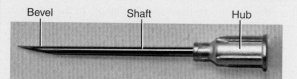

Fig. 2.10 A needle consists of three parts: hub, shaft, and bevel.

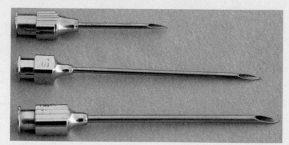

Fig. 2.12 Stainless steel bleeding needles. (From Sonsthagen, T. [2019]. *Veterinary instruments and equipment.* St. Louis: Elsevier.)

TABLE 2.1   Commonly Used Needle Gauges for Different Animals.

Animal	Needle Gauge
Swine	16, 18
Cattle	16, 18
Horses	16, 18, 20
Dogs	20, 21, 22, 25
Cats	22, 25
Small exotics	23, 25, 27

DRUG ADMINISTRATION

A veterinarian initiates administration of drugs for therapeutic purposes. (It is unlawful for a veterinary technician to prescribe drugs for an animal patient.) The role of the technician is to administer drugs to the patient on the order of a veterinarian. When doing this, a technician must always follow the *six rights:*

1. Right patient
2. Right drug—check label three times before administering the drug
3. Right dose
4. Right route
5. Right time and frequency
6. Right documentation

By following these rules, a technician will efficiently and effectively medicate a patient.

Oral Medications

The most common forms of drug therapy are tablets and capsules. These are easily administered (Procedure 2.2) and are sometimes used in conjunction with other drug forms.

In large animals, a balling gun (Fig. 2.16) is used to administer boluses. Proper restraint and careful use of the instrument are necessary for proper administration and avoidance of injury to the patient.

PROCEDURE 2.2 Oral Administration of Tablets or Capsules for Dogs and Cats

Materials Needed

Medication in tablet or capsule form
Pilling gun (optional) (Fig. 2.13)

Procedure

1. Hold the animal's upper jaw with one hand and apply pressure against the upper premolars to cause the mouth to open.
2. Push the medication over the tongue of the animal with the other hand or with the pilling gun (Fig. 2.14).
3. Close the animal's mouth.
4. Initiate swallowing by blowing into the animal's nose and/or rubbing its throat (Fig. 2.15).

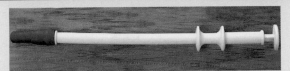

Fig. 2.13 Example of a small-animal pilling gun. (Sonsthagen, T. [2019]. *Veterinary instruments and equipment*. St. Louis: Elsevier.)

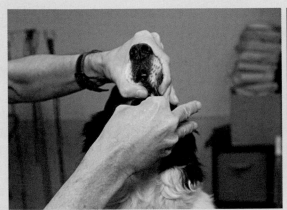 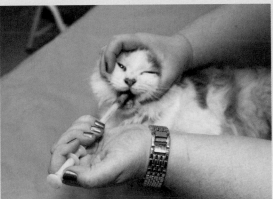

Fig. 2.14

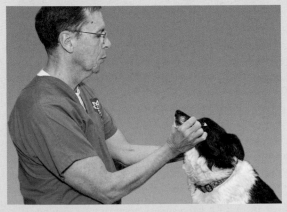

Fig. 2.15

🗒 TECHNICIAN NOTES

Coating the tablet or capsule with a palatable substance such as Cat Lax, peanut butter, or canned food may help in pilling difficult animals.

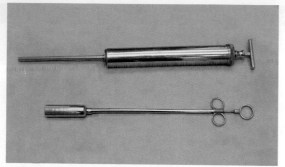

Fig. 2.16 A balling gun used to administer a bolus to large animals and a dose syringe used to administer small volumes of liquids.

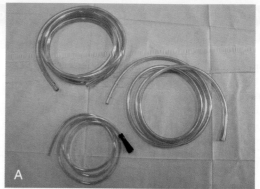

A

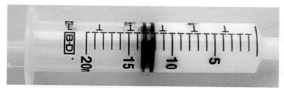

Fig. 2.17 A syringe without a needle may be used to administer oral liquid medication. (From Macklin, D., Chernecky, C., & Infortuna, H. [2011]. *Math for clinical practice*. [2nd ed.]. St. Louis: Mosby.)

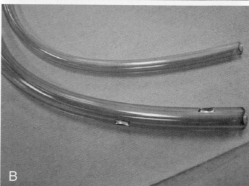

B

Liquid oral medications may be administered to small animals through a syringe with the needle removed (Procedure 2.3 and Fig. 2.17) or, in some instances, through an orogastric or nasogastric tube. Medications may be made more palatable for these patients by mixing with a vitamin mixture or food to ease administration. Oral liquid medications used in exotic animals may be administered through the drinking water or an orogastric tube. In large animals, a dose syringe (see Fig. 2.16) is used to give small amounts of liquids and a stomach tube is used to administer large amounts of oral liquid medications. In horses, the tube is passed via the nasogastric route (Fig. 2.18A–C). In cattle, the stomach tube is passed through a Frick **speculum** (Fig. 2.19) via the orogastric route.

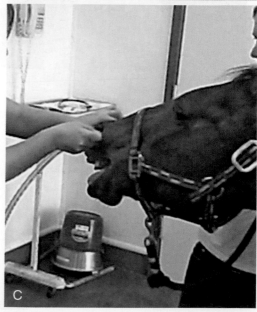

C

Fig. 2.18 (A–C) A large-animal stomach tube may be used to administer liquid medications to horses via the nasogastric route. (A and B, From Hanie, E. A. [2006]. *Large animal clinical procedures for veterinary technicians*. St. Louis: Mosby. C, From Sirois, M. [2011]. *The principles and practices of veterinary technology*. St. Louis, Elsevier.)

TECHNICIAN NOTES

- Remember when administering oral medications that it takes longer for a drug to be absorbed into the bloodstream by this route than by parenteral injection.
- Do not use oral administration in animals that are vomiting.
- Care must be taken when drawing up oral medication in a parenteral syringe so that it is not inadvertently given by a parenteral route (injection).

Parenteral Medications

Parenteral administration (i.e., injection) of liquid medications may be used alone or in conjunction with other forms of medication. Some conditions are unfavorable for oral administration (e.g., in vomiting patients), and some drugs are available only for parenteral administration.

Approximately 10 routes are used commonly for **parenteral administration** of drugs; the most commonly used are the intramuscular, subcutaneous, and IV routes

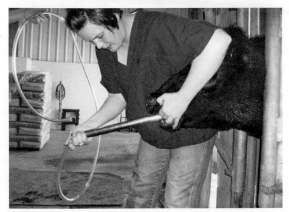

Fig. 2.19 A Frick speculum can be used to facilitate passage of the stomach tube through the mouths of cattle. (From Holtgrew-Bohling, K. [2020]. *Large animal clinical techniques.* St. Louis, Elsevier.)

(Figs. 2.21 to 2.23). A veterinary technician must be aware of the proper route of administration for each drug. For those in doubt, the route of administration usually is listed on the drug label or the package insert. Sometimes, complications may result after parenteral administration of a drug. Common complications include irritation, necrosis, and infection of the injection site. Sometimes, allergic reactions to medications may occur. Clinical signs of an allergic reaction after a parenteral drug has been administered include swelling around the face or extremities, raised bumps or swellings on the skin's surface, edema, and salivation. If any complications are observed, these should be reported immediately to the veterinarian. Care should be exercised when an intramuscular injection is administered so that nerve damage or accidental injection into a vein or artery can be avoided. Negative pressure should be applied to the plunger of the syringe before an intramuscular (or subcutaneous) injection is performed. Should any blood be observed in the hub of the needle, the needle should be redirected or removed. Care should also be exercised when intraperitoneal injections are provided so that peritonitis does not develop and damage the abdominal viscera. Proper administration involves knowing (1) what equipment is needed, (2) how the dose should be calculated, and (3) the proper method for withdrawing and administering medication (Procedure 2.4).

Intravenous administration allows the most rapid and effective drug administration (Procedure 2.5). IV therapy

---

PROCEDURE 2.3 Oral Administration of Liquid Medication With a Syringe for Dogs and Cats

Materials Needed
Syringe with the needle removed or oral dose syringe
Oral medication in liquid form

Procedure
1. Fill syringe with the calculated amount of medication.
2. Tilt the animal's head up slightly.
3. Insert the tip of the syringe into the animal's cheek pouch (Fig. 2.20).
4. Administer the medication slowly.

 TECHNICIAN NOTES

Attachment of a J-12 Teat Infusion Cannula (Jorgensen Laboratories, Loveland, CO) is helpful for administering oral liquid medications.

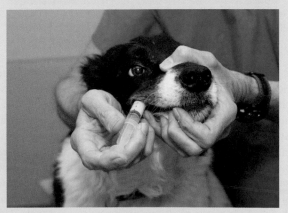

Fig. 2.20

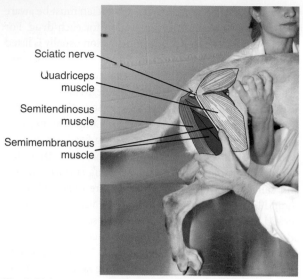

Fig. 2.21 Intramuscular injections in the pelvic limb should be given in an area that avoids the large sciatic nerve. (From Meric Taylor, S. [2016]. *Small animal clinical techniques*. Elsevier.)

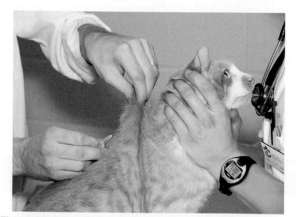

Fig. 2.22 Subcutaneous injection. (From Meric Taylor, S. [2016]. *Small animal clinical techniques*. St. Louis, Elsevier.)

is used most commonly to maintain and restore fluid and electrolyte balance, to administer drugs, and to transfuse blood. IV administration also is used when the medication is contraindicated for other routes of administration. Intravenous injections can be given as an **IV bolus** in which a single, precise amount of medication is given one time, or as an **IV infusion** or constant rate infusion which is given at a slower rate over an extended period of time using an infusion pump. Sites for IV administration include the cephalic vein, the jugular vein, the lateral saphenous vein, and sometimes the femoral veins.

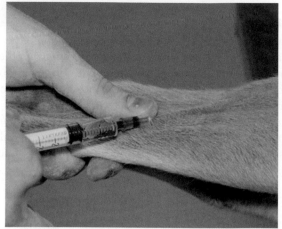

Fig. 2.23 Intravenous injection. (From Meric Taylor, S. [2016]. *Small animal clinical techniques*. Elsevier.)

Long-term IV therapy is best achieved with the cephalic or jugular veins.

In some cases, an animal may need repeated IV injections. The veterinarian may order the placement of an indwelling IV catheter in an effort to lessen vein damage and pain for the animal (Procedures 2.6 and 2.7).

> **📋 TECHNICIAN NOTES**
>
> Intravenous catheters should be inspected frequently and changed if signs of phlebitis or other complications appear. Time of placement can be accounted for by writing (e.g., use a permanent marker) placement time on the adhesive bandage that secures the IV catheter in the animal's vein. Intravenous and extension sets should be changed out on a schedule in accordance with clinic policy.

If the patient is receiving IV fluids, the Y-injection site (see Fig. 2.28)—located on the IV tubing—may be used to administer medications by direct bolus (Procedure 2.8). When medications are to be administered continuously and for long periods, the IV tubing may be changed after a 48- to 72-hour period (AAHA, 2018) or in accordance with clinic policy. Once the medication bottle or bag has been emptied, replacement is necessary to facilitate care of the patient. An indwelling catheter must be inspected frequently and changed if phlebitis or other complications occur. Recent studies have shown that catheter complications are related more to the lack of sterile technique

PROCEDURE 2.4 Parenteral Administration of Medications—Intramuscular or Subcutaneous

Materials Needed

Syringe and needle (Fig. 2.24)
Parenteral medication
Cotton swabs
70% isopropyl alcohol

Procedure

1. If the syringe is not supplied ready to use, firmly attach the needle to the syringe.
2. Swab the bottle's rubber diaphragm with cotton that is saturated with alcohol.
3. Remove the needle cap, insert the needle at an angle into the rubber diaphragm, and withdraw the calculated amount of the drug.
4. Hold the syringe with the needle pointing upward, and remove the large air bubbles by briskly tapping the barrel of the syringe.
5. Release the air bubbles by slightly pushing on the syringe plunger. Carefully replace the needle cap if the medication is not to be given immediately. Avoid contamination.
6. Swab the injection site with another cotton swab that is saturated with alcohol.

7. Insert the needle into the appropriate site and pull slightly on the plunger. If no blood is seen, inject the medication and remove the needle from the site. Blood indicates that a vessel has been entered. Withdraw the needle and continue with the same procedure at a different site.
8. Massage the injection site to aid distribution and decrease pain.
9. Properly dispose of the syringe and needle.

Guidelines for Parenteral Doses

- Round up to the nearest tenth if the amount is greater than 1 mL, and measure in a 3-mL syringe.
- Measure amounts less than 1 mL in a tuberculin syringe.
- In cats weighing less than 9 lb (4.09 kg), 0.5 to 1 mL is an appropriate amount for intramuscular injection.
- In cats weighing more than 9 lb (4.09 kg), 1 to 1.5 mL is an appropriate amount for intramuscular injection.
- In dogs weighing up to 10 lb (4.55 kg), 0.5 to 1 mL is an appropriate amount for intramuscular injection.
- In dogs weighing 10 (4.55 kg) to 30 lb (13.64 kg), 1 to 2 mL is an appropriate amount for intramuscular injection.
- In dogs weighing more than 30 lb (13.64 kg), 2 to 4 mL is an appropriate amount for intramuscular injection.

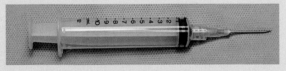

Fig. 2.24

TECHNICIAN NOTES

Injecting multidose vials with air sometimes allows easier withdrawal of medication.

---

in placement than the length of time it has been in place, although 72 to 96 hours generally should not be exceeded, depending on the catheter type (Veterinary Information Network Discussion Boards, 2013). If the IV catheter is not used continuously, it should be flushed with saline or heparinized saline every 4 to 6 hours.

A Simplex (i.e., gravity set) IV set may be used to administer medications or fluids intravenously to large animals (Fig. 2.29). This administration set may be disinfected and reused. Disposable IV sets and large-volume fluid bags are available for large animals that require continuous IV therapy.

In pediatric patients and small exotics, IV medications may be administered by intraosseous cannulation. This route also may be used in larger patients when rapid administration of fluids or drugs is necessary and a vein is not readily available. If needed, large volumes of fluid may be administered in this manner.

In some veterinary hospitals, the use of an infusion pump may facilitate continuous IV administration. Once the necessary flow rate is known (the rate is ordered by the veterinarian), the technician can set the infusion pump to deliver a constant amount of solution per minute or hour. To determine the pump settings, the technician considers

PROCEDURE 2.5   Parenteral Administration of Medication—Intravenous Direct Bolus

Materials Needed

Syringe containing calculated dose with needle attached

Cotton swabs

70% isopropyl alcohol or surgical scrub

Butterfly catheter (scalp vein needle, Fig. 2.25)—optional

Syringe containing 3 mL of flushing solution (e.g., heparinized saline: 500 IU sodium heparin in 250 mL of normal saline) or sterile saline alone

Tape (optional)

Procedure Without Catheter

1. Select the proper site for administration.
2. Clip the area over the venipuncture site, if desired.
3. Prepare the area with alcohol swabs or surgical scrub.
4. Occlude the vein with digital pressure or use a tourniquet.
5. Introduce the needle into the vein with the bevel of the needle facing up.
6. Aspirate to check for blood prior to injecting the medication.

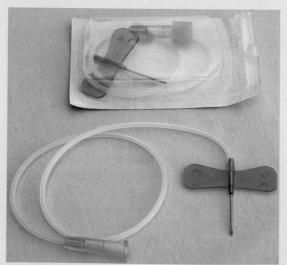

Fig. 2.25 Butterfly catheter. (From Sonsthagen, T. [2019]. *Veterinary instruments and equipment.* St. Louis, Elsevier.)

7. Release pressure from the vein but still hold leg in position and inject the medication over the recommended time interval.
8. Remove the needle and apply pressure to the site to stop bleeding.
9. A bandage made of tape and cotton may be applied, if needed.
10. Properly dispose of all syringes and needles in an approved sharps container.

Procedure with a Butterfly Catheter

Proceed with steps **1 through 4** as described in the previous section.

5. Remove the cap from the catheter tubing and needle cover.
6. Perform venipuncture with the catheter. If this is successful, blood will enter into the catheter tubing.
7. Release pressure from the vein, and allow the blood to fill the catheter tubing.
8. Remove the needle from the medication syringe and attach the syringe hub to the catheter tubing.
9. Administer the medication at the recommended time interval.
10. Remove the needle from the syringe containing the flushing solution. Remove the medication syringe from the catheter and attach the syringe containing the flushing solution.
11. Flush the catheter with 1 to 2 mL of heparinized saline or just sterile saline to ensure administration of all medication.
12. Remove the catheter and apply pressure to the site to stop the bleeding.
13. A bandage may be applied as described earlier.
14. Properly dispose of all syringes and needles in an approved sharps container.

 TECHNICIAN NOTES

Watch for swelling at the injection site. Swelling may signal extravascular injection. Notify the veterinarian immediately if this should occur.

PROCEDURE 2.6   Administration by Bolus With an Indwelling Intravenous Catheter

Materials Needed

Syringe containing flushing solution (about 3 mL)

70% isopropyl alcohol

Cotton swabs

Syringe with medication and attached needle or needle-free connector

Procedure

1. Clean the cap of the indwelling catheter with an alcohol swab.
2. Insert into the catheter cap the needle of the syringe containing the flushing solution. (Use the smallest gauge needle possible to help prevent a leak in the catheter cap.)
3. Gently aspirate to determine correct placement of the catheter (blood entering the hub shows proper placement).
4. Inject half the flushing solution into the catheter. Observe the area over the vein for swelling.
5. Remove the syringe and needle, and carefully replace the cap to prevent contamination.
6. Insert into the catheter cap the needle of the syringe containing the medication, and inject the medication over the recommended time interval.
7. Remove the syringe and needle from the catheter.
8. Flush the catheter with the remaining flushing solution.
9. Observe the area for swelling and look for signs of discomfort. Report any abnormal observations to the veterinarian.
10. Properly dispose of syringes and needles.

 TECHNICIAN NOTES

Some hospitals may require that, with flushing solution, two syringes should be used instead of the same syringe and needle for both flushes. Keep additional male adapter plugs (catheter caps) (Fig. 2.26) in stock to replace a leaky cap.

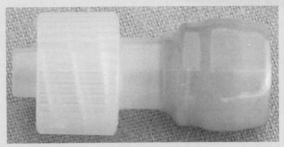

Fig. 2.26 Example of a male adapter plug. (From Sonsthagen, T. [2019]. *Veterinary instruments and equipment*. St. Louis, Elsevier.)

the total amount of solution to be given and the time interval for infusion. The operating instructions for the infusion pump should be followed because each model may operate in a slightly different manner.

 TECHNICIAN NOTES

It should be remembered that any patient receiving IV fluid therapy should be monitored every 15 to 30 minutes.

Monitoring involves evaluating drip rate, ensuring that the IV catheter is properly placed in the vein, making sure the patient has not moved around in the cage to such an extent that the IV tubing has become kinked, and, most importantly, ensuring that the patient has not chewed on and thus dislodged the IV catheter. Animals can do surprising things, and it is up to the technician to provide an excellent level of nursing to ensure that no harm comes to the patient.

 TECHNICIAN NOTES

- Some liquid medications for parenteral administration may "settle out" or precipitate (e.g., penicillin G procaine, triamcinolone acetonide [Vetalog]). Therefore, these medications should be shaken gently to mix the solution before it is injected into the patient.
- Drugs that may cause tissue irritation are administered by the IV route (e.g., vincristine). Therefore, be sure to check the drug's package insert to identify the correct way to administer the drug.

Intramuscular Injections

- Ketamine (Ketaset) can be administered by intramuscular injection. Ketamine has a tendency to burn on injection, and careful restraint methods, along with rapid injection of this drug, should be used in cats.

PROCEDURE 2.7   Administration of Intravenous Fluids

Materials Needed

Indwelling catheter (Fig. 2.27)

Tape

70% isopropyl alcohol or surgical scrub

Infusion set

Intravenous fluids

Clippers

Procedure

1. Remove the IV tubing from the container and the protective covering from the medication bottle or bag.
2. Remove the covering of the diaphragm of the medication bag or bottle.
3. Close the clamp on the IV tubing. Remove the cap of the IV tubing spike and insert it into the diaphragm of the medication bag or bottle using aseptic technique.
4. Squeeze the drip chamber to allow fluid to collect in the chamber. Fill to the designated line or about half full.

5. Remove the protective cap from the end of the IV tubing and slowly open the roller clamp to allow the fluid to clear the tubing of air, then reclamp the tubing. Replace the protective cap and hang the medication bag or bottle on the IV pole near the patient.
6. Clip and scrub the chosen site for catheter placement.
7. After successful catheter placement, cap the catheter, wipe away any blood, and quickly tape in place. The time of placement should be recorded on the adhesive tape with a permanent marker.
8. Remove the catheter cap and the protective cap of the IV tubing and insert the end of the tubing directly into the end of the catheter. Or, if desired, a needle may be placed on the end of the tubing and inserted into the catheter cap.
9. Open the clamp to begin a slow drip and lower the medication bag or bottle to below the IV site to confirm correct placement.
10. Return the bottle or bag to the IV pole and set at desired flow rate or use a fluid pump to set the rate.
11. Tape the tubing to the patient at the catheter site.

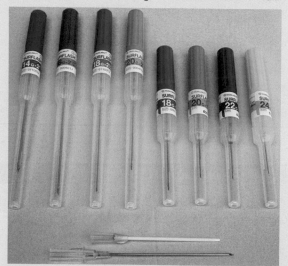

Fig. 2.27 An assortment of indwelling catheters. (From Sonsthagen, T. [2019]. *Veterinary instruments and equipment.* St. Louis, Elsevier.)

TECHNICIAN NOTES

- Mark the fluid level and time on tape placed on the bag with a permanent marker (tape can be used on bottles). Use this procedure each time the patient is checked.
- If any medications are added to the fluids, write the medication, time, and amount on the medication bag or tape.
- Tape the catheter cap to the bag or bottle so that it will be ready when needed.
- Use fluid or syringe pumps whenever possible; they must be monitored regularly for proper functioning as catheter positioning can affect the rate. The use of IV fluid pumps is the safest and most accurate way to deliver fluids to a patient.

- On insertion of the needle into the chosen muscle, always apply negative pressure to the syringe's plunger to be certain that the needle has not entered a blood vessel. If blood is seen in the hub of the syringe, remove and redirect the needle.

Subcutaneous Injections

- Most vaccines can be administered subcutaneously. However, the intrascapular area should always be avoided when subcutaneous injections are given.

Inhalation Medications

In veterinary medicine, inhalation is used primarily to produce anesthesia. The inhalant gas is placed into the anesthetic machine in liquid form and then is vaporized through the machine and delivered to the patient via an endotracheal tube, an anesthetic gas mask, or an induction chamber (Figs. 2.30 to 2.32). Medications occasionally may be nebulized to treat an upper respiratory tract problem, and oxygen may be delivered to a patient with dyspnea with the use of inhalation techniques.

BOX 2.3   Case Scenario

A healthy, 9-month-old, intact female, German Short-haired Pointer was presented to the veterinary hospital for an OVH (ovariohysterectomy). The attending veterinarian preformed a preanesthetic patient assessment on the patient. The veterinary technician prepared the materials needed to place the catheter including clippers with a #40 blade, surgical scrub, alcohol, the appropriate indwelling catheter size, saline for flushing the catheter, tape, ± antiseptic ointment, and male adapter. The technician clipped and prepared the site using standard aseptic technique and placed a 20-gauge IV catheter in the cephalic vein. The IV catheter serves as an important access point for delivering IV fluids, pain medications, anesthetic drugs, and emergency drugs.

The patient was premedicated with drugs, subcutaneously, to provide sedation and analgesia prior to induction. This was performed by observing the syringe to confirm the contents with the correct drug. Loose skin was pinched over the shoulder blades, the bevel of the needle was facing up and the needle was inserted under the skin, the plunger was pulled back slightly to be sure no blood was drawn back, and the contents of the syringe containing the drug was given subcutaneously.

The induction drugs were administered as an IV bolus which allowed for endotracheal intubation. This was achieved by flushing the catheter with saline prior to giving the induction drug. The needle was inserted into the catheter cap and the plunger was gently aspirated to determine correct placement of the catheter (blood should appear in the hub of the needle), the needle was removed and the cap replaced to prevent contamination. The syringe containing the induction drug was observed to confirm the contents of the syringe with the correct drug. The needle was inserted into the catheter cap and was injected over the recommended time interval. The syringe and needle were removed and recapped and the catheter was flushed with saline to ensure administration of all medication. The endotracheal tube was placed.

Postoperatively, pain medication (buprenorphine) was given subcutaneously. The patient was continuously monitored throughout the recovery period; temperature, respiratory rate, heart rate and rhythm, blood pressure, oxygenation, level of sedation, and level of pain.

This illustrates the importance of preparation prior to a procedure, understanding proper administration of subcutaneous injections, and intravenous bolus injections via a catheter.

PROCEDURE 2.8   Administration by Bolus Using the Y-Injection Site

Materials Needed

Syringe with medication and the needle attached
Cotton swabs
70% isopropyl alcohol

Procedure

1. Close the clamp on the infusion set.

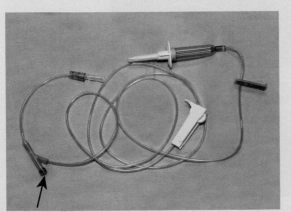

Fig. 2.28 Intravenous set with roller clamp and Y-injection site.

2. Clean the Y-injection site (Fig. 2.28) with an alcohol swab.
3. Insert the needle of the medication syringe into the Y-injection site.
4. Inject the medication over the recommended time interval.
5. Remove the medication syringe and needle.
6. Open the clamp on the infusion set. Allow enough fluid to flow through the infusion set to ensure that all medication is received. Then return to the desired flow rate.
7. Properly dispose of the syringe and needle.
8. *Note:* No flushing solution is required for this procedure.

📋   TECHNICIAN NOTES

To check for proper placement of the IV catheter, remove the bag of fluids from the IV pole and hold the bag and tubing below the level of the catheter (do not close the clamp on the infusion set). If blood returns into the tubing, the catheter is properly placed. Return the bag to the IV pole and continue fluid administration.

Topical Medications

Topical administration of medicine involves application of drugs (creams, ointments, and drops) to the body's surface. Topical preparations usually provide local effects instead of systemic ones. Clipping hair from the affected area provides better visualization during treatment and makes application easier and absorption faster. The technician should observe the area after treatment and should report adverse reactions to the veterinarian. The technician should provide client education regarding skin medications, including information on frequency and number of applications. Many clients apply too much medication, which not only is unnecessary but also can be quite costly with some medications.

Ophthalmic drugs are supplied as an ointment or a solution. The eyes have the ability to remove foreign substances rapidly. Therefore, these preparations usually are applied several times a day. Application frequency depends on the disease or disorder, the drug, and the type of formulation. When ophthalmic preparations are applied, the hand that is holding the medication should rest on the animal's head above the affected eye (Fig. 2.33). Drops should be placed at the inner canthus of the eye. If application of ointment is necessary, a small strip should be applied along the lower palpebral border; the applicator tip should not come into contact with the eye or conjunctiva. When you are demonstrating to a client how to apply eye medications, point out that the applicators have blunt tips. Therefore if the applicator tip inadvertently touches the eye, no harm should occur.

Drugs may be applied topically to the ears for local effect to soften cerumen and ease its removal or to treat a superficial infection or ear mites. Cleaning of the ears before otic medication is applied aids the effectiveness of treatment. The veterinary technician should provide instruction to the client regarding the correct ways to clean ears and to apply ear medication. By explaining the ear's anatomy, the technician can assure the client that it is difficult to reach the animal's eardrum when one is swabbing the ear clean.

MEDICATION ORDERS

In a veterinary hospital, most medication orders are written or verbal. A written order may be provided in prescription form or may be noted in the medical record. Verbal orders are given directly to the technician by the veterinarian. When filling a prescription, the technician must be familiar with abbreviations frequently applied to the medical record to describe drug therapy. Appendix A lists abbreviations commonly used in veterinary medicine. The technician must

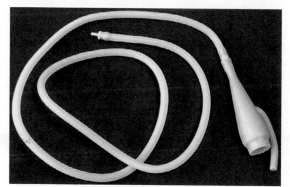

Fig. 2.29 A large-animal intravenous set (Simplex). (Courtesy Jorgensen Laboratories, Inc., Loveland, CO. In Sonsthagen, T. [2019]. *Veterinary instruments and equipment.* St. Louis, Elsevier.)

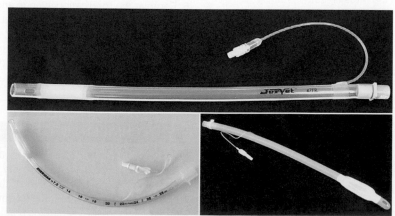

Fig. 2.30 Endotracheal tube with cuff. (Courtesy Jorgensen Laboratories, Inc., Loveland, CO. In Sonsthagen, T. [2019]. *Veterinary instruments and equipment.* St. Louis, Elsevier.)

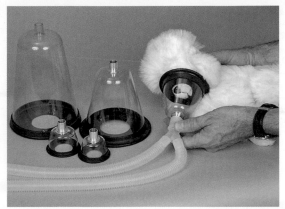

Fig. 2.31 A small-animal anesthetic mask. (From Thomas, J. [2017]. *Anesthesia and analgesia for veterinary technicians*. St. Louis, Elsevier.)

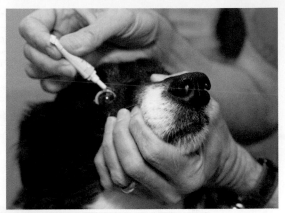

Fig. 2.33 Ointment is applied to a dog's eye on the lower palpebral border.

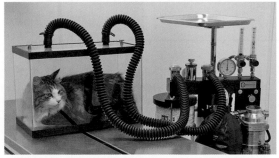

Fig. 2.32 A small-animal induction chamber. (From Sonsthagen, T. [2019]. *Veterinary instruments and equipment*. St. Louis, Elsevier.)

know the patient being treated, the route of administration used, and the frequency of administration. This information is described in the medication order. After the medication has been administered to the patient, a notation should be made in the medical record describing when, what, how, and by whom the medication was administered. Observations of the patient's progress should be noted in the medical record (Fig. 2.34). If the medication order is a prescription (Fig. 2.35) to be filled, the order should be dated and noted in the medical record (Fig. 2.36). If the owner picks up the prescription at the veterinary hospital, the medical record should be retrieved and presented to the veterinarian for approval of the refill. The same procedure as described earlier should be followed for dispensing medication.

DISPENSED MEDICATION LABELING

When a drug is prescribed for a patient, the drug label is an important part of the dispensing process. It is important that the label contain the following information:

- The veterinary facility's name, address, and telephone number.
- The veterinarian's name.
- The client's name and address.
- The patient's name and species.
- The name of the drug.
- The strength of the drug.
- The quantity being dispensed.
- Instructions to the client about how the drug should be administered.
- The amount to be given for each dose.
- The manner in which the drug should be administered.
- How often the drug should be given.
- Information that includes the duration of administration.
- The number of refills permitted.
- The expiration date of the drug being dispensed.
- The statement "for veterinary use only" should be included on the label.
- Optional statement to include is "keep out of reach of children."
- Any necessary warning and precautionary statements including withdrawal times.

CONTROLLED SUBSTANCES

Substances that have the ability to become habit-forming for humans are labeled as *controlled substances or scheduled drugs*. Every veterinarian who orders, dispenses, prescribes, or administers controlled substances must be registered with the DEA. This registration is valid for 3 years. The DEA further requires that the upper right corner of the original container of

4/6/2019 10:00 AM Patient is bright, alert and responsive

Temp – 102° F, HR – 120 bpm, RR – panting

Gave 100 mg Amoxicillin tablet PO, flushed IV catheter with 1 ml

of heparinized saline, continue IV lactated ringers fluids at 15

gtt/min and continue to monitor vital signs   L Johnson, DVM

Fig. 2.34 After medication is administered to a patient, a notation should be made in the patient's medical record.

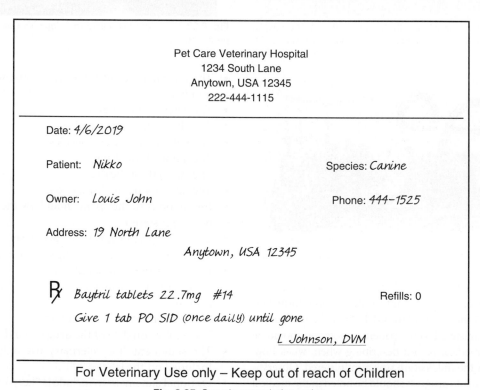

Pet Care Veterinary Hospital
1234 South Lane
Anytown, USA 12345
222-444-1115

Date: 4/6/2019

Patient: Nikko   Species: Canine

Owner: Louis John   Phone: 444–1525

Address: 19 North Lane

Anytown, USA 12345

℞ Baytril tablets 22.7mg #14   Refills: 0

Give 1 tab PO SID (once daily) until gone

L Johnson, DVM

For Veterinary Use only – Keep out of reach of Children

Fig. 2.35 Sample prescription order.

4/6/2019 Rx per Dr Johnson

Baytril tablets 22.7mg 1 tab PO SID x 14 days

L Johnson, DVM

Fig. 2.36 Prescriptions should be written in the patient's medical record.

controlled substances should show a code containing a capital C (controlled), followed by a Roman numeral indicating one of the five schedules defined by the *Code of Federal Regulations* (Fig. 2.37). The higher the value of the Roman numeral, the lesser the abuse potential of the drug. Drugs classified as C-I have the highest abuse potential and drugs classified as C-V have the least. Because some of these drugs may be misused, the DEA requires that they be stored in an unmovable locked safe or cabinet and that an inventory log be kept to report amounts used (administered or dispensed) and on hand (Fig. 2.38). Records must also show the flow of controlled substances into and out of the practice including when drugs are acquired, inventoried, stolen, lost, or distributed. These records must be readily retrievable

and may be computerized. An inventory of all controlled substances must be completed at least every 2 years.

Each time a controlled drug is administered or dispensed to a patient, this event must be reported in the controlled substance inventory log, as well in the patient's medical record. This documentation should include the following: (1) date, (2) owner's name, (3) patient's name, (4) drug name, (5) amount administered or dispensed, and (6) the names of veterinary personnel who dispensed the drug.

TECHNICIAN NOTES

- Controlled drugs must be kept in a securely locked cabinet of substantial construction or safe to prevent unauthorized personnel access.
- Inventory logs must be kept, for 2 years, to show the flow of controlled drugs into and out of the hospital including acquired, inventoried, lost, stolen or distributed controlled substances.

Some of the common controlled substances used in veterinary clinics include analgesics and anesthetics like ketamine, tiletamine (Telazol), diazepam, pentobarbital, morphine, and butorphanol tartrate (Torbugesic). Others include diphenoxylate, hydrocodone, and phenobarbital. Anabolic steroids such as stanozolol, testosterone, mibolerone, and boldenone are also controlled.

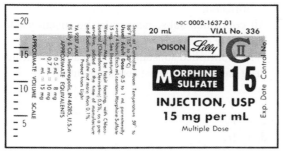

Fig. 2.37 Label showing schedule II-controlled substance designation. (From Mulholland, J. [2011]. *The nurse, the math, the meds.* Elsevier.)

Record of controlled substances administered/dispensed

Name of controlled substance: *Ketamine*   Form: *Injection*   Strength: *100 mg/mL*   Size: *10mL*

Date	Patient/Animal name and address	Species of Animal	Initials of Person Administering/ Dispensing	Previous Balance	Amount Administered/ Dispensed (or purchased)	New Balance
1/10/13	Tim Smith / Toby	K-9	BD	10.0mL	1mL	9mL
1/15/13	Bill Potts / Prissy	Feline	LW	9mL	0.5mL	8.5mL
2/3/13	Chris Pettes / Gilbert	K-9	KM	8.5mL	2mL	6.5mL
2/8/13	Elaine Curtis / TJ	Feline	BD	6.5mL	0.4mL	6.1mL

Fig. 2.38 Example of a controlled substance log.

See Appendix F for more details on DEA regulations.

> ### TECHNICIAN NOTES
>
> **Drug Storage**
> - The manufacturer's instructions should be followed closely to facilitate safe storage.
> - Some drugs are sensitive to light and humidity.
> - The location of the pharmacy in a veterinary hospital should not be accessible to the public.

CLIENT EDUCATION

Veterinary technicians should make themselves familiar with all administered and dispensed drugs. Often, it is the technician's duty to educate clients about how a medication should be administered, why it has been prescribed, and what adverse reactions may occur, if any. Technicians should consult the veterinarian to gather information about any questions that they cannot answer. If needed, written information about the medication should be available for the client's reference purposes.

▌ REVIEW QUESTIONS

1. Name four common drug preparations.
2. Boluses are used in the treatment of large animals and are administered with a _____.
3. Name two types of parenteral injection forms.
4. Vials may be either _____ dose or _____ dose.
5. All used needles should be discarded in a _____.
6. Name the six rights of drug administration.
7. Oral drugs should never be administered in animals that are _____.
8. Intravenous administration of drugs allows the most _____ and effective drug administration.
9. If you are having difficulty administering oral medications by hand to a cat, what device can be used as an effective method of delivery?

10. A Simplex (i.e., gravity set) IV system is used to administer fluids to _____ animals.
11. Name six items that should be recorded in the controlled substance log.
12. Why should drugs given by injection not be stored in syringes for any length of time before administration?
13. List four types of syringe tips that are available for use.
14. A tuberculin syringe holds up to _____ mL of medication.
15. What type of syringe is divided into units rather than milliliters?
16. What is meant by the term "enteric coated tablets?"
17. Describe the difference between an elixir and an emulsion.
18. Explain the difference between an IV bolus and an IV infusion.
19. All controlled substances must be inventoried, at least once every _____.
20. What controlled substance classification indicates a drug having the highest abuse potential?
    a. C-I
    b. C-V
    c. C-IV
    d. C-III
21. A veterinarian who orders, dispenses, prescribes, or administers controlled substances must be registered with the _____; this registration is valid for a period of _____ years.
22. Clearly interpret each of the following drug orders into Layman's terms.
    * 2 gtt AD TID × 7d
    * 1t PO EOD PRN
    * Amoxicillin 100 mg tabs PO BID × 10d
    * Baytril 2.5 mg/kg IM
23. What is the maximum amount of time that an indwelling catheter can be left in the vessel?
24. An in-hospital patient receiving IV fluid therapy should be monitored every 15 to 30 minutes. What parameters are monitored to ensure safety of the patient?
25. Describe two different techniques in which liquid medications can be administered orally to a large animal patient.

REFERENCES

American Animal Hospital Association (website). https://www.aaha.org/aaha-guidelines/infection-control-configuration/protocols/intravenous-catheter-placement-and-maintenance2/. Accessed March 26, 2020.

Bassert, J. M., Samples, O., & Beal, A. (Eds.). (2018). *McCurnin's clinical textbook for veterinary technicians* (9th ed.) St. Louis: Elsevier.

https://www.deadiversion.usdoj.gov/schedules/index.html#define. Accessed 6.4.19.

https://www.fda.gov/animal-veterinary/resources-you/fda-regulation-animal-drugs#dispensing. Accessed April 6, 2019.

Veterinary Information Network. Reuse of intravenous extension tubing or giving sets (website). http://www.vin.com/Members/Boards/DiscussionViewer.aspx?documentid=3995391&ViewFirst=1. Accessed February 9, 2013.

Practical Calculations

OBJECTIVES

After studying this chapter, you should be able to

1. List and understand common abbreviations used in drug orders.
2. Exhibit an understanding of the systems of measurement.
3. Explain how to perform conversions while using the metric system and other systems of measurement.
4. Demonstrate how to accurately calculate a variety of dosage calculations needed for an individual dose, as well as accurately calculate the amount needed for a complete drug order.
5. Understand how percent concentrations are prepared and accurately perform calculations using percentage solutions.
6. Accurately calculate constant rate infusions based on the patient's needs.

OUTLINE

KEY TERMS

Concentration of a drug
Dilution
Dosage
Dosage form
Dosage range
Dose
Equivalent weight
Milliequivalent

Percent concentration
Quantity sufficient
Regimen
Ratio concentration
Solute
Solution
Solvent
Stock solution

INTRODUCTION

Veterinary technicians often are asked to prepare and administer medications to animal patients. A veterinarian's orders may ask for administration of a specific number of milligrams or units of medication (dose). The veterinary technician then must identify the appropriate dosage form (tablets, capsules, liquid) of the preparation prescribed and calculate the appropriate quantity (tablets, capsules, milliliters) of the preparation that contains the appropriate dose for the patient. In other instances, the technician may be asked to calculate the dose on the basis of a drug's dosage (found in the insert or in reference books) and the animal's weight. The drug's dosage may be listed as a dosage range (2–5 mg/kg) rather than a single amount per unit of body weight. This range allows the veterinarian some flexibility to adjust the dose to the available size of the tablet or capsule (5, 100, 250 mg) so that the tablet does not need to be split in half. The veterinary technician then must administer the prescribed medication in the correct amount (dose), by the correct route, at the correct frequency (how often the drug is administered), and at the correct duration (how long the drug is to be given). This is also known as the regimen. When medications are being dispensed the veterinary technician must accurately calculate the total amount of the dosage form (tablet, liquid, etc.) needed to complete the entire duration of the dosage regimen prescribed. An example would be 14 tablets total, for a duration of 7 days. This chapter provides the background information and applications needed by the veterinary technician to accurately carry out a veterinarian's medication orders.

Refer to Appendix A for common abbreviations used in veterinary medicine.

Refer to Appendix B for additional weights and measurements.

Abbreviations are commonly used in prescriptions, drug orders, and medical records as a standardized form of communication in veterinary medicine.

Table 3.1 provides commonly used abbreviations in prescriptions and drug orders.

MATHEMATIC FUNDAMENTALS

It is assumed that the student who uses this text has a basic understanding of fractions and decimals. With these fundamentals as a background, the concepts of percent, ratio, and proportion should be reviewed before the practice

---

TABLE 3.1 Commonly Used Abbreviations in Prescriptions and Drug Orders.

AD	right ear	mEq	milliequivalent
ad lib	as much as desired	mg	milligram
AS	left ear	mL	milliliter
AU	both ears, each ear	npo	nothing by mouth
bid	twice daily	OD	right eye
caps	capsule	OS	left eye
cc	cubic centimeter	OU	both eyes, each eye
d	day	oz	ounce
disp	dispense	po	by mouth
eod	every other day	prn	as needed/necessary
gr	grain	q	every
g	gram	q6h	every 6 hours
gt	drop	qd	every day
gtt	drops	qh	every hour
h	hour	qid	four times daily
IC	intracardiac	qod	every other day
ID	intradermal	SC or SQ	subcutaneous
IM	intramuscular	sid	once daily
IO	intraocular	stat	immediately
IP	intraperitoneal	tab	tablet
IV	intravenous	Tbsp (TBL)	tablespoon
L	liter	tid	three times daily
lb	pound	tsp	teaspoon

problems are solved. It is also important to remember to always include a zero in front of a decimal for any decimal number less than one (e.g., 0.5); this will prevent the risk of errors in reading drug orders and performing calculations.

Percent is defined as parts per hundred. Percent is a fraction with the percent as the numerator and 100 the denominator (e.g., 5% = 5/100). Percentages may be written as decimals, fractions, or whole numbers.

Example 1: Decimal: 0.3%

> (three-tenths percent [3/10 ÷ 100])
> Fraction: 1/5%
> (one-fifth percent [1/5 ÷ 100])
> Whole number: 5%
> (five percent [5 ÷ 100])

Percent may be changed to fractions or decimals.

Example 2: Change to a fraction:

$$5\% = 5/100 = 1/20$$

Change to a decimal:

$$5\% = 5/100 = 0.05$$

Note that a percent can be changed to a decimal quickly by dropping the percent sign and moving the decimal two places to the left.

Example 3:

$$5\% = 0.05$$

A *ratio* is a way of expressing the relationship of a number, quantity, substance, or degree between two components. In reality, ratios are fractions, with the first number in the ratio the numerator and the second number the denominator. The numbers may be placed side by side, separated by a colon, or they may be set up as a numerator/denominator (e.g., 1:5, 1/5). In mathematics, a ratio may be expressed as a quotient, a fraction, or a decimal, per the following:

Example 4:

$$1 \div 5, \ \frac{1}{5}, \ 5\overline{)1.0} = 0.2$$

A *proportion* shows the relationship between two ratios. When a proportion is set up, the two ratios usually are separated by an = (equals) sign.

Example 5:

$$8:16 \text{ as } 1:2 \text{ or } \frac{8}{16} = \frac{1}{2}$$

The proportions above read "8 is to 16 as 1 is to 2." The two inner numbers in the first example (16 and 1) are called the *means,* and the two outer numbers (8 and 2) are called the *extremes.* In a true proportion, the product of the means equals the product of the extremes (16 × 1 = 16, 8 × 2 = 16). This fact makes the proportion a useful mathematical tool. When a part of the problem is unknown, X can be substituted for the unknown part in the proportion and the equation solved for X. Care must be taken to ensure that the proportion is set up correctly, and that the same unit of measure is used on both sides of the equation.

Example 6:

$$8:16 = 1:X \text{ or } \frac{8}{16} = \frac{1}{X}$$
$$8X = 16$$
$$X = 2$$

Example 7: To convert 0.2 g to milligrams, calculate the following:

$$1000 \text{ mg}:1 \text{ g} = X \text{ mg}:0.2 \text{ g or } \frac{1000 \text{ mg}}{1 \text{ g}} = \frac{X \text{ mg}}{0.2 \text{ g}}$$
$$X = 200 \ (1000 \times 0.2)$$

To convert grams to milligrams using an equation:

$$0.2 \ \cancel{g} \times \frac{1000 \text{ mg}}{1 \ \cancel{g}} = 200 \text{ mg}$$

The units for grams (g) will cancel out, leaving milligrams (mg) as the final unit.

SYSTEMS OF MEASUREMENT

The first step in the successful calculation of doses is to develop an understanding of the units of measure used to carry out the calculations. These units are components of the following three separate systems:

1. Metric system
2. Apothecary system
3. Household system

All three systems are expressed in the fundamental units of weight, volume, and length. Technicians should be able to convert values within each system and between the three systems.

Metric System

The fundamental units of measurement in the metric system are the gram (weight), the liter (volume), and the meter (length). Gram is abbreviated *g,* liter is abbreviated *L,* and meter is abbreviated *m.* The usefulness of the metric system is that all units are powers of the fundamental units. Prefixes are used in combination with fundamental units to denote smaller or larger quantities. Table 3.2 illustrates the units of measurement used in the biologic sciences.

TABLE 3.2	Units of Measure for the Biologic Sciences.		
Weight	**Volume**	**Length**	**Multiple Power of 10**
Gram (g)	Liter (L)	Meter (m)	1
Kilogram (kg)	Kiloliter (kL)	Kilometer (km)	1000
Decigram (dg)	Deciliter (dL)	Decimeter (dm)	1/10
Centigram (cg)	Centiliter (cL)	Centimeter (cm)	1/100
Milligram (mg)	Milliliter (mL)	Millimeter (mm)	1/1000
Microgram (μg)	Microliter (μL)	Micrometer (μm)	1/1,000,000
Nanogram (ng)	Nanoliter (nL)	Nanometer (nm)	1/1,000,000,000
Picogram (pg)	Picoliter (pL)	Picometer (pm)	1/1,000,000,000,000

The units that are used most commonly in dosage calculations include the gram, the kilogram (kg; 1000 g), the milligram (mg; 1/1000 g), and the milliliter (mL; 1/1000 L). It should be noted that a milliliter is equivalent to the quantity of water contained in 1 cubic centimeter (cc), which is also equivalent to 1 g of weight. Therefore, for practical purposes, it may be said that 1 mL = 1 cc = 1 g.

On occasion, the microgram (μg) may be used. (It should be noted that this unit also may be abbreviated as *mcg*.) Care should be taken to differentiate this abbreviation from *mg*, which looks very similar when written orders are used.

Conversion Between Metric Units

The most fundamental way to convert between metric units is to multiply the units given by the conversion factor involving the units desired. If the desired conversion is from milligrams (mg) to grams (g), the number of milligrams given should be multiplied by the factor 1 g/1000 mg because 1 g = 1000 mg. The following steps would be involved in this conversion:

1. Write down the number of milligrams to be converted to grams.
2. To the right of that number, write down the number of milligrams in 1 g, with the milligrams as the denominator. (The numerator should always contain the unit to which you wish to convert.)
3. Multiply the two numbers together.

Example 1: Convert 3000 mg to grams.

$$\text{Step 1. } 3000 \text{ mg}$$

$$\text{Step 2. } 3000 \text{ mg } \frac{1 \text{ g}}{1000 \text{ mg}}$$

$$\text{Step 3. } 3000 \text{ mg} \times \frac{1 \text{ g}}{1000 \text{ mg}} = 3 \text{ g}$$

Note that the units for milligrams (mg) will cancel out, leaving grams (g) as the final unit.

Fig. 3.1 illustrates the stairstep method of converting from one unit to another within the metric system. When converting measurements in the metric system via the stairstep method, divide by 10 for each step up to the desired measurement, and multiply by 10 for each step down to the desired measurement.

You also may think of converting measurements with this method by remembering that for each step up, the decimal point is moved one place to the left. For each step down, the decimal point is moved one place to the right.

Example 2:

$$500 \text{ mL} = \underline{\hspace{2cm}} \text{ L}$$

Conversion of milliliters to liters requires three steps upward. Therefore, divide 500 by 10 three times (or 500 ÷ 1000). This moves the decimal point three places to the left, and the answer is 500 mL = 0.5 L.

To convert milliliters to liters using an equation:

$$500 \text{ mL} \times \frac{1 \text{ L}}{1000 \text{ mL}} = 0.5 \text{ L}$$

The units for milliliters (mL) will cancel out, leaving liters (L) as the final unit.

Example 3:

$$2 \text{ g} = \underline{\hspace{2cm}} \text{ mg}$$

To convert grams to milligrams, go down three steps. Multiply 2 by 10 three times (or 2 × 1000). This moves the decimal point three places to the right, and the answer is 2 g = 2000 mg.

To convert grams to milligrams using an equation:

$$2 \text{ g} \times \frac{1000 \text{ mg}}{1 \text{ g}} = 2000 \text{ mg}$$

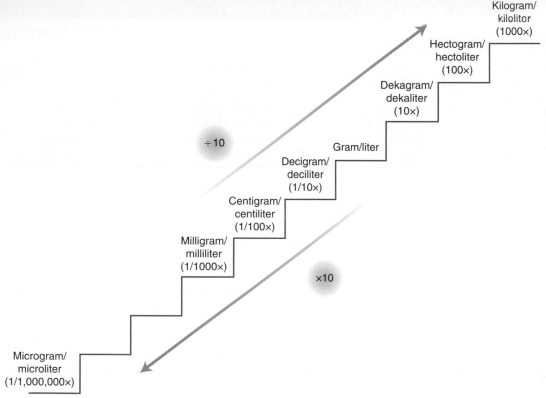

Fig. 3.1 The stairstep method for converting within the metric system. For each step up the stairs, divide the given amount by 10. For each step down the stairs, multiply the given amount by 10.

The units for grams (g) will cancel out, leaving milligrams (mg) as the final unit.

A second method for performing conversions in the metric system can be called the *arrow method*. When this method is used, it is paramount to remember which units of measure are larger. Conversions between the commonly used units of kilograms, grams, milligrams, and micrograms are illustrated in the following text.

A kilogram is 1000 times larger than a gram (g), a gram is 1000 times larger than a milligram (mg), and a milligram is 1000 times larger than a microgram (mcg). This relationship can be abbreviated as follows with the use of the "greater than" symbol (>):

$$kg > g > mg > mcg$$

Many times, the veterinary technician will have to calculate the amount of drug to be given when the supply on hand is not measured in the same units as the order calls for. For example, the order is for 0.3 g of drug A, and the supply on hand is in milligram

(mg) tablets. Before it can be determined how many tablets should be given, 0.3 g must be converted to milligrams. The 0.3 g can be changed to milligrams by multiplying 0.3 g by 1000 mg/g because it is known that 1 g = 1000 mg.

$$0.3\ \cancel{g} \times \frac{1000\ mg}{1\ \cancel{g}} = 300\ mg$$

The units for grams will cancel out, leaving milligrams (mg) as the final unit.

The conversion could have been made very quickly by simply moving the decimal point three places to the right $(0.3 \rightarrow 3_{\uparrow 1}\ 0_{\uparrow 2}\ 0_{\uparrow 3})$.

To know which direction to move the decimal, one should determine which way the arrow is pointing (e.g., kg > g > mg > mcg).

Any time the conversion is made between two adjacent units in the relationship of kg > g > mg > mcg, the decimal point will be moved three places.

The steps for converting grams to milligrams with the use of this method are as follows:

1. Write down the order first, using the units called for (0.3 g).
2. Write down the equivalent units (on hand) needed next to the order units (0.3 g = __ mg).
3. Place an arrow between the two units, with the closed part of the arrow pointing toward the smaller unit (g > mg).
4. Move the decimal point three places in the direction the arrow points ($0.3 \text{ g} \rightarrow 3_{\uparrow1}\, 0_{\uparrow2}\, 0_{\uparrow3}$).

If the order had been for 300,000 mcg of drug A, and the supply on hand is in milligram (mg) tablets, micrograms would have to be converted to milligrams through the following steps:

1. Write the order (300,000 mcg).
2. Write down the equivalent units needed next to the order units (300,000 mcg = ___ mg).
3. Place an arrow between the two units, with the closed part of the arrow pointing toward the smaller units (mcg < mg).
4. Move the decimal three places in the direction the arrow points ($300 \text{ mg} \leftarrow 300_{\uparrow3}\, 0_{\uparrow2}\, 0_{\uparrow1}\, 0.\text{ mcg}$).

Using an equation:

$$300{,}000 \; \cancel{\text{mcg}} \times \frac{1 \text{ mg}}{1000 \; \cancel{\text{mcg}}} = 300 \text{ mg}$$

The units for micrograms (mcg) will cancel out, leaving milligrams (mg) as the final unit.

Additional problems for converting within the metric system are provided at the end of this chapter.

Apothecary and Household Systems

The apothecary and household systems of measurement are older systems than the metric system. The apothecary system is seldom used, but the household system is used for giving clients instructions about dosage.

The units most often encountered in the apothecary system are the minim, abbreviated *m* or *min;* the dram, abbreviated *dr;* the ounce, abbreviated *oz;* and the grain, abbreviated *gr.* A minim is equal to 1 drop (it is always expressed as a whole number), a fluid dram is equal to 4 mL, an ounce is equal to 30 mL, and a grain is equal to 65 mg (64.8, sometimes rounded to 65). When quantities related to grains are written, the symbol *gr* should be placed before the number, and common fractions are used when appropriate (e.g., gr

---

BOX 3.1 Weight Equivalents

1 kg = 1000 g = 2.2 lb
1 g = 1000 mg
1 mg = 1000 µg (mcg) – 0.001 g
65 mg = 1 gr (grain)
1 µg (mcg) = 0.001 mg = 0.000001 g
1 lb = 453.6 g = 0.4536 kg = 16 oz
1 oz = 28.35 g

BOX 3.2 Volume Equivalents

1 L = 1000 mL ≈ 1 qt (946.4 mL)
1 mL = 1 cc
1 mL = 1000 µl (mcl)
500 mL = 1 pt (473 mL) = 2 cups (equivalent to 1 lb of water)
15 mL = 1 Tbsp (TBL)
1 Tbsp (TBL) = 3 tsp
5 mL = 1 tsp
30 mL = 1 oz
240 mL = 1 cup/glass
1 mL = 15 gtt/min[a]

[a] The number of drops/minim in 1 mL depends on the size of the dropper. With a standard-size dropper, 1 mL equals 15 drops.

1/50) or writing out the word grain after the number (1 grain) to prevent confusion with the abbreviation g for gram. The apothecary pound (12 oz) is not used when doses are calculated. Instead, the avoirdupois pound (16 oz) is used.

Units commonly used in the household system include the drop, abbreviated *gtt;* the tablespoon, abbreviated *TBL* or *Tbsp;* and the teaspoon, abbreviated *tsp.* One drop is equivalent to 1 min, 1 Tbsp is equivalent to 15 mL, and 1 tsp is equivalent to 5 mL. The pint, quart, and gallon are other units that are sometimes encountered. Boxes 3.1 and 3.2 illustrate equivalent values that are useful in dosage calculations. Veterinary technicians must be proficient in converting between the systems of measure; memorizing equivalents is necessary. Veterinary technicians are responsible for administering medications to patients, involved in discharging and ensuring that the client can safely administer medications to their animals correctly. Practice problems for converting within and between the apothecary and household systems are found at the end of this chapter.

DOSAGE CALCULATIONS

The drug **dose** (mass of the drug) is the amount of medication, in milligrams (mass), that has been calculated to be given one-time to a patient. An example of a dose is 20 mg of drug X, which is the mass of the drug. The drug **dosage** (conversion factor) is based on the mass of the drug in milligrams (mg) per unit of body weight in kilograms (kg) or pounds (lb). It is very important to know whether the dosage of the drug is based on the animal's weight in kilograms or pounds. An example of a dosage is 2 mg/kg of drug X or 5 mg/lb of drug X. An error in calculation can seriously affect the health of a patient. The **dosage range** of a drug (2–5 mg/kg) may be listed in the drug formulary rather than a single amount per unit of body weight; this allows the veterinarian some flexibility to adjust the dose of the drug to the available size of the tablet or capsule so that the tablet would not need to be split in half. The **concentration of the drug** or strength must be recorded, by the manufacturer, on the container and is listed as a mass (milligrams, grams, grains, etc.) per volume (milliliters, liters, etc.) unit such as milligrams per milliliter (mg/mL) and milligrams per tablet (mg/tab); it may also be listed as a percentage (10%) or percent solution. The **dosage form** of the drug includes solids, liquids, ointments, etc. The total amount or volume of the drug is also listed on the container (e.g., 50 tablets, 50 mL).

To calculate the drug dose, the animal's body weight in kilograms or pounds is multiplied by the dosage expressed in milligrams per kilogram (mg/kg) or milligrams per pound (mg/lb). It is important to understand that the animal's weight and the dose per unit weight must be the same so that the units cancel out and you are only left with the mass of the drug (mg).

$$\text{Animal's body weight} \times \frac{\text{Mass of the drug}}{\text{Unit of weight}} = \text{Dose}$$
$$\text{(Dosage)}$$

Example 1: If an animal weighs 10 lb and the dosage to be given is 5 mg/lb then we can plug these values into the formula and multiply to determine the animal's dose.

$$10 \text{ lb} \times \frac{5 \text{ mg}}{\text{lb}} = 10 \times 5 \text{ mg} = 50 \text{ mg}$$

Therefore, 50 mg is the dose (mass) of the drug needed to be given to this 10 lb animal using a dosage of 5 mg/lb.

Example 2: If an animal weighs 10 kg and the dosage to be given is 2 mg/kg, the animal's dose would be as follows:

$$10 \text{ kg} \times \frac{2 \text{ mg}}{\text{kg}} = 10 \times 2 \text{ mg} = 20 \text{ mg}$$

Therefore, 20 mg is the dose of the drug needed to be given to this 10 kg animal using a dosage of 2 mg/kg.

Example 3: If an animal weighs 200 g and the dosage to be given is 10 mg/kg, the animal's dose in mg would be as follows:

$$200 \text{ g} \times \frac{1 \text{ kg}}{1000 \text{ g}} = 0.2 \text{ kg}$$

$$0.2 \text{ kg} \times \frac{10 \text{ mg}}{\text{kg}} = 2 \text{ mg}$$

Therefore, 2 mg is the dose of the drug needed to be given to this 200 g animal using a dosage of 10 mg/kg. In this problem, the dosage and the animal's weight are expressed in different units.

So, we need to first convert the animal's weight from grams to kilograms so that the dosage of the drug (10 mg/kg) and the animal's weight are in the same units. We can then incorporate, into the equation, the animal's weight in kilograms with the dosage of the drug in mg/kg and kilograms will cancel out giving the dose in milligrams.

Conversion of Kilograms and Pounds

A conversion must be made from pounds to kilograms because most scales used to weigh animals for drug dosage calculation provide the weight in pounds. The animal's weight may be recorded in pounds, kilograms, or grams. Doses are usually calculated based on the animal's weight in kilograms.

> ### 📋 TECHNICIAN NOTES
>
> - It is extremely important for veterinary technicians to convert the animal's weight to match the dose per unit of weight so that the units cancel out and you are only left with the mass of the drug (e.g., milligrams).
> - When converting from pounds to kilograms, the weight in kilograms is always a lower number. Think of it as preferring to be weighed in kilograms as you seem to weigh less.

To convert pound to kilograms (if the dosage is provided in milligrams per kilogram), divide the weight in pounds by 2.2.

To convert kilograms to pounds (if the dosage is provided in milligrams per pound), multiply the weight in kilograms by 2.2.

The conversion factor is 1 kg = 2.2 lb.

Example 1: 44 lb = _____ kg

$$44 \ \cancel{lb} \times \frac{1 \ kg}{2.2 \ \cancel{lb}} = 20 \ kg$$

So, 44 lb is divided by 2.2 which equals 20 kg. In the above equation pounds cancel out giving the answer in kilograms.

Example 2: 20 kg = _____ lb

$$20 \ \cancel{kg} \times \frac{2.2 \ lb}{1 \ \cancel{kg}} = 44 \ lb$$

So, 20 kg is multiplied by 2.2 which equals 44 lb. In the above equation kilograms cancel out giving the answer in pounds.

Conversion of Ounces to Pounds

If an animal is weighed in pounds and ounces (3 pounds 8 ounces) it must be converted to a weight in pounds. The ounces (oz) must be converted to tenths of a pound and added to the pounds.

Example: 3 lb 8 oz = _____ lb

$$8 \ \cancel{oz} \times \frac{1 \ lb}{16 \ \cancel{oz}} = 0.5 \ lb$$

$$3 \ lb + 0.5 \ lb = 3.5 \ lb$$

So, there are 16 oz in 1 lb. You must first convert the ounces into tenths of a pound and add it to the pounds to get the amount in one unit (pounds).

When performing calculations, you must double or even triple check your work and refer back to the drug order and the dosage prescribed. The bottle or container, should be looked at, at least three times, to be sure of the drug's concentration and that it is the correct drug before administering the medication to the animal. Veterinary technicians must possess critical thinking skills when calculating doses and administering medication. Choosing the correct type of syringe to administer a dose of medication, asking for clarification of a drug order that you do not understand, considering what would be a reasonable answer based on the drug order, understanding that tablets and capsules are available in different strengths, and tablets that are scored can be broken down into halves or quarters unlike unscored tablets that cannot be broken, are all examples of critical thinking.

When a dosage form is a liquid, the concentration of the drug will be expressed as a drug mass per volume (100 mg/mL) or as a percentage (10%). Once the dose in milligrams is determined, you must determine the concentration of the drug so that you can determine the volume needed to be administered. The volume is calculated by multiplying the dose of the medication (milligrams) and the concentration of the drug (mass of drug per volume); they must be expressed in the same units. The following example shows how the concentration of the drug in inverted so that the units will cancel out leaving the volume in milliliters.

BOX 3.3   Case Scenario

The veterinarian wants to start a 10-year-old Beagle on a low dose of furosemide to help relieve his congestion. The dog weighs 27 lb and the dose is 2 mg/kg PO once daily for 2 weeks. The concentration of furosemide is 12.5 mg/tablet.

First the weight needs to be converted to kilograms.

27 lb = 12.27 kg

How many mg of furosemide does the dog need at each dose?

12.27 $\cancel{kg}$ × 2 mg/$\cancel{kg}$ = 24.54 mg

How many tablets will he receive at each dose?

24.54 $\cancel{mg}$ × 1 tab/12.5 $\cancel{mg}$ = 1.96 tabs = 2 tabs

The veterinarian wants to re-check him in 2 weeks to re-assess his condition. How many tablets will the owner need in order to maintain the regimen for 2 weeks?

2 tablets/$\cancel{day}$ × 14 $\cancel{days}$ = 28 tablets

He returns to the hospital 2 weeks later for his follow-up examination. The veterinarian is not satisfied with his response to the diuretic and decides to increase the dose to 3 mg/kg once daily.

How many mg of furosemide will he receive in each dose?

12.27 $\cancel{kg}$ × 3 mg/$\cancel{kg}$ = 36.81 mg

How many tablets will he receive in each dose?

36.81 $\cancel{mg}$ × 12.5 $\cancel{mg}$ = 2.94 tabs = 3 tabs

How many tablets will the owner need in order to maintain the new regimen for 2 weeks?

3 tablets/$\cancel{day}$ × 14 $\cancel{days}$ = 42 tablets

Example 1: If an animal needs 50 mg of drug X and the concentration of the drug X is 100 mg/mL, the equation would be as follows:

$$\text{Dose (mg)} \times \text{Concentration (mg/mL)}$$
$$= \text{Volume of fluid to be administered}$$

$$50 \text{ mg} \times \frac{1 \text{ mL}}{100 \text{ mg}} = 0.5 \text{ mL}$$

OR

To determine the volume, the calculation is performed by dividing the dose in milligrams by the concentration (mg/mL). The equation is as follows:

$$\frac{\text{Dose (mg)}}{\text{Concentration (mg/mL)}}$$
$$= \text{Volume of fluid to be administered}$$

$$\frac{50 \text{ mg}}{100 \text{ mg/mL}} = 0.5 \text{ mL}$$

Both calculations are correct; however, it is best to be consistent with which equation you use to prevent errors from occurring and allowing you to be more comfortable and confident in your calculations.

To calculate a dose, the following information must be used:
1. The weight of the animal
2. The dosage of the drug
3. The concentration of the drug

Example 2: A dog weighs 44 lb and needs drug X given, subcutaneous (SC), at a dosage of 10 mg/kg and the label of the drug lists the concentration at 100 mg/mL. Determine the amount of the drug form to be administered.

You need to first determine if the units are the same for the weight and dosage.

We must first convert pounds to kg:

$$44 \text{ lb} = 20 \text{ kg}$$

$$44 \text{ lb} \times \frac{1 \text{ kg}}{2.2 \text{ lb}} = 20 \text{ kg}$$

Note that in this step, pounds cancel out and leave only kilograms in the numerator.

The dosage of the drug is 10 mg/kg; now that we have the weight in kg, the units are the same.

$$20 \text{ kg} \times \frac{10 \text{ mg}}{\text{kg}} = 200 \text{ mg}$$

Note that in this step, kilograms cancel out and leave only milligrams in the numerator.

Once the dose is calculated, you will need the concentration of the drug.

$$200 \text{ mg} \times \frac{1 \text{ mL}}{100 \text{ mg}} = 2 \text{ mL}$$

Therefore, the animal needs 2 milliliters of the drug to be administered subcutaneously.

In this step, milligrams cancel out and leave milliliters.

If the drug order to the veterinary technician is to "give a dog 300 mg of amoxicillin," then the ordered amount (dose) is simply multiplied with the concentration of the drug to determine the amount to be administered. Remember, the dose units and the concentration units need to be the same in order to cancel out.

Example 3: If the order is to give a dog 300 mg of amoxicillin (concentration 100 mg/mL), the calculation would be as follows:

$$300 \text{ mg} \times \frac{1 \text{ mL}}{100 \text{ mg}} = 3 \text{ mL}$$

Example 4: A dog weighs 22 kg and needs drug X to be given at a dosage of 20 mg/kg and the label of the drug lists the concentration at 50 mg/tablet. Determine the amount of the drug form to be administered.

You need to first determine if the units are the same for the weight and dosage. Now you figure out the dose:

$$22 \text{ kg} \times \frac{20 \text{ mg}}{\text{kg}} = 440 \text{ mg}$$

Then:

$$440 \text{ mg} \times \frac{\text{tablet}}{50 \text{ mg}} = 8.8 \text{ tablets} = 9 \text{ tablets}$$

Since the tablet amount does not equal an even number, you must round to the nearest half or whole tablet. When rounding to the nearest half or whole tablet the veterinarian must decide the risks of causing side effects and may round down to the nearest half or whole tablet. When the number of tablets per dose is a decimal fraction, choose the fraction of a tablet (¼, ½, or ¾) that is closest to the dose, when the tablets are scored. You should always check with the veterinarian before dispensing the medication.

The general rule for rounding is if the required number of the tablet is 0.5 then it will equal ½ a tablet. If the required number of tablets calculated is 2.23 then it would round down to 2 tablets. If the number of tablets calculated is 6.77 then it would round up to 7 tablets.

Other examples include:
0.59 tablets are rounded down to 0.5 tablets
1.2234 = 1.2 tablets are rounded down to 1 tablet
1.376 = 1.4 tablets are rounded up to 1.5 tablets
2.65 tablets are rounded down to 2.5 tablets
3.2456 = 3.3 rounds up to 3.5 tablets
4.789 = 4.8 rounds up to 5 tablets

Example 5: A dog weighing 25 kg is prescribed drug X at a dosage of 20 mg/kg and the label of the drug lists the concentration at 250 mg/tablet. The drug order states that the animal is going to receive the dose twice daily for 7 days. Determine the total amount of the drug to be dispensed.

Since the weight of the animal is in kilograms and the dosage is in milligrams per kilogram, the units are the same and can continue with the calculation.

Calculate the dose of the drug using the animal's weight:

$$25 \text{ kg} \times \frac{20 \text{ mg}}{\text{kg}} = 500 \text{ mg}$$

Next, you will calculate the number of tablets per dose:

$$500 \text{ mg} \times \frac{1 \text{ tablet}}{250 \text{ mg}} = 2 \text{ tablets/dose}$$

Next, the total number of doses was determined in the order to be twice daily for 7 days.

$$\frac{2 \text{ doses}}{\text{day}} \times 7 \text{ days} = 14 \text{ total doses}$$

Next, you will calculate the total number of tablets needed to complete the order.

$$14 \text{ doses} \times \frac{2 \text{ tabs}}{\text{dose}} = 28 \text{ tablets}$$

You can also use the following equation for the total amount of tablets to be dispensed:

$$\frac{\text{Amt of tablets}}{\text{dose}} \times \frac{\text{\# of times administered}}{\text{day}}$$
$$\times \text{ \# of days given} = \text{Total number of tablets}$$

$$\frac{2 \text{ tablets}}{\text{dose}} \times \frac{2 \text{ doses}}{\text{day}} \times 7 \text{ days} = 28 \text{ tablets}$$

TECHNICIAN NOTES

Because drugs are manufactured in different concentrations, always record the dose (milligrams, units, mEq) of active ingredient in the medical record rather than the number of milliliters, tablets, etc.

It should be noted that the dose of most drugs used to treat neoplasms is calculated according to the total body surface area of the patient. Body surface area is correlated with the weight of the animal. A table is available in Chapter 16 (see Table 16.2) for converting an animal's weight to surface area in square meters (sq M or m²). In these cases, the formula for dosage calculation becomes the following:

$$\text{Dose} = \text{mg/m}^2 \text{ (from insert)} \times \text{m}^2 \text{ (from table)}$$

Dosage calculation problems are provided at the end of this chapter.

SOLUTIONS

To understand dosage calculation problems and how to prepare dilutions of substances (e.g., allergy injections and disinfectants), a technician must have a basic understanding of solutions. *Solutions* are mixtures of two or more substances (solvent and solute) that are combined with each other. In most cases the solvent will be a liquid, but it can also be a solid. A *solvent* is a solution capable of dissolving other substances. A *solute* is a substance that is dissolved in a liquid (solution). A *dilution* is a process of reducing the concentration of a substance in a solution. Not all substances form solutions with each other. Those that form solutions are called *miscible,* and those that do not are called *immiscible.* A solution is referred to as *saturated* if it contains the maximum amount of solute at a particular temperature and pressure. Under some circumstances, a solution can become supersaturated. Mixtures of substances in which the solute is made up of very large particles are called *suspensions.* The particles in suspensions settle on standing, and the mixture must be agitated before it is administered. True solutions do not settle and remain mixed without agitation.

When working with solutions, it is important to know the amount of solute in the solvent or to be able to measure it. The amount of solute dissolved in the solvent is referred to as the *concentration (strength)* of the substance. Concentrations may be expressed in a number of ways, including the following:

- Parts ratio
- Weight per volume (w/v) for liquids
- Volume per volume (v/v) for liquids
- Weight per weight (w/w) for solids

Solutions can be described in terms of parts without any reference to units of measurement. The parts simply refer to the relationship between the solvent and the solute. For example, instructions may call for a 1-to-32 (1:32) dilution of a disinfectant. The first number of the ratio refers to the amount of the disinfectant and the second number refers to the amounts of solvent and disinfectant combined. This strength of the mixture is expressed as a parts ratio or **ratio concentration**.

 TECHNICIAN NOTES

A 1:32 dilution means that 1 mL of the drug is added to 31 mL of the solvent to produce 32 total mL of the solution.

Another unit that describes the relationship of parts (parts ratio) is called *parts per million* (ppm). Parts per million is equal to 1 mg of a solute in a kilogram or liter of solvent. One part per million is also equivalent to 1 µg (mcg) in a gram or milliliter. Upson (1988) reports that 1 ppm is equivalent to 1 minute in approximately 2 years or 1 oz of sand in approximately 31 tons of cement. Parts per billion is a ratio unit that is used occasionally. It is equivalent to 1 µg (mcg) in a kilogram or liter, or 1 nanogram in a gram or milliliter.

A ratio concentration can be converted to a percentage concentration by using a ratio and proportion equation:

Example: Express 1:32 as a percent concentration (parts per hundred).

Answer:

$$1 : 32 = Y : 100 \text{ or } \frac{1}{32} = \frac{Y}{100}$$
$$32Y = 100$$
$$Y = 3.1\%$$

PERCENT CONCENTRATIONS

The term *percent concentration* may be used when weight per volume (w/v), weight per weight (w/w), or volume per volume (v/v) concentrations are described.

Percent (percentage) means parts of solute per 100 parts of the solution. Percent w/v means the number of grams of solute in 100 mL of solution; percent w/w describes the number of grams of solute in 100 g of diluent (liquid or solid); and v/v expresses the number of milliliters of solute in 100 mL of the solution.

A 100% solution (w/v) contains 100 g of solute per 100 mL of solution. Another way to say this is that it contains 1 g (1000 mg) of solute per 1 mL of solution (1000 mg/mL).

- To convert from a percent solution to mg/mL, multiply the percentage by 10 (e.g., a 5% Lasix solution contains 50 mg/mL; a 20% solution contains 200 mg/mL).
- To convert mg/mL to a percent, divide the milligrams per milliliter by 10 (e.g., a Lasix solution containing 50 mg/mL is a 5% solution; a 200 mg/mL solution is a 20% solution).

Sometimes, the term *milligrams percent* (mg%) is encountered. This term is used to refer to the number of milligrams in 100 mL of solution. It is an expression of concentration but not of percent concentration (g/100 mL). A more accurate description of mg% would be milligrams per deciliter (mg/dL) because a deciliter is equal to 100 mL.

A 100% solution (w/w) contains 100 g of solute in 100 g of solid or liquid. A 5% solution (w/w) of sodium chloride would contain 5 g of sodium in 100 g of solution. To make this preparation, weigh out 5 g of sodium chloride and mix it with 95 g of water.

A 100% solution (v/v) would simply be pure drug or chemical. A 10% solution would contain 10 mL of the chemical in 100 mL of solution. When a w/v solution or a v/v solution is prepared, the desired amount of solute is added to a container, and enough solvent is added to create the desired volume. This process is called *diluting up,* or it may be said that you *q.s.* to the desired volume. The abbreviation *q.s.* means to add a "**quantity sufficient**" to arrive at the desired volume. For example, to make 100 mL of a 10% formalin solution, place 10 mL of formaldehyde (100% formalin) in a container and q.s. (quantity sufficient) to 100 mL (10 mL formalin, 90 mL distilled water).

The most common way of expressing drug concentration when the solute is a solid and the solvent is a liquid is weight per volume (w/v). For example, the concentration of most pharmaceutic preparations is expressed as milligrams per milliliter (mg/mL); the concentration for ketamine (Ketaset) for example is 100 mg/mL.

To convert a percent concentration to a ratio concentration, set up a ratio and proportion equation:

Example: Convert a 3.1% (parts per 100) solution to a ratio concentration.

Answer:

$$3.1:100 = 1:Y \text{ or } \frac{3.1}{100} = \frac{1}{Y}$$
$$3.1\,Y = 100$$
$$Y = 32$$

Calculations Involving Concentrations

To determine the amount of solute needed to make a desired amount of solution, you may use the following formula:

$$\text{Grams of solute to q.s. to desired volume} = \frac{\% \times \text{desired volume}}{100}$$

Example 1: How many grams of sodium chloride are needed to make 1 L of 0.9% sodium chloride?

Answer:

$$\text{Grams needed} = \frac{0.9 \times 1000\text{ mL}}{100} = 9\text{ g}$$

This can also be calculated using the following equation:

$$\text{The total volume of the final drug solution} \times \text{concentration} = \text{Amount}$$

So, for the same example above, the equation would be as follows:

You will first need to change: 1 L to 1000 mL

0.9% is equal to 90 mg/mL or 0.9 g/100mL

Since we want to know the number of grams then we would use 0.9% as 0.9 g/100 mL

$$1000\text{ mL} \times \frac{0.9\text{ g}}{100\text{ mL}} = 9\text{ g}$$

Nine grams of sodium chloride are added to a container and is diluted up to 1000 mL. When the amount of solute and the volume of solution are known, the percent solution may be calculated as follows:

$$\text{Percent solution} = \frac{\text{grams of solute} \times 100}{\text{volume of solution}}$$

Example 2: What percentage is a solution that contains 9 g of sodium chloride?

Answer:

$$\text{Percent solution} = \frac{9 \times 100}{1000} = \frac{900}{1000} = 0.9\%$$

To solve problems involving a change in concentration of the solution (dilution), the following formula may be used:

V1 (Volume 1) × C1 (Concentration 1) = V2 (Volume 2) × C2 (Concentration 2)

V1 (Vol of stock) × C1 (Stock concentration) = V2 (Desired Vol) × C2 (Desired Concentration)

So, V1C1 is **what you have** on hand and V2C2 is **what you want** to make.

Volume (V's): may be in milliliters or liters but must be the same for both.

Concentration (C's): may be in % or mg/mL but must be the same for both.

- **Volume one (V1):** the volume of stock solution to be used; or "amount to use" to prepare the new volume.
- **Concentration one (C1):** the original concentration of the stock solution; or "available strength" of solution on hand.
- **Volume two (V2):** the desired final volume of the new solution; or "amount to make."
- **Concentration two (C2):** the desired final concentration of the new solution (what you are making).

Example 3: How would you prepare 100 mL of a 5% dextrose solution from a 50% dextrose solution?

So, the 100 mL is V2 (the final volume of the new solution), the 5% is C2 (the final concentration of the new solution); this is what you want or trying to make and the 50% is C1; this is what you have on hand. Therefore, you are solving for V1 and this volume is diluted (q.s.) up to the desired volume.

Answer:

$$V1 \times C1 = V2 \times C2$$
$$V1 \times 50\% = 100\text{ mL} \times 5\%$$
$$V1 \times 50 = 500\text{ mL}$$
$$V1 = 10\text{ mL}$$

You can also set up the equation in which you convert the percentages (%) to, in this case, milligrams per milliliter (mg/mL).

A 5% solution = 50 mg/mL and a 50% solution = 500 mg/mL.

Answer:

$$V1 \times C1 = V2 \times C2$$

$$V1 \times 500 \text{ mg/ml} = 100 \text{ mL} \times 50 \text{ mg/mL}$$

$$V1 \times 500 \text{ mg/mL} = 5000 \text{ mg}$$

$$V1 = \frac{5000 \text{ mg}}{500 \text{ mg/mL}}$$

$$V1 = 10 \text{ mL}$$

This formula demonstrates that you would take 10 mL of the 50% dextrose solution and q.s. to 100 mL (10 mL stock + 90 diluent) to prepare the 5% solution.

MILLIEQUIVALENTS

When electrolytes are involved, the concentration of a solution is often expressed in terms of milliequivalents (mEq). One milliequivalent is equal to 1/1000 of an equivalent. Potassium chloride and sodium bicarbonate are drugs that are expressed in milliequivalents (mEq). An equivalent weight is equal to (for practical applications) 1 g molecular weight divided by the total positive valence of the material in question (Blankenship & Campbell, 1976). The concentration of an electrolyte solution is expressed as milliequivalents per liter (mEq/L), which can be calculated when the concentration of the solution is known by using the following formula:

$$mEq/L = \frac{mg/dL \times 10}{eqwt}$$

Example 1: How many milliequivalents per liter is found in a sodium chloride solution that contains 700 mg/dL?

For this problem you would need to know the atomic weights for sodium and chloride. The atomic weight of sodium is 23 and the atomic weight of chlorine is 35.5.

$$NaCl \text{ eq wt} : 23(Na) + 35.5(Cl) = 58.5$$

$$mEq/L = \frac{700 \times 10}{58.5} = 119.66$$

The number of milligrams per deciliter also can be calculated when the number of milliequivalents per liter is known by manipulating the previous formula as follows:

$$mg/dL = \frac{mEq/L \times eqwt}{10}$$

BOX 3.4 Chart for Determining the Amount of Potassium

Serum K* (mEq/L)	Maximum Rate* (mL/kg/h)	Total mEq KCl needed per 1 L
<2.0	6	80
2.1–2.5	8	60
2.6–3.0	12	40
3.1–3.5	18	28
3.6–5.0	25	20

*Do not exceed 0.5 mEq/kg/hr. DiBartola SP. Fluid Therapy in Small Animal Practice. 3rd ed. Philadelphia, WB Saunders. From American Animal Hospital Association. (2013). AAHA/AAFP Fluid Therapy Guidelines for Dogs and Cats Implementation Toolkit (Supplemental information). https://www.aaha.org/globalassets/02-guidelines/fluid-therapy/fluidtherapy_tipsheet.pdf.

Example 2: How many milligrams per deciliter is contained in a solution that has 119.66 mEq/L?

Answer:

$$mg/dL = \frac{119.66 \times 58.5}{10} = \frac{7000}{10} = 700 \text{ mg/dL}$$

A veterinarian may ask you to add potassium chloride (KCl) to intravenous (IV) fluids for an animal patient that is hypokalemic and you would need to understand how to calculate the volume of potassium to add to the fluids. A chart is commonly used to determine the amount of potassium to add. The dose is determined by the serum potassium levels of the patient (Box 3.4).

The equation is as follows:

$$\text{Volume needed} = \frac{\text{Dose}}{\text{Concentration}}$$

Example: The drug order is to add 20 mEq of potassium (KCl) to a bag of IV fluids containing 1 L (1000 mL). The concentration of potassium is 40 mEq/20 mL. How much KCl will you add to the bag of IV fluids?

The first step is to break down 40 mEq/ 20 mL into a smaller concentration. This is equal to 20 mEq/10 mL or 2 mEq/1 mL.

Using the equation:

$$\text{Volume needed} = \frac{20 \text{ mEq}}{2 \text{ mEq/mL}}$$

$$\text{Volume needed} = 10 \text{ mL}$$

Therefore, 10 mL of potassium would be added to 1000 mL of IV fluids.

CALCULATIONS INVOLVING INTRAVENOUS FLUID ADMINISTRATION

Calculations for determining the volume of fluid to administer are covered in Chapter 15. Veterinary technicians must be able to calculate fluid drip rates and set the appropriate rate, with or without, the use of an infusion pump. The rate at which to run IV fluids (in drops per minute) can be determined by dividing the volume of fluids to be given by the time in minutes during administration, and then multiplying that number by the drops per milliliter delivered by the administration set. The drops per milliliter (drops/mL) calibration is listed on the package material that contains the IV administration set. The most common forms of IV administration sets are calibrated at 15 drops per mL (known as a "standard" drip set) or 60 drops per mL (known as a "micro drip set"). The "micro drip" administration set is more often used for smaller patients when lower drip rates are required.

$$\frac{\text{Volume of infusion (mL)}}{\text{Time of infusion (min)}} \times \text{drop factor (gtt/mL)}$$
$$= \text{drops per minute}$$

The drip rate in drops per minute can be divided by 60 to determine the rate in drops per second—a number that is easier to work with when one is actually adjusting the flow.

Example 1: Give 480 mL of lactated Ringer's solution to Dog A over a 4-hour period using a standard 15 gtt/mL administration set.

$$\frac{480 \text{ mL}}{240 \text{ min}} = \frac{2 \text{ mL}}{\text{min}} \times \frac{15 \text{ gtt}}{\text{mL}} = \frac{30 \text{ gtt}}{\text{min}} \times \frac{1 \text{ min}}{60 \text{ sec}} = \frac{1 \text{ gtt}}{2 \text{ sec}}$$

Giving one drop every 2 seconds will deliver 30 drops in a minute.

Calculations for Constant Rate Infusion Problems

Sometimes, medications given by IV infusion have to be administered at a dose delivered at a constant flow rate over a specified period of time; this is known as a constant rate infusion (CRI). All CRIs require an IV catheter. Constant rate infusions are commonly used in veterinary medicine to treat seizures, to control pain, to supplement electrolytes, to minimize and treat cardiac arrhythmias, etc. Drugs commonly used include fentanyl, morphine, lidocaine, etc.

The dosage is often ordered in micrograms per kilogram per minute, micrograms per kilogram per hour, milligrams per kilogram per day, milligrams per kilogram per hour, etc. These dosages can be confusing because most drugs are available in a concentration expressed as milligrams/milliliter (mg/mL) and are delivered through infusion pumps at a rate expressed as milliliters/hour (mL/h).

There are multiple steps required for calculating a CRI. You will need the animal's weight, the dose of the drug, the concentration of the drug, the rate of infusion, and the volume of fluid.

- Convert the animal's weight to match the dose units, usually kilograms.
- Units for the concentration of the drug and the dose of the drug need to be in the same units.
- Calculate the dose of the drug for the animal's weight. The kilograms will cancel out. The answer is the dose (mass) per time (e.g., mg/hour).
- Calculate the volume of the drug per hour or minute.
- Calculate how many hours the bag of fluids will last.

$$\frac{\text{Fluid volume in mL}}{\text{hourly rate in mL/h}}$$
$$= \text{The number of hours the bag will last}$$

It is important to remove as much fluid from the IV bag to equal the amount of drug(s) to be added. This is done so that you do not dilute the concentration further. Be sure to place a label on the bag of fluids with the name of the drug(s) added, concentration of the drug(s), amount of the drug(s) added, date, time, and animal's name.

Example 1: A 44-lb dog with acute heart failure is ordered to receive 10 mcg/kg/min of dopamine. You will add a 200-mg vial of dopamine to a 1-L bag of D_5W (dextrose 5% in water) solution (0.2 mg/mL). At what rate in drops per minute will you administer this solution to deliver the correct dosage?

Step 1: Convert to the same units. The dose is expressed in mcg/kg, so the patient's weight must be converted from pounds to kilograms, and the drug concentration must be expressed in mcg/mL.

$$44 \text{ lbs} \times \frac{1 \text{ kg}}{2.2 \text{ lbs}} = \frac{44 \text{ kg}}{2.2} = 20 \text{ kg}$$

$$\frac{0.2 \text{ mg}}{1 \text{ mL}} \times \frac{1000 \text{ mcg}}{1 \text{ mg}} = \frac{200 \text{ mcg}}{1 \text{ mL}}$$

Step 2: Determine the number of micrograms per minute.

$$20 \, \cancel{kg} \times \frac{10 \text{ mcg}}{\cancel{kg}/\text{min}} = \frac{200 \text{ mcg}}{\text{min}}$$

Step 3: Determine the number of milliliters per minute.

$$\frac{200 \, \cancel{mcg}}{1 \text{ min}} \times \frac{1 \text{ mL}}{200 \, \cancel{mcg}} = \frac{1 \text{ mL}}{1 \text{ min}}$$

Step 4: Determine the number of drops per minute using a micro drip (60 gtt/mL) administration set.

$$\frac{1 \, \cancel{mL}}{\text{min}} \times \frac{60 \text{ gtt}}{1 \, \cancel{mL}} = \frac{60 \text{ gtt}}{1 \text{ min}} \text{ or } 1 \text{ gtt/sec}$$

Example 2: A lidocaine CRI is ordered for a 20 kg dog at a rate of 40 mcg/kg/min at 4 mL/h. Lidocaine is a 2% solution. The dog is expected to be on the CRI for 5 hours. How will you prepare the IV fluids?

Weight of the animal: 20 kg

Dose of the medication: 40 mcg/kg/min = 0.04 mg/kg/min

Concentration of the drug: 2% = 20 mg/mL

Rate of infusion: 4 mL/h

Volume of fluids: 20 mL (4 mL/h × 5 hours)

$$20 \, \cancel{kg} \times \frac{0.04 \text{ mg}}{\cancel{kg}/\text{min}} = \frac{0.8 \text{ mg}}{\cancel{min}} \times \frac{60 \, \cancel{min}}{1 \text{ h}}$$

$$= \frac{48 \text{ mg}}{\cancel{h}} \times 5 \, \cancel{h} = 240 \text{ mg total}$$

$$240 \, \cancel{mg} \times \frac{1 \text{ mL}}{20 \, \cancel{mg}} = 12 \text{ mL of lidocaine}$$

$$\frac{4 \text{ mL}}{\cancel{h}} \times 5 \, \cancel{h} = 20 \text{ mL}$$

Therefore, 20 mL total volume of fluids minus 12 mL of lidocaine = 8 mL of fluids.

Example 3: A dog weighing 40 kg is ordered to have a Reglan (metoclopramide) CRI at 1 mg/kg/24 hours. You have a 1-liter bag LRS (Lactated Ringers solution) and the fluid rate is 160 mL/h. The concentration of Reglan is 5 mg/mL. How many mgs will you add to the bag? How many mLs?

Figure out how many mgs are needed in 24 hours. Then, how many mgs are needed in a single hour.

$$40 \, \cancel{kg} \times \frac{1 \text{ mg}}{\cancel{kg}/\text{day}} = \frac{40 \text{ mg}}{\cancel{day}} \times \frac{1 \, \cancel{day}}{24 \text{ h}} = \frac{1.67 \text{ mg}}{\text{h}}$$

Now, figure out how many hours the bag will last.

$$\frac{\text{Volume of fluids}}{\text{Fluid rate}} = \text{Number of hours the bag will last}$$

$$\frac{1000 \, \cancel{mL}/\text{L}}{160 \, \cancel{mL}/\text{h}} = 6.25 \text{ h/L}$$

Now, calculate the mg needed for the number of hours the bag will last and the mL of Reglan to be added.

$$\text{Drug dose per hour} \times \text{hours of fluids per liter} = \text{Amount of medication needed per liter}$$

$$\frac{1.67 \text{ mg}}{\cancel{h}} \times \frac{6.25 \, \cancel{h}}{\text{L}} = 10.44 \text{ mg/L}$$

$$\text{Drug dose per liter} \times \text{concentration of drug} = \text{Drug dose needed in total amount of fluids}$$

$$\frac{10.44 \, \cancel{mg}}{\text{L}} \times \frac{1 \text{ mL}}{5 \, \cancel{mg}} = 2.09 \text{ mL}$$

Another way to calculate the mg, if all of the units are the same is the following:

$$\frac{0.04 \text{ mg}}{\cancel{kg}/\text{h}} \times \frac{40 \, \cancel{kg}}{1} \times \frac{6.25 \, \cancel{h}}{1} = 10 \text{ mg Reglan}$$

Now, calculate the mount of drug in milliliters.

$$\frac{10 \, \cancel{mg}}{1} \times \frac{1 \text{ mL}}{5 \, \cancel{mg}} = 2 \text{ mL reglan}$$

Therefore, 2 mL of fluid is removed from the bag of fluids and add 2 mL of Reglan.

If the fluid rate changes then you would need to determine how many milligrams of Reglan are in each milliliter of fluid.

$$\frac{\text{mg of drug added}}{\text{Volume of fluid (mL) it was added to}} = \text{Dose of drug per mL of fluid}$$

$$\frac{10 \text{ mg}}{1000 \text{ mL}} = 0.01 \text{ mg Reglan/mL}$$

Formulas and recipes have been devised to simplify the CRI calculations (Macintire & Tefend, 2004). The

---

BOX 3.5 Case Scenario

A 5 kg DSH cat is prescribed a fentanyl CRI for pain management at a rate of 3 mcg/kg/h (0.003 mg/kg/h) at 3 mL/h. The fentanyl CRI will continue for 12 hours postoperatively. The total fluid volume is 36 mL. The concentration of fentanyl is 50 mcg/mL (0.05 mg/mL).

36 mL × 1 h/3 mL = 12 hours (this is the number of hours that the fluids will run)

How many mgs of fentanyl is needed?

5 kg × 0.003 mg/kg/h = 0.015 mg/h

0.015 mg/h × 12 hours = 0.18 mg fentanyl

How many mL of fentanyl is needed?

0.18 mg × 1 mL/0.05 mg = 3.6 mL of fentanyl

How many mL of diluent (fluid) will be needed?

36 mL total volume of fluid − 3.6 mL of fentanyl = 32.4 mL of diluent (fluid)

Therefore, 3.6 mL of fentanyl will be added to 32.4 mL of fluid.

---

following formula can also be used to determine the number of milligrams of drug that must be added to a bag of fluids to deliver a predetermined dosage rate to a patient. A volume of the delivery fluid equal to the volume of the drug added should be removed before the drug is added, to keep the dose and volume accurate.

$$M = \frac{(D)\,(W)\,(V)}{(R)\,(16.67)}$$

M = number of milligrams of drug to add to delivery fluid

D = dosage of drug in micrograms per kilogram per minute

W = patient body weight in kilograms

V = volume in milliliters of delivery fluid

R = rate of delivery in milliliters per hour

16.67 = conversion factor

The next formula can be used to adjust the dosage (mcg/kg/min) in accordance with the response of the animal.

$$R = \frac{(D)\,(W)\,(V)}{(M)\,(16.67)}$$

Another formula allows rapid calculation of the amount of drug to be added to a standard volume of 250 mL of fluid at a standard delivery rate of 15 mL/h.

Drug dosage (mcg/kg/min) × Body weight (kg) = milligrams of drug to add to 250 mL fluid and run at 15 mL/h.

Some CRI drugs are dosed in milligrams per kilogram per hour rather than micrograms per kilogram per minute.

A combination of morphine and ketamine (MK) sometimes is delivered as a CRI for pain control in dogs and cats. A recipe (Ortel, 2006) for this combination calls for adding to a single 500-mL bag of fluids the following:

60 mg of ketamine (100 mg/mL)

60 mg of morphine (15 mg/mL)

When the two drugs are added, the patient's weight in kilograms becomes the infusion rate in milliliters per hour that is set on the infusion pump. The delivery dose is 1 mL/kg/h or 2 mcg/kg/min ketamine and 2 mcg/kg/min morphine.

For dogs, lidocaine (500 mg of a 20 mg/mL concentration) can be added to the MK recipe previously mentioned to make the MLK mixture. The MLK mixture also is run at a delivery rate of 1 mL/kg/h, delivering 17 mcg/kg/min of lidocaine, in addition to the ketamine and morphine.

REVIEW QUESTIONS

Problems Using Ratios and Proportions

Ratios

1. Express 1/4 as a ratio and as a decimal.
2. Express 0.75 as a ratio and as a fraction.
3. Express 1:80 as a fraction and as a decimal.
4. Express 9/1000 as a ratio and as a decimal.
5. Express 0.50 as a ratio and a fraction.
6. Express 2:3 as a fraction and decimal.

Proportions (Solve for X)

1. 25:X = 5:10
2. 1/2:100=X:500
3. $\dfrac{1/4}{X} = \dfrac{20}{400}$
4. If a drug concentration is labeled 5 mL = 250 mg, how many milligrams are in three-fourths of a milliliter?

$$\frac{250\,mg}{5\,mL} = \frac{X}{3/4\,mL}$$

5. How much bleach would you use to prepare 1 gallon (3784 mL) of a 1:32 sol

$$1 : 32 = X : 3784$$

6. If a 10-lb dog gets one-fourth of a tablet of an antibiotic, how many tablets will a 50-lb dog get?

$$\frac{1}{4} : 10 = X : 50$$

7. What is the percentage concentration of a 1/5000 solution?

$$\frac{1}{5000} = \frac{X}{100}$$

8. If a 10-lb dog gets 0.5 mL of an anthelmintic, how many milliliters does a 60-lb dog get?

$$0.5 : 10 = X : 60$$

Problems Using the Metric System

1. 150 mg = _____ g
2. 2 L = _____ mL
3. 2250 mg = _____ g
4. 5 g = _____ mg
5. 3000 mL = _____ L
6. 2 kg = _____ g
7. 0.5 kg = _____ g
8. 5000 mg = _____ kg
9. 1.25 mg = _____ g
10. 0.004 g = _____ mg
11. 2050 µg = _____ mg
12. How many grams would you administer if the veterinarian ordered 10 mg of acepromazine?
13. If the medical order is for 0.5 L of sodium chloride 0.9%, how many milliliters would be administered?
14. How many liters would you give to the patient if the order called for 750 mL to be administered?
15. If the veterinarian orders 300 µg of vitamin B_{12}, how much is this in milligrams?
16. If the order is for 2.5 mg of vitamin B_{12}, how many micrograms are administered?
17. A 1% solution of ivermectin contains how many micrograms per milliliter?
18. How many millimeters wide is a lesion 0.5 cm in diameter?
19. What is the weight in grams of a parrot weighing 0.9 kg?
20. How many kilograms does a 20g mouse weigh?

Problems Using the Apothecary and Household Systems

1. 1.5 qt = _____ pt
2. 12 pt = _____ gal
3. 3 tsp = _____ Tbsp
4. 3 qt = _____ cups
5. 12 cups = _____ pt
6. 2 oz = _____ Tbsp
7. 1 gal = _____ oz
8. 1 pt = _____ oz
9. 6 pt = _____ qt
10. 48 oz = _____ lb

Problems Combining the Two Systems

1. 1 pt = _____ mL
2. 2 Tbsp = _____ mL
3. 15 mL = _____ cc
4. 2 cups = _____ oz
5. 6.5 mL = _____ pt
6. 125 mL = _____ tsp
7. 1.5 oz = _____ mL
8. 15 kg = _____ lb
9. 250 mL = _____ pt
10. 5 oz = _____ mL
11. 35 lb = _____ kg
12. 3 cups = _____ mL
13. 4 Tbsp = _____ oz
14. 90 mL = _____ oz
15. 260 mg = _____ gr

Problems Measuring Oral Medications

1. The order is for 500 mg of amoxicillin, and tablets on hand are 250 mg. How many tablets will be administered?
2. The order is for 15 mg of prednisone, and 10-mg (scored) tablets are on hand. How many tablets will be administered?
3. The order is for enrofloxacin to be given once daily at 5 mg/kg to a 10-lb cat for 7 days. How many 22.7-mg tablets should be dispensed to the client?
4. The veterinarian prescribes 15 mg of prednisone every other day for 10 days. The tablets on hand are 10 mg.
   How many tablets per dose will be administered?
   How many tablets will be dispensed?
5. The veterinarian prescribes sulfadimethoxine (Albon) for Coccidia. Your patient is a puppy that weighs 8 lbs and needs treatment for 21 days. The dose

for Albon is a 25-mg/lb loading dose and 12.5-mg/lb maintenance dose to be given once daily (s.i.d.). The drug is supplied at 250 mg/5 mL.

How many milligrams does your patient need for a loading dose?

A maintenance dose?

How many milligrams per milliliter are there in Albon?

How many milliliters will be dispensed?

6. The veterinarian orders 4.4 mg/kg of carprofen for pain control divided into two equal daily doses for a 50-lb dog. On hand are 100-mg scored tablets. How many tablets are administered each morning and afternoon?

7. The veterinarian prescribes 2.5 mg of acepromazine three times a day (t.i.d.) for 3 days, and tablets on hand are 5 mg (scored).

How many tablets will be administered?

How many will be dispensed?

8. The veterinarian prescribes aminophylline to be given three times daily for 14 days to a 15-lb dog. The dose for aminophylline is 10 mg/kg.

How many kilograms does your patient weigh?

How many milligrams have to be administered to your patient?

Because the tablets on hand are 100 mg (scored), how many tablets per dose will you give to the patient?

How many tablets will be dispensed?

9. A farmer has 10 calves that weigh approximately 100 lbs each. A microscopic fecal examination reveals Coccidia. The veterinarian chooses to treat all 10 calves with Corid powder (20% amprolium) by drenching daily for 10 days. To make a drench solution, mix 3 oz of Corid powder in 1 qt of water (1 oz of powder = 3.5 Tbsp). The dose of Corid for drenching is 1 oz of solution per 100 lb of body weight. How much solution should be mixed to drench these 10 calves for 10 days?

10. The veterinarian orders clenbuterol syrup for a 200-lb foal. The dosage is 0.8 mcg/kg twice daily for 3 days. The syrup contains 72.5 mcg/mL. How many milliliters is given at each dose?

Problems Measuring Parenteral Medications

1. The veterinarian orders an injection of desoxycorticosterone pivalate (Percorten-V) for a 20-lb dog at the dosage rate of 2.2 mg/kg. The concentration of desoxycorticosterone pivalate is 25 mg/mL. How much of the drug should be injected?

2. The veterinarian orders phenylbutazone to be administered to a 1500-lb horse at a dose of 5 mg/kg intravenously. The vial is labeled 200 mg/mL. How many milliliters will be administered?

3. The veterinarian orders penicillin G procaine for a 25-lb dog to be administered at a dose of 40,000 U/kg IM. The vial is labeled 300,000 U/mL. How many milliliters will be administered?

4. The veterinarian orders cefazolin to be given to a 23-lb dog at a dosage of 20 mg/kg IV for surgical prophylaxis. The concentration of cefazolin on hand is 100 mg/mL. How much (mL) of the drug should be given?

5. A microscopic fecal examination reveals a *Giardia* infection in a 500-g African gray parrot. The veterinarian chooses to treat the infection with injectable metronidazole at a dosage of 30 mg/kg daily for 3 days. How many milligrams will the parrot receive at each treatment?

6. A 45-lb dog is to be treated for lymphosarcoma with vincristine sulfate, 1 mg/mL. The dose is 0.5 mg/m^2.

How many square meters of body surface area does this patient have?

How many milligrams will be given to the patient?

How many milliliters?

7. The veterinarian orders lincomycin HCl for a 500-lb Yorkshire boar. The dosage to be administered is 5 mg/lb/day intramuscular (IM) for 5 days. The medication on hand is 100 mg/mL in a 50-mL multidose vial.

How many milligrams will be administered to the boar each day?

How many milliliters will be administered to the boar each day?

How many bottles of medication does the owner have to purchase to treat the boar for 5 days?

8. The veterinarian orders 7 mEq of potassium chloride to be added to the IV fluids. The vial is labeled 20 mEq in 10 mL. How many milliliters will be added to the fluids?

9. The veterinarian orders testosterone propionate for a 475-lb Landrace boar. The dose to be administered is 1 mg/10 lb. The label on the vial is 25 mg/mL.

How many milligrams will be administered?

How many milliliters will be administered?

10. The veterinarian orders 15 mg of vitamin K_1. The vial is labeled 10 mg/mL. How many milliliters will be administered?
11. The order is for meloxicam at 0.2 mg/kg to control postsurgical pain in a 4.5-kg cat. The concentration of the drug is 5 mg/mL. What volume of the drug should be given?
12. A rabbit weighing 12 lb is to be given 0.02 mg/kg of buprenorphine subcutaneously for pain control. The concentration of the drug is 0.3 mg/mL. How much of the drug should be given?
13. The veterinarian orders enrofloxacin at 5 mg/kg IM for a 7-kg python with respiratory disease. The product contains 100 mg/mL. How much should be injected?
14. The order is for an injection of metoclopramide at 0.4 mg/kg for a 15-kg dog. The concentration of available product is 5 mg/mL. How much should be injected?

Injection Problems

Order	Give	Stock
1.	0.5 g IM	250 mg/mL
2.	20 mEq IV	40 mEq/10 mL
3.	0.75 mg IM	0.50 mg/mL
4.	150 mg IM	0.2 g/5 mL
5.	25 mg IM	100 mg/mL
6.	0.5 mg IM	0.5 mg/2 mL
7.	0.3 mg IV	0.4 mg/mL
8.	300,000 U SC	40,000 U/mL
9.	0.3 mg IM	0.5 mg/mL
10.	55 mg SC	250 mg/mL

Preparing Solutions

1. Order: 100 mL of 10% formalin solution
   On hand: formaldehyde 37% (considered as 100% formalin) and water
   Amount needed: _____
2. Order: 1000 mL 0.9% NaCl and 5% dextrose
   On hand: 1000 mL 0.9% NaCl and 500 mL 50% dextrose
   Amount of each needed: _____
3. Order: 100 mL 5% dextrose
   On hand: 500 mL 50% dextrose and 250 mL sterile water for injection
   Amount needed: _____

4. Order: 2000 mL lactated Ringer's solution and 2.5% dextrose
   On hand: two containers of 1000 mL lactated Ringer's solution and 250 mL 50% dextrose
   Amount of each needed: _____
5. Order: 500 mL 2.5% dextrose and 0.45% NaCl
   On hand: 1000 mL 0.45% NaCl and 500 mL 50% dextrose
   Amount of each needed: _____
6. Order: 1000 mL of 10% glyceryl guaiacolate solution
   On hand: packets containing 50 g guaifenesin (GG) powder and 1000 mL sterile water for injection
   Amount of each needed: _____
7. Order: 8% thiamylal sodium solution
   On hand: one 5-g vial of powder and 1 mL of sterile water for injection
   Amount of sterile water needed: _____
8. Order: 5 mL of 2% cyclosporine ophthalmic solution
   On hand: 50 mL cyclosporine (Sandimmune Oral Solution) 100 mg/mL and 16 oz of extra virgin olive oil
   Amount of each needed: _____
9. Order: 50 mL of 2% formalin for Knott's heartworm test
   On hand: 100% formaldehyde and water
   Amount of each needed: _____
10. Order: Prepare 1 L of a 1:32 sodium hypochlorite (bleach) solution
    On hand: distilled water and 5% sodium hypochlorite (bleach)
    Amount of each needed: _____
11. Order: Prepare 50 mL of a 0.5 mEq/mL KCl solution.
    On hand: sterile water for injection and KCl (2 mEq/mL)
    Amount of each needed: _____
12. Order: Prepare 15 mL of a 5 mg/mL enrofloxacin solution.
    On hand: 22.7 mg/mL enrofloxacin and sterile water for injection.
    Amount of each needed: _____

Problems Calculating Intravenous (IV) Drip Rates

1. What drip rate will you use to administer 500 mL of lactated Ringer's solution over a 3-hour period with a standard (15 gtt/mL) administration set?
2. What drip rate would you use to deliver 120 mL 0.9% NaCl over a 2-hour period using a microdrip (60 gtt/mL) administration set?

3. What drip rate would you use to deliver 1.2 L of Normosol over a 10-hour period using a standard (15 gtt/mL) administration set?

4. What drip rate would you use to deliver 8 mcg/kg/min of drug C (500 mg/250 mL) to an 83-lb dog using a microdrip (60 gtt/mL) administration set?

5. What drip rate would you use to deliver 10 mcg/kg/min of dopamine (0.2 mg/mL) to a 22-lb dog using the microdrip (60 gtt/mL) administration set?

6. Using the formula

$$M = \frac{(D)\,(W)\,(V)}{R\,(16.67)}$$

how much nitroprusside (25 mg/mL) would you add to 1000 mL of 5% dextrose to deliver 2 mcg/kg/min of nitroprusside at a delivery rate of 12 mL/h to a 3.8-kg dog?

7. Using the formula

$$M = \frac{(D)\,(W)\,(V)}{R\,(16.67)}$$

how much dobutamine (12.5 mg/mL) would you add to 100 mL of a 5% dextrose solution to administer 15 mcg/kg/min to a 28-kg dog at a delivery rate of 10 mL/h?

8. How much furosemide (10 mg/mL) would you add to a 250-mL fluid bag to deliver 3 mcg/kg/min to a 5-kg patient with the fluid pump set at 15 mL/h?

9. How much morphine (15 mg/mL) would you add to a 250-mL fluid bag to deliver 0.2 mg/kg/h to a 10-kg animal with the pump set on 10 mL/h?

REFERENCES

American Animal Hospital Association. (2013). *AAHA/AAFP fluid Therapy Guidelines for dogs and cats Implementation Toolkit (supplemental information)*. https://www.aaha.org/globalassets/02-guidelines/fluid-therapy/fluidtherapy_tip-sheet.pdf. Accessed August 2019.

Blankenship, J., & Campbell, J. B. (1976). Solutions. In J. Blankenship, & J. B. Campbell (Eds.), *Laboratory mathematics: Medical and biological applications*. St. Louis: Mosby.

Macintire, D. K., & Tefend, M. (2004). Constant rate infusions: Practical use. *North American Veterinary Conference Clinician's Brief*, Orlando, FL, April 25–28.

Ortel, S. O. (2006). Constant-rate infusions. *Veterinary Technician*, 27(1), 47–50.

Upson, D. W. (1988). General principles. In D. W. Upson (Ed.), *Handbook of clinical veterinary pharmacology* (3rd ed.). Manhattan, KS: Dan Upson Enterprises.

4

Drugs Used in Nervous System Disorders

OBJECTIVES

After studying this chapter, you should be able to

1. Define terms related to the pharmacology of the nervous system.
2. Develop a basic understanding of the anatomy and physiology of the nervous system.
3. Describe the subdivisions, functions, and primary neurotransmitters of the autonomic nervous system (ANS).
4. Describe how drugs affect the ANS.
5. List and discuss the different classes of ANS drugs.
6. Discuss the central nervous system (CNS) and list the categories of CNS drugs.
7. List the major classification schemes of barbiturates, including a discussion on the indications and precautions for each.
8. Describe dissociative anesthesia and list three dissociative agents.
9. List the opiate receptors and the basic function of each.
10. List the indications for the use of narcotics, as well as discuss the potential side effects of narcotic use or overdose.
11. Describe how opioid antagonists exert their effects, and list three examples of this category of drug.
12. Define *neuroleptanalgesics* and give an example.
13. List examples of drugs used to prevent or control seizures.
14. List commonly used inhalant anesthetic agents and compare their characteristics. Also, define *minimum alveolar concentration (MAC)*, *partition coefficient*, and *vapor pressure* as the terms relate to the use of inhalant anesthetics.
15. Describe the primary uses of CNS stimulants and discuss neuromuscular blocking drugs.
16. List drugs used in behavioral pharmacotherapy.
17. Describe the characteristics of a good euthanasia agent.

OUTLINE

KEY TERMS

Acetylcholine
Acetylcholinesterase
Adrenergic
Analgesia
Anesthesia
Autonomic nervous system
Catalepsy
Catecholamine
Cholinergic
Effector
Ganglionic synapse
Minimum alveolar concentration (MAC)
Muscarinic receptors

Neuroleptanalgesia
Nicotinic receptors
Parasympathetic nervous system
Parasympatholytic
Parasympathomimetic
Precision vaporizer
Sedative
Sympathetic nervous system
Sympatholytic
Sympathomimetic
Tranquilizer
Vapor pressure

INTRODUCTION

The nervous system is the body's primary communication and control center. It functions in harmony with the endocrine system to allow an animal to respond and adapt to its environment and to maintain a relatively constant internal environment (homeostasis) through control of the many internal organ systems. In broad terms, the nervous system serves three functions: (1) sensory, (2) integrative (analysis), and (3) motor (action). It senses changes within the environment and within the body, interprets the information, and responds to the interpretation by bringing about an appropriate action. The nervous system carries out this complex activity very rapidly by sending electric-like messages over a network of nerve fibers. The endocrine system

works much more slowly by sending chemical messengers (hormones) through the bloodstream to target structures. The two systems are very closely interrelated functionally and anatomically. The nervous system exerts control over the endocrine system through the influence of the hypothalamus (brain) on the pituitary gland.

ANATOMY AND PHYSIOLOGY

The nervous system has two main divisions, the central nervous system (CNS) and the peripheral nervous system, as well as their related subdivisions (Fig. 4.1). The CNS is composed of the brain and the spinal cord and serves as the control center of the entire nervous system. All sensory

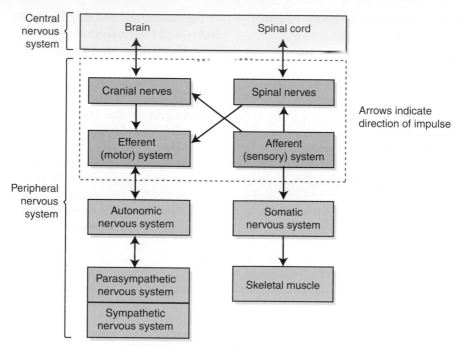

Fig. 4.1 Organization of the nervous system.

information must be relayed to the CNS before it can be interpreted and acted on. Most impulses that stimulate glands to act and muscles to contract originate in the CNS.

The nerve processes that connect the CNS with the various glands, muscles, and receptors in the body make up the peripheral nervous system. Functionally, the peripheral nervous system is divided into afferent and efferent portions. The afferent portion is composed of nerve cells that carry information from receptors in the periphery of the body to the CNS. The efferent system consists of nerve cells that carry impulses from the CNS to muscles and glands. Anatomically, the peripheral nervous system is composed of cranial nerves and spinal nerves.

The peripheral nervous system is also subdivided into a somatic nervous system and an **autonomic nervous system (ANS)**. The somatic nervous system consists of efferent nerves that carry impulses from the CNS to skeletal muscle tissue. It is under conscious control and is therefore called *voluntary*. The ANS consists of efferent nerve cells that carry information from the CNS to cardiac muscle, glands, and smooth muscle. It is under unconscious control and is called *involuntary*. The ANS has two subdivisions, the **sympathetic nervous system** and the **parasympathetic nervous system**. Most tissues innervated by the ANS receive both sympathetic and parasympathetic fibers. In general, one division stimulates an activity by

a receptor and the other inhibits the activity to serve as a method of checks and balances.

The fundamental unit of all branches and divisions of the nervous system is the neuron (nerve cell). Neurons have the amazing ability to transmit information from point to point. The second point may be nearby or at a great distance. Similar to all cells in the body, neurons have a nucleus surrounded by cytoplasm. Different from other cells, however, neurons have cellular extensions or processes called *axons* and *dendrites*. Axons carry electric-like messages away from the nerve cell, and dendrites carry electric-like messages toward the nerve cell (Fig. 4.2). Transmission of these messages along nerve fibers occurs through a wave of charge reversal that moves down the fiber (Fig. 4.3). The resting (polarized) fiber has positive charges lined up on the outside of its membrane and negative charges lined up on the inside of its membrane. When a stimulus of sufficient magnitude reaches the fiber, depolarization or charge reversal (positive in, negative out) occurs in a progressive wave down the fiber toward the synapse. Repolarization is the movement of charges back to their original positions.

Axons may be short or long (up to 4 feet in humans), and they terminate, or end, in as many as 10,000 nerve endings called *telodendra* (Snyder, 1986). The large number of nerve endings allows for great variety in the number and type of connections made with other neurons.

The synaptic end-bulbs of the telodendra pass nerve impulses to an adjacent structure (another neuron, gland, or muscle) by emitting a chemical messenger called a *neurotransmitter* into the gap or junction (synapse) between the nerve ending and the adjacent structure (Fig. 4.4). Neurotransmitters then combine with receptors on the dendritic side of the synapse and cause a stimulatory or inhibitory effect. Dendrites may respond to neurotransmitters by generating a nerve impulse, which is conducted via the axon to the adjacent structure (neuron, gland, or muscle). Neurotransmitters can be mimicked or blocked by the use of appropriate drugs (Fig. 4.5).

Nerve fibers (nerves) may have a large diameter (A fibers), a medium diameter (B fibers), or a small diameter (C fibers; Boothe, 2012). Fibers with large diameters conduct nerve impulses faster than those with small diameters. Fibers that are surrounded by the insulating substance called *myelin* also transmit impulses faster than nonmyelinated fibers. Type A and B fibers are generally myelinated fibers.

The most basic impulse conduction system through the nervous system is the reflex arc (Fig. 4.6). The reflex arc is composed of the following:

- A receptor
- A sensory neuron
- A center in the CNS for a synapse
- A motor neuron
- An effector

The receptor of the reflex arc may be located in a peripheral site—such as the skin—or in a central area—such as a muscle, tendon, or visceral organ. The sensory neuron carries the impulse from the receptor to the CNS. In the CNS, the sensory neuron synapses with interneurons in the spinal cord. These interneurons send the impulse to the brain for interpretation or send the

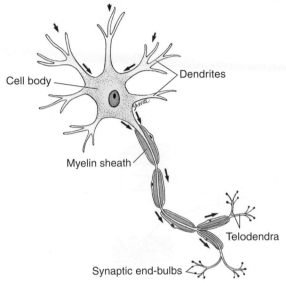

Fig. 4.2 Impulse transmission through the neuron.

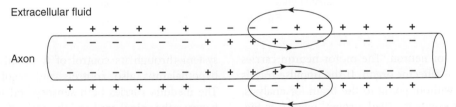

Fig. 4.3 Electric impulse transmission along a nerve fiber.

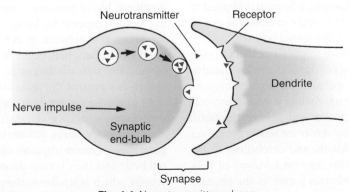

Fig. 4.4 Neurotransmitter release.

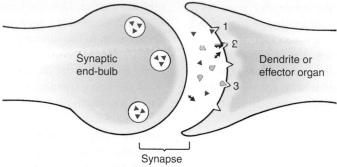

1. Normal neurotransmitter   ▸ Neurotransmitter
2. Neurotransmitter blockade   ⇥ Drug that blocks neurotransmitter
3. Neurotransmitter mimicry   ◦ Drug that mimics neurotransmitter

Fig. 4.5 Neurotransmitter activity.

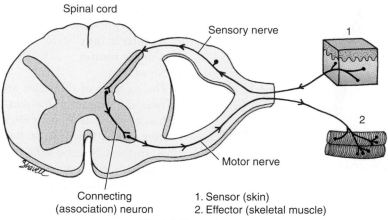

1. Sensor (skin)
2. Effector (skeletal muscle)

Fig. 4.6 The reflex arc.

impulse to a motor neuron. The motor neuron carries the message to an effector organ. If the impulse travels around the arc without going to the brain for analysis, the sequence of events is called a *spinal reflex* (see Fig. 4.6). A spinal reflex can occur even if the spinal cord is completely severed. For example, a hemostat applied to the toe of a dog with a severed cord can cause the dog to withdraw its leg by means of the spinal reflex.

Areas of the brain that have importance to an understanding of the pharmacology of the CNS are illustrated in Fig. 4.7. The cerebrum is responsible for higher functions of the brain, such as learning, memory, and interpretation of sensory input (e.g., vision and pain recognition). The thalamus serves as a relay center for sensory impulses from the spinal cord, brainstem, and cerebellum to the cerebrum. The thalamus also may be involved in pain interpretation. The hypothalamus serves as the primary mediator between the nervous system and the endocrine system through its control of the pituitary gland. The hypothalamus also controls and regulates the ANS. The medulla carries both sensory and motor impulses between the spinal cord and the brain. It contains centers that control vital physiologic activities, such as breathing, heartbeat, blood pressure, vomiting, swallowing, coughing, body temperature, hunger, and thirst. The reticular formation is a network of nerve cells scattered through bundles of fibers that begin in the medulla and extend upward through the brainstem. The reticular activating system is a part of the reticular formation, which functions to arouse the cerebral cortex and is responsible for consciousness, sleep, and wakefulness (DeLahunta, 1983).

In summary, nerve activity is usually described as the generation of nerve impulses that occurs in a dendrite or cell body and then travels down an axon by electric-like activity, which is similar to the passage of an electric current down a wire. When this current reaches a synapse, a

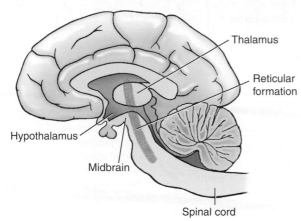

Fig. 4.7 Pharmacologically important areas of the brain.

chemical "bridge" or neurotransmitter allows the message to be passed to one or as many as thousands of other neurons. Neurotransmitter substances include acetylcholine, norepinephrine, dopamine, serotonin, and gamma-aminobutyric acid (GABA). These other neurons then carry the message to an interpretation center or a structure that takes appropriate action. The CNS drugs act by mimicking or blocking the effects of neurotransmitters.

AUTONOMIC NERVOUS SYSTEM

The ANS is that portion of the nervous system that controls unconscious body activities. The ANS fibers innervate smooth muscle, heart muscle, salivary glands, and other viscera. This system operates automatically and involuntarily to control visceral functions, such as gastrointestinal (GI) motility, rate and force of the heartbeat, secretion by glands, sizes of the pupils, and various other involuntary functions and characteristics. In contrast to the somatic nervous system, the ANS has two subdivisions: parasympathetic (cholinergic) and sympathetic (adrenergic). The sympathetic division regulates energy-expending activities (fight-or-flight responses), and the parasympathetic division regulates energy-conserving activities.

The ANS has two neurons that carry impulses to target structures (in contrast to the somatic nervous system, which has only one). The cell body of the first neuron arises in the CNS—in the thoracolumbar cord for the sympathetic nervous system and in the craniosacral cord for the parasympathetic nervous system (Fig. 4.8). The axon of the first neuron leaves the CNS and travels to a ganglion, where it synapses with dendrites of the second neuron. This second neuron then travels to the target structure (Fig. 4.9). Axons of the first neuron are called *preganglionic*, and

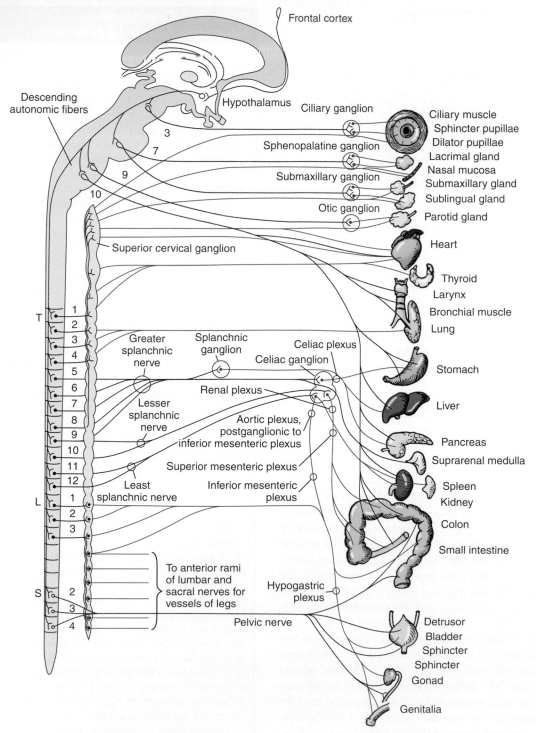

Fig. 4.8 Schematic of the autonomic nervous system. (From Thibodeau, J. A. [1987]. *Anatomy and physiology*. St. Louis: Mosby.)

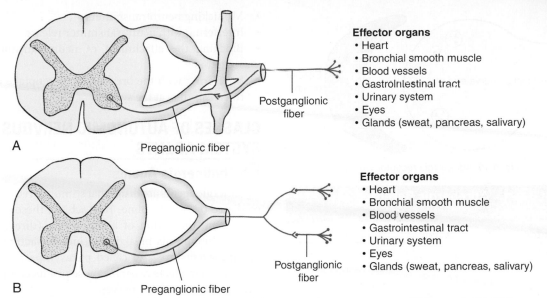

Fig. 4.9 Preganglionic and postganglionic fibers of the autonomic nervous system. (A) Sympathetic. (B) Parasympathetic.

those of the second are called *postganglionic*. The synapse between the preganglionic neuron and the postganglionic neuron is called the **ganglionic synapse.**

Preganglionic fibers of the sympathetic nervous system are short. They end in ganglia adjacent to the spinal cord. The only exception is the preganglionic fiber to the adrenal medulla. The adrenal medulla itself is analogous to a postganglionic fiber because it releases epinephrine and norepinephrine directly into the bloodstream when stimulated by preganglionic fibers. Postganglionic sympathetic fibers are long.

Preganglionic fibers of the parasympathetic nervous system are generally long. They travel to ganglia located in the wall of the target organ. Postganglionic fibers are consequently short.

Normally, target sites of the ANS have both sympathetic and parasympathetic innervation. The physiologic functions of the two systems usually oppose each other, thereby bringing about a state of balance. When this balance is disrupted, drug therapy may be indicated to restore the balance. The adrenal medulla, sweat glands, and hair follicles have only sympathetic fibers.

Stimulation of the sympathetic nervous system causes an increase in heart rate and respiratory rate, a decrease in GI activity, dilation of the pupils, constriction of blood vessels in smooth muscle, dilation of blood vessels in skeletal muscle, dilation of bronchioles, and an increase in blood glucose levels. These actions prepare an animal to fight or to flee. On the other hand, stimulation of the parasympathetic nervous system causes a decrease in heart rate and respiratory rate, an increase in GI activity, constriction of the pupils, and constriction of the bronchioles.

Receptors of the sympathetic (adrenergic) nervous system are subdivided as follows (Fig. 4.10):

- Alpha-1
- Alpha-2
- Beta-1
- Beta-2
- Dopaminergic

Generally, alpha receptors are stimulatory and beta receptors are inhibitory (Table 4.1). The parasympathetic (cholinergic) nervous system has **nicotinic** and **muscarinic receptors. Effector** organs have one or a combination of these receptors. A drug's effect is determined by the number of receptors in the effector and the drug's specificity for the receptor (Williams & Baer, 1990).

The primary neurotransmitters for adrenergic sites are norepinephrine, epinephrine, and dopamine. Epinephrine equally stimulates alpha and beta receptors and is therefore a potent stimulator of the heart and an equally powerful dilator of bronchioles. Acetylcholine is the neurotransmitter at sympathetic postganglionic fibers to sweat glands and the smooth muscle of blood vessels (muscarinic sites).

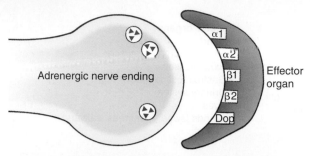

Fig. 4.10 Adrenergic receptor types.

TABLE 4.1 **Adrenergic Receptor Responses.**

Receptor	Target Organ	Response
Alpha-1	Arterioles	Constriction
	Urethra	Increased tone
	Eye	Dilation of pupil
Alpha-2	Skeletal muscle	Constriction
Beta-1	Heart	Increased rate, conduction, and contractility
	Kidneys	Renin release
Beta-2	Skeletal blood vessels	Dilation
	Bronchioles	Dilation
Dopaminergic	Kidneys	Dilation of blood vessels
	Heart	Dilation of coronary vessels
	Mesenteric blood vessels	Dilation

The neurotransmitter for cholinergic sites is acetylcholine. Acetylcholine combines with both nicotinic and muscarinic receptors.

Cholinergic sites are found in both the sympathetic and parasympathetic nervous systems. Nicotinic receptors are found in all autonomic ganglia, in the adrenal medulla, and at the neuromuscular junction of the somatic nervous system. Muscarinic receptors are found at the synapse of postganglionic fibers of the parasympathetic nervous system and at a few of the sympathetic postganglionic fibers.

How Drugs Affect the Autonomic Nervous System

Autonomic drugs bring about their effects by influencing the sequence of events that involve neurotransmitters. Most autonomic drugs bring about this alteration of events by doing the following:

- Mimicking neurotransmitters
- Interfering with neurotransmitter release
- Blocking the attachment of neurotransmitters to receptors
- Interfering with the breakdown or reuptake of neurotransmitters at the synapse

CLASSES OF AUTONOMIC NERVOUS SYSTEM AGENTS

℞ Cholinergic Agents

Cholinergic agents are drugs that stimulate receptor sites mediated by acetylcholine. They achieve these effects by mimicking the action of acetylcholine (direct-acting) or by inhibiting its breakdown (indirect-acting). Cholinergic agents are also called parasympathomimetic because their effects resemble those produced by stimulating parasympathetic nerves.

Clinical Uses. Cholinergic agents do the following:
- Aid in the diagnosis of myasthenia gravis
- Reduce the intraocular pressure of glaucoma
- Stimulate GI motility
- Treat urinary retention
- Control vomiting
- Act as an antidote for neuromuscular blockers

Direct-Acting Cholinergics

- **Acetylcholine**: Acetylcholine is seldom used clinically because it is broken down so rapidly by acetylcholinesterase.
- **Carbamylcholine**: This product has been used to treat atony of the GI tract and to stimulate uterine contractions in swine.
- **Bethanechol**: Bethanechol is used to treat GI and urinary tract atony.
- **Pilocarpine** (Isopto Carpine): Pilocarpine reduces intraocular pressure associated with glaucoma and is used to treat keratoconjunctivitis sicca.
- **Metoclopramide** (Reglan): Metoclopramide is used to control vomiting and to promote gastric tract emptying.

Indirect-Acting Cholinergic (Anticholinesterase) Agents

- **Edrophonium**: Edrophonium is primarily used in the presumptive diagnosis of myasthenia gravis.
- **Neostigmine** (Prostigmine): These products are used to treat urine retention and GI atony and are used as an antidote to neuromuscular blocking agents.

- **Physostigmine** (Antilirium): Uses of this product are similar to those of neostigmine.
- **Organophosphate compounds**: These are commonly used as insecticide dips and may result in toxicity if used inappropriately. See pralidoxime under Dosage Forms for Cholinergic Blocking Agents later in this chapter.
- **Demecarium** (Humorsol): This drug is used in the preventive management of glaucoma.
- **Pyridostigmine** (Mestinon): This drug is used for the treatment of myasthenia gravis.

Adverse Side Effects. Adverse side effects of the cholinergic drugs may include bradycardia, hypotension, heart block, lacrimation, diarrhea, vomiting, increased intestinal activity, intestinal rupture, and increased bronchial secretions.

Ⓡ Cholinergic Blocking Agents (Anticholinergic)

Cholinergic blocking agents are drugs that block the action of acetylcholine at muscarinic receptors of the parasympathetic nervous system. Anticholinergic agents are also called parasympatholytic because their effects reduce the activity of the parasympathetic nervous system.

Clinical Uses. Clinical uses of these drugs include the following:

- Treatment of diarrhea and vomiting via a decrease in GI motility
- Drying of secretions and prevention of bradycardia before anesthesia
- Dilation of the pupils for ophthalmic examination
- Relief of ciliary spasm of the eye
- Treatment of sinus bradycardia

The belladonna alkaloids of the deadly nightshade family of plants have been used as drugs for centuries and represent the prototype for this category of agents.

Dosage Forms

- **Atropine**: Numerous generic and trade name products are available for parenteral or ophthalmic administration. Atropine is used as a preanesthetic to dry secretions and prevent bradycardia; to counteract organophosphate poisoning; to dilate the pupils for ophthalmic examination; to control ciliary spasms of the eye; to treat sinus bradycardia; and to slow a hypermotile gut.
- **Methscopolamine** is an ingredient of Biosol-M. Methscopolamine is used to control diarrhea.

- **Glycopyrrolate**: Glycopyrrolate is a quaternary ammonium compound with actions similar to atropine. It provides longer duration of action than atropine and is used primarily as a preanesthetic.
- **Aminopentamide**: Aminopentamide is used to control vomiting and diarrhea in dogs and cats.
- **Propantheline**: Propantheline is used to treat diarrhea, urinary incontinence, and bradycardia and to reduce colonic peristalsis in horses to allow rectal examination. Propantheline, similar to glycopyrrolate, is a quaternary ammonium compound.
- **Pralidoxime** (Protopam, 2-PAM): Pralidoxime is a cholinesterase reactivator used to treat organophosphate intoxication.

Adverse Side Effects. Adverse side effects of the cholinergic blockers are dose related. Overdoses can cause drowsiness, disorientation, tachycardia, photophobia, constipation, anxiety, and burning at the injection site.

📋 TECHNICIAN NOTES

- Atropine administered as a preanesthetic causes dilation of the pupils. It dries secretions and prevents bradycardia.
- Atropine is packaged in small-animal and large-animal concentrations. Care should be taken not to confuse the two preparations.

Ⓡ Adrenergic (Sympathomimetic) Agents

Adrenergic (sympathomimetic) agents bring about action at receptors mediated by epinephrine or norepinephrine; mimic the "fight or flight" response. Adrenergic agents may be classified as catecholamines or noncatecholamines, and either category can also be classified according to the specific receptor types activated (alpha-1, alpha-2, beta-1, beta-2). In most cases, alpha receptor activity causes an excitatory response (except in the GI tract), and beta stimulation causes an inhibitory response (except in the heart). Adrenergic activity is a complex subject, and more advanced texts should be consulted for a thorough explanation.

Clinical Uses. Adrenergic agents are used for the following purposes:

- To stimulate the heart to beat during cardiac arrest
- To reverse the hypotension and bronchoconstriction of anaphylactic shock
- To strengthen the heart during congestive heart failure
- To correct hypotension through vasoconstriction
- To reduce capillary bleeding through vasoconstriction
- To treat urinary incontinence

- To reduce mucous membrane congestion (vasoconstriction) in allergic conditions
- To prolong the effects of local anesthetic agents by causing vasoconstriction of blood vessels at the injection site, thereby prolonging their absorption
- To treat glaucoma (alpha stimulation increases the outflow of and beta stimulation decreases the production of aqueous humor)

Dosage Forms

- **Epinephrine**: Epinephrine stimulates all receptors to cause an increase in heart rate and cardiac output, constriction of the blood vessels in the skin, dilation of the blood vessels in muscle, dilation of the bronchioles, and an increase in metabolic rate.
- **Norepinephrine**: Norepinephrine is mostly an alpha stimulator with some beta stimulation. Its primary influence is that of a vasopressor (to raise blood pressure).
- **Isoproterenol** (Isuprel): Isoproterenol is a pure beta stimulator. Its primary use is for bronchodilation.
- **Phenylephrine** (Neo-Synephrine): Phenylephrine is an alpha stimulator that is used as a nasal vasoconstrictor. It also increases blood pressure.
- **Dopamine**: Dopamine is a precursor of epinephrine and norepinephrine. Its action is dose dependent. It is used to treat shock and congestive heart failure and to increase renal perfusion. It increases blood pressure and cardiac output.
- **Phenylpropanolamine**: Phenylpropanolamine is used to treat urinary incontinence in dogs. It is also used as a decongestant and bronchodilator.
- **Dobutamine**: Dobutamine is a beta-1 agonist that is used for short-term treatment of heart failure.
- **Albuterol**: Albuterol is a beta agonist and the main use is bronchodilation.

Adverse Side Effects. These may include tachycardia, hypertension, nervousness, and cardiac arrhythmias. Hypertension, arrhythmia, and pulmonary edema may occur with an overdose.

> **📋 TECHNICIAN NOTES**
>
> Epinephrine is available in two concentrations: 1 mg/mL (1:1,000) and 0.1 mg/mL (1:10,000).

Adrenergic (Sympatholytic) Blocking Agents

Adrenergic blocking (sympatholytic) agents are used to disrupt/inhibit the activity of the sympathetic nervous system. They are classified according to the site of their action as an alpha blocker, beta blocker, or ganglionic blocker. Drugs usually block only one category of receptor.

Alpha Blockers

Alpha blockers have had limited use in veterinary medicine. Phenoxybenzamine has been advocated by some clinicians for the treatment of laminitis in horses and urethral obstruction in cats. Yohimbine is used for xylazine antagonism.

Clinical Uses. See section, Dosage Forms.

Dosage Forms

- **Phenoxybenzamine**: Phenoxybenzamine is a hypotensive (vasodilator) agent.
- **Acepromazine**: This tranquilizer acts as an alpha blocker and causes vasodilation. It is used as a sedative, tranquilizer, and preanesthetic adjunct.
- **Prazosin**: Prazosin is a hypotensive agent. It is also used to treat urethral spasms in cats and dogs secondary to urethral obstruction.
- **Yohimbine** (Yobine): Yohimbine is used as an antidote for xylazine toxicity.
- **Atipamezole** (Antisedan): Atipamezole is a reversal agent for dexmedetomidine.

Adverse Side Effects. Adverse side effects may include hypotension (phenoxybenzamine, tranquilizers, prazosin), tachycardia (phenoxybenzamine), muscle tremors (yohimbine), and seizures (acepromazine).

Beta Blockers

Beta blockers are used to treat glaucoma, arrhythmias, and hypertrophic cardiomyopathy.

Clinical Uses. See section, Dosage Forms.

Dosage Forms

- **Propranolol**: Propranolol is used to treat cardiac arrhythmias and hypertrophic cardiomyopathy. It decreases the heart rate, decreases blood pressure, and decreases cardiac output.
- **Timolol**: Timolol is an ophthalmic preparation used to treat glaucoma.
- **Atenolol**: Used in a similar way to propranolol.

Adverse Side Effects. These include bradycardia, hypotension, worsening of heart failure, bronchoconstriction, heart block, and syncope.

Ganglionic Blockers

Ganglionic blockers are seldom used in veterinary medicine.

CENTRAL NERVOUS SYSTEM

The CNS drugs have various uses in veterinary medicine. Depressant drugs are used to tranquilize or sedate animals to facilitate restraint or anesthetic procedures. They are also used to control pain, to induce **anesthesia**, and to prevent or control seizures. The CNS drugs are also available to antagonize (reverse) the effects of some depressant drugs. Another group of CNS agents is used to stimulate the CNS to treat cardiac or respiratory depression or arrest. Euthanasia drugs allow veterinarians to provide a quick and painless end to hopeless medical situations.

Drugs that affect the CNS generally cause depression or stimulation. They are thought to generate these changes by altering nerve impulse transmissions between the spinal cord and the brain or within the brain itself. Altering impulse transmissions within the thalamus could prevent messages regarding painful stimuli from reaching interpretation centers within the cerebrum. Interfering with impulses within the reticular activating system could alter levels of consciousness or wakefulness (Ganong, 2003). The changes that occur in the transmission of nerve impulses as a result of administration of CNS drugs are probably brought about by altered neurotransmitter activity.

The categories of CNS drugs that are covered in this chapter include the following:

- Tranquilizers
- Barbiturates
- Dissociatives
- Opioid/antagonists
- Neuroleptanalgesics/antagonists
- Drugs to prevent or control seizures
- Inhalants
- Miscellaneous CNS drugs
- CNS stimulants
- Euthanasia agents

® Tranquilizers

Tranquilizers and sedatives play an important role in veterinary medicine. They are used to calm patients, produce muscle relaxation, decrease dose of anesthetic requirements, ease of placing an intravenous catheter, and promote smooth induction and recovery. **Tranquilizers** decrease anxiety without causing excessive sedation or drowsiness; animals are usually aware of their surroundings but do not appear to care. Tranquilizers do not provide analgesia. **Sedatives** are used to suppress brain activity and awareness to prevent movement for some short medical procedures; animals are usually unaware of their surroundings and are drowsy. Sedatives offer some analgesia.

Phenothiazine Derivatives

The mechanism of action of the phenothiazine derivatives on the CNS is not well understood. However, it has been proposed that they are dopamine blockers (Muir, Hubbell, Bednarski, & Lerche, 2013). The effects on the cardiovascular system are a result of alpha-adrenergic blockade.

Phenothiazine derivative tranquilizers produce sedation and allay fear and anxiety without producing significant analgesia. Sudden painful stimuli arouse the animal. Phenothiazine derivative tranquilizers produce an antiemetic effect by depressing the chemoreceptor trigger zone in the brain and have a mild antipruritic effect. These agents also reduce the tendency of epinephrine to induce cardiac arrhythmias.

Clinical Uses. Phenothiazine derivatives are used for prevention or treatment of vomiting, relief of mild pruritus, and sedation/tranquilization.

Dosage Forms
- **Acepromazine maleate** (PromAce)
- **Chlorpromazine hydrochloride** (Thorazine-human label)
- **Promazine hydrogen chloride** (HCl)
- **Prochlorperazine**

Adverse Side Effects. Phenothiazine derivative tranquilizers can cause hypotension and hypothermia through their vasodilator effects (alpha blockade). Acepromazine has been avoided in epileptic animals as it was previously cautioned that it lowered the seizure threshold and caused seizures. However, there is no clinical evidence to support this claim and some studies have shown that it has some anticonvulsant activity (Plumb, 2015).

TECHNICIAN NOTES

- Phenothiazine derivatives should not be used within 1 month of worming with an organophosphate anthelmintic.
- The tranquilizing effect may be reduced in an excited animal.

Phenothiazine derivative tranquilizers are approved for use in a wide variety of animals and for administration by almost any route. They generally are relatively safe drugs to use when administered appropriately. They should be given with care when used with other CNS depressants because of the additive effect. Most pheno-thiazine derivative tranquilizers are metabolized by the liver and excreted by the kidneys.

Benzodiazepine Derivatives

The mechanism of action of diazepam occurs through depression of the thalamic and hypothalamic areas of the brain. This drug produces sedation, muscle relaxation, appetite stimulation (especially in cats), and anticonvulsant activity. Diazepam also produces minimal depression of the cardiovascular and respiratory systems when compared with other CNS depressants. It sometimes is used in combination with ketamine to induce short-term anesthesia. Diazepam is very useful for treating seizures in progress. Diazepam is painful if administered intramuscularly. Midazolam is very similar to diazepam but has a greater potency. Midazolam is water soluble and absorbed well after intramuscular injection unlike diazepam, which is not water soluble. Zolazepam (Telazol) is a short-acting anesthetic that produces mild to moderate analgesia and is used for minor procedures of short duration.

Several potential drug interactions can occur when diazepam is administered simultaneously with other drugs, and appropriate references should be consulted.

Clinical Uses. Clinical uses include sedation, relief of anxiety and behavioral disorders, treatment of seizures, and appetite stimulation. Diazepam can be used as an injectable anesthetic.

Dosage Forms
- **Diazepam** (Valium, Diastat)
- **Midazolam** (Versed)
- **Zolazepam** (Telazol)
- **Alprazolam** (Xanax)

Adverse Side Effects. These are limited when used as directed. Dogs can exhibit excitement. An overdose may cause excessive CNS depression.

📋 TECHNICIAN NOTES

- Diazepam should be stored at room temperature and protected from light.
- Diazepam should not be stored in plastic syringes or in solution bags because it can be absorbed into the plastic.
- Manufacturers recommend that it not be mixed with other medications or solutions.
- Diazepam is painful if administered intramuscularly.
- Diazepam is metabolized by the liver and eliminated by the kidneys.
- Alprazolam is also used as an appetite stimulant.

Alpha-2 Agonists

Alpha-2 agonists are sedative analgesics used commonly in veterinary medicine. They provide sedation, analgesia, muscle relaxation, and antianxiety. The CNS effects of alpha-2 agonists can be antagonized by alpha-2 receptor antagonists such as yohimbine, tolazoline, and atipamezole.

Xylazine Hydrochloride

Xylazine is an alpha-2 agonist with sedative, analgesic, and muscle relaxant properties. It is approved for use in dogs, cats, horses, deer, and elk. This agent causes vomiting in a large percentage of cats and in some dogs. Xylazine is antagonized by yohimbine. It produces effective analgesia in horses and is often used for treating the pain associated with colic and for sedation for minor procedures. It is also used in combination with ketamine for short-term field procedures in horses, such as castration and suturing of extensive wounds, because this combination usually produces 15 to 20 minutes of recumbency. Extralabel use of xylazine for cesarean sections in cattle and other surgical procedures is common. Xylazine is used in cats and dogs as a tranquilizer and in combination with other injectable agents for surgical procedures.

Clinical Uses. Clinical uses include sedation, analgesia, short-term anesthesia (when combined with other agents), and induction of vomiting.

Dosage Forms
- **Rompun**
- **AnaSed**
- **Sedazine**
- **Cervizine** (labeled for deer and elk)

Adverse Side Effects. These include bradycardia, hypotension, respiratory depression, and increased sensitivity to epinephrine, resulting in cardiac arrhythmias. An overdose increases the potential for these effects.

📋 TECHNICIAN NOTES

- Because of the potential of xylazine to cause bradycardia or heart block in dogs, atropine should be used as a premedicant in this species.
- Xylazine is used in cattle at one-tenth of the equine dose.
- Horses may appear heavily sedated with xylazine and still respond to painful stimuli by kicking.
- Small-animal (20 mg/mL) and large-animal (100 mg/mL) concentrations are available. Care should be taken not to confuse them when administering a drug dose to an animal.

Yohimbine is used as the reversal agent for xylazine.

Detomidine Hydrochloride

Detomidine, similar to xylazine, is an alpha-2 agonist. It is approved as a sedative/analgesic for horses, and some clinicians report excellent analgesic properties in their patients when using this product. Some animals may respond to stimuli by kicking even when they appear heavily sedated with this drug. Atipamezole is used as the reversal agent for this drug.

Clinical Uses. Detomidine is used for sedation and analgesia in horses.

Dosage Form
- **Dormosedan** injectable
- **Dormosedan gel** (for sublingual administration)

Adverse Side Effects. These may include sweating, muscle tremors, penile prolapse, bradycardia, and heart block.

 TECHNICIAN NOTES

The manufacturer warns that detomidine should be used very carefully with other sedative drugs and that it should not be used with potentiated sulfa drugs such as trimethoprim/sulfamethoxazole.

Medetomidine

Medetomidine is an alpha-2-adrenergic agonist labeled for use as a sedative and analgesic in dogs older than 12 weeks. Atipamezole (Antisedan) is the reversal agent for this drug.

Clinical Uses. Uses include facilitating clinical examination, minor surgical procedures, and minor dental procedures that do not require intubation.

Dosage Form. Domitor (not currently available in the U.S. market but still available in Canada).

Adverse Side Effects. Side effects include bradycardia (product insert states that hemodynamics are maintained), atrioventricular heart block, decreased respirations, hypothermia, urination, vomiting, hyperglycemia, and pain at the injection site.

Dexmedetomidine

Dexmedetomidine is an alpha-2-adrenergic agonist labeled for use as a sedative and analgesic in dogs and cats. It is a "right-handed" enantiomer (isomer) of medetomidine (Plumb, 2015). It is considered to be more potent than medetomidine in terms of its ability to produce analgesia and sedation. Atipamezole is the reversal agent for dexmedetomidine.

BOX 4.2 Alpha 2 Agonist and Reversal Drugs

Drug	Reversal Drug
Xylazine	Yohimbine
Detomidine (Dormosedan)	Atipamezole
Medetomidine (Domitor)	Atipamezole
Dexmedetomidine (Dexdomitor)	Atipamezole
Romifidine	Yohimbine or Atipamezole

Clinical Uses. Dexmedetomidine is used as a sedative, preanesthetic, and analgesic in dogs and cats. It may be combined with other agents such as opioids and ketamine to produce surgical anesthetic levels. A combination of these three products for cats is sometimes called "kitty magic."

Dosage Form
- **Dexdomitor**

Adverse Side Effects. These include bradycardia, hypertension, vomiting, atrioventricular block, muscle tremors, and others.

 TECHNICIAN NOTES

- Dexmedetomidine should not be used in dogs or cats with cardiovascular, respiratory, kidney, or liver disease or in patients with shock or severe debilitation or stress due to heat, cold, or fatigue.
- Atipamezole may be used for treatment of dexmedetomidine-induced effects (Plumb, 2015).
- Before the use of dexmedetomidine in combination with other sedatives is attempted, references should be consulted for potential side effects and dosages.

Romifidine

Romifidine is an alpha-2-adrenergic agonist labeled for use in horses.

Clinical Uses. Romifidine is used as a sedative to facilitate handling, examination, and treatment and as premedication before general anesthesia.

Dosage Form
- **Sedivet**

Box 4.2 alpha 2-agonist and reversal drugs.

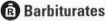 Barbiturates

The barbiturates are one of the oldest categories of CNS depressants used in veterinary medicine. They are derived from the parent compound barbituric acid and cause various responses ranging from

TABLE 4.2	Barbiturate Classifications.		
Generic Name	Proprietary Name	Classification	Duration of Action
Phenobarbital	Luminal	Long-acting oxybarbiturate	4–8 hours
Pentobarbital	Nembutal	Short-acting oxybarbiturate	½–2 hours
Thiopental	Pentothal	Ultrashort-acting thiobarbiturate	10–30 minutes

sedation to death, depending on the dose and the circumstances of use. Barbiturates are used in veterinary medicine as sedatives, anticonvulsants, general anesthetics, and euthanasia agents. They are easy and cheap to administer. They have great potential for complications because of their potent depressing effects on the cardiac and pulmonary systems (especially in cats) and because they are nonreversible and must be metabolized by the liver before elimination can occur. Individual patients with poor liver function, little body fat, or preexisting illnesses that cause acidosis may be at risk when receiving barbiturates. The ultrashort-acting barbiturates can cause necrosis of the tissue if administered outside the vein in the subcutaneous space because of their alkalinity. Barbiturates are metabolized by the liver and are potent depressors of the respiratory system.

Barbiturates are classified according to their duration of action as long-acting, short-acting, and ultrashort-acting. Alternatively, they are classified according to the chemical side chain on the barbituric acid molecule as an oxybarbiturate or a thiobarbiturate (Table 4.2). The long- and short-acting barbiturates have a side chain that is connected by oxygen; they are therefore called *oxybarbiturates*. The thiobarbiturates have a side chain connected by a sulfur. The thiobarbiturates are highly soluble in fat and tend to move rapidly out of the CNS into the fat stores of the body, thus accounting for their ultrashort activity.

Clinical Uses. Clinical uses include the prevention and treatment of seizures, as well as sedation, anesthesia, and euthanasia.

Long-Acting Barbiturates (Oxybarbiturates, 8 to 12 Hours)

Phenobarbital's proprietary and generic products are numerous. Phenobarbital is used primarily as an anticonvulsant and is the drug of choice for long-term control of epileptic seizures. It is administered by the oral route. Phenobarbital is a Class IV controlled substance.

Short-Acting Barbiturates (Oxybarbiturates, 45 Minutes to 1.5 Hours)

Pentobarbital sodium has numerous generic products, and Nembutal is a proprietary product. Pentobarbital is given by intravenous injection (the intraperitoneal route also may be used) and provides 1 to 2 hours of general anesthesia. In the early days of veterinary anesthesia, it was the general anesthetic that was routinely used in dogs. Today, pentobarbital is used primarily for controlling seizures in progress and as a euthanasia agent. Intravenous administration of glucose or concurrent use of chloramphenicol may prolong the recovery period. Pentobarbital is a Class II controlled substance.

Ultrashort-Acting Barbiturates (Thiobarbiturates, 5 to 30 Minutes)

Thiobarbiturates are very alkaline (especially at the higher concentrations) and must be given intravenously to avoid necrosis and subsequent sloughing of tissue. Thiobarbiturates are redistributed into the fat stores of the body within 5 to 30 minutes.

Extreme care should be taken when a thiobarbiturate is administered to a thin animal because of the lack of fat stores. Thiobarbiturates are prepared as a sterile powder in vials for dilution up to the desired concentration. They are stable for long periods in undiluted form. Sterile water for injection should be used as the diluent because solutions with electrolytes hasten precipitate formation. Solutions should not be administered if precipitates are present.

Thiobarbiturates can cause a period of apnea when they are rapidly administered intravenously. If spontaneous respirations do not resume in a short time, controlled respirations should be started. Barbiturates can also cause a period of CNS excitement when administered intravenously if they are given too slowly. It is often recommended to give one-third to one-half of the calculated dose rapidly to avoid the excitement phase. The remainder of the dose is administered in increments until the desired effect is achieved.

Dosage Forms. Thiobarbiturates (thiamylal and thiopental) are currently not available in the United States.

- **Methohexital**

Adverse Side Effects. These include excessive CNS depression, paradoxical CNS excitement, severe respiratory depression, and cardiovascular depression. Tissue irritation may occur when barbiturates are injected perivascularly.

TECHNICIAN NOTES

- Recovery from pentobarbital is often prolonged, and dogs exhibit padding limb movements during this time.
- Thiobarbiturates should not be used in sighthounds or in any very thin animal.
- Giving additional doses of thiobarbiturates may prolong recovery.
- Barbiturates are potent depressors of the respiratory system.

Ⓡ Dissociative Agents

The dissociative agents belong to the cyclohexylamine family, which includes phencyclidine, ketamine, and tiletamine. Involuntary muscle rigidity (catalepsy), amnesia, and analgesia characterize dissociative anesthesia. Pharyngeal/laryngeal reflexes are maintained, and muscle tone is increased. Because deep abdominal pain is not eliminated (surgical stage III is not usually reached) with dissociative anesthesia, it is recommended only for restraint, diagnostic procedures, and minor surgery. Dissociative agents, however, often are combined with other agents for abdominal surgery. Dissociative drugs produce minor cardiac stimulation, and respiratory depression can occur with higher doses. These agents act by altering neurotransmitter activity, causing depression of the thalamus and cerebral cortex, and activating the limbic system (Plumb, 2015).

Some species are often ataxic and hyperresponsive during induction and recovery with dissociative agents (Muir, Hubbell, Bednarski, & Lerche, 2013). Tremors, spasticity, and convulsions can occur at higher doses. Hallucinations have been reported in humans and are suspected in cats.

Clinical Uses. Dissociative agents are used for sedation, restraint, analgesia, and anesthesia.

Dosage Forms

- **Ketamine HCl** (Ketaset): Ketamine is approved for use in humans, primates, and cats but has extralabel uses in various species, including dogs, horses, birds, small ruminants, and reptiles. Tranquilizers, such as acepromazine, dexmedetomidine, xylazine, and diazepam,

are often used concurrently with ketamine to enhance muscle relaxation and to deepen the level of anesthesia. Oral, ocular, and laryngeal reflexes are maintained when ketamine is used alone (except at high doses). Occasional spastic jerking movements can occur in cats that are administered ketamine. Ketamine also produces analgesic effects by acting as an *N*-Methyl-D-aspartate (NMDA) receptor antagonist (see Chapter 14).

- **Increased salivation** may accompany administration of this drug and can be controlled or prevented with the use of atropine or glycopyrrolate. An ophthalmic lubricant should be used because cats' eyes remain open after administration of ketamine. Ketamine is a Class III controlled substance.
- **Tiletamine HCl** (Telazol [tiletamine plus zolazepam HCl]): Telazol is an injectable anesthetic that consists of a combination of tiletamine (chemically related to ketamine) and zolazepam (a benzodiazepine). Telazol is approved for use in dogs and cats. The pharmacokinetics and pharmacotherapeutics of tiletamine are similar to those of ketamine. Additional agents are not needed for muscle relaxation because of the zolazepam in this product. Tiletamine should only be used for restraint and minor procedures of short duration requiring mild to moderate analgesia. Ocular lubrication should be used in cats receiving Telazol. Telazol is a Class III controlled substance.
- **Phencyclidine**: This dissociative agent is no longer available. It was originally used as an immobilizing agent for nonhuman primates. Its street name is "PCP" or "angel dust" (Upson, 1988).

Adverse Side Effects. These are usually associated with high doses and include spastic jerking movement, convulsions, respiratory depression, burning at the intramuscular injection site, and drying of the cornea.

TECHNICIAN NOTES

- Both ketamine and tiletamine may cause burning at the injection site. Adequate restraint should be used to ensure injection of all medication.
- Tiletamine has a longer duration of action and produces better analgesia than ketamine.
- Metabolites of the dissociative agents are excreted through the kidneys. These drugs may be contraindicated in animals with compromised kidney function.
- Use in animals with certain cardiac conditions (potentially hypertensive) may be dangerous.

℞ Opioid Agonists

An opioid is any compound derived from opium poppy alkaloids and synthetic drugs with similar pharmacologic properties. These drugs produce analgesia and sedation (hypnosis) while reducing anxiety and fear. Narcotic effects are produced in combination with opiate receptors at deep levels of the brain (e.g., thalamus, hypothalamus, limbic system). Opioid receptors are grouped into the following four classes (Paddleford, 1999):

1. **Mu**—found in pain-regulating areas of the brain; contribute to analgesia, euphoria, respiratory depression, physical dependence, and hypothermic actions.
2. **Kappa**—found in the cerebral cortex and spinal cord; contribute to analgesia, sedation, depression, and miosis.
3. **Sigma**—may be responsible for struggling, whining, hallucinations, and mydriatic effects.
4. **Delta**—modify mu receptor activity; contribute to analgesia.

Opioids are used as preanesthetics or postanesthetics because of their sedative and analgesic properties. Sedation is more pronounced at higher doses. They are sometimes used alone or in combination with tranquilizers as anesthetics for surgical procedures, for relief of colic pain in horses, and for restraint/capture of wild/zoo animals. At low doses, the opioids have antitussive (cough suppression) properties because of depression of the cough center in the brain; they also have antidiarrheal action because of a reduction in peristalsis or segmental contractions. Several potential adverse side effects are associated with narcotics. Opioids are potent respiratory depressants and because they affect the thermoregulatory centers in the brain (the body's thermostat), they may cause panting. They may also cause defecation, flatulence, vomiting, or sound sensitivity. Excitement may occur in dogs if the narcotic is rapidly given intravenously. Cats and horses are reported to be sensitive to the opioids and may exhibit excitatory effects at high doses. Opioids can be useful when cesarean section is performed because they cross the placenta fairly slowly and their effects can be antagonized. The liver metabolizes opioids, and resultant metabolites are eliminated in the urine. Many opioid preparations are Class II controlled substances, and narcotic-antagonists can block their effects.

Clinical Uses. Opioid agonists are used for analgesia, sedation, restraint, anesthesia, treatment of coughing, and treatment of diarrhea.

Naturally Occurring Narcotics

- **Opium** (laudanum—10% opium), paregoric: Opium is derived from the seed capsule of the opium poppy. Paregoric, also called *camphorated tincture of opium*, has been used for longer than 100 years for the treatment of diarrhea. It has been used in veterinary medicine for treating diarrhea, primarily in calves and foals.
- **Morphine sulfate** (Duramorph): Morphine is an opium derivative used to treat severe pain. Occasionally, it is used as a preanesthetic or anesthetic agent (e.g., cesarean section in dogs). It is also used to relieve anxiety associated with acute congestive heart failure. It exerts its effects primarily on mu receptors. Morphine is a Class II controlled substance that should be used under strict supervision because of its potential for abuse. It is the standard opioid with which all others are compared in terms of analgesic effect.

Synthetic Narcotics

- **Meperidine** (Demerol): Meperidine is a mu agonist that is approximately one-eighth as potent an analgesic as morphine. It is used for relief of acute pain, such as that occurring after orthopedic procedures. It also may be combined with a tranquilizer for use as an anesthetic agent (neuroleptanalgesic). No meperidine products carry a veterinary label. However, human products often have extralabel uses in animals. Naloxone is the preferred antagonist.
- **Oxymorphone** (Numorphan and Opana): Oxymorphone is a semisynthetic opioid that is a mu agonist. It is approximately 10 times more potent an analgesic than morphine. This drug is used primarily in dogs for restraint, for diagnostic procedures, and for minor surgical procedures. It may be combined with tranquilizers to produce neuroleptanalgesia; naloxone is the antagonist.
- **Butorphanol tartrate** (Torbutrol, Torbugesic): Butorphanol is a synthetic, opioid agonist/antagonist. Its opioid agonist activity is exerted on kappa and sigma receptors while its antagonist activity occurs at the mu receptor. It is a Class IV controlled substance. Butorphanol has four to seven times the analgesic properties of morphine and significant antitussive effects (Plumb, 2015). Torbutrol is a product that is approved as an antitussive agent in dogs. It is also used in dogs and cats as an analgesic and preanesthetic. Torbugesic is approved for the treatment of pain associated with colic in horses. It is also

used in combination with other sedatives/tranquilizers in horses, dogs, and cats as a preanesthetic or for minor surgical procedures. Butorphanol should not be used as the only analgesic agent (Claude, 2013).

- **Fentanyl** (Recuvrya, Sublimaze, and Duragesic-human labels): Fentanyl is an opioid agonist that has approximately 100 times the analgesic properties of morphine. Fentanyl is a Class II controlled substance. Fentanyl transdermal patches are sometimes used in animals to control chronic pain (see Chapter 14).
- **Hydrocodone bitartrate** (Hycodan, Tussigon): Hydrocodone is an opioid agonist that is used as an antitussive agent in dogs. It is a Class III controlled substance.
- **Etorphine** (M-99): Etorphine is an opioid that produces analgesic effects 1000 times those of morphine. It is restricted to use by veterinarians in zoo or exotic animal practice (Upson, 1988). It is lethal to people who accidentally inject themselves (it also can be absorbed through intact skin) if the antagonist (diprenorphine) is not administered immediately. Etorphine is a Class II controlled substance.
- **Pentazocine** (Talwin): Pentazocine is a partial opioid agonist that is approved for pain relief in horses and dogs. It is a Class IV controlled substance.
- **Diphenoxylate** (Lomotil): Diphenoxylate is a synthetic opioid agonist that is combined with atropine for use as an antidiarrheal agent. This drug is a Class V controlled substance.
- **Apomorphine** (Apokyn-human label and generic products): Apomorphine is a dopamine agonist derived from morphine with the principal effect of inducing vomiting by stimulating the chemoreceptor trigger zone in the brain. This drug is often administered by placing a portion of a tablet in the conjunctival sac for absorption (see Chapter 8).
- **Methadone** (Dolophine): Methadone is a synthetic opioid that was developed as a treatment for morphine and heroin addiction in humans. Its primary use in veterinary medicine is in the treatment of colic pain in horses. Methadone is a Class II controlled substance.
- **Codeine**—generic labeling or in combination: Codeine is an opioid that is available in human label products for use as an antitussive in dogs. Codeine is a Class II agent when used alone but a Class III or Class V when used in combination products.
- **Carfentanil** (Wildnil): Carfentanil is used to induce wildlife anesthesia. It has 10,000 times the potency of morphine and is a Class II agent that should be used with care to avoid accidental exposure to the users.
- **Buprenorphine** (Buprenex): Buprenorphine is a human label, partial mu agonist–antagonist. It is a potent analgesic that is used in several small animal species with especially good results in the cat. Buprenorphine has a longer duration of action than butorphanol. Buprenorphine is a Class III controlled substance.
- **Buprenorphine** (Simbadol): Simbadol is Food and Drug Administration (FDA) approved for subcutaneous injection once daily, for up to 3 days in cats. It provides 24 hours of continuous pain control; indicated for the control of postoperative pain associated with surgical procedures in cats (Zoetis, 2017).
- **Tramadol**: (see Chapter 14)

Adverse Side Effects. These can include respiratory depression, excitement (cats and horses), nausea, vomiting, diarrhea, defecation, panting, and convulsions. Overdose causes profound respiratory depression.

Ⓡ Opioid Antagonists

Opioid antagonists block the effects of opioids by binding with opiate receptors, displacing narcotic molecules already present, and preventing further narcotic binding at the sites. These antagonists are classified as pure antagonists or as partial antagonists. The partial antagonists may have some agonist activity (analgesic and respiratory depressant effects).

These drugs usually are administered by the intravenous route and exert their effects very rapidly (15–60 seconds).

Clinical Uses. Opioid antagonists are used to antagonize (reverse) the effects of opioid agonists.

Dosage Forms
- **Naloxone** (Naloxone HCl injection, Narcan): Naloxone is a pure opioid antagonist that is chemically similar to oxymorphone, with high affinity for mu receptors. It has no agonist activity. It is commonly used to reverse the CNS and respiratory depression caused by administration of opioid drugs.
- **Nalorphine** (Nalline): Nalorphine is a partial antagonist that may produce unpleasant analgesic and respiratory depressant effects.
- **Butorphanol**: This is a mu antagonist used primarily as a sedative or analgesic. It is rarely used as an antagonist.

Adverse Side Effects. Nalorphine may induce respiratory depression. Naloxone usually has few adverse effects if given in the correct dose.

℞ Neuroleptanalgesics

A neuroleptanalgesic agent consists of an opioid and a tranquilizer. Animals that receive neuroleptanalgesics may or may not remain conscious (Muir, Hubbell, Bednarski, & Lerche, 2013). They often defecate and are highly responsive to sound stimuli. The opioid effects of the neuroleptanalgesics can be antagonized with the opioid antagonists.

Clinical Uses. Neuroleptanalgesics are used for sedation, restraint, and anesthesia. They are commonly used in patients undergoing short procedures including wound suturing, porcupine quill removal, and radiographs.

Dosage Forms
- Fentanyl and droperidol (Innovar-Vet). Innovar-Vet is no longer commercially available, although its components are available; therefore, a similar compounded product could be formulated.

Any combination of an opioid analgesic such as morphine, butorphanol, buprenorphine, and hydromorphone and a tranquilizer such as acepromazine, dexmedetomidine, diazepam, midazolam, and xylazine.
- Other neuroleptanalgesics may be prepared by a clinician and include the following:
  - Acepromazine and morphine
  - Acepromazine and oxymorphone
  - Xylazine and butorphanol

Adverse Side Effects. These can include panting, flatulence, personality changes, increased sound sensitivity, and bradycardia. An overdose may cause severe depression of the CNS, respiratory system, and cardiovascular system.

📋 **TECHNICIAN NOTES**

- It is important to understand the side effects of both drugs when a patient is given a neuroleptanalgesic combination.

℞ Drugs Given to Prevent or Control Seizures

Seizures occur in animals for various reasons, which include but are not limited to unknown (idiopathic), infectious (postdistemper), traumatic (head injury), toxic (strychnine poisoning), and metabolic (heatstroke) factors. Prolonged seizures in progress require emergency action with intravenous therapy. Periodic, recurring seizures require preventive oral medication. Oral preventive therapy often must be titrated to the individual patient and reviewed regularly for the appropriate dose adjustment that controls seizure activity.

Clinical Uses. These drugs are used to prevent seizures or to control seizures in progress.

Dosage Forms
- **Diazepam** (Valium): Diazepam is a tranquilizer with potent antiseizure properties. It is administered intravenously and has a 3- to 4-hour duration of action.
- **Pentobarbital** (Nembutal and generic products): Pentobarbital is a short-acting barbiturate that is effective for controlling seizures. It is administered intravenously and has a 1- to 3-hour duration.
- **Phenobarbital** (Luminal, Solfoton, generic formulations): Phenobarbital is an effective antiseizure drug that is available in oral and parenteral formulations. The oral route is the usual means of administering this drug to dogs and cats. The injectable form is used in horses (foals) by some clinicians. Drowsiness is a potential side effect of phenobarbital. Phenobarbital is a Class IV controlled substance.
- **Primidone** (Mylepsin and Neurosyn): Primidone is similar chemically to phenobarbital, and a portion of the primidone dose is metabolized to phenobarbital by the liver. It is administered orally to dogs and cats, although its use in cats is controversial. Adverse side effects may include agitation, anxiety, polyuria, polydipsia, and dermatitis.
- **Bromide**: Bromide is an old anticonvulsant that has sparked renewed interest, mainly as an adjunct to phenobarbital or primidone therapy.
- **Gabapentin** (Neurontin): Gabapentin may be used as an adjunctive treatment of seizures that are difficult to control, as well as for partial complex seizures or pain control.
- **Levetiracetam** (Kappra): May be useful as an adjunct for refractory canine epilepsy.
- **Zonisamide** (Zonegran): Use is similar to levetiracetam.

Adverse Side Effects. These may include drowsiness, CNS depression, anxiety, agitation, polyuria, polydipsia, and hepatotoxicity (phenobarbital and primidone). Consult product inserts or appropriate references for specific effects.

TECHNICIAN NOTES

- Inadequate compliance is a frequent cause of failure of anticonvulsant therapy. Clients should be advised about the importance of following medication instructions carefully.
- Reserpine and phenothiazine drugs should not be given to epileptic animals.

Inhalant Anesthetics

Inhalant anesthetic agents are used to produce general anesthesia. They are converted from a liquid to a gaseous phase by an anesthetic vaporizer and are delivered to the lungs with the use of an oxygen source and a patient breathing circuit. From the alveoli of the lungs, they are absorbed into the bloodstream and delivered to the CNS, where they produce unconsciousness, analgesia, and muscle relaxation through mechanisms not fully understood.

Inhalants generally require little biotransformation for elimination from the body. They enter and exit the body through the lungs, and this facilitates a rapid induction and recovery from the effects of the agent compared with injectable anesthetic agents. It also permits a quicker alteration of the depth of anesthesia.

The amount (partial pressure) of inhalant anesthetic in the brain is proportionate to the alveolar concentration of the agent. Alveolar concentration depends on the amount of agent delivered to the lungs compared with the amount removed from the lungs. Delivery of the agent to the lungs can be increased by increasing the vaporizer setting, increasing the fresh gas (oxygen) flow, increasing minute ventilation, or decreasing mechanical and physiologic dead space. Factors that influence removal of the agent from the lungs include the solubility (blood–gas partition coefficient) of the agent, the molecular weight of the agent, the partial pressure difference between the agent in the alveolus and the agent in the blood, the amount of alveolar surface available for exchange (absence of lung pathology), and cardiac output.

Uptake by tissue of an anesthetic agent depends mainly on the degree of tissue perfusion and the solubility of the agent in the tissue. Vessel-rich tissue (e.g., brain, heart, lungs, liver, kidneys, intestine, and endocrine glands) receives the greatest percentage of cardiac output and is consequently the first to reach equilibrium during uptake of an anesthetic gas and the first to download an agent. Lipid-rich cells, similar to brain cells, absorb more agent than do lipid-poor cells.

Characteristics important to the understanding of inhalant agents include the minimum alveolar concentration (MAC), partition coefficient, and vapor pressure (Table 4.3). The MAC value of an anesthetic agent is a measure of potency and is the alveolar concentration that prevents gross purposeful movement in 50% of patients in response to a standardized painful stimulus. Lower numbers indicate more potent agents. An agent with a low MAC is a more potent anesthetic than an agent with a high MAC. Therefore, the lower the MAC the less gas it takes to produce anesthesia. Also, an agent with a high MAC is a less potent anesthetic and therefore more gas is needed to produce anesthesia, and values may vary slightly between species. The partition coefficient is the ratio of the number of molecules of an anesthetic gas that exist in two phases (blood/gas). It indicates the solubility of an inhalation agent in blood as compared with alveolar gas. The key factor determining the speed of induction and recovery from inhalation anesthesia is the blood-gas partition coefficient. Therefore, the lower the blood-gas partition coefficient, the faster the induction and recovery. The vapor pressure of an agent indicates how volatile it is and the maximum concentration that can be achieved. Vapor pressure of an inhalant anesthetic is a measure of its tendency to evaporate. Higher numbers indicate greater volatility and the need for a precision vaporizer. Most precision vaporizers have temperature compensating mechanisms; therefore, temperature does not affect the concentration delivered (Thomas & Lerche, 2017). Precision vaporizers are located out of the circuit and are designed for use with only one specific anesthetic agent (Fig. 4.11). The function of a precision vaporizer is to convert a liquid anesthetic to a gas state and produce a precise concentration of anesthetic vapor in the carrier gas (oxygen) passing through the vaporizer and delivered to the patient.

Exposure to anesthetic waste gases can pose a health hazard to the veterinary technician if improper scavenging of waste is not performed. Reproductive, hepatic, and renal effects have been noted. Toxicity is likely due to the biotransformation of byproducts of the agents. Inhalant agents are biodegraded to various degrees (methoxyflurane, 50%; halothane, 25%; isoflurane, <0.2%; sevoflurane, 3%; nitrous oxide, 0.0004%).

TABLE 4.3 Physical Properties of Inhalation Anesthetics.

Property	Sevoflurane	Desflurane	Isoflurane	Halothane	Methoxyflurane	Nitrous Oxide
Formula	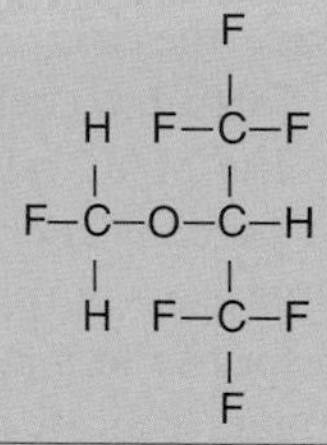	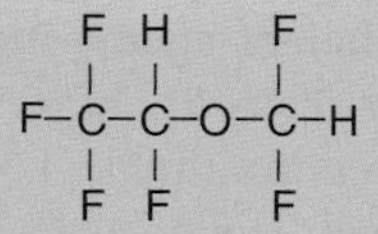	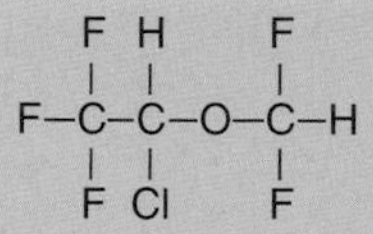	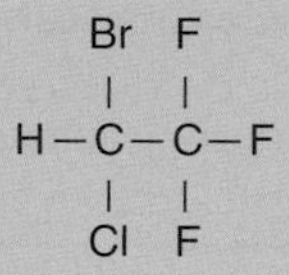	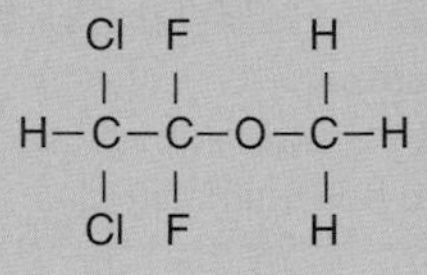	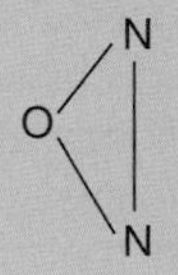
Molecular weight	200	168	184.5	197.4	165.3	44
Specific gravity (20°C)	1.52	1.47	1.49	1.86	1.41	–
Boiling point (°C)	59	23.5	48.5	50.2	104.7	–
Vapor pressure at 20°C (mm Hg)	160	664	239.5	244.1	22.8	–
mL Vapor/mL liquid at 20°C	182.7	209.7	194.7	227	207	–
Preservative	None	None	None	0.01% thymol	0.01% butylhydroxytoluene	None
Stability soda lime	No?	Stable	Stable	Decomposes	Decomposes	Stable
UV light	–	–	Stable	Decomposes	Decomposes	–

From Paddleford, R. R. (1999). *Manual of small animal anesthesia* (2nd ed.). Philadelphia: WB Saunders.

Clinical Uses. Inhalant anesthetics are used to induce and maintain general anesthesia in animal patients.

Dosage Forms

- **Isoflurane** (IsoFlo, Isothesia): Isoflurane was synthesized in 1968 and was used clinically in people by 1970. Isoflurane is a colorless liquid with a pungent odor. It is stable and does not require a preservative. A halogenated ether, it is one of the least soluble of the inhalant agents. It is less potent than halothane and methoxyflurane but has very rapid induction and recovery times. Isoflurane allows a stable heart rhythm and does not decrease cardiac output at clinically used levels. It is metabolized at a very low rate (<0.2%) This agent is used in a wide variety of species.
- **Sevoflurane** (SevoFlo): Sevoflurane is a halogenated ether with little odor, which makes it a good choice for mask induction. This agent is characterized by very rapid induction and recovery times. Its cardiovascular and respiratory effects are similar to those of isoflurane. Sevoflurane is often used in high-risk, small-animal patients because of its safety and rapid, smooth induction. Only 3% of sevoflurane is metabolized. The disadvantage of the use of this agent is its cost compared with that of isoflurane.

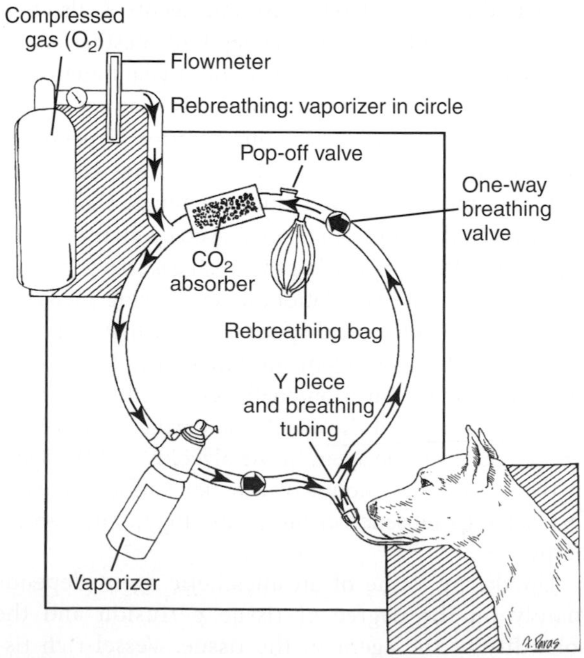

Fig. 4.11 Precision vaporizer out of circuit (VOC). The vaporizer is located outside the circle; which contains the CO_2 absorbent, one-way breathing valves and reservoir bag. (From Muir, W. W., Hubbell, J. A., Bednarski, R. M., & Lerche, P. [2013]. *Handbook of veterinary anesthesia* [5th ed.]. St. Louis: Mosby, Elsevier.)

- **Halothane** (Fluothane): Halothane is a halogenated hydrocarbon that was first used clinically in human anesthesia in 1956. Halothane decomposes when exposed to ultraviolet light and for this reason has thymol added as an antioxidant. Halothane sensitizes the heart to the catecholamines; this may result in cardiac dysrhythmias. Similar to isoflurane and sevoflurane, halothane has a high vapor pressure and must be used in precision vaporizers. "Halothane hepatitis" has been reported in humans but is a very rare occurrence. This agent is metabolized at the rate of 25%, a considerably higher rate than that of the previous two agents. Halothane is no longer available in the United States.
- **Methoxyflurane** (Metofane): Methoxyflurane has been used since 1959. It is a methyl-ethyl-ether that is highly soluble in blood and other tissues. It consequently has a very slow induction and recovery time. Methoxyflurane is the most potent (MAC, 0.23%–0.27%) of the agents considered in this section. It has a relatively low vapor pressure, making 3% the maximum level that can be vaporized. Also, because of this low vapor pressure, it can be used in nonprecison, in-circuit vaporizers or precision, out-of-circuit vaporizers. Methoxyflurane undergoes the greatest biotransformation (50%) of any of the inhalants. It has been associated with renal toxicity in human patients. Methoxyflurane has not been available in the U.S. for many years.
- **Nitrous oxide**: Nitrous oxide is a colorless inorganic gas. It was discovered to have anesthetic properties in the late 1700s. Nitrous oxide may be used as an adjunct to more potent agents during mask induction to speed the induction of anesthesia. General anesthesia cannot be produced with nitrous oxide alone. It is compressed to form a liquid and is supplied in blue cylinders. It has the lowest solubility coefficient of any of the inhalants, which means that it enters and exits the blood and tissue rapidly. Nitrous oxide displaces nitrogen from the alveoli, blood, and gas-filled cavities of the body because it is 30 times more soluble than nitrogen. This means that it will diffuse into and potentially cause distention of the intestines and other gas-filled areas (e.g., pneumothorax). Nitrous oxide is delivered through a flowmeter and must always be given with oxygen to prevent hypoxia. Oxygen should always be administered for several minutes after the nitrous oxide is turned off to prevent diffusion hypoxia. (The rapid exit of nitrous oxide from the blood will dilute the oxygen in the alveoli.)

TECHNICIAN NOTES

- Exposure to anesthetic waste gas can pose a health hazard if improper scavenging of waste is not performed or waste gas is leaking from the machine.
- Halothane and methoxyflurane are no longer available in the United States; however, their physical properties are used for comparison with current inhalant anesthetics.

℞ Miscellaneous Central Nervous System Drugs

Propofol

Propofol is a short-acting hypnotic that is unrelated to other general anesthetic agents. Its mechanism of action is not well understood. Chemically, it is an alkylphenol derivative. Propofol products are commercially available either as a milky white macroemulsion or as a clear microemulsion. Because most propofol products are white in color, some clinicians call these products "milk of amnesia." Propofol produces a rapid and smooth anesthetic induction in dogs when given slowly intravenously. It produces sedation, restraint, or unconsciousness, depending on the dose. A single bolus lasts 2 to 5 minutes, making it particularly useful when rapid recovery is important. Some of the products contain no preservative (Rapanofal, PropoFlo), must be refrigerated after opening, and should be discarded after 6 hours. PropoFlo-28 contains preservatives, need no refrigeration, and have a shelf life of 28 days.

Clinical Uses. Propofol is useful for anesthetic induction before administration of an inhalant anesthetic, for outpatient procedures, as a substitute for barbiturates in sighthounds, and for patients with preexisting cardiac arrhythmia. It is also useful as an anesthetic agent for dogs undergoing a cesarean section because it does not cross the placental barrier.

Dosage Forms
- **Rapanofal** for dogs and cats.
- **PropoFlo** for dogs and cats.
- **PropoFlo-28** (with preservatives) for dogs.

Adverse Side Effects. Apnea may occur if propofol is given too rapidly intravenously. Occasional seizure-like signs may be seen. Prolonged recovery and/or Heinz body production may be seen in cats with repeated use.

Glyceryl Guaiacolate or Guaifenesin (Guailaxin)

Guaifenesin is a skeletal muscle relaxant that exerts its effects on the connecting neurons of the spinal cord and brainstem (Plumb, 2015). It is used primarily in equine medicine to induce general anesthesia, extend the anesthetic activity of other injectable field anesthetics, or enhance muscle relaxation of anesthetized patients. It may be used as a 5% or 10% solution in 5% dextrose. Some clinicians use it as an adjunct to anesthesia and add other agents like ketamine and xylazine (GKX) to the solution before administering it intravenously. Relatively large amounts are required to induce general anesthesia/recumbency, and small increments are given to maintain or extend the anesthetic effects of other agents.

Clinical Uses. These include induction or prolongation of general anesthesia in large animals and occasional use as an expectorant.

Dosage Forms
- **Guaifenesin** Injection
- **Guailaxin**
- Various others

Adverse Side Effects. Adverse side effects are limited. Hemolysis has been reported when greater than 5% solutions are used.

TECHNICIAN NOTES

- Guaifenesin is packaged as a soluble powder. It may be difficult to dissolve when the diluent is added. Warming 5% dextrose before mixing may aid solution preparation. It should be mixed only immediately before use because a precipitate forms if the solution is allowed to stand for several hours.
- When increments of guaifenesin are administered to maintain or extend anesthesia, one should communicate thoroughly with the veterinarian to understand the quantity of this drug that should be administered.

℞ Central Nervous System Stimulants

The primary medical use of the CNS stimulants is for treatment of respiratory depression or arrest. Many of the other uses of CNS stimulants are illegal or unethical (e.g., to enhance athletic performance).

Doxapram

Doxapram activates the respiratory system by stimulating respiratory centers in the medulla. It is labeled for use in dogs, cats, and horses. Its main indications are to stimulate respirations during or after general anesthesia; it is used in newborns and may be used in cases of cardiopulmonary arrest; however, it should not be used as a substitute for artificial respiratory support in instances of severe respiratory depression (Plumb, 2015) and may be contraindicated in states of apnea. It is labeled for intravenous use, but it may be administered under the tongue (one to two drops) or into the umbilical vein of the newborn.

Clinical Uses. These include use to stimulate respiration in newborns and use during or after anesthesia in which the respiratory rate and depth of respirations need to be increased.

Dosage Forms
- **Dopram-V**

Adverse Side Effects. Adverse side effects are rare and usually are associated with overdoses. Hypertension, seizures, and hyperventilation may occur.

TECHNICIAN NOTES

One to two drops of doxapram may be placed under the tongue or injected into the umbilical vein of the newborn to stimulate respirations.

 ## Neuromuscular Blocking Drugs

Neuromuscular blocking drugs, sometimes called *muscle relaxants,* interfere with neuromuscular transmission of impulses and are used as an adjunct to general anesthesia. These drugs provide no analgesia or sedation. However, they do stop ventilation, and this makes ventilation and constant patient monitoring necessary (Muir, Hubbell, Bednarski, & Lerche, 2013).

Neuromuscular blocking drugs are classified as depolarizing agents or nondepolarizing agents. Depolarizing agents act in a way that is similar to that of acetylcholine at the neuromuscular synapse, but the effects last longer, leading to muscle paralysis (phase I block). These drugs are not broken down by acetylcholinesterase and have no antagonist. Nondepolarizing agents prevent (competitive inhibition) acetylcholine from binding to receptor sites (phase II block). These drugs are not degraded by cholinesterase, but they can be antagonized by edrophonium or neostigmine.

Clinical Uses. Neuromuscular blocking agents are used as an adjunct to general anesthesia (e.g., ophthalmic/orthopedic surgery) and to facilitate endotracheal intubation.

Dosage Forms
- **Depolarizing**
  - Succinylcholine chloride (Anectine-human label)
  - Decamethonium (Syncurine)
- **Nondepolarizing**
  - Gallamine (Flaxedil)
  - Pancuronium bromide (Pavulon)
  - Vecuronium bromide (Norcuron)
  - Atracurium (Tracrium)

BEHAVIORAL PHARMACOTHERAPY

The use of drugs to treat behavioral problems in animals is a relatively new but rapidly growing area of veterinary medicine. Behavior problems—such as separation anxiety, fears and phobias, unruliness, hyperactivity, compulsive disorders, cognitive dysfunction in older dogs, and inappropriate elimination in cats—are being diagnosed in increasing numbers. Many animals with behavioral disorders are taken in desperation to animal shelters, but a growing number of clients are willing to attempt to correct these conditions with environmental management, behavior modification, and/or pharmacotherapy.

Informed consent should be obtained from the client before these drugs are used (Seibert, 2013) because many of the drugs used in behavioral pharmacotherapy are human psychiatric drugs that have not been approved for use in animals. The technician or veterinarian should explain to the animal owner the extralabel status of the drug, its possible side effects or precautions, and the medical effects to be expected in the pet. Owners should also be aware that pharmacotherapy may not be a cure-all for problems of behavior and that these problems may return after therapy is discontinued.

All drugs used in psychotherapy are thought to produce their effects through alteration of neurotransmitter activity in the brain (Simpson & Simpson, 1996a, 1996b). The five neurotransmitters of clinical importance in behavioral pharmacotherapy are acetylcholine, dopamine, norepinephrine, serotonin, and GABA.

Dopamine, norepinephrine, and serotonin are called *monoamine neurotransmitters* because they have similar chemical structures. Monoamines are found in large quantities in areas of the brain often associated with expression and control of emotions. The primary method by which monoamines are inactivated is through their reuptake from the synapse back into synaptic vesicles in nerve endings (see Fig. 4.4). Drugs that block or inhibit their reuptake increase their activity. Acetylcholine is the most widely distributed neurotransmitter in the body. It is associated with a variety of behavioral effects and is inactivated by cholinesterase at the synapse. Some of the most common side effects of drugs used in behavioral psychotherapy are related to their anticholinergic effects, such as dry mouth, increased heart rate, urine retention, and constipation. The GABA is considered to be an inhibitory neurotransmitter and is widely distributed in the brain.

Pharmacotherapeutic Agents

Drugs most commonly used in treating behavioral problems in veterinary medicine include antianxiety medications, antidepressants, and miscellaneous agents—such as synthetic progestins. All drugs listed in the following section carry a human label, except those that are otherwise indicated.

℞ Antianxiety Medications
Benzodiazepines

The benzodiazepines most commonly used in veterinary medicine include diazepam, alprazolam, and lorazepam. All the benzodiazepines are similar in structure and mechanism of action. They are thought to bind with and promote GABA activity in the cerebral cortex and in subcortical areas, such as the limbic system.

Clinical Uses. Behavioral uses of benzodiazepines include the treatment of fears and phobias, separation anxiety, aggression, anxiety-induced stereotypes, urine marking in cats, and appetite stimulation.

Dosage Forms
- **Diazepam** (Valium)
- **Alprazolam** (Xanax)
- **Lorazepam** (Ativan)

Adverse Side Effects. These may include lethargy, ataxia, polyuria and polydipsia (PUPD), hyperexcitability, and hepatic necrosis (cats).

Azapirones

Buspirone is the azapirone agent that is used in behavioral pharmacotherapy. In contrast to the benzodiazepines, it possesses no muscle relaxant, anticonvulsant, or sedative effects. Its antianxiety effect is thought to be caused by blocking serotonin receptors.

Clinical Uses. Veterinary uses include the control of urine spraying/marking and the control of fearfulness and anxiety.

Dosage Form
• **Buspirone**

Adverse Side Effects. Few serious side effects appear to exist.

Dexmedetomidine Oromucosal Gel

Dexmedetomidine is the active substance of Sileo and is a highly potent and selective alpha-2 adrenoceptor agonist (Zoetis, 2017). It binds with the alpha-2 receptors in the brainstem, preventing release of norepinephrine and reducing the levels. Decreased levels of norepinephrine reduce the levels of anxiety and fear.

Clinical Uses. It is used for noise aversion (thunder and fireworks) to relieve anxiety without inducing sedation. The oral gel is administered between the cheek and gum area in the mouth. A multi-dose oral syringe is used for dosing the medication.

Dosage Form
• **Sileo** (oromucosal gel)

Adverse Side Effects. Temporary pale mucous membranes may occur at the site of application. It may also cause hypotension, bradycardia, and drowsiness.

TECHNICIAN NOTES

• Once Sileo is opened, the multi-dose syringe is good for up to 4 weeks.
• Sileo should be given 30 minutes to one hour before noise is expected and additional doses should be 2 hours apart; up to five doses can be given for one noise event (Zoetis, 2017).
• The ring-stop, on the Sileo multi-dose syringe, must be locked into position before dosing to avoid an overdose.
• Gloves should be worn when handling the syringe to avoid direct contact with skin.

℞ Antidepressants

Tricyclics

Tricyclics used commonly in veterinary medicine include amitriptyline, imipramine, and clomipramine. These drugs are thought to exert their effects by preventing reuptake of norepinephrine and serotonin.

Clomipramine is apparently a selective inhibitor of serotonin reuptake. The tricyclic group is often used on a long-term basis and may take several weeks of use to become effective. Some of the tricyclics are available in the generic form and are relatively inexpensive to use.

Clinical Uses. Uses include the treatment of separation anxiety, obsessive disorders (e.g., lick granuloma, tail chasing), fearful aggression, hyperactivity, hypervocalization, and urine marking.

Dosage Forms
• **Amitriptyline** (Elavil, generic forms)
• **Imipramine** (Tofranil)
• **Clomipramine** (Clomicalm–veterinary label)

Adverse Side Effects. Side effects may include sedation, tachycardia, heart block, mydriasis, dry mouth, reduced tear production, urine retention, and constipation.

Serotonin Reuptake Inhibitors

Serotonin reuptake inhibitors include fluoxetine, sertraline, and paroxetine. As their name indicates, these drugs increase the amount of serotonin in the synapse by inhibiting its reuptake back into the nerve terminal. Serotonin reuptake inhibitors have fewer potential side effects than the tricyclics but are usually more expensive.

Clinical Uses. These drugs are used for a variety of behavioral syndromes, including obsessive disorders, phobias, aggression, inappropriate urine marking, and separation anxiety. Fluoxetine can be compounded by a specialty pharmacy.

Dosage Forms
• **Fluoxetine** (Prozac, human label) (Reconcile, labeled for use in dogs)
• **Sertraline** (Zoloft)
• **Paroxetine** (Paxil)

Adverse Side Effects. Side effects are relatively few but include anorexia, nausea, lethargy, anxiety, and diarrhea.

Trazodone. Trazodone is a serotonin antagonist and reuptake inhibitor used in behavioral disorders such as anxiety and noise aversion. Trazodone causes serotonin to remain in the brainstem longer allowing for less anxiety.

Clinical Uses. Trazodone is used to manage short-term anxiety in dogs and cats. In dogs it has been used for noise aversion and to calm anxious dogs to restrict their activity after orthopedic surgery. In cats it has been used for temporary sedation during transportation (Papich, 2016). It may also be used as a supplemental therapy when animals are not responding to conventional therapies.

Dosage Form
- **Desyrel**
  Adverse Side Effects. Adverse effects may include sedation, aggression, and nausea (Papich, 2016).

Monoamine Oxidase-B Inhibitors

The neurotransmitter dopamine is broken down by the enzyme monoamine oxidase-B (MAO-B). Substances such as selegiline (a MAO-B inhibitor) block or inhibit MAO-B and allow dopamine levels to increase. Decreased dopamine levels may be associated with certain types of dementia that are seen in older dogs (canine cognitive dysfunction). Canine cognitive dysfunction is characterized by disorientation, decreased activity level, abnormal sleep–wake cycles, loss of house training, decreased or altered responsiveness, and decreased or altered greeting behavior.

Clinical Uses. Uses include treatment of old-dog dementia and treatment of canine Cushing's disease (hyperadrenocorticism).

Dosage Form
- **Selegiline** (Anipryl)
  Adverse Side Effects. Side effects include vomiting, diarrhea, anorexia, restlessness, lethargy, salivation, shaking, and deafness.

Synthetic Progestins

Synthetic progestins are sometimes used to treat behavioral problems through mechanisms associated with changing hormonal levels (reduced gonadotropins) or through some direct effect on the cerebral cortex.

Clinical Uses. Uses include the treatment of urine spraying/marking, intermale aggression, and dominance aggression.

Dosage Forms
- **Megestrol acetate** (Megace, Ovaban [veterinary label])
- **Medroxyprogesterone** (Depo-Provera)
  Adverse Side Effects. Transient diabetes mellitus (cats), PUPD, increased weight gain, personality changes, endometritis, endometrial hyperplasia, mammary hypertrophy, mammary tumor, adrenal atrophy, and lactation are side effects.

Miscellaneous Behavioral Agents
- **Gabapentin.** Gabapentin may be used for anxiety or social phobias.

- **Clorazepate** (Tranxene-SD). Clorazepate is used for anxiety or social phobias; it is a Class IV controlled substance
- **Methylphenidate** (Ritalin). Methylphenidate has been used for hyperactivity in dogs; it is a Class II controlled substance

℞ Euthanasia Agents

Euthanasia agents should have several properties that make them effective medically and aesthetically for this emotion-laden procedure. These drugs should rapidly produce unconsciousness without struggling, vocalizations, or excessive involuntary movement. Death should follow quickly as a result of the cessation of all vital functions, such as respiratory and cardiac functions.

The main component of most of the euthanasia agents is pentobarbital. Pentobarbital may also be combined with other agents, such as propylene glycol and alcohol. Pentobarbital alone is a Class II controlled substance, and pentobarbital combinations usually are Class III controlled substances.

Clinical Uses. These agents are used to produce a rapid, humane death.

Dosage Forms
- **Pentobarbital sodium** (Socumb, Fatal Plus, pentobarbital generic). These products are Class II controlled substances for intravenous use.
- **Pentobarbital sodium** (Beuthanasia-D, Euthasol, SomnaSol). These drugs are Class III controlled substances for intravenous use. These products are different from the pentobarbital sodium described previously in that they contain rhodamine B, a bluish-red dye that helps to distinguish them from other parenteral pentobarbital solutions, as well as phenytoin and preservatives.

Adverse Side Effects. These may include muscle twitching; death may be delayed if the drug is injected outside the vein.

▌ REVIEW QUESTIONS

1. Define the difference between an agonist and an opioid antagonist.
2. Define *neurotransmitter.*
3. Most CNS drugs act by _____ or _____ the effects of neurotransmitters.
4. What are the primary neurotransmitters for adrenergic receptors?

5. List the four primary ways in which drugs affect the ANS.
6. List five indications for the use of cholinergic agents.
7. Atropine, scopolamine, glycopyrrolate, and aminopentamide are examples of what specific drug class?
8. Propranolol is an example of what category of drug?
   a. Alpha agonist
   b. Beta agonist
   c. Alpha blocker
   d. Beta blocker
9. What are some adverse side effects of xylazine, and what drug may be used to antagonize its effects?
10. Why would you be concerned about using a thiobarbiturate to induce anesthesia in a very thin dog?
11. What are some of the characteristics of a cat anesthetized with ketamine?
12. List some of the signs of a narcotic overdose.
13. List two narcotic antagonists.
14. Why should glyceryl guaiacolate not be mixed until just before use?
15. Why are euthanasia solutions that contain only pentobarbital classified as Class II controlled substances, whereas those that contain pentobarbital and other substances are classified as Class III controlled substances?
16. All psychotherapy drugs are thought to produce their effects by altering _____ activity in the brain.
17. Dissociative agents, such as ketamine and tiletamine, may cause _____ at the injection site.
18. A hypnotic (anesthetic) known for its very short duration and its white color is _____.
19. A benzodiazepine that is used as an antianxiety medication and as an appetite stimulant in cats is _____.
20. An example of a tricyclic antidepressant used in veterinary medicine for separation anxiety in dogs is _____.
21. _____ is used to treat old-dog dementia.
22. The _____ nervous system is under voluntary control.
   a. somatic
   b. autonomic
23. The neurotransmitter for cholinergic sites is _____.
   a. atropine
   b. scopolamine
   c. pralidoxime
   d. acetylcholine
24. The direct-acting cholinergic metoclopramide is ordered for a 50-lb dog to control vomiting and promote gastric emptying. The dosage of metoclopramide is 0.25 mg/kg and the concentration of the drug is 5 mg/mL. How many milliliters would you prepare?
25. Dexmedetomidine will be given to an 8-lb cat as a preanesthetic at a dosage of 30 mcg/kg. The concentration of Dexdomitor is 0.5 mg/mL. What quantity would you draw up?

REFERENCES

Boothe, D. M. (2012). Control of pain in small animals: Opioid agonists and antagonists and other locally and centrally acting analgesics. In D. M. Boothe (Ed.), *Small animal clinical pharmacology and therapeutics.* Philadelphia: WB Saunders.

Claude, A. (2013). Acute pain management in the small animal practice: Pharmaceutical options. *Murfreesboro, Tenn: Music City Vet Conf.*

DeLahunta, A. (1983). Diencephalon. In A. DeLahunta (Ed.), *Veterinary neuroanatomy and clinical neurology.* Philadelphia: WB Saunders.

Ganong, W. F. (2003). *Review of medical physiology* (21st ed.). New York: McGraw-Hill.

Muir, W. W., Hubbell, J. A., Bednarski, R. M., & Lerche, P. (2013). *Handbook of veterinary anesthesia* (5th ed.). St. Louis: Mosby Elsevier.

Package insert for Simbadol. (July, 2017). Zoetis United States.

Package insert for Sileo. (November, 2017). Zoetis, United States.

Paddleford, R. R. (1999). *Manual of small animal anesthesia.* Philadelphia: WB Saunders.

Papich, M. G. (2016). *Saunders handbook of veterinary drugs* (4th ed.). Philadelphia: Elsevier.

Plumb, D. C. (2015). *Veterinary drug handbook* (8th ed.). Ames, IA: Wiley-Blackwell.

Seibert, L. M. (2013). Behavior drug protocols. *Murfreesboro, Tenn: Music City Vet Conf.*

Simpson, B. S., & Simpson, D. M. (1996a). Behavioral pharmacotherapy part I: antipsychotics and antidepressants. *The Compendium on Continuing Education for the Practicing Veterinarian, 18*(10), 1067–1081.

Simpson, B. S., & Simpson, D. M. (1996b). Behavioral pharmacotherapy part II: anxiolytics and mood stabilizers. *The Compendium on Continuing Education for the Practicing Veterinarian, 18*(11), 1203–1210.

Snyder, S. (1986). Mood modifiers. In S. Snyder (Ed.), *Drugs and the brain*. New York: Scientific American Library.

Thomas, J. A., & Lerche, P. (2017). *Anesthesia and analgesia for veterinary technicians* (5th ed.). St. Louis: Elsevier.

Upson, D. W. (1988). Central nervous system. In D. W. Upson (Ed.), *Handbook of clinical veterinary pharmacology* (3rd ed.). Manhattan, KS: Dan Upson Enterprises.

Williams, B. R., & Baer, C. (1990). Drugs affecting the autonomic nervous system. In B. R. Williams, & C. Baer (Eds.), *Essentials of clinical pharmacology in nursing*. Springhouse, PA: Springhouse Corp.

Drugs Used in Respiratory System Disorders

KEY TERMS

Aerosolization
Antitussive
Bronchoconstriction
Bronchodilation
Decongestant
Expectorant
Humidification
IgA

Inspissated
Mucolytic
Nebulization
Nonproductive cough
Productive cough
Reverse sneeze
Surfactant
Viscid

INTRODUCTION

Veterinary references list a wide variety of diseases of the respiratory system. A partial listing of general origins includes the following:
- Allergies
- Aspiration
- Bacteria
- Congenital defects
- Fungi
- Immunologic factors
- Neoplasia
- Neurologic conditions
- Parasites
- Trauma
- Viruses

The respiratory system has a series of defense mechanisms by which it protects itself from disease. These natural defenses can be damaged by management practices such as those that cause a buildup of ammonia in enclosed, poorly ventilated housing. They can also be suppressed by inappropriate therapy, such as the use of cough suppressants for a productive cough. It is very important that technicians have a basic understanding of respiratory anatomy and physiology, respiratory defense mechanisms, and respiratory therapeutics because it is essential that these defense mechanisms function optimally for prompt recovery from respiratory disease.

RESPIRATORY ANATOMY AND PHYSIOLOGY

The respiratory system consists of the lungs and the passageways that carry air to and from the lungs (Figs. 5.1A,B). These passageways include the nostrils, nasal cavity, pharynx, larynx, trachea, bronchi, and bronchioles.

The passageways that lead to the lungs are referred to as the *upper respiratory system*. The upper respiratory system begins with the nostrils, which open into the nasal cavity. The nasal cavity contains turbinates that are covered with mucous membranes. These turbinates increase the surface area of the nasal cavity to allow humidification and warming of inspired air. Air that passes out of the nasal cavity moves, in turn, through the pharynx and the larynx into the trachea. The trachea bifurcates into right and left bronchi, which lead to the right and left lungs, respectively. Each bronchus then divides into a series of passageways of decreasing size, called *bronchioles*.

Smooth muscle fibers are found in the walls of the bronchioles. Contraction of smooth muscle fibers decreases the diameter of the bronchioles, and relaxation of fibers allows the diameter to return to normal size (Fig. 5.2).

The upper respiratory tract is lined with ciliated, pseudostratified columnar epithelial cells. Interspersed between the epithelial cells are goblet cells capable of secreting mucus. Mucus is secreted onto the surface of the epithelial cells and is moved toward the pharynx by movement of the cilia (mucociliary apparatus).

Sympathetic stimulation results in decreased production of mucus by the goblet cells and relaxation of smooth muscle in the walls of the bronchioles, leading to **bronchodilation**.

Parasympathetic stimulation causes increased secretion of mucus and constriction of smooth muscle (**bronchoconstriction**) (Fig. 5.3).

The bronchioles terminate in small, saclike structures called *alveoli*. The alveoli are arranged in grapelike clusters and are lined with a chemical substance called **surfactant,** which reduces the surface tension of the alveoli and helps to keep them from collapsing. The alveoli are surrounded by capillaries; this makes it possible for the blood to unload its carbon dioxide into the alveoli and to pick up oxygen from the alveoli.

Functions that the respiratory system serves include the following:
- Oxygen–carbon dioxide exchange
- Regulation of acid–base balance
- Body temperature regulation
- Voice production

The work of the respiratory system can be divided into the following four parts:
1. Ventilation—movement of air into and out of the lungs. The inspiratory portion of ventilation is usually an active process, whereas expiration is usually a passive process. Forced inspiration may be associated with upper airway obstruction, and active expiration may be related to intrathoracic airway obstruction (Tilley & Smith, 2004).
2. Distribution—distributing of inspired gases throughout the lungs.
3. Diffusion—movement of gases across the alveolar membrane.
4. Perfusion—supply of blood to the alveoli. The ratio of perfusion to ventilation of the alveoli is normally close to 1:1.

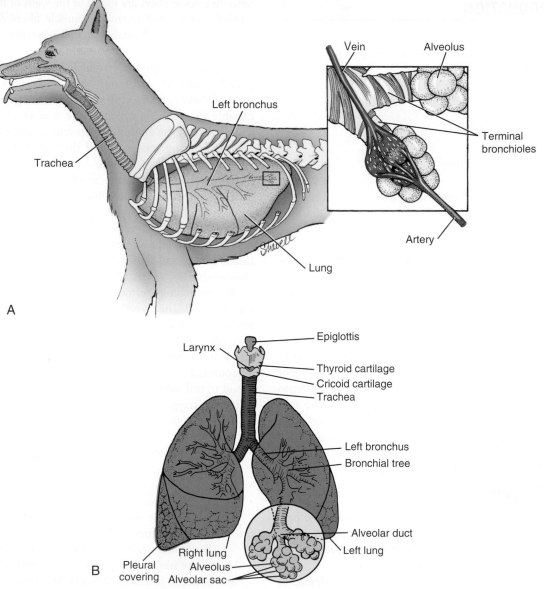

Fig. 5.1 (A) Anatomy of the respiratory system. (B) Lower respiratory tract. (B, From Summers, A. [2020]. *Common diseases of companion animals* [4th ed.]. St. Louis: Elsevier.)

RESPIRATORY DEFENSE MECHANISMS

The respiratory system has several effective methods of defense against disease processes, including the following:
- Nasal cavity: The turbinates of the nasal cavity provide a large surface area for warming and humidifying inspired air. Hair in the nasal passages also may help to filter out larger particulate matter.

- Protective reflexes: The cough, the sneeze, and perhaps the **reverse sneeze** respond to stimulation of receptors on the surfaces of air passageways to forcefully expel foreign material. Laryngospasm and bronchospasm also help to prevent introduction of materials into the lung tissue.
- Mucociliary clearance: The layer of mucus secreted onto the surface of the epithelial lining of the respiratory tract

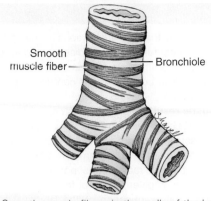

Fig. 5.2 Smooth muscle fibers in the walls of the bronchioles relax to allow bronchodilation and contract to cause bronchoconstriction.

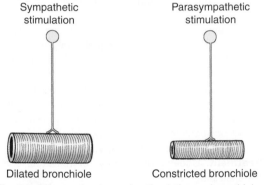

Fig. 5.3 Effects of autonomic stimulation on bronchioles.

helps to trap foreign debris that enters the respiratory passages. Wavelike actions of the cilia then move the debris up the passages ("escalator" action) to the pharynx, where it can be swallowed or expelled. Macrophages and immunoglobulin (**IgA**) also contribute to the defensive qualities of the mucociliary apparatus by immobilizing or phagocytizing foreign material.

PRINCIPLES OF RESPIRATORY THERAPEUTICS

It is important that a specific diagnosis be made through radiology, cytology, or appropriate culture before treatment of respiratory disease is initiated because the correct treatment for one type of disease may be contraindicated for another. Once the diagnosis has been made, treatment for respiratory disease is divided into the following three general goals (McKiernan, 1988):

1. Control of secretions: Secretions may be reduced by decreasing their production or increasing their

elimination. Removing the cause of the secretions by means of antibiotic, antifungal, antiparasitic, or other appropriate therapy is of vital concern. Methods are also aimed at making the secretions less **viscid** through the use of expectorants or through **nebulization** of **mucolytics** (aerosol therapy).

2. Control of reflexes: Coughing may be suppressed through the use of antitussives or bronchodilators if the cough is **nonproductive.** Sneezing is controlled by removal of the offending agent or through the use of vasoconstrictors. Bronchospasms may be controlled with bronchodilators and corticosteroids.

3. Maintaining normal airflow to the alveoli: Airflow to the alveoli may be maintained by reversing bronchoconstriction, by removing edema or mucus from alveoli and air passages, and by providing oxygen therapy. Intermittent positive-pressure ventilation and other ventilation strategies are often used in humans and may have application in selected animal cases.

INHALATION THERAPY FOR RESPIRATORY DISEASE

Although drugs used to treat respiratory disease are often administered by the oral or parenteral route, inhalation therapy may also be useful. **Aerosolization** (nebulization) of drugs allows their delivery at high concentrations directly into the airways while minimizing their blood levels—a feature that may reduce the chance of a toxic reaction. The efficacy of an inhaled drug depends on the dose and on how well it is distributed in the lungs. Distribution of an aerosol depends on several factors such as the size, shape, and pattern of the airways and the breathing pattern of the animal. The size of the inhaled particle plays a significant role in its distribution. The optimum particle size for entry into the peripheral airways is 1 to 5 microns (Lavoie, 2001). Particles smaller than 0.5 micron are likely to be exhaled, and those larger than 5 microns could be deposited in the upper airways. Airway pathology (e.g., excessive mucus or exudate) can interfere with distribution of the drug, causing some clinicians to assert that inhalation therapy should always be accompanied by systemic treatment (Boothe, 2012). Concurrent use of a bronchodilator and/or a mucolytic may be a helpful adjunct to inhalation therapy.

Two basic types of aerosol delivery systems are available for inhalation therapy: nebulizers and metered dose inhalers (MDI). Generally, nebulizers produce and deliver smaller particles that reach deep into the respiratory system whereas MDIs deliver particles to the upper

---

BOX 5.1   Case Scenario Laryngeal Paralysis

Coco, an 8-year-old neutered male Lab rador was presented for examination and diagnostic workup after collapoing on a walk with his owner.

History: The owner stated that over the past few weeks he had a voice change with a hoarse bark, an intermittent dry nonproductive cough, and occasionally gags after eating. He seems to be slower and weaker in his legs but the owner attributed this to his increasing age. He is currently on glucosamine supplements for arthritis but no other medications.

Additional history: Up to date on vaccines. No travel history aside from visiting relatives nearby.

Physical examination findings: Coco was anxious; Temperature: 103.8°F; Heart rate: 100 bpm with good pulse quality; Respiratory rate: panting with abdominal effort and inspiratory stridor; auscultation of the lungs: revealed no abnormal lung sounds; mucous membranes: dark pink-muddy; cathode-ray tube (CRT): <2 seconds.

Based on the history and initial findings considerations for diagnosis can be upper airway obstruction, congestive heart failure, pericardial effusion, or heat stroke.

The patient was stabilized with supplemental oxygen via a mask, given butorphanol as a sedative, provided active cooling by placing a fan directed toward the patient, and applied cool water to the skin. An intravenous catheter was placed and crystalloid fluids were administered as a bolus to expand the intravascular volume, increase blood flow to the periphery, aiding in the cooling process.

Diagnostic workup: The veterinarian ordered an SpO2, electrocardiograph (ECG), and blood pressure to help further assess stability and the need for emergent intervention such as the need for antiarrhythmics, etc. A complete blood count (CBC) and chemistry panel were ordered as well as thoracic radiographs including the cervical region to help rule out heart disease and assess for any concurrent lower airway disease such as aspiration pneumonia, foreign body, or mass contributing to upper airway obstruction.

Diagnostic results: SpO$_2$: 93% on room air but 98% on oxygen; ECG: revealed normal sinus rhythm; Systolic blood pressure: 120 mm Hg; CBC and Chemistry: revealed an inflammatory leukogram but otherwise within normal limits; thoracic radiographs: normal.

The patient was given propofol for a light anesthetic plane and an oral examination of the laryngeal area revealed lack of abduction of the arytenoid during inspiration. This was obtained by the veterinary technician noting each inhalation for the vet so that normal opening of the cartilages during inspiration can be differentiated from abnormal.

The patient responded well to sedation and oxygen.

Coco was diagnosed with laryngeal paralysis.

The vet discussed possible complications that could occur after surgery including life-long risk of aspiration pneumonia, difficult breathing if suture breaks, and coughing/gagging postoperatively, which may be reduced by feeding dry food at the floor level or trying different food bowl positions to slow down food intake.

The owner agreed to the surgery.

Treatment: Underwent surgery for unilateral arytenoid lateralization.

The patient was monitored for respiratory distress 24 hours after surgery.

Coco went home the next day with exercise restrictions for 1 to 2 months. The owner reported back a month later, stating that Coco was doing well.

---

airways. Nebulizers use compressors to create an aerosol that can be inhaled without the necessity of using positive pressure to force the aerosol into the airways. Nebulizers produce the aerosol using a jet or ultrasonic mechanism. In jet nebulizers, compressed air or oxygen is forced through a small orifice to create the aerosol. Drugs in solution are drawn from a fluid reservoir and shattered into droplets by the gas stream. Ultrasonic nebulizers use high-frequency vibrations from a piezoelectric crystal to create the aerosol. Ultrasonic nebulizers are more efficient at creating smaller aerosol droplets and are gentler on drug molecules than the jet nebulizers. Aerosolized drugs can be delivered to cats and dogs in a tent-like structure, closed container, or face mask, but a tight-fitting face mask, endotracheal tube, or tracheostomy tube probably delivers the most efficient concentration of the drug to the patient (Reinero & Selting, 2010). Nebulizers must be kept meticulously clean to avoid iatrogenic infection of a patient already compromised with an airway pathology. Small inexpensive nebulizers are available for adaption for veterinary use (Omron) (Fig. 5.4).

Metered dose inhalers are designed for home use by animal owners. The aerosol of an MDI is driven by a propellant. Older MDIs used chlorofluorocarbons (CFCs) as the propellant, but CFCs are being replaced by hydrofluoroalkanes (HFAs), which contain no chlorine and do not affect the ozone. Hydrofluoroalkane propellants allow drugs to be delivered as a solution rather than a microsuspension,

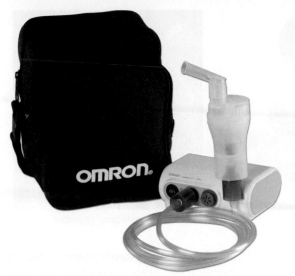

Fig. 5.4 Omron nebulization device.

which, in turn, allows the production of a smaller particle that can reach deeper in the airways (Boothe, 2012). The use of spacers and holding chambers with the MDIs makes delivery to the patient more efficient and directed.

Nebulizers have been used primarily in the treatment of respiratory infections. Nebulizers are used to provide airway humidification (saline), mucolytics, bronchodilators, and antimicrobials. Mucolytics and saline can help treat pneumonia and other airway infections by decreasing the viscosity of airway secretions and improving their clearance from the airway. Bronchodilators increase flow through the airways, and antimicrobials counter infectious agents. A potential use of nebulizer therapy may be for inhaled chemotherapy, which would take advantage of the concept that high doses of the agents may be delivered to the lung while avoiding the potential side effects of intravenous use.

Metered dose inhaler therapy has been used primarily for feline lower airway disease (asthma), lower airway disease in horses (heaves or recurrent airway obstruction [RAO]), and, occasionally, in lower airway disease (bronchitis) in dogs. Metered dose inhalers frequently contain bronchodilators like albuterol or clenbuterol and/or corticosteroids.

Box 5.2 lists drugs frequently used in inhalation therapy.

Metered dose inhaler units for inhalation therapy are available for use in small animals (Opti-Chamber, Aero-Chamber, AeroKat, AeroDawg) and in horses (AeroMask) (Fig. 5.5).

BOX 5.2 Drugs Administered by Aerosolization

Bronchodilators
Isoproterenol
Isoetharine
Albuterol
Atropine
Glycopyrrolate
Glucocorticoids
Beclomethasone
Triamcinolone
Mucokinetics
Water
Saline
Bicarbonate
N-Acetylcysteine
Antimicrobials
Ceftriaxone (40 mg/mL in water or dimethyl sulfoxide)
Chloramphenicol (13 mg/mL)
Enrofloxacin (10 mg/mL)
Gentamicin, amikacin (5 mg/mL)
Kanamycin
Polymyxin B (66,600 IU/mL)
Amphotericin B (7 mg/mL in 5% dextrose)
Nystatin
Clotrimazole (10 mg/mL in polyethylene glycol)
Enilconazole (10 mg/mL in water)
Other
Alcohol

From Boothe, D. (2012). *Small animal clinical pharmacology and therapeutics* (2nd ed.). St. Louis: Elsevier.

CATEGORIES OF RESPIRATORY DRUGS

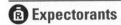 Expectorants

Expectorants are drugs that liquefy and dilute viscid secretions of the respiratory tract, thereby helping in evacuation of those secretions. Most expectorants are administered orally, although a few are given by inhalation or parenterally. Expectorants are thought to act directly on the mucus-secreting glands or by reducing the adhesiveness of mucus. Expectorants are indicated when a productive cough is present and are often combined with other substances, such as ammonium chloride, antihistamines, or dextromethorphan.

Guaifenesin

Guaifenesin is found in a few veterinary-label products and in many human-label over-the-counter

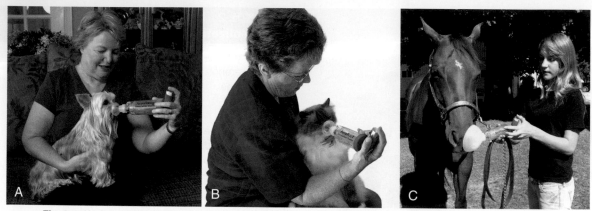

Fig. 5.5 (A) AeroDawg metered dose inhaler (MDI) device. (B) AeroKat MDI device. (C) AeroHippus chamber.

cough preparations. Guaifenesin is more commonly used in equine practice to induce or maintain general anesthesia.

Clinical Uses. These include relief of cough symptoms related to upper respiratory tract conditions.

Dosage Forms. These are primarily liquid (syrup) and tablet preparations.

- **Guaifenesin oral tablets**
- **Guaifenesin syrup/liquid**
- **Guaifenesin powder**
- **Robitussin-AC**
- **Triaminic expectorant**

Adverse Side Effects. Adverse side effects of guaifenesin are rare, although mild drowsiness or nausea may occur.

Iodide Preparations

Ethylenediamine dihydriodide is an expectorant that may be useful in treating mild respiratory disease of horses and cattle. Iodide preparations should not be used in pregnant or hyperthyroid animals.

Hypertonic Saline

Aerosolized hypertonic saline has been used as an expectorant in humans and may have potential for use in veterinary patients. It is thought to work by exerting an osmotic pull of fluid into the airway lumen, which helps to liquefy the contents for easier removal.

Ⓡ Mucolytics: Acetylcysteine

Mucolytics, such as acetylcysteine, decrease the viscosity of respiratory secretions by altering the chemical composition of the mucus through the breakdown of

chemical (disulfide) bonds. Acetylcysteine is the only mucolytic of clinical significance in veterinary medicine. It is administered by nebulization for pulmonary uses. This drug is also administered intravenously or orally as an antidote for acetaminophen (Tylenol) toxicity.

Clinical Uses. Acetylcysteine is used to break down thick or inspissated (dry) respiratory mucus and to treat acetaminophen toxicity.

Dosage Forms. Dosage forms with a human label include a 10% solution and a 20% solution in 4-, 10- and 30-mL vials (Plumb, 2015).

- **Acetylcysteine** (Mucomyst)
- **Dembrexine** (Sputolysin)—veterinary label

Adverse Side Effects. Adverse side effects are few when acetylcysteine is nebulized. However, the drug may cause nausea or vomiting when administered orally.

Ⓡ Antitussives: Centrally Acting Agents

Antitussives are drugs that inhibit or suppress coughing. They are commonly used to treat dry, nonproductive coughs such as tracheobronchitis (kennel cough) in dogs. Antitussives are classified as centrally acting or peripherally acting (Fig. 5.6). Centrally acting agents suppress coughing by depressing the cough center in the brain, whereas peripherally acting agents depress cough receptors in the airways. Peripherally acting antitussives are seldom used in veterinary medicine because they are usually prepared as cough drops or lozenges, which are not practical for administration to animal patients.

Butorphanol Tartrate

Butorphanol is a synthetic opiate, agonist/antagonist with significant antitussive activity. It is a class

Hydrocodone Bitartrate

Hydrocodone is a schedule II opiate agonist used for the treatment of nonproductive coughs in dogs.

Clinical Uses. Hydrocodone is used primarily as an antitussive for harsh, nonproductive coughs.

Dosage Forms. Dosage forms include human-label combination products in syrup and tablet form.

- **Hycodan** (hydrocodone and homatropine) tablets
- **Hycodan** (hydrocodone and homatropine) syrup
- **Hydrocodone/acetaminophen combination**; contraindicated in cats

Adverse Side Effects. These include potential sedation, constipation, and gastrointestinal upset.

Codeine

Codeine containing cough syrups are a schedule V, III, II (depending on the amount of codeine contained in the product) opiate agonist that is used as an antitussive in human-label combination products.

Clinical Uses. Clinical uses of codeine are to help manage moderate pain and may be used in some cases as a cough suppressant and antidiarrheal.

Dosage Forms. Dosage forms include human-label combination products.

- **Codeine phosphate** oral tablets, 30 and 60 mg
- **Codeine sulfate** oral tablets (15, 30, and 60 mg)
- **Codeine with aspirin** or acetaminophin

Adverse Side Effects. Adverse side effects include sedation and constipation.

> **TECHNICIAN NOTES**
>
> - Codeine-only products are class II (C-II).
> - Codeine with aspirin or acetaminophen is C-III.
> - Orally administered codeine is poorly absorbed in the dog and not commonly used.

Dextromethorphan

Dextromethorphan is a nonnarcotic antitussive that is chemically similar to codeine. It has no analgesic or addictive properties. It acts centrally and elevates the cough threshold. Similar to the two drugs previously mentioned, it is available primarily in human-label combination products. Dextromethorphan may be used in cats, without acetaminophen (Boothe, 2012). Pharmacokinetic studies in dogs indicated that

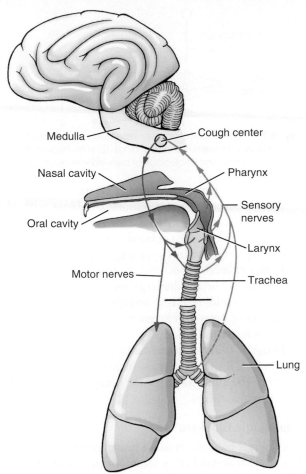

Fig. 5.6 Antitussives act peripherally on sensory nerve endings or centrally on cough centers.

Labels: Medulla, Cough center, Nasal cavity, Pharynx, Sensory nerves, Oral cavity, Larynx, Motor nerves, Trachea, Lung

IV-controlled substance. It is also used as a preanesthetic and as an analgesic.

Clinical Uses. Butorphanol tartrate is used for the relief of chronic nonproductive coughs in dogs and for analgesia and preanesthesia in dogs and cats.

Dosage Forms. Dosage forms include injectable and tablet forms.

- **Butorphanol (Torbutrol)** injection; approved for use in dogs
- **Butorphanol (Torbugesic-SA)**; approved for use in cats
- **Butorphanol (Torbugesic)** injection; approved for use in horses
- **Butorphanol (Torbutrol)** tablets

Adverse Side Effects. Adverse side effects may include sedation and ataxia.

dextromethorphan is poorly absorbed and does not attain effective concentrations after oral administration and is not recommended for use to control coughing (Papich, 2016).

Clinical Uses. Dextromethorphan is used to suppress a nonproductive cough.

Dosage Forms. The primary dosage form is the syrup product.

- **Dimetapp DM** (dextromethorphan, phenylpropanolamine, and brompheniramine)
- **Robitussin DM** (dextromethorphan and guaifenesin)

Adverse Side Effects. Adverse side effects are rare when this drug is given in the correct dose but can include drowsiness and gastrointestinal upset.

TECHNICIAN NOTES

Technicians who administer combination products to cats should take special precautions to ensure that the product does not contain acetaminophen.

Temaril-P

Temaril-P is a combination product that contains a centrally acting antitussive (trimeprazine tartrate) and a corticosteroid (prednisolone).

Clinical Uses. Temaril-P is used as an antitussive, an antipruritic and an antiinflammatory.

Dosage Forms. Dosage forms include tablets.

- **Temaril-P tablets** 5 mg trimeprazine tartrate, 2 mg prednisolone

Adverse Side Effects. These include sedation, depression, hypotension, and minor central nervous system signs.

Bronchodilators

Contraction of the smooth muscle fibers that surround the bronchioles results in bronchoconstriction and often corresponding dyspnea. Contraction of these smooth muscle fibers can result from the following three basic mechanisms (Bill, 2017) (Fig. 5.7):

1. Release of acetylcholine at parasympathetic nerve endings or inhibition of acetylcholinesterase. Increased acetylcholine levels also tend to increase secretions of the respiratory tract, thus reducing airflow and adding to the level of dyspnea.

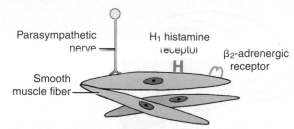

Fig. 5.7 Bronchoconstriction may result from (1) acetylcholine release at parasympathetic nerve endings, (2) stimulation of H_1 histamine receptors, and (3) blockade of beta$_2$-adrenergic receptors.

2. Release of histamine through allergic or inflammatory mechanisms. Histamine combines with H_1 receptors on smooth muscle fibers to cause bronchoconstriction. Histamine also increases the inflammatory response in the airways, further leading to increased levels of secretion and viscosity.

3. Blockade of beta$_2$-adrenergic receptors by drugs such as propranolol results in bronchoconstriction. Stimulation of beta$_2$-adrenergic receptors, however, produces bronchodilation.

Drugs that cause bronchodilation are of four basic categories. Those categories include the cholinergic blockers, the antihistamines, the beta$_2$ adrenergics, and the methylxanthines.

Cholinergic Blockers

Cholinergic blockers produce bronchodilation by combining with acetylcholine receptors on smooth muscle fibers and preventing the bronchoconstrictive effects of acetylcholine. Cholinergic blockers such as atropine, aminopentamide (Centrine), and glycopyrrolate (Robinul-V) have limited use in treating bronchoconstriction, except in cases of organophosphate or carbamate toxicity. Ipratropium bromide, a synthetic anticholinergic, may be of some value in treating equine pulmonary obstructive disease (Hoffman, 2001) and may have potential for use in dogs and cats as an inhalant.

Antihistamines

Antihistamines are discussed later in this chapter.

Beta$_2$-Adrenergic Agonists

Beta$_2$-adrenergic agonists combine with appropriate receptors on the smooth muscle fibers and effect relaxation of those fibers. They also stabilize mast cells and reduce the amount of histamine released (Bill, 2017). It is preferred that these drugs have limited beta$_1$ activity because beta$_1$ stimulation can produce tachycardia.

Clinical Uses. Beta$_2$-adrenergic agonists are used as bronchodilators.

Dosage Forms

- **Epinephrine**: This drug is a potent bronchodilator that is used only in life-threatening situations (e.g., anaphylactic shock) because it also produces significant tachycardia.
- **Pseudoephedrine/pyrilamine** (EquiPhed) is approved for horses not intended for food.
- **Isoproterenol** (Isuprel): This drug also causes beta$_1$ stimulation and has limited use as a bronchodilator in veterinary medicine.
- **Albuterol** (salbutamol) (Ventolin, Proventil)
- **Clenbuterol** (Ventipulmin syrup and clenbuterol HCl oral syrup): Ventipulmin is approved for horses not intended for food.
- **Terbutaline**
- **Metaproterenol** (Alupent)

Adverse Side Effects. These include tachycardia and hypertension.

Methylxanthines

Methylxanthine derivatives that are used therapeutically include aminophylline and theophylline. These two products are very similar in their chemistry and pharmacologic effects. Both inhibit an enzyme in smooth muscle cells called *phosphodiesterase*. When beta$_2$ receptors are stimulated, a chemical messenger called *cyclic adenosine monophosphate (cyclic AMP)*, which is released in the smooth muscle cell, completes the relaxation response to allow dilation. Phosphodiesterase inhibits cyclic AMP in the cell, thereby tending to promote bronchoconstriction. By inhibiting the inhibitor (phosphodiesterase) and allowing cyclic AMP to accumulate, the methylxanthines tend to promote bronchodilation.

Methylxanthines also cause mild stimulation of the heart and respiratory muscles and minor diuresis.

Caffeine and theobromine (found in chocolate) are methylxanthines.

Aminophylline is an ethylenediamine salt of theophylline. It is available in various human-label products. One hundred milligrams of aminophylline contains approximately 79 mg of theophylline (Plumb, 2015). Aminophylline is currently available in the injectable form and theophylline is available in a timed-release tablet/capsule.

Clinical Uses. Methylxanthines are used for bronchodilation in respiratory and cardiac conditions and for mild heart stimulation (positive inotropic effect). They are used for inflammatory airway disease in cats (feline asthma), dogs, and horses.

Dosage Forms

- **Theophylline**—timed release tablets/capsules
- **Aminophylline**—injectable

Adverse Side Effects. These may include gastrointestinal upset, central nervous system stimulation, tachycardia, ataxia, and arrhythmia.

 TECHNICIAN NOTES

Because theophylline may interact adversely with many drugs, including phenobarbital, cimetidine, erythromycin, thiabendazole, clindamycin, and lincomycin, appropriate precautions should be taken before this drug is administered.

Decongestants

Decongestants are drugs that reduce the congestion of nasal membranes by reducing associated swelling. Decongestants may be administered as a spray or nose drops, or may be given orally as a liquid or a tablet. These drugs act directly or indirectly to reduce congestion through vasoconstriction of nasal blood vessels. Phenylephrine (Neo-Synephrine) drops is an example. These products have limited use in veterinary medicine as their effectiveness has not been demonstrated.

Antihistamines

Antihistamines are substances that are used to block the effects of histamine. Histamine is released from mast cells by the allergic response and combines with H$_1$ receptors on bronchiole smooth muscle to cause bronchoconstriction. Antihistamines may be useful in treating respiratory disease because they prevent mast cell degranulation and block H$_1$ receptors on smooth muscle. Antihistamines are thought to be more effective when used prophylactically because they apparently do not replace histamine that has already combined with receptors (Bill, 2017).

Respiratory conditions that may be treated with antihistamines include "heaves" in horses, pneumonia in cattle, feline asthma, and insect bites.

Generic names for antihistamines often are easily recognized because most end in the suffix "-amine" (e.g., pyrilamine, diphenhydramine, chlorpheniramine).

Veterinary-label antihistamines for treating respiratory conditions are available in injectable and oral preparations.

Clinical Uses. Antihistamines are used in the treatment of allergic and respiratory conditions. They also may be used for their antiemetic effects.

Dosage Forms
- **Pyrilamine** (Hist-Eq, Histall)
- **Tripelennamine**
- **Diphenhydramine** (Benadryl)
- **Hydroxyzine** (Atarax)
- **Cyproheptadine**; may be used in cats to block bronchoconstriction and also as an appetite stimulant
- **Cetirizine** (Zyrtec)

Adverse Side Effects. These include sedation and, occasionally, gastrointestinal effects.

® Corticosteroids

Corticosteroids are used primarily in the treatment of allergic respiratory conditions. They are considered the most effective drugs in the treatment of equine chronic obstructive pulmonary disease (Lavoie, 2001). Corticosteroids prepared for inhalation therapy have strong antiinflammatory effects locally in the lungs and are rapidly biodegraded when absorbed into the general circulation. Oral corticosteroids (prednisone or prednisolone) are considered the drugs of choice in the treatment of chronic airway inflammation in dogs and cats (Dowling, 2001). Oral prednisolone should be used in cats as they do not absorb or convert prednisone to prednisolone as well as in dogs (Plumb, 2015). Corticosteroid therapy controls the signs of respiratory disease, not the cause; good short-term effects often ensue with few of the residual effects that may accompany long-term use.

Clinical Uses. Corticosteroids are used in the treatment of equine heaves, feline asthma, acute respiratory distress syndrome, and allergic pneumonia.

Dosage Forms
- **Prednisolone sodium succinate** (Solu-Delta-Cortef)
- **Prednisolone** (Temaril-P, generic forms)
- **Prednisone tablets and syrup**
- **Dexamethasone** (Dexasone, Dexamethasone Solution, Azium)
- **Beclomethasone dipropionate** (Vanceril) (for inhalation)

- **Fluticasone propionate** (Flovent) (for inhalation)
- **Triamcinolone** (Vetalog)

Adverse Side Effects. Adverse side effects are associated with long-term use of the drug. Some of the effects include polyphagia, polydipsia/polyuria, behavior changes, gastrointestinal ulceration, delayed wound healing, and immunosuppression.

® Miscellaneous Respiratory Drugs

Many other drugs are used to treat respiratory disorders. These include antimicrobials, mast cell stabilizers, and diuretics. Antimicrobials are used in cases of bacterial infection of the respiratory tract and may be administered parenterally or by nebulization. Mast cell stabilizers, such as cromolyn, are most effective if used before inflammatory activation. Diuretics are used to treat respiratory disease in which pulmonary edema is a major problem.

Respiratory Stimulants

Doxapram Hydrochloride. Doxapram is a general central nervous system stimulant that is used primarily as a stimulant for the respiratory system.

Clinical Uses. Doxapram is used for stimulation of respiration during and after anesthesia and to speed awakening and restoration of reflexes after anesthesia. In neonatal animals, doxapram is used to stimulate respiration after dystocia or cesarean section.

Dosage Form
- **Dopram-V** for injection.

Adverse Side Effects. These include hypertension, arrhythmia, hyperventilation, central nervous system excitation, and seizures. These effects are most likely to occur at high doses (Plumb, 2015). The safety of doxapram in pregnant animals has not been established.

Mast Cell Stabilizers

Cromolyn (Cromolyn Sodium for Inhalation) is a substance that inhibits the release of histamine and leukotrienes from sensitized mast cells found in nasal and lung mucosa and in the eyes. It may also inhibit bronchospasm. It is used primarily in the treatment of horses with RAO (recurrent airway obstruction—heaves).

Leukotriene Antagonists

Montelukast sodium (Singulair tablets) and zafirlukast (Accolate tablets) are leukotriene receptor antagonists. Leukotrienes are proinflammatory products of arachidonic acid released from mast cells and eosinophils. Montelukast has been used in veterinary medicine to treat feline asthma, inflammatory bowel disease (IBD), heartworm respiratory disease syndrome, and upper respiratory infection. Zafirlukast has been used to treat feline asthma, feline IBD, and canine atopic dermatitis. Both of these products have produced marginal efficacy (Plumb, 2015).

Naloxone

Naloxone is used to stimulate respirations in narcotic overdose.

Yobine

Yobine is used to stimulate respirations in xylazine overdose.

▮ REVIEW QUESTIONS

1. What structures would a molecule of oxygen pass over or through as it travels from the environment to the alveoli?
2. What are the four primary functions of the respiratory system?
3. Describe the function of the three basic defense mechanisms of the respiratory system.
4. What are three important principles of respiratory therapeutics?
5. Expectorants are indicated when what type of cough is present?
6. Mucolytics decrease the viscosity of respiratory mucus by what mechanism?
7. What is the term for administering a liquid drug into a mist so it can be more easily inhaled into the lungs.
8. Match the following drugs with the correct category.

A. Guaifenesin	_____ Respiratory stimulant
B. Mucomyst	_____ Antitussive
C. Albuterol	_____ Beta$_2$-Adrenergic agonist
D. Butorphanol	_____ Expectorant
E. Theophylline	_____ Mucolytic
F. Dopram	_____ Methylxanthine

9. What is the mechanism of action of most antitussives used in veterinary medicine?
10. List three mechanisms that can cause smooth muscle contraction in the bronchioles.

11. List two bronchodilators that are beta$_2$-adrenergic agonists.
12. The bronchioles terminate in small, saclike structures in the lung called _____ which are arranged in grape-like clusters.
13. The methylxanthines bring about bronchodilation by inhibiting what cellular enzyme?
14. _____ is used as an antitussive, an antipruritic, and an antiinflammatory drug.
15. List two potential uses for antihistamines in veterinary medicine.
16. What suffix is found at the end of many antihistamine names?
17. List two potential uses for Dopram.
18. Maxi Jones is being treated for canine infectious tracheobronchitis. Dr. Ladd has instructed you to dispense Hycodan tablets at 0.22 mg/kg b.i.d. for 7 days. Maxi weighs 50 lb and 5-mg tablets are available. What dose of Hycodan does Maxi require? How many tablets will you dispense?
19. List two uses of acetylcysteine in veterinary medicine.
20. Which of the following is *not* an example of a methylxanthine?
    a. Aminophylline
    b. Theophylline
    c. Caffeine
    d. Theobromine
    e. These are all examples of methylxanthines.
21. Particles of what size are capable of reaching the alveoli?
22. Give an example of a beta$_2$-adrenergic agonist bronchodilator.
23. _____ are drugs that inhibit or suppress coughing.
    a. Antitussives
    b. Decongestants
    c. Bronchodilators
    d. Expectorants
24. _____ is used for the relief of chronic nonproductive coughs in dogs, and for analgesia and preanesthesia in dogs and cats.
    a. Hydrocodone bitartrate
    b. Butorphanol tartrate
    c. Temaril P
    d. Doxapram HCl
25. An 8-lb cat with feline asthma will be treated with Singulair at a dosage of 0.5 mg/kg daily for 3 days. Singulair tablets (4 mg) are available. How many tablets will you dispense? _____

REFERENCES

Bill, R. (2017). Drugs affecting the respiratory system. In R. Bill (Ed.), *Pharmacology for veterinary technicians* (4th ed.). St. Louis: Mosby.

Boothe, D. M. (2012). Drugs affecting the respiratory system. In *Small animal clinical pharmacology and therapeutics*. Philadelphia: WB Saunders.

Dowling, P. M. (2001). Respiratory drugs. In *Proceedings. Annual meeting of the American Veterinary Medical Association*, Boston.

Hoffman, A. M. (2001). What's new with aerosol medications in the horse. In *Proceedings. Annual meeting of the American Veterinary Medical Association*, Boston.

Lavoie, J. P. (2001). Inhalation therapy for equine heaves. *Compendium on Continuing Education for the Practising Veterinarian*, *23*(5), 475–477.

McKiernan, B. (1988). *Respiratory therapeutics in proceedings. 17th Las Vegas: Semin for vet tech, west vet conf.*

Papich, M. G. (2016). *Saunders handbook of veterinary drugs* (4th ed.). Philadelphia: Elsevier.

Plumb, D. C. (2015). *Veterinary drug handbook* (8th ed.). Ames, IA: Wiley-Blackwell.

Tilley, L. P., & Smith, W. K. (2004). *The 5-minute veterinary consult: Canine and feline* (3rd ed.). Baltimore: Lippincott Williams & Wilkins.

Veterinary Information Network. (2010). VIN Proceedings Library (website). In C. N. Reinero, & K. A. Selting (Eds.), *Inhalational therapies in dogs and cats*. http://www.vin.com/members/proceedings.plx?CID=ACVIM2010&PID=559. Accessed March 19, 2013.

6

Drugs Used in Renal and Urinary Tract Disorders

KEY TERMS

Agonist
Antagonist
Atony
Catecholamine
Detrusor
Detrusor areflexia
Erythropoiesis

Erythropoietin
Hematuria
Hypertension
Hypertonus
Hypokalemia
Lower motor neurons
Nephrology

KEY TERMS—CONT'D

Nephron
Polydipsia
Polyuria
Retroperitoneal

Upper motor neurons
Uremia
Urinary incontinence
Urinary tract infection

INTRODUCTION

The urinary system (i.e., the renal system) is composed of two kidneys, two ureters, a urinary bladder, and a urethra (Figs. 6.1 to 6.4). The medical study of the renal system is known as **nephrology** because the basic functional unit of the kidney is the **nephron.** The kidneys work in the body similar to the way in which a fish aquarium filter works. All the water in an aquarium is sent through the filter to capture waste products in the water so that the tank is kept clean. Thus, the kidneys filter all waste products from the bloodstream but allow those elements needed by the body to remain. The kidneys are bean shaped and lie on each side of the spine. They are also **retroperitoneal.**

The nephron regulates water and soluble matter (especially electrolytes) in the body. Nephrons filter the blood under pressure and then reabsorb necessary fluid and molecules back into the blood. The kidneys thus excrete a variety of waste products produced by metabolism such as urea, uric acid, and water. The kidneys are involved in factors of homeostasis such as acid-base balance, regulation of electrolyte concentrations, blood volume control,

and regulation of blood pressure. The kidneys communicate with other organs in the body through hormones that are secreted into the bloodstream.

Veterinary technicians should educate clients about the importance of nutrition, especially in those dog breeds

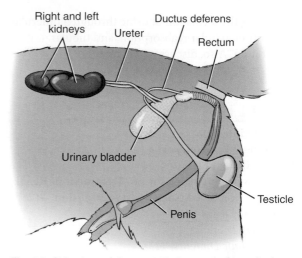

Fig. 6.2 Side view of the urogenital system of a male dog.

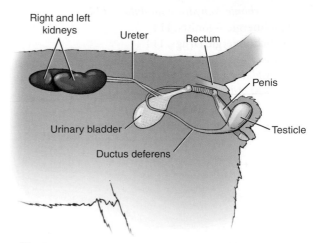

Fig. 6.1 Side view of the urogenital system of a female dog.

Fig. 6.3 Side view of the urogenital system of a male cat.

predisposed to developing urinary bladder stones (e.g., dalmatians, miniature schnauzers). Fresh water should be available for animals at all times. Companion animals observed straining to urinate or with bloody urine (i.e., **hematuria**) should be brought to the veterinary hospital immediately.

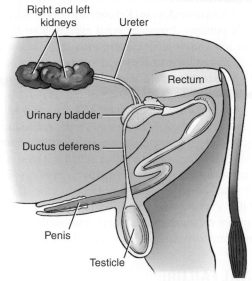

Fig. 6.4 Side view of the urogenital system of a bull.

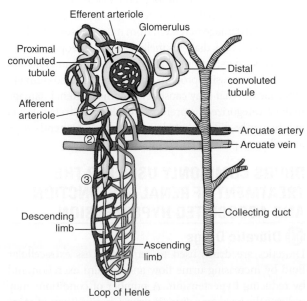

Fig. 6.5 Shown are the direction and location of glomerular filtration: *1*, tubular reabsorption; *2*, tubular secretion; and *3*, as they would occur in the glomerulus and the proximal tubule.

PHYSIOLOGIC PRINCIPLES

The formation of urine is a rather complex process that involves glomerular filtration, tubular reabsorption, and tubular secretion (Fig. 6.5). The glomerular filtrate is composed of water and dissolved substances, which pass from the plasma into the glomerular capsule. The formation of glomerular filtrate is controlled by effective filtration pressure (EFP = arterial blood pressure – [plasma osmotic pressure + capsule pressure]). The amount of glomerular filtrate is directly proportional to the EFP (Fig. 6.6). Changes in blood flow through the glomerulus, glomerular blood pressure, plasma osmotic pressure, and capsule pressure affect glomerular filtration.

The kidney tubules are responsible for the reabsorption or the secretion of specific substances. Substances needed by the body are reabsorbed from the filtrate, pass through the tubular cell wall, and reenter the plasma. This process filters needed substances and returns them to the body. Reabsorbed materials include water, glucose, amino acids, urea, and ions such as Na, K, Ca^{2+}, Cl^-, HCO_3^-, and HPO_4^{2-}. Any excess of these substances or of substances that are not useful remain in the filtrate and are excreted in the urine.

Tubular secretion occurs when substances are carried to the tubular lumen. This involves the active transport

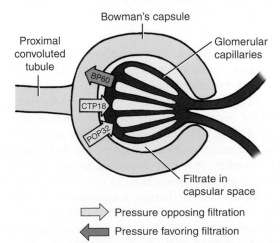

⇨ Pressure opposing filtration

⬅ Pressure favoring filtration

Fig. 6.6 Filtration occurs through the glomerular membrane within Bowman's capsule. The amount of filtrate produced is determined by the difference between the pressures favoring filtration and those opposing filtration. This diagram shows that filtration occurs because 60 − (32 + 18) = 10 mm Hg. Values greater than or less than 10 mm Hg would correlate with more or less filtration, respectively. Pressure values (60, 32, 18) are measured in mm Hg. *BP,* Blood pressure; *CTP,* capsular tissue pressure; *POP,* plasma osmotic pressure.

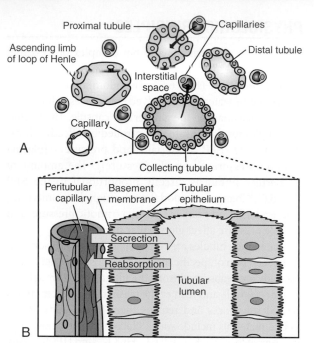

Fig. 6.7 Tubular reabsorption and secretion. (A) Cross-section of nephron tubules and peritubular capillaries. Interstitial fluid occupies the interstitial space. Reabsorption is represented by substance *X* going from tubule to capillary, and secretion is represented by substance *Y* going from capillary to tubule. (B) Longitudinal section of nephron tubule. Shown is the relationship among the tubular lumen, epithelial cell, and capillary.

of certain endogenous substances and many exogenous substances. These secreted substances include potassium and hydrogen ions, ammonia, creatinine, and some drugs. The main effects of tubular secretion are to rid the body of certain materials and to help control blood pH (Fig. 6.7). The kidneys are active in the metabolism and excretion of many drugs and their metabolites. Therefore, it is very important to remember that these actions may be inhibited in cases of renal failure or dysfunction. Drug therapy in animals with renal dysfunction has increased risks. Renal failure can impair a drug's absorption from an administration site, affect a drug's distribution in the body, and affect the elimination of the drug from the body.

If the kidneys' functionality is decreased, **erythropoiesis** may not occur correctly. Erythropoiesis is the formation of erythrocytes. **Erythropoietin** is a hormone secreted by the healthy kidney that communicates with the bone marrow to make more red blood cells. In diseased kidneys, this hormone is secreted in reduced amounts or not at all, and the animal may develop a nonregenerative anemia as

a result. Injections of human recombinant erythropoietin may be given to animals to treat this anemia.

Uremia can increase the sensitivity of some tissues to certain drugs. For example, sensitivity to central nervous system depressants is increased; therefore, the dose of opiates, barbiturates, and tranquilizers should be reduced in uremic patients. Xylazine (Rompun) and ketamine hydrochloride (Ketaset) are contraindicated in uremic patients. Impaired renal excretion or biotransformation causes delayed elimination of many drugs and enhances their toxicity and duration of action.

Dosage regimen adjustments may be required in renal-impaired conditions. Modifications can be made by measuring the plasma concentration of a drug and adjusting the dose accordingly. However, this is impractical in most clinical settings, so a veterinarian may use the normal dose but lengthen the time intervals at which it is administered or give a smaller dose at normal time intervals. Technicians may be responsible for administering anesthesia, and it is important to remember that patients with renal failure are at greater anesthetic risk and require even closer monitoring than patients with normal renal function.

RENAL FAILURE

Renal failure is among the major causes of nonaccidental death in dogs and cats. Although the disease is most common in older animals, it may be diagnosed in younger animals. Renal damage may stem from many causes including: infectious disease, diabetes mellitus, toxins, neoplasia, congenital disorders, immunologic problems, and amyloidosis. Diets with excessive protein, phosphorus, and sodium are other factors that may cause renal damage. Renal damage may be categorized as prerenal, renal, or postrenal. Renal failure may be differentiated as acute, chronic, or end-stage, according to parameters common to each stage.

DRUGS COMMONLY USED FOR THE TREATMENT OF RENAL DYSFUNCTION AND ASSOCIATED HYPERTENSION

℞ Diuretic Drugs

Diuretics are drugs used to remove excess extracellular fluid by increasing urine flow and sodium excretion and by reducing **hypertension**. A number of conditions may indicate the need for a diuretic drug. Classifications of commonly used diuretics include loop diuretics, osmotic diuretics, thiazide and thiazide-like diuretics, potassium-sparing diuretics, and carbonic anhydrase inhibitors.

Loop Diuretics

Loop diuretics are highly potent diuretics that inhibit the tubular reabsorption of sodium. Once these drugs are administered, their actions are generally rapid. Additionally, loop diuretics promote the excretion of chloride, potassium, and water. Some patients receiving long-term loop diuretic therapy may also need potassium supplementation.

Clinical Uses. Loop diuretics are useful in the treatment of congestive heart failure (CHF) in canines and felines, pulmonary edema, udder edema, hypercalcemic nephropathy, and uremia, as an adjunct in the treatment of hyperkalemia, and sometimes as an antihypertensive agent (Plumb, 2015).

Dosage Forms
• **Furosemide** (Lasix, Salix)

Adverse Side Effects. These include hypokalemia (because of the increased excretion of potassium), other fluid and electrolyte abnormalities, ototoxicity, gastrointestinal distress, hematologic effects, weakness, and restlessness (Plumb, 2015).

 TECHNICIAN NOTES

A potassium supplement may be given to patients who are receiving long-term potassium-depleting diuretic therapy to prevent hypokalemia.

Osmotic Diuretics

Osmotic diuretics can be administered intravenously to promote diuresis by exerting high osmotic pressure in the kidney tubules and limiting tubular reabsorption. Water is drawn into the glomerular filtrate, which reduces its reabsorption rate and increases the excretion of water. These drugs may be used to treat oliguric acute renal failure and to reduce intracranial pressure.

Clinical Uses. These drugs are used for oliguric renal failure, reduction of intraocular and cerebrospinal fluid (intracerebral) pressure, and rapid reduction of edema or ascites (Plumb, 2015).

Dosage Forms
• **Mannitol 20%**
• **Glycerine** (oral)

Adverse Side Effects. These drugs should not be used in patients with anuria secondary to renal disease, in patients that are severely dehydrated, or in patients with pulmonary congestion or edema. Osmotic diuretics may cause fluid and electrolyte imbalances (Plumb, 2015).

Thiazide Diuretics

Thiazide diuretics reduce edema by inhibiting reabsorption of sodium, chloride, and water. Their duration of action is longer than that of loop diuretics.

Dosage Forms
• **Chlorothiazide**
• **Hydrochlorothiazide**

Clinical Uses. Chlorothiazide may be used for the treatment of nephrogenic diabetes insipidus and hypertension in dogs. Hydrochlorothiazide may be used in the treatment of calcium oxalate uroliths, hypoglycemia, and as a diuretic for patients with heart failure (Plumb, 2015).

Adverse Side Effects. These include hypokalemia if therapy is prolonged. Hypersensitivity may be a side effect in some individuals. These drugs should not be used during pregnancy or in patients with severe renal disease, preexisting electrolyte/water balance abnormalities, hepatic disease, or diabetes mellitus. The drugs may cause gastrointestinal upset (Plumb, 2015).

 TECHNICIAN NOTES

• Similar to loop diuretics, thiazide diuretics cause an increase in potassium excretion. A potassium supplement may be necessary to prevent hypokalemia.
• These drugs cross the placental border.

Potassium-Sparing Diuretics

Potassium-sparing diuretics have weaker diuretic and antihypertensive effects than other diuretics; therefore, they conserve potassium. These agents are also referred to as *aldosterone antagonists*. They work by antagonizing aldosterone, an adrenal mineralocorticoid. This action enhances the excretion of sodium and water and reduces the excretion of potassium. Aldosterone secretion may be a factor in edema associated with heart failure.

Clinical Uses. Potassium-sparing diuretics are used to help manage edema or fluid retention due to congestive heart failure, ascites, hypertension and other conditions where the body retains excess fluids. It may be used along with furosemide, digoxin, or angiotensin-converting enzyme (ACE) inhibitors in cases of congestive heart failure or fluid retention due to liver failure (Papich, 2016). It is also used in conditions in which hypokalemia is a concern.

Dosage Forms
• **Spironolactone**
• **Triamterene**

Adverse Side Effects. These are uncommon, but hyperkalemia may result if these drugs are administered concurrently with potassium supplements or ACE inhibitors, such as captopril or enalapril. They should not be prescribed for patients with hyperkalemia, Addison's disease, anuria, acute renal failure, or significant renal impairment (Plumb, 2015).

Carbonic Anhydrase Inhibitors

A carbonic anhydrase inhibitor is a substance that decreases the rate of carbonic acid and hydrogen production in the kidney, thereby promoting the excretion of solutes and increasing the rate of urinary output (O'Toole, 2017). These drugs also reduce intraocular pressure by reducing the production of aqueous humor and may be used in the treatment of glaucoma.

Dosage Forms
- **Acetazolamide** (Diamox)
- **Dichlorphenamide** (Daranide)
- **Methazolamide**

Clinical Uses. Acetazolamide may be used in metabolic alkalosis, glaucoma, and hyperkalemic periodic paralysis (HYPP) in horses. Dichlorphenamide is used primarily for open angle glaucoma. Methazolamide is also used primarily for open angle glaucoma (Plumb, 2015).

Adverse Side Effects. These include the ability to cause hypokalemia. Acetazolamide is contraindicated in patients with hepatic, renal, pulmonary, or adrenocortical insufficiency; hyponatremia; hypokalemia; or electrolyte imbalances. Dichlorphenamide and methazolamide are contraindicated in patients with hyperchloremic acidosis (Plumb, 2015).

> **TECHNICIAN NOTES**
>
> Carbonic anhydrase inhibitors have the least efficacy when compared with the other tubular inhibitors and are not commonly used to treat edema.

Cholinergic Agonists

Cholinergic agents act directly or indirectly to promote the function of acetylcholine. Cholinergic agents also may be referred to as *parasympathomimetic agents* because their effects mimic stimulation of the parasympathetic nervous system. Cholinergic agonists mimic the action of natural acetylcholine by directly stimulating cholinergic receptors. Once the cholinergic agonist binds with receptors on the cell membrane of smooth muscles, the permeability of the cell membrane changes, permitting calcium and sodium to enter into the cells. Depolarization of the cell membrane occurs, and muscle contraction is achieved.

Clinical Uses. These drugs are used primarily to increase the contractility of the urinary bladder.

Dosage Form
- **Bethanechol** (Urecholine)

Adverse Side Effects. These include the potential for cholinergic toxicity. They should not be used in patients with gastrointestinal obstructions or if the integrity of the urinary bladder wall is unknown. Other side effects may include salivation, lacrimation, urination, and defecation (SLUD). A cholinergic crisis may occur if this drug is injected intravenously or subcutaneously, so atropine should be readily available (Plumb, 2015).

> **TECHNICIAN NOTES**
>
> - Observe the patient for signs of cholinergic toxicity (e.g., vomiting, defecation, dyspnea, and tremors).
> - Atropine is antidotal.

® Anticholinergic Drugs

The action of anticholinergic drugs is the opposite of that of cholinergic agents. They block the action of acetylcholine at receptor sites in the parasympathetic nervous system. These drugs may also be described as parasympatholytic because of their ability to block the passage of impulses through the parasympathetic nerves. Their action produces muscle relaxation.

Clinical Uses. Anticholinergic drugs can be used for treating urge incontinence by promoting the retention of urine in the urinary bladder.

Dosage Forms
- **Propantheline**
- **Butylhyoscine** (Buscopan)

Adverse Side Effects. These include decreased gastric motility and delayed gastric emptying, which may decrease the absorption of other medications.

® Adrenergic Antagonists

Adrenergic blocking agents disrupt the sympathetic nervous system by blocking impulse transmission at adrenergic neurons, adrenergic receptor sites, or adrenergic ganglia. These agents also may be described as sympatholytic agents because of their ability to block sympathetic nervous system stimulation. The classification of adrenergic antagonists is based on their site of action (i.e., alpha blockers, beta blockers, or autonomic ganglionic blockers).

Alpha-Adrenergic Antagonists

Alpha-adrenergic antagonists relax vascular smooth muscle, enhance peripheral vasodilation, and decrease blood pressure by interrupting the actions of sympathomimetic agents at alpha-adrenergic receptor sites.

Clinical Uses. In the urinary system, these drugs reduce internal sphincter tone when the urethral sphincter is in hypertonus. This action is useful in the treatment of urinary retention because of detrusor areflexia or functional urethral obstruction. Prazosin is effective in controlling moderate to severe hypertension, which may be a complicating factor in chronic renal failure.

Dosage Forms
- **Phenoxybenzamine** (Dibenzyline)
- **Nicergoline** (Sermion)
- **Prazosin** (Minipress)

Adverse Side Effects. These include a rapid decrease in blood pressure, resulting in weakness or syncope after the first dose of prazosin. This is usually self-limiting. Phenoxybenzamine hydrogen chloride (HCl) should not be used in horses exhibiting clinical signs of colic. Phenoxybenzamine HCl may cause increased intraocular pressure, tachycardia, nasal congestion, inhibition of ejaculation, weakness/dizziness, gastrointestinal effects, and constipation in equines. Phenoxybenzamine HCl may have to be obtained through a compounding pharmacy (Plumb, 2015).

> **TECHNICIAN NOTES**
>
> - Prazosin may be used alone or combined with a diuretic to produce the desired effect.
> - Because the liver metabolizes alpha-adrenergic antagonists, dosage modification is not necessary in patients with renal dysfunction.

Beta-Adrenergic Antagonists

Beta-adrenergic antagonists inhibit the action of catecholamines and other sympathomimetic agents at beta-adrenergic receptor sites, thereby inhibiting stimulation of the sympathetic nervous system.

Clinical Uses. These include control of mild to moderate hypertension associated with chronic renal failure.

Dosage Form
- **Propranolol**

Adverse Side Effects. These include decreased cardiac output and the promotion of bronchospasm. Therefore, caution should be exercised with their use in patients with cardiac or pulmonary disease (Cowgill, 1991).

> **TECHNICIAN NOTES**
>
> Combination with a diuretic is common because of the tendency of beta-adrenergic antagonists to cause salt and fluid retention.

Angiotensin-Converting Enzyme Inhibitors

Blood pressure and fluid balance is regulated by the kidneys via the renin-angiotensin system. Cells in the kidney release an enzyme called renin; renin converts angiotensinogen (produced in the liver) to angiotensin I. Angiotensin I is converted into angiotensin II by ACE. Angiotensin II stimulates the release of aldosterone from the adrenal glands and causes retention of sodium and water. This retention causes the fluid volume to increase, which raises the blood pressure. ACE inhibitors block the conversion of angiotensin I to angiotensin II, decrease aldosterone secretion, reduce peripheral arterial resistance, and alleviate vasoconstriction (Fig. 6.8).

Clinical Uses. ACE inhibitors are used to treat heart failure, hypertension, chronic renal failure, and protein-losing glomerulonephropathies in dogs and cats.

Dosage Forms
- **Benazepril**
  - **Fortekor** (veterinary label)
  - **Benazepril** (Lotensin)
- **Captopril** (Capoten)
- **Enalapril** (Enacard)
- **Lisinopril**
- **Ramipril**

Adverse Side Effects. These include complications in patients with renal insufficiency caused by excretion by the kidneys.

Vasodilators and Calcium Channel Blockers

A vasodilator or calcium channel blocker may be substituted for or used in combination with other medications if previous drug therapy to control hypertension fails.

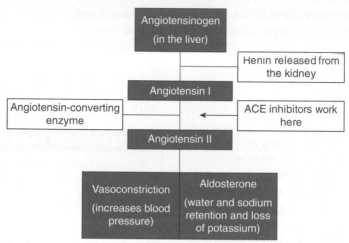

Fig. 6.8 The site of action of angiotensin-converting enzyme *(ACE)* inhibitors on the Renin-Angiotensin-Aldosterone system.

Clinical Uses. These drugs are used to treat non-responding hypertension. Dopamine may be used to promote diuresis in patients unresponsive to loop or osmotic diuretics.

Dosage Forms
- **Vasodilators**
  - **Hydralazine** (Apresoline)
  - **Dopamine** (Intropin)
- **Calcium channel blockers**
  - **Diltiazem** (Cardizem)
  - **Verapamil** (Isoptin)
  - **Amlodipine** (Norvasc)

Adverse Side Effects. These include hypotension, edema, conduction disturbances, heart failure, and bradycardia (Cowgill, 1991). Hydralazine is excreted by the kidneys and requires dosage modification when used to treat hypertension in patients with renal failure.

 Antidiuretic Hormone

Antidiuretic hormone (ADH) is normally secreted by the posterior pituitary gland. This secretion regulates fluid balance in the body. In some conditions, such as pituitary diabetes insipidus, this hormone fails to be synthesized or excreted properly, and **polyuria** and **polydipsia** may occur.

Clinical Uses. ADH is used to treat diabetes insipidus.

Dosage Form
- **Vasopressin** (Pitressin)

Adverse Side Effects. These are uncommon.

TECHNICIAN NOTES

Chlorpropamide (Diabinese, Glucamide) is a human product that is used to control type II diabetes mellitus. It potentiates the action of ADH and may be used to treat mild diabetes insipidus.

 Urinary Acidifiers

Urinary acidifiers are used to produce acid urine, which assists in dissolving and preventing formation of struvite uroliths. Since the introduction of urinary acidifying diets, urinary acidifiers have not been routinely prescribed.

Dosage Forms
- **Methionine** (Methigel, Methio-Tabs)
- **Ammonium chloride** (Uroeze)

Adverse Side Effects. These include gastrointestinal disturbances. These products should not be administered to patients with severe liver, kidney, or pancreatic disease or to those who exhibit acidosis.

TECHNICIAN NOTES

It is very important to inform clients who may change from using an acidifier to one of the available acidifying diets that while the diet is being administered, no acidifiers, salt, vitamin or mineral supplements, or any other food items—other than what is allowed in the diet—should be given to the patient.

BOX 6.1   Case Scenario Urethral Obstruction

A 6-year-old neutered male indoor cat was presented for oliguria and lethargy.

History: The owner stated that he was vocalizing while in the litter box and no clumps of litter was noticed. He is the only cat in the household and she explained that she just cleaned the litter box last night. She also noted that he had been licking at his penis. He is not interested in food or water since yesterday.

Additional history: Up to date on vaccines.

Physical examination findings: The patient was quiet, alert, and responsive. Temperature: 101°F, pulse: 180 bpm, respiration: 48 bpm. A large firm bladder was palpated and could not be expressed with gentle pressure; he had abdominal discomfort. The penis was red and no hard plug was palpable. He was approximately 7%–8% dehydrated.

The veterinary technician anticipated the need of the veterinarian and began to get all supplies ready for an intravenous (IV) catheter, IV fluids (lactated Ringers), 12 mL and 30 mL syringes, sterile water for flushing, urethral catheterization supplies including a tomcat catheter, lube, tape, suture material, etc. Treatment almost begins in conjunction with the diagnostic procedures.

An IV catheter was placed and the patient was premedicated with buprenorphine and midazolam, induced with propofol and maintained on isoflurane. A bolus of dextrose was given IV to drive potassium into the cells and correct the hyperkalemia and cardiac dis-

turbances. The obstruction was alleviated by passage of an open-ended polypropylene urinary catheter into the urethra and sutured into place. Approximately 40 mL of bloody urine was removed from the bladder, and a sample was collected for urinalysis. The urinary bladder was flushed with sterile water. A closed collection urinary system was attached and taped into place. An e-collar was placed on the cat. Recovery from anesthesia was uneventful.

Diagnostic results: Hyperkalemia, hyponatremia, metabolic acidosis. BUN and creatinine were elevated, ECG revealed diminished P waves.

The patient was maintained on IV fluids and given buprenorphine and prazosin (to treat urethral spasm and decrease urethral sphincter tone). The veterinary technician took abdominal radiographs which revealed no opaque uroliths, a small bladder, and no free fluid. The veterinary technician closely monitored urinary output and urinary catheter care every 4 hours. She also palpated the bladder every 2 hours to assess the volume. An ECG was hooked up to the patient to monitor the rate and rhythm. Approximately 3 hours later, the patient was resting quietly. The electrolytes (sodium and potassium) were down to normal range.

Veterinary technician's "hands-on" skills of observing, interpreting, and monitoring are extremely important. The ability to critically think and interpret their observations correctly to provide immediate and complete care is essential in a critically ill patient.

Xanthine Oxidase Inhibitors

Xanthine oxidase inhibitors decrease the production of uric acid and are used in combination with a urate calculolytic diet for the dissolution of ammonium acid urate uroliths. Once dissolution occurs, a urine-alkalizing, low-protein, low-purine, low-oxalate diet is usually prescribed to prevent recurrence of uroliths.

Dosage Form
- **Allopurinol** (Zyloprim)

Clinical Uses. These are used as a uric acid reducer in dogs, cats, reptiles, and birds.

Adverse Side Effects. These are uncommon, but because excretion occurs via the kidneys, the dosage may be altered in patients with renal insufficiency. Xanthine oxidase inhibitors should not be used in red-tailed hawks (Plumb, 2015). Hypersensitivity and hepatic and renal effects can occur.

TECHNICIAN NOTES

In cases of recurrence, allopurinol may once again be prescribed.

Urinary Alkalizers

Urinary alkalizers may be used in the management of ammonium acid urate, calcium oxalate, and cystine urolithiasis.

Dosage Forms
- **Potassium citrate** (Urocit-K)
- **Sodium bicarbonate,** administered orally
- **Tiopronin tablets** (Thiola)

Adverse Side Effects. These include possible fluid and electrolyte imbalance with the use of sodium bicarbonate.

PHARMACOTHERAPY OF RENAL FAILURE COMPLICATIONS

Chronic renal failure can cause an absolute or relative deficiency in erythropoietin production because it is produced by the renal cortex. The resultant complication is normocytic, normochromic anemia that is classified as nonregenerative. Parenteral androgens, such as nandrolone (Durabolin) and testosterone enanthate, are capable of stimulating the production of red blood cell precursors and may increase the level of erythropoietin. Injections of recombinant human erythropoietin (Epogen, Procrit) have been shown to correct anemia associated with chronic renal failure (Ettinger, 2017). Human recombinant erythropoietin (rHuEPO) has been used to treat dogs and cats for anemia associated with chronic renal failure. Because of the expense of the drug and the potential risk of the formation of antibodies to erythropoietin, this drug is considered today to be a "last ditch effort" and the hematocrit level (i.e., packed cell volume [PCV]) should be in the "teens" before its therapy is considered. Hopefully, canine and feline recombinants will be developed in the future to reduce autoantibody formation. In addition, it is hoped that in the future, erythropoietin (EPO) may be demonstrated to have benefits in reducing the number of blood transfusions (Plumb, 2015).

Epoetin Alpha (Epogen, Procrit)

Adverse Side Effects ese include local or systemic allergic reactions in animals and pain occurring at the injection site.

PHARMACOTHERAPY OF URINARY INCONTINENCE

Ettinger (2017) states: "Pharmacologic agents are selected for management of urinary incontinence when urinary tract infection, morphologic abnormalities, and mechanical types of excessive outlet resistance have been excluded as possible causes of the problem." Urinary incontinence may be described as a neurogenic disorder or a nonneurogenic disorder. A neurogenic disorder is evidenced by a neurologic lesion that affects the upper motor neuron segments or the lower motor neuron segments. When upper motor neuron segments are affected, the result is a spastic neuropathic urinary bladder.

Detrusor muscle contractions are normal, but bladder and urethral functions are abnormal. Therefore, as the bladder fills with urine, contractions occur more frequently (hypercontractility) and bladder capacity decreases. In addition, contraction of the detrusor muscle and relaxation of the urethral sphincter often are not coordinated. This results in interrupted, incomplete, and involuntary urination.

Functional urinary obstruction and urinary retention may also be present. When lower motor neuron segments are affected, the result is an atonic, neuropathic urinary bladder. With this disorder, detrusor muscle contractions are abnormal and the sensation of fullness is absent when the urinary bladder fills (hypocontractility). This causes the urinary bladder to distend, and eventually capacity increases. Urinary bladder distention may cause damage to the tight junctions between smooth muscle fibers. Urination eventually occurs when pressure inside the urinary bladder exceeds urethral outlet resistance.

Nonneurogenic disorders occur as a result of some type of anatomic anomaly of the lower urinary tract. In the young dog, this is usually a congenital anomaly. A congenital anomaly seen in young female dogs is ectopic ureter, which causes constant dribbling of urine. This occurs when the ureters end in abnormal places rather than at normal sphincters. In the older dog, acquired anatomic anomalies are usually responsible for nonneurogenic disorders. Conditions that commonly cause such problems include chronic cystitis, chronic urethritis, neoplasia, urolithiasis, and postsurgical adhesions. Other nonneurogenic disorders include functional abnormalities such as urethral incompetence and partial urethral obstruction. One type of nonneurogenic urethral incompetence is often seen in spayed female dogs and is usually responsive to hormonal therapy. Once the cause of the urinary incontinence has been identified, medical or surgical management begins. If a morphologic abnormality is causing urinary incontinence, surgical correction of the problem is necessary.

Medical management may include treatment for infection, if present, and treatment for the cause of the urinary incontinence (e.g., urethral incompetence, urinary bladder hypercontractility or hypocontractility). Drugs used in the medical management of urinary incontinence and urinary retention include the previously mentioned cholinergic agonists, anticholinergics, alpha-adrenergic antagonists, smooth muscle relaxants, skeletal muscle relaxants, tranquilizers, alpha-adrenergic agonists, and hormones such as estrogen and testosterone. Table 6.1 outlines these drugs for easy reference.

Dosage Forms

- **Baclofen** (Lioresal)
- **Diethylstilbestrol** (DES)
- **Estradiol and Estriol** (Incurin)
- **Ephedrine sulfate**
- **Flavoxate HCl** (Urispas)
- **Imipramine** (Tofranil)
- **Oxybutynin** (Ditropan, Oxytrol)
- **Phenylpropanolamine (PPA)** – (Proin)
- Various others

Clinical Uses. Baclofen is used as a muscle relaxant for treating urinary retention in dogs. Ephedrine is a sympathomimetic used for the treatment of urinary incontinence. Estradiol and Estriol are short-acting estrogen drugs used to treat urinary incontinence in spayed female dogs. Flavoxate is a medication used to treat hyperactive urinary bladder and urge incontinence in dogs. Imipramine is a tricyclic antidepressant used to treat urinary incontinence in dogs and cats. Diethylstilbestrol (DES) is a synthetic estrogen hormone used to treat urinary incontinence in spayed females; it is available through compounding pharmacies. Oxybutynin chloride is a genitourinary smooth muscle relaxant used as a urinary antispasmodic in dogs or cats. Phenylpropanolamine HCl is a sympathomimetic used primarily for urethral sphincter hypotonus (Plumb, 2015).

Adverse Side Effects. Baclofen should not be used in cats. It may cause sedation, weakness, pruritis, salivation, and gastrointestinal upset. Ephedrine sulfate is contraindicated in patients with severe cardiovascular disease, glaucoma, prostatic hypertrophy, hyperthyroidism, diabetes mellitus, and hypertension. Diethylstilbestrol should be used at very low doses to avoid toxicity and bone marrow suppression. Flavoxate HCl is not commonly used in veterinary medicine, but the most likely adverse effect is weakness. Imipramine HCl may cause tachycardia, hyperexcitability, and tremors. Phenylpropanolamine HCl should be used cautiously in patients with glaucoma, prostatic hypertrophy, hyperthyroidism, diabetes mellitus, cardiovascular disorders, or hypertension (Plumb, 2015).

Ⓡ Miscellaneous Renal Drugs

Urinary Tract Analgesics

Phenazopyridine. Phenazopyridine is used in humans as a urinary tract analgesic. It can be bought over-the-counter. It can be used alone or with sulfa drugs. Its use is contraindicated in felines because they are quite susceptible to dose-related methemoglobinemia, and oxidative changes in hemoglobin may be irreversible, causing formation of Heinz bodies and anemia (Osborne, 2001).

Tricyclic Antidepressants

Amitriptyline

Amitriptyline (Elavil). Amitriptyline has many properties and has been used in treating interstitial cystitis in humans. Its mechanism is not fully understood. Amitriptyline is a tricyclic antidepressant and anxiolytic

TABLE 6.1	Pharmacotherapy of Urinary Incontinence and Urinary Retention.	
Drug	**Action**	**Examples of Indications**
Bethanechol (Urecholine)	Cholinergic agonist	Bladder hypocontractility
Propantheline	Anticholinergic agent	Urge incontinence, bladder hypercontractility
Phenoxybenzamine (Dibenzyline)	Alpha-adrenergic antagonist	Urethral hyperreflexia
Nicergoline (Sermion)	Alpha-adrenergic antagonist	Urethral hyperreflexia
Aminopropazine (Jenotone)	Smooth muscle relaxant	Urge incontinence, bladder hypercontractility
Dantrolene (Dantrium)	Skeletal muscle relaxant	Urethral hyperreflexia
Diazepam (Valium)	Tranquilizer/skeletal muscle relaxant	Urethral hyperreflexia
Phenylpropanolamine	Alpha-adrenergic agonist	Urethral incompetence
Diethylstilbestrol (DES) (available through a compounding pharmacy)	Antineoplastic, estrogen (hormone)	Hormone-responsive urethral incompetence
Estradiol and Estriol (Incurin)	Estrogen hormone	Hormone-responsive urethral incompetence
Testosterone cypionate	Hormone	Hormone-responsive urethral incompetence
Testosterone propionate	Hormone	Hormone-responsive urethral incompetence

drug with anticholinergic, antihistaminic, anti–alpha-adrenergic, antiinflammatory, and analgesic properties. It has been used extensively for the treatment of interstitial cystitis in humans. Although it is a popular drug, its exact mechanism of action and therapeutic value in managing patients with interstitial cystitis remain unknown. This drug has been used recently for symptomatic treatment of idiopathic feline lower urinary tract disease (FLUTD) (Plumb, 2015).

Adverse Side Effects. Many side effects such as dry mouth, rapid heart rate, and sedation (i.e., antihistamine effects) are associated with this drug. High doses can cause heart toxicity. Sometimes it may cause cats to be less interested in grooming themselves. Additionally, weight gain may occur (Papich, 2016).

Glycosaminoglycans

Glycosaminoglycans (GAGs) are found covering the transitional epithelium of the urinary tract. These urothelial GAGs have the ability to keep microorganisms and crystals from adhering to the urinary bladder wall and limit the transepithelial movement of urine proteins and solutes (ionic or nonionic). Defects in surface GAGs and subsequent urothelial permeability are believed to be a factor in the pathogenesis of idiopathic FLUTD (Osborne, 2001).

Pentosan Polysulfate Sodium (Elmiron)

Clinical Uses. This drug is often used to manage human interstitial cystitis and has been used to reinforce urothelial GAGs and to reduce transitional cell injury. It has been used in the adjunctive treatment of feline interstitial cystitis or FLUTD. However, studies using pentosan for FLUTD have shown that it is not effective for short-term acute FLUTD (Plumb, 2015).

Adverse Side Effects. The safety and efficacy of pentosan polysulfate or other GAGs for the treatment of FLUTD have not been reported. In canines, vomiting, anorexia, lethargy, or mild depression are possible. Pentosan has some anticoagulant effects, so bleeding is possible in any species (Plumb, 2015).

Other Agents

Epakitin. Epakitin is a chitosan-based nutritional supplement made from a polysaccharide extracted from crab and shrimp shells.

Clinical Uses. The product information states that Epakitin binds phosphorus in the intestine, causing phosphorus to be eliminated through the intestinal tract. Reducing the amount of phosphorus absorbed then helps to lower the elevated levels of phosphorus noted in renal failure

Azodyl. Azodyl is a nutritional supplement that has the potential to reduce the azotemia of renal failure by flushing out uremic toxins and slowing down uremic toxin buildup to help prevent further damage to the kidney.

TECHNICIAN'S ROLE

Veterinary technicians have a vital role in the care of patients with problems that affect the urinary system. This role includes providing client support and education, carrying out patient nursing care, performing necessary laboratory or radiologic examinations, providing surgical assistance, and understanding the various drugs and diets available for the treatment of renal disease.

▌ REVIEW QUESTIONS

1. What structures constitute the urinary system?
2. Name two drugs that are contraindicated in uremic patients.
3. Renal damage may be categorized as _____, _____ _____, or _____.
4. Explain how diuretics work.
5. What supplement may be administered in conjunction with loop diuretics?
6. What drug is a potassium-sparing diuretic?
7. Which one of the following is an osmotic diuretic?
   a. Chlorothiazole
   b. Mannitol
   c. Furosemide
   d. Spironolactone
8. ACE inhibitors block the conversion of angiotensin I to _____.
9. Urinary acidifiers are used to produce acid urine, which assists in dissolving and preventing the formation of _____ uroliths.
10. The renal cortex produces_____; thus chronic renal failure can cause an absolute or relative _____ in its production.
11. Why is furosemide referred to as a loop diuretic?

12. Name a beta-adrenergic blocker drug that is used to control mild to moderate hypertension associated with chronic renal failure?

13. Enalapril is a(n) _____.
    a. anticholinergic
    b. vasoconstrictor
    c. cholinergic agonist
    d. ACE inhibitor

14. Where is ADH secreted? _____

15. The ureters ____.
    a. originate from the urinary bladder and lead to the outside of the body.
    b. originate from the kidneys and connect with the urinary bladder.
    c. are found inside the nephrons.
    d. are found inside the glomerulus.

16. Persistently high blood pressure is known as _____.
    a. hypertonus
    b. hyperkalemia
    c. hypertension
    d. atony

17. Diuretics are used to remove ____ fluid.
    a. intracellular
    b. extracellular

18. Antidiuretic hormone (ADH) is normally secreted by the _____ pituitary gland.
    a. anterior
    b. posterior

19. What supplement may be administered in conjunction with loop diuretics?
    a. Calcium
    b. Phosphorus
    c. Aluminum hydrochloride
    d. Potassium

20. Urinary acidifiers are used to produce acid urine, which assists in dissolving and preventing the formation of ____.
    a. calcium
    b. uroliths
    c. urinary casts
    d. bacteria

21. Patients with renal failure are at a lesser anesthetic risk than patients with normal renal function.
    a. True
    b. False

22. Loop diuretics inhibit the tubular reabsorption of _____.
    a. calcium
    b. phosphorus
    c. sodium
    d. potassium

23. A border collie named Sam is presented to the veterinarian and diagnosed with CHF, chronic kidney failure, and clinical signs of pulmonary edema. Sam weighs 40 lb and the veterinarian prescribes furosemide at 3.5 mg/kg once a day for a month. The pharmacy has on hand 50-mg, 20-mg, and 12.5-mg furosemide tablets. What is the dose that Sam should receive each day? What milligram tablets should be dispensed and how many?
    a. 64 mg/day; furosemide (50 mg × 30 tablets) and furosemide (12.5 mg × 30 tablets)
    b. 140 mg/day; furosemide (50 mg × 90 tablets)
    c. 70 mg/day; furosemide (50 mg × 30 tablets) and furosemide (20 mg × 30 tablets)
    d. 35 mg/day; furosemide (20 mg × 30 tablets) and furosemide (12.5 mg × 30 tablets) and furosemide (12.5 mg × 7.5 tablets [cut in quarter-size tablets])

24. The veterinarian orders a prescription of furosemide at 2.5 mg/kg b.i.d. for a patient that weighs 55 lb. How many milligrams should the patient receive for one dose?
    a. 25 mg
    b. 62.5 mg
    c. 61.5 mg
    d. 18.3 mg

25. A dog weighing 33 lb with protein-losing nephropathy is presented to the veterinarian who orders enalapril 0.5 mg/kg PO once daily. What is the dose this dog requires?
    a. 5.5 mg daily
    b. 7.5 mg daily
    c. 9.5 mg daily
    d. 2.5 mg daily

REFERENCES

Cowgill, L. D. (1991). Clinical significance, diagnosis, and management of systemic hypertension in dogs and cats. In L. D. Cowgill (Ed.), *Managing renal disease and hypertension*. Kansas City: Harmon-Smith.

Ettinger, S. J. (2017). *Textbook of veterinary internal medicine expert consult* (8th ed., Vols. I and II). St. Louis, MO: Elsevier.

O'Toole, M. T. (2017). (8th ed.). *Mosby's pocket dictionary of medicine, nursing and health professionals*. St. Louis, Missouri: Elsevier.

Osborne, C. A. (2001). Idiopathic lower urinary tract diseases: Therapeutic rights and wrongs. In *Proceedings. Annual meeting of the American Veterinary Medical Association*. Boston.

Papich, M. G. (2016). *Saunders handbook of veterinary drugs* (4th ed.). Philadelphia: Elsevier.

Plumb, D. C. (2015). *Veterinary drug handbook* (8th ed.). Ames, IA: Wiley-Blackwell.

7

Drugs Used in Cardiovascular System Disorders

OBJECTIVES

After studying this chapter, you should be able to

1. Describe the basic anatomy and physiology of the cardiovascular system.
2. List four compensatory mechanisms of the cardiovascular system.
3. List five basic objectives of the treatment of cardiovascular disease.
4. List and describe the indications, physiologic effects, and toxic side effects of the cardiac glycosides.
5. List the four categories of antiarrhythmic drugs, give an example from each category, and list potential adverse side effects of antiarrhythmic drugs.
6. Describe the actions and potential side effects of the vasodilator drugs.
7. Describe the actions and potential side effects of the angiotensin-converting enzyme (ACE) inhibitors.
8. Describe the actions and potential side effects of the diuretics used to treat cardiovascular disease.
9. Describe the purpose of dietary sodium restriction in the therapy of cardiovascular disease.
10. List ancillary drugs or procedures that may be used in the treatment of cardiovascular disease.

OUTLINE

KEY TERMS

Afterload

Arrhythmia (dysrhythmia)

Automaticity

Bradyarrhythmia

Bradycardia

Cardiac output

Cardiac remodeling

Chronotropic

Depolarization

Diastole

Inotropic

Preload

Premature ventricular contraction

Repolarization

Stroke volume

Systole

Tachyarrhythmia

Tachycardia

INTRODUCTION

Heart disease has a relatively high incidence in veterinary medicine. Studies have found that approximately 11% of all dogs presented to veterinary clinics exhibited some degree of heart disease (Roudebush et al., 2000). Heart disease may be congenital or acquired. However, the acquired form accounts for most cases. The incidence and cause may vary from location to location. Heartworm disease accounts for a large percentage of heart disease in some parts of the country, whereas acquired disease of the atrioventricular valves or myocardium has a more uniform distribution. Acquired disease is encountered more often in older animals, and congenital disease is more prevalent in younger ones.

Whatever the cause, treatment of heart disease is often individualized to the particular patient according to cause, degree of progression, and owner cooperation. The response to treatment must be monitored carefully and adjusted while the disease progresses, which may cause poor liver or kidney function, or while toxic side effects develop. Some cardiovascular drugs have a narrow margin of safety (i.e., they are potentially toxic at low doses), and failing liver and kidney function may reduce the body's ability to metabolize or eliminate these drugs.

Veterinary technicians are often the persons who monitor the progress of hospitalized patients, thus they must be aware of the signs of cardiovascular disease and of normal and abnormal responses to drugs used to treat this disease.

ANATOMY AND PHYSIOLOGY OF THE HEART

The heart is a four-chambered pump that is responsible for moving blood through the vascular system. The

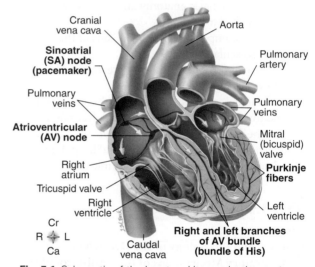

Fig. 7.1 Schematic of the heart and its conduction system.

two dorsal chambers are called *atria*, and the two ventral chambers are called *ventricles* (Fig. 7.1). Each of the chambers is composed primarily of strong muscle tissue called *myocardium*, which contracts to eject the blood. Even though the heart is considered one organ, it functions as two pumps (Spinelli & Enos, 1978).

The right atrium and ventricle constitute the "right-side pump," and the left atrium and ventricle make up the "left-side pump." Blood from the general circulation returns by way of the vena cava to the right atrium, enters the right ventricle through the right atrioventricular valve (tricuspid valve), and is pumped through the pulmonary artery to the lungs. In the lungs, the blood gives up carbon dioxide and picks up oxygen. The oxygenated blood returns to the heart via the pulmonary veins, where it fills the left atrium, passes through the left atrioventricular valve (mitral valve), and enters the left ventricle. The mitral and tricuspid valves swing open when the atria contract and snap shut when the ventricles contract. The closing of the valves as the ventricles contract prevents blood from flowing back into the atria. The left ventricle then contracts and ejects the oxygenated blood through the aorta into the branching arteries. These arteries divide into arterioles and end in the thin-walled capillaries throughout the body, where carbon dioxide is loaded to the blood and oxygen is unloaded to the tissue. The left ventricular wall is thicker than the right ventricular wall because the left ventricle must work harder to pump blood throughout the body compared with the right ventricle that pumps blood to the lungs.

The pumping action of the heart is divided into two phases—systole and diastole. **Systole** is the period of contraction of the chambers, and **diastole** represents the relaxation phase when the chambers are filling with blood. Because each cell in the heart is capable of contracting spontaneously, the interaction of these two phases must be carefully coordinated to create an efficient pumping action. Diastolic time must be adequate to allow the atria to fill completely, and atrial systole must occur shortly before ventricular systole to allow the ventricles to fill maximally. Coordination of these two phases is achieved primarily through a wave of electric activity that arises in a specialized group of cells in the right atrium and then is conducted throughout the myocardium by a special conduction system.

The structures that make up the cardiac conduction system (see Fig. 7.1) include the sinoatrial node, the atrioventricular node, the bundle of His and its branches, and the Purkinje system. Under abnormal conditions, parts of the myocardium and conduction system are capable of spontaneous discharge. Normally, however, the sinoatrial node discharges most rapidly and spreads a wave of depolarization over remaining areas of the heart before they can depolarize spontaneously. The rate of discharge of this node therefore controls the heart rate and is called the *cardiac pacemaker.* Impulses generated by the sinoatrial node travel over the atria to the atrioventricular node, face a brief delay (about 0.1 second) in the atrioventricular node, travel down the bundle of His to its left and right branches, and pass into the ventricular muscle via the Purkinje fibers (located at the apex of the heart). Myocardial cells are joined together by structures called *intercalated disks* and by fusing of cell membranes into an interconnected mass of cells

called a *syncytium.* The syncytium of cells in the atria is separate and is insulated from the syncytium in the ventricles (Ganong, 2003). An electric stimulus from the sinoatrial node is transmitted over the entire atrial mass by the syncytial arrangement of cells. The impulse is not, however, transmitted directly into the ventricular syncytium. The impulse first must be picked up and transmitted by the atrioventricular node through its conduction system to the ventricular syncytium. Stimulation of a single atrial or ventricular muscle fiber causes the entire atrial or ventricular muscle mass to contract as a unit. When situations cause spontaneous depolarization of cardiac muscle or abnormalities of the conduction system, **arrhythmias** may occur.

When a cardiac cell is stimulated by electric activity that arises in the sinoatrial node, it undergoes depolarization and contracts. **Depolarization** is characterized by the rapid influx of sodium ions into the cell through channels or "gates," the slower influx of calcium ions, and the outflow of potassium ions (Fig. 7.2). Until the sodium, potassium, and calcium ions have returned to the positions they had before depolarization, the cell is in a refractory period (Fig. 7.3). A cell in an absolute refractory state cannot normally depolarize. In a relative refractory period, however, a cardiac cell can depolarize again, but the stimulus must be stronger than normal. A refractory period is essential for a cardiac cell to prevent it from remaining in a constant state of contraction as the result of stimulation by recycling impulses. The return of the ions to their original positions is brought about in part by the sodium-potassium pump and is an essential part of the **repolarization** process. Summed electric activity arising from the contraction of all heart cells represents the electrocardiogram (Fig. 7.4A,B), and each of its waves signifies activity in a particular area. An electrocardiogram (EKG or ECG) is a recording of the electrical activity of the heart and evaluates the rhythm of the heart. The P wave reflects depolarization of the right and left atrium and atrial contraction. The PR interval is the distance between the onset of the P wave to the onset of the QRS complex. The QRS complex refers to depolarization of the ventricles and ventricular contraction. The T wave follows the QRS complex and reflects repolarization of the ventricles (see Fig. 7.4).

Even though the heart establishes its own inherent rate of beating, this rate is subject to outside influences through the autonomic nervous system. The sympathetic portion of the autonomic nervous system, through beta$_1$ receptors, produces positive **chronotropic** and **inotropic** effects on the heart. The parasympathetic

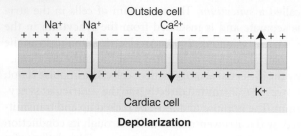

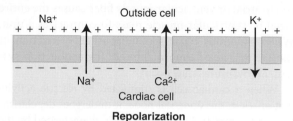

Fig. 7.2 Depolarization and repolarization of a cardiac cell. Repolarization: the sodium–potassium–adenosine triphosphate pump restores electrolytes to their resting sites.

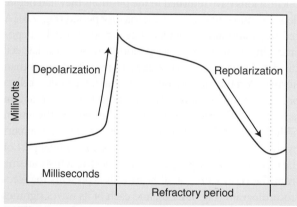

Fig. 7.3 Schematic of the refractory period of a cardiac cell. After depolarization (contraction), cardiac muscle cells are unable to contract again until they have undergone repolarization. The time during which they are unable to contract is the refractory period.

branch of the autonomic nervous system causes negative chronotropic effects through cholinergic receptors.

The heart pumps blood through a series of arteries (arterial tree) to deliver it to the tissues. The larger of these arteries have elastic properties, which allow them to stretch and recover when blood is pumped into them, thereby serving as a second pump (Upson, 1988). The smaller arteries are capable of changing their diameter (constricting or dilating) through the action of smooth

muscle in their walls to increase or decrease the resistance against which the heart must pump. Stimulation of alpha-1 receptors causes vessels to constrict, and stimulation of beta$_2$ receptors causes vessels to dilate.

The amount of blood that the heart is capable of pumping per minute is called *cardiac output*; this value is calculated by multiplying the heart rate by the stroke volume. The stroke volume is determined in part by the amount of blood that fills the ventricle during diastole, called the *preload*, and the arterial resistance that the ventricle must pump against, called the *afterload*.

COMPENSATORY MECHANISMS OF THE CARDIOVASCULAR SYSTEM

The cardiovascular system has a built-in reserve capacity, which allows it to increase its output during times of need (e.g., athletic performance) and to compensate for cardiac disease. The four basic factors of cardiac reserve or compensation are described as follows:

1. Increasing the heart rate. Increasing the rate of contraction increases cardiac output up to the point at which the rate is so fast that there is inadequate time for ventricular filling.
2. Increasing the stroke volume. Up to a point, an increased force of contraction results in an increase in the amount of blood that is pumped.
3. Increasing the efficiency of the heart muscle.
4. Cardiac remodeling. The heart is composed of muscle that responds to work by increasing its size and becoming stronger. This change usually precedes the development of heart failure signs by months or years.

Many disorders can result in cardiac disease. However, most that respond to pharmacologic therapy fall into one of the following categories:

- **Valvular disease.** Valvular insufficiency, a backflow or leakage of blood backward through the valve, is a relatively common acquired heart disorder of dogs. If the tricuspid valve is affected, ascites may occur. If the mitral valve is involved, pulmonary edema may result. Valvular disease may result from progressive bacterial endocarditis. Inadequate opening of valves may also occur and cause disease. Insufficiency or stenosis may be accompanied by a murmur.
- **Cardiac arrhythmias.** If a focus of cardiac tissue depolarizes out of sequence with the sinoatrial node, an arrhythmia may result. Various types of arrhythmias, including **tachyarrhythmias** (arrhythmias

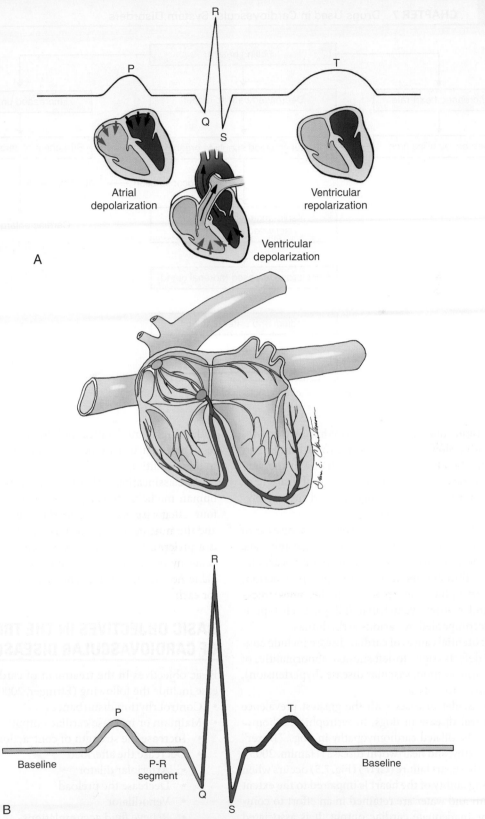

Fig. 7.4 (A and B) Cardiac events as depicted on an electrocardiogram. Electrical signal patterns of the heart. (B, From Christenson, D. E. [2020]. *Veterinary medical terminology* [2nd ed.]. St. Louis: Elsevier.)

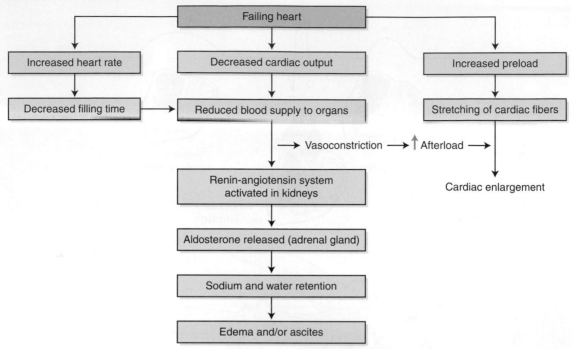

Fig. 7.5 Pathophysiology of congestive heart failure.

with a rapid rate) and bradyarrhythmias (arrhythmias with a slow rate), may occur. Arrhythmias may occur in the atria (supraventricular) or in the ventricles (ventricular). Several categories of drugs (e.g., catecholamines, xylazine, digoxin, and others) predispose the heart to arrhythmias.

- **Myocardial disease.** Cardiomyopathy, a disease of the myocardium, primarily affects dogs and cats. It may be classified as congestive (the myocardium becomes thin and ineffective in its pumping action) or hypertrophic (the myocardium becomes thickened and restricts ventricular filling). Each type is often accompanied by various arrhythmias.
- Other potential causes of cardiac disease include congenital defects (right-to-left shunts), abnormalities of cardiac innervation, vascular disease (hypertension), and heartworm disease.

Cardiovascular diseases with the greatest prevalence include mitral disease in dogs, hypertrophic cardiomyopathy in cats, dilated cardiomyopathy in dogs, "Boxer" cardiomyopathy, and heartworm disease (Hamlin, 2003).

Congestive heart failure (CHF) (Fig. 7.5) occurs when the pumping ability of the heart is impaired to the extent that sodium and water are retained in an effort to compensate for inadequate cardiac output. It is associated with exercise intolerance, pulmonary edema, and ascites. The heart usually becomes structurally remodeled in this condition.

A classification scheme has been adapted from human medicine to categorize veterinary patients into four categories according to the course of the disease and the treatment for each stage because cardiac disease is a progressive condition in which structural changes occur before clinical signs appear (DeFrancesco, 2013). Table 7.1 lists these stages and general treatment options for each.

BASIC OBJECTIVES IN THE TREATMENT OF CARDIOVASCULAR DISEASE

Basic objectives in the treatment of cardiovascular disease include the following (Ettinger, 2000):
- Control rhythm disturbances
- Maintain or increase cardiac output
  - Increase the strength of contraction
  - Decrease the afterload
    - Arteriolar dilator
    - Decrease the preload
    - Venodilator
    - Relieve fluid accumulations

TABLE 7.1	Stages and Treatment of Cardiac Disease.	
Stage	**Description/Signs**	**Treatment**
A	High risk for development of heart failure but no structural abnormality of the heart	None
B	Structural abnormality present but no signs of heart failure	ACEI Beta blockers Restricted sodium diet
C	Structural abnormality present, and current or previous signs of heart failure/coughing, reduced exercise tolerance	Dog: diuretic, pimobendan ACEI, sodium restricted diet Cat: diuretic, ACEI
D	End stage signs of heart failure resistant to standard treatment/dyspnea at rest	Multimodal therapy

ACEI, Angiotensin-converting enzyme inhibitor.

- Diuretics
- Dietary salt restriction
- Increase the oxygenation of the blood
  - Bronchodilation
- Ancillary treatment
  - Narcotics/sedatives
  - Oxygen

CATEGORIES OF CARDIOVASCULAR DRUGS

℞ Positive Inotropic Drugs

The general principle involved in the use of drugs that improve the strength of contraction is that the heart, even in the presence of disease, has reserve capacity for contraction that can be called on to improve cardiac output. Some clinicians advise cautious use of positive inotropic drugs because these can increase the oxygen demand of cardiac muscle, can potentially damage the contractile apparatus, and can increase the tendency for arrhythmias. Proof of clinical efficacy of positive inotropic drugs is lacking, and their use is controversial (Boothe, 2012). Their popularity has waxed and waned through the years as newer, more effective products have come into use.

Cardiac Glycosides (Digitalis)

The digitalis compounds (digoxin and digitoxin) are obtained from the dried leaves of the plant *Digitalis purpurea.* The beneficial effects of these compounds have been known for hundreds of years and include (1) improved cardiac contractility, (2) decreased heart rate, (3) antiarrhythmic effects, and (4) decreased signs of dyspnea.

Digitalis increases the strength of contraction by increasing the level of calcium ions available in the

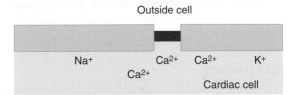

Outside cell

Fig. 7.6 Effect of digitalis on the sodium–potassium–adenosine triphosphate (ATPase) pump. Digitalis compounds block the sodium–potassium–ATPase enzyme, reduce the amount of Ca^{2+} pumped from the cell during repolarization, and increase the amount of Ca^{2+} available for depolarization.

contractile filaments within cardiac muscle cells. This action occurs as a result of inhibition of sodium–potassium–adenosine triphosphatase (Fig. 7.6). The heart rate is slowed by prolonging atrioventricular conduction time and by increasing parasympathetic, autonomic stimulation. The primary actions of the digitalis drugs are to (1) increase the force of contraction, (2) decrease the rate of contraction, and (3) improve baroreceptor function (Hamlin, 2003).

Digitalis use is indicated in patients with cardiac disease that results from impaired cardiac contraction or atrial arrhythmias as suggested by clinical signs such as exercise intolerance, weak peripheral pulses, pulmonary edema, and coughing—or by electrocardiographic diagnosis.

Clinical Uses. Clinical uses of the digitalis compounds include the treatment of CHF, atrial fibrillation, and supraventricular tachycardia.

Dosage Forms. Dosage forms include tablets and elixirs.

- **Digoxin tablets** (Lanoxin)
- **Digoxin oral solution** (Lanoxin)

Adverse Side Effects. Adverse side effects from the use of digitalis compounds are often associated with high or toxic serum levels of drugs and can include anorexia, vomiting, diarrhea, and various arrhythmias. Cats are relatively more sensitive than dogs to toxic effects (Plumb, 2015). Animals with kidney dysfunction must receive lower doses to avoid accumulating toxic concentrations. Digitalis compounds are adversely affected when given concurrently with many drugs (e.g., cimetidine, metoclopramide, diazepam, anticholinergics, and others). Consult appropriate references for suitability.

> **TECHNICIAN NOTES**
>
> • The bioavailability of digoxin varies from 60% in tablet form to 75% in elixir form, and adjustments are likely needed if the dosage form is changed.
> • Clients should be advised to monitor their pets carefully for signs of toxicity and to advise the veterinarian if any arise.

Catecholamines

Catecholamines include a group of sympathomimetic (adrenergic) compounds that (1) increase the force and rate of muscular contraction of the heart (increase in cardiac output), (2) constrict peripheral blood vessels (increase blood pressure), and (3) elevate blood glucose levels. Catecholamines increase cardiac contractility primarily by stimulating beta$_1$ receptors. Catecholamines are used mainly for short-term management of severe heart failure because of their short serum half-lives.

Epinephrine. Epinephrine is the preferred drug for providing stimulation for contraction of the heart and for supporting the circulatory system after cardiac arrest. It may be administered by the intracardiac, intratracheal, or intravenous route. Epinephrine is not used for therapy of chronic heart failure because it greatly increases the workload of the heart and increases the tendency for arrhythmias.

Clinical Uses. Epinephrine is used in veterinary medicine for cardiac resuscitation and for the treatment of anaphylaxis.

Dosage Forms
• **Epinephrine hydrogen chloride** (HCl) for injection
Adverse Side Effects. These include hypertension, arrhythmias, anxiety, and excitability.

> **TECHNICIAN NOTES**
>
> • Epinephrine is available in two concentrations: 1 mg/mL (1:1,000) and 0.1 mg/mL (1:10,000).

Isoproterenol. Isoproterenol is seldom used in the treatment of cardiac disease. It is indicated in atropine-resistant bradycardia.

Clinical Uses. Isoproterenol is used in the treatment of cardiac arrhythmias and acute bronchial constriction. It is not commonly used in veterinary medicine.

Dosage Forms
• **Isuprel**
Adverse Side Effects. These include tachycardia and ventricular arrhythmias.

Dopamine. Dopamine is a biosynthetic precursor of norepinephrine. It stimulates dopaminergic receptors in coronary, mesenteric, renal, and cerebral vascular beds. It also is capable of stimulating alpha- and beta-adrenergic receptors to increase heart contractility, heart rate, and blood pressure. Dopamine use in cardiac cases is mainly limited to heart failure associated with anesthetic emergencies or after cardiac resuscitation.

Clinical Uses. Dopamine is used for adjunctive treatment of acute heart failure and oliguric renal failure and for the supportive treatment of shock.

Dosage Forms
• **Dopamine HCl**
• **Dopamine HCl in 5% dextrose**
Adverse Side Effects. These include vomiting, tachycardia, dyspnea, and blood pressure variations (hypotension or hypertension).

Dobutamine. Dobutamine is a synthetic inotropic agent related structurally to dopamine. It causes increased cardiac contractility, as does dopamine, but does not produce dilation of selected vascular beds. Dobutamine is a direct beta$_1$-adrenergic agent. It produces increased cardiac output with little tendency to cause arrhythmias or increased heart rate. It is available only as a human label product and is administered in diluted form by intravenous infusion. Consult the *Veterinary Drug Handbook* (Plumb, 2015) for directions on preparation of the solution for infusion.

Clinical Uses. Dobutamine is used in patients with acute signs of heart failure such as dilated cardiomyopathy.

Dosage Forms
• **Dobutrex**
Adverse Side Effects. These include tachycardia and ventricular arrhythmias.

TECHNICIAN NOTES

- Dopamine and dobutamine must be diluted before use and are given as a constant rate infusion.

Bipyridine Derivatives

Amrinone and milrinone are representatives of a new class of positive inotropic drugs that appear to work by inhibiting enzymes that ultimately lead to an increase in cellular calcium. Amrinone (Inocor) is given intravenously and is limited to short-term inpatient use, whereas milrinone is given orally and has potential for long-term use.

Inotropic, Mixed Dilator

Pimobendan. Pimobendan was approved for use in veterinary medicine in April, 2007. It is a positive inotropic drug that increases the calcium sensitivity of cardiac myofilaments and inhibits the enzyme phosphodiesterase. Pimobendan produces balanced vasodilation (combination of venous and arterial dilation) leading to a reduction of both cardiac preload and afterload (Gordon, 2019).

Clinical Uses. Pimobendan is labeled for the treatment of atrioventricular insufficiency, CHF, and dilated cardiomyopathy in dogs.

Dosage Form
- **Vetmedin** Chewable Tablets

Adverse Side Effects. Side effects may include anorexia, lethargy, diarrhea, atrial fibrillation, and others.

Contraindication. Pimobendan is contraindicated in cases of hypertrophic cardiomyopathy, aortic stenosis, or any other condition when cardiac augmentation is inappropriate for anatomic reasons.

Ⓡ Antiarrhythmic Drugs

An arrhythmia is a variation from the normal rhythm of the heart. Such a variation may result from an abnormality of impulse generation (increased **automaticity**) or from abnormalities of impulse conduction. Many arrhythmias arise when a local group of cells begin to depolarize faster than the sinoatrial node (pacemaker), which causes disruption of the normal depolarization pattern of the heart. The location of this group of cells is called an *ectopic focus* (foci if more than one location is involved). Arrhythmias usually result in reduced cardiac output caused by poorly coordinated pumping activity.

Some arrhythmias may be auscultated by an experienced ear, but arrhythmias more often are diagnosed through their production of abnormal waveforms seen on an electrocardiogram.

Factors that may cause or predispose the heart to arrhythmias include the following:
- Conditions that cause hypoxemia
- Electrolyte imbalances
- Increased levels of or increased sensitivity to catecholamines
- Drugs such as digitalis compounds, xylazine, and others
- Cardiac trauma or disease that results in altered cardiac cells

Arrhythmias are classified in relation to heart rate as tachyarrhythmias or bradyarrhythmias. Tachyarrhythmias are further classified into ventricular or atrial, depending on their location, and can lead to rapid contraction rates in corresponding chambers. At these rapid rates, pumping efficiency is greatly reduced because of decreased filling time. Rapid, uncoordinated activity called *flutter* or *fibrillation* may also result.

Pharmacologists classify antiarrhythmic drugs into the following four basic categories (Boothe, 2012):
1. Class IA includes quinidine, procainamide, and others.
   Class IB includes lidocaine, tocainide, and mexiletine.
   Class IC includes flecainide and encainide.
2. Class II includes the beta-adrenergic blockers (propranolol).
3. Class III includes bretylium and amiodarone.
4. Class IV includes the calcium channel blockers (verapamil, nifedipine, amlodipine, and diltiazem).

Class IA

Class IA drugs include quinidine and procainamide. Drugs in Class IA depress myocardial excitability, prolong the refractory period, decrease automaticity, and increase conduction times. Class IA drugs are used to treat atrial and ventricular arrhythmias and may be given orally on a long-term basis.

Quinidine. Quinidine is an alkaloid that is obtained from cinchona plants or is prepared from quinine (Plumb, 2015).

Clinical Uses. Quinidine is used to treat ventricular arrhythmias and atrial fibrillation in small animals and horses.

BOX 7.1   **Case Scenario Left Sided Congestive Heart Failure**

A 12-year-old female spayed Chihuahua mix named Mimi presented with the chief complaint of difficulty breathing.

History: The owner stated during the last 3 weeks Mimi seems to be coughing more, especially at night or when laying down. She seems to be quiet and lethargic, and seems to tire easily while on walks. She has not eaten for the past 2 days. There is no vomiting or diarrhea. History of heart murmur, but owner said it was a "soft" murmur. Mimi is not on any medication. Up to date on vaccinations. No travel history.

Physical examination findings: Quiet, alert, and responsive. Temperature: 98.5°F, pulse: 170 bpm with pulse deficits, respiratory rate: 80 bpm with cheek puffing and abdominal component, mucous membranes: cyanotic, CRT: 4 sec. A grade IV/VI apical holosystolic heart murmur was heard on auscultation of the chest. The veterinary technician hooked up the pulse ox to get an SpO_2 (room air): 90%.

The veterinary technician prepared the anesthesia machine for delivery of oxygen via a mask. Other supplies for IV catheter, blood tubes, syringes and needles, pulse ox, blood pressure machine and ECG were obtained.

Mimi was stabilized with oxygen via a mask and butorphanol was given intramuscularly. The patient calmed down and an IV catheter was placed without causing further stress.

The veterinary technician obtained blood for a complete blood count (CBC) and chemistry, hooked up the ECG, blood pressure machine, and pulse ox. The veterinary technician took note if Mimi was becoming stressed while performing these procedures.

Diagnostic results: The ECG revealed a sinus tachycardia, blood pressure: 80 mm Hg, SpO_2: 97% on oxygen. CBC and chemistry were unremarkable.

Once stabilized the veterinary technician took thoracic radiographs and set up for an ultrasound. Thoracic radiographs revealed cardiomegaly with left atrial enlargement, enlarged pulmonary vasculature, interstitial pattern most prominent in the caudodorsal lung fields. The ultrasound revealed no pleural or pericardial effusion, left atrial enlargement, and fluid lines in the caudal and dorsal lung fields.

Diagnosis: Left sided congestive heart failure

The veterinary technician set up the oxygen cage and placed Mimi inside and set the oxygen flow rate at 40% per doctor's instruction. Mimi was started on a furosemide CRI (constant rate infusion) to be given for 4 hours. She closely monitored the respiratory rate and effort, mucous membrane color, and CRT. She started Mimi on pimobendan per the doctor's instruction.

An ECHO (electrocardiograph) was scheduled for Mimi.

Veterinary technicians play an important role in the day-to-day procedures in veterinary practice. Having the knowledge of normal physiology of the cardiovascular system, how cardiac drugs alter this physiology and how these drugs work is imperative. Understanding the patient's needs, monitoring (physically and device-based), and how the patient is responding to treatment are a critical part of complete patient care.

Dosage Forms
- **Quinidine sulfate** (Cin-Quin, Quinora)
- **Quinidine gluconate** (Duraquin)
- **Quinidine polygalacturonate** (Cardioquin)

Adverse Side Effects. These include anorexia, vomiting, diarrhea, weakness, and laminitis (horses).

 TECHNICIAN NOTES

Do not allow animals to chew or crush quinidine oral dosage forms.

Procainamide. Procainamide is an antiarrhythmic that is chemically related to procaine.

Clinical Uses. Procainamide is used to treat premature ventricular contractions (PVCs), ventricular tachycardia, and some forms of atrial tachycardia.

Dosage Forms
- **Procainamide** (Pronestyl)

Adverse Side Effects. These include anorexia, vomiting, diarrhea, hypotension, tachycardia, and others. However, these effects are generally dose related.

Class IB

Class IB drugs include lidocaine, tocainide, and mexiletine. Drugs in this category exert their influence by stabilizing myocardial cell membranes. By blocking the influx of sodium into the cell, these drugs prevent depolarization and decrease cell automaticity (Fig. 7.7). They are used to treat ventricular arrhythmias, but they have not been approved for this use by the U.S. Food and Drug Administration (FDA).

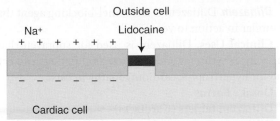

Fig. 7.7 Effect of lidocaine on sodium channels. Lidocaine blocks sodium channels and reduces the automaticity of cardiac cells.

Lidocaine. Lidocaine is a local anesthetic and antiarrhythmic. It is prepared only in injectable form and is administered intravenously; it may be used intravenously in some anesthesia protocols. It is used frequently in emergency medicine and acute care.

Clinical Uses. Lidocaine is primarily used for the control of PVCs and for the treatment of ventricular tachycardia.

Dosage Forms
- Various veterinary brand name forms are available in 1% and 2% intravenous solutions such as lidocaine and xylocaine.

Adverse Side Effects. These are rare but may include drowsiness, depression, ataxia, and muscle tremors. Cats are potentially sensitive to the central nervous system effects of lidocaine and require lower doses than what is used in dogs. These should be monitored carefully when a patient is receiving this drug.

 TECHNICIAN NOTES

When administering lidocaine for an arrhythmia, make certain that it is lidocaine without epinephrine. Epinephrine (a catecholamine) predisposes the heart to arrhythmia.

Tocainide and Mexiletine. Tocainide (Tonocard) and mexiletine (Mexitil) are other class IB agents that may be given orally for long-term control of PVCs and other arrythmias. Adverse side effects include vomiting and ataxia.

Class IC

Class IC agents are seldom used in veterinary medicine.

Class II

Class II antiarrhythmics are the beta-adrenergic blockers, propranolol and atenolol. Propranolol was the prototype agent in this class for veterinary therapeutics, although atenolol and other agents are now generally favored. Beta blockers may block only beta$_1$ receptors or only beta$_2$ receptors (selective), or they may block both types (nonselective). They also are thought to upregulate or increase adrenergic receptors to improve cardiac efficiency (Hamlin, 2003). These drugs may be used to treat atrial or ventricular arrhythmias, decrease cardiac conduction, reduce cardiac output, and decrease blood pressure.

Propranolol. Propranolol reduces automaticity of cardiac conduction cells by blocking beta$_1$ and beta$_2$ receptor sites. Myocardial oxygen demand is reduced by propranolol. Reducing myocardial oxygen demand reduces the tendency for ischemia, which in turn reduces automaticity (Williams & Baer, 1990). Propranolol reduces heart rate, cardiac output, and blood pressure. It also may improve cardiac performance in animals with hypertrophic cardiomyopathy.

Clinical Uses. In veterinary medicine, propranolol is used to treat hypertrophic cardiomyopathy and various atrial and ventricular arrhythmias. It is used in cats to treat systemic hypertension and hyperthyroidism (Plumb, 2015).

Dosage Forms
- **Propranolol HCl tablets** (Inderal)
- **Propranolol for injection** (Inderal)
- **Propranolol oral solution**

Adverse Side Effects. These include bradycardia, hypotension, worsening of heart failure, lethargy, bronchospasm, and depression.

 TECHNICIAN NOTES

- Propranolol is contraindicated in patients with overt heart failure, greater than first-degree heart block, and sinus bradycardia (Plumb, 2015).
- Do not discontinue therapy abruptly because tachycardia or hypertension may occur.

Atenolol. Atenolol is a selective beta$_1$ blocker (Papich, 2016). Atenolol decreases heart rate, slows cardiac conduction, decreases myocardial oxygen demand, reduces blood pressure, and diminishes cardiac output. Atenolol may be safer to use in animals prone to bronchospasm because of its selective beta$_1$ effect.

Clinical Uses. Atenolol is used in the treatment of supraventricular tachyarrhythmias, PVCs, hypertension, and cardiomyopathy.

Dosage Forms

- **Atenolol tablets** (Tenormin)

Adverse Side Effects. Bradycardia, lethargy and depression, hypotension, syncope, or heart failure is most commonly reported in older animals.

Other Beta Blockers

- **Carvedilol** (Dilatrend)
- **Esmolol** (Brevibloc). Selective beta$_1$ blocker for short-term use.
- **Metoprolol** (Lopressor). Metoprolol is a beta$_1$ blocker otherwise similar to propranolol.

Class III

Class III antiarrhythmics bretylium (Bretylol) and amiodarone (Cordarone) are not commonly used in veterinary medicine. Some clinicians have reported that Bretylol has promise for treating ventricular fibrillation in the absence of a defibrillation unit. These drugs are used in human medicine to treat ventricular arrhythmias. Sotalol (Betapace) is nonselective with action similar to propranolol. This drug is replacing quinidine as the antiarrhythmic drug of choice by some clinicians. Sotalol is the most commonly used long-term treatment for hemodynamically significant ventricular arrhythmias in dogs and cats (Gordon, 2019).

Class IV

Class IV antiarrhythmic drugs work by blocking the channels that permit entry of calcium ions through the cardiac cell membrane. This effect causes depression of the contractile mechanism in myocardial and smooth muscle cells and depresses automaticity and impulse transmission (Williams & Baer, 1990).

Verapamil Hydrochloride. Verapamil is a channel-blocking agent and is available in oral and injectable forms. It has had limited use in veterinary medicine and has diminished because of adverse effects.

Clinical Uses. Verapamil is used to treat supraventricular tachycardia, atrial flutter, and atrial fibrillation.

Dosage Forms

- **Verapamil HCl tablets** (Calan, Isoptin)
- **Verapamil HCl for injection** (Calan, Isoptin)

Adverse Side Effects. These include hypotension, bradycardia, tachycardia, pulmonary edema, and worsening of CHF.

Diltiazem. Diltiazem is a channel-blocking agent that is similar in action to verapamil.

Clinical Uses. Diltiazem is used for supraventricular tachyarrhythmias and hypertension in dogs and cats and for hypertrophic cardiomyopathy in cats.

Dosage Forms

- **Diltiazem tablets** (Cardizem)
- **Diltiazem oral capsules** extended/sustained release (Cardizem)

Other Class IV Antiarrhythmics

Other channel blockers include nifedipine (Adalat) and amlodipine (Norvasc). These agents are used primarily for the treatment of hypertension rather than as antiarrhythmics.

Ⓡ Vasodilator Drugs

When heart failure occurs, cardiac output is reduced, which results in hypotension and poor perfusion of tissue. As a reaction to this poor perfusion of tissue, the body activates compensatory mechanisms to increase blood pressure and improve blood supply to tissues. The first compensatory activity is stimulation of the sympathetic nervous system to increase the heart rate and to cause constriction of small arteries, which in turn raises blood pressure. Next, the renin–angiotensin–aldosterone system (RAAS) is activated by the release of renin from poorly perfused kidneys (Fig. 7.8). Renin causes angiotensinogen to be converted to angiotensin I. Angiotensin I then is converted by ACE to angiotensin II. Angiotensin II causes further vasoconstriction and stimulates the adrenal glands to release aldosterone. Aldosterone acts on the kidney tubules to cause reabsorption of sodium ions and osmotic retention of water. The water that is retained helps to expand the circulating blood volume to improve tissue perfusion.

In the short term, these compensatory mechanisms are beneficial. In the long term, however, they become harmful because the heart must work harder to pump blood through vessels constricted by sympathetic nervous stimulation and by the effects of angiotensin II (increased afterload). The ever-increasing blood volume (increased preload) caused by aldosterone release and water retention also necessitates more strenuous activity by the heart, which in a weakened state initiates the preceding chain of events.

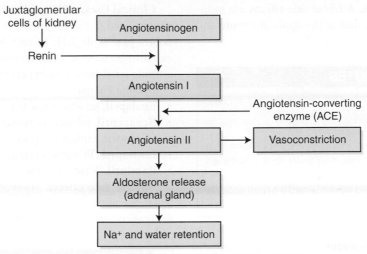

Fig. 7.8 The renin-angiotensin-aldosterone system.

Vasodilator drugs act by dilating arteries (arteriolar dilator), veins (venodilator), or both (combined vasodilator). Dilatory activity may be brought about by direct action on vessel smooth muscle, through blockage of sympathetic stimulation, or by preventing conversion of angiotensin I to angiotensin II. Dilation of constricted arteries tends to decrease the afterload and improve cardiac output. The preload is also reduced because of pooling of blood in dilated veins.

Many forms of CHF are improved by the use of vasodilators, which can be used in conjunction with other heart medications.

Hydralazine—Arterial Vasodilator

Hydralazine is primarily an arteriolar dilator. It acts directly on smooth muscle in the arterial wall by interfering with calcium movement and inhibiting the contractile state allowing smooth muscle relaxation to occur (Plumb, 2015). The net result is that peripheral resistance is reduced and cardiac output is often greatly improved in animals with CHF. Some clinicians recommend that hydralazine be used with a diuretic because it may activate the renin–angiotensin system and cause water retention (Bill, 1994).

Clinical Uses. Hydralazine is used for afterload reduction associated with CHF, especially CHF caused by mitral valve insufficiency.

Dosage Forms. Human forms are used.
- **Hydralazine HCl tablets** (Apresoline)
- **Hydralazine for injection**

Adverse Side Effects. Adverse side effects in small animals include hypotension, vomiting, diarrhea, sodium and water retention, and tachycardia.

Amlodipine—Arterial Vasodilator

Amlodipine (Norvasc), as stated previously, is classified as a calcium channel blocker but it also acts as a peripheral arteriolar vasodilator on smooth muscle to reduce vascular resistance thereby decreasing afterload. Adverse side effects include hypotension and bradycardia.

Nitroglycerin Ointment—Venous Vasodilator

Nitroglycerin is primarily a venodilator that reduces preload as the result of pooling of blood in peripheral vessels and decreased venous return to the heart. Some arteriolar dilation may occur at higher doses. Nitroglycerin is applied topically on hairless areas of small animal patients. Gloves must be worn when applying ointment to the skin. The medical vehicle of nitroglycerin causes it not to be explosive.

Clinical Uses. In small animal medicine, nitroglycerin is used as a vasodilator to improve cardiac output and reduce associated pulmonary edema. In equine medicine, nitroglycerin is used as a leg sweat to reduce swelling and to treat laminitis.

Dosage Forms
- **Nitroglycerin topical ointment** (Nitro-Bid)
- **Nitroglycerin transdermal patch**

Adverse Side Effects. Adverse side effects are minimal and may include rashes at the application site and hypotension.

> **TECHNICIAN NOTES**
>
> • Gloves should be worn when nitroglycerin is applied.
> • Rotate application sites.
> • Do not pet animals at application sites.
> • The dose is measured in inches by application of a strip of ointment to measuring paper that is supplied with the product.
> • The veterinarian should be contacted if a rash appears at the application site.

Prazosin—Mixed Vasodilator

Prazosin is a combined vasodilator. It reduces blood pressure and peripheral vasoconstriction by blocking alpha$_1$-adrenergic receptor sites. Prazosin apparently does not activate the renin–angiotensin system.

Clinical Uses. Prazosin is used for adjunctive treatment of CHF, dilated cardiomyopathy in dogs, systemic hypertension, and pulmonary hypertension.

Dosage Forms
• **Prazosin capsules** (Minipress)

Adverse Side Effects. These include hypotension, syncope, vomiting, and diarrhea.

Nitroprusside—Mixed Vasodilator

Nitroprusside is a potent mixed vasodilator that is used as a short-term drug in patients with acute, severe hypertension and acute pulmonary edema. Nitroprusside must be diluted before being administered intravenously. The patient's blood pressure must be monitored continuously.

Angiotensin-Converting Enzyme Inhibitors—Mixed Vasodilators

Benazepril, captopril, and enalapril are potent mixed vasodilators that exert their effects on blood vessels by preventing formation of the potent vasoconstrictor angiotensin II. They prevent the conversion of angiotensin I to angiotensin II by inhibiting angiotensin-converting enzyme (ACE) (see Fig. 7.8). They are combined vasodilators that produce mild preload and significant afterload reduction. ACE inhibitors also influence several other mediators associated with cardiac remodeling (Boothe, 2012). The drugs in this category are called ACE inhibitors.

Clinical Uses. ACE inhibitors act as vasodilators and may be used in the treatment of Stage B, C, and D heart failure (see Table 7.1). In cats, benazepril and enalapril can also be used to treat hypertension associated with chronic renal failure or hypertrophic cardiomyopathy.

Dosage Forms
• **Enalapril,** tablets (Enacard, Vasotec)
• **Benazepril,** tablets (Lotensin)
• **Captopril,** tablets (Capoten)
• **Lisinopril** (Prinivil, Zestril)
• **Ramipril** (Vasotop, Altace)

Adverse Side Effects. These include hypotension, azotemia, vomiting, diarrhea, hyperkalemia, and others. The safety of enalapril in breeding dogs has not been established.

> **TECHNICIAN NOTES**
>
> • Care should be taken when captopril or enalapril is administered with other vasodilators and certain diuretics because of potential hypotension.
> • Concurrent use of nonsteroidal antiinflammatory drugs may reduce the effectiveness of captopril.
> • Captopril may cause a false-positive urine acetone finding.

Other Vasodilators

• **Isosorbide** (Isordil)
• **Isoxsuprine** (Vasodilan)
• **Sildenafil** (Viagra); may have use in the treatment of pulmonary hypertension in small animals
• **Tadalafil** (Cialis); may be useful in treating pulmonary hypertension in dogs

Diuretics

Diuretics have been some of the most commonly used drugs in the treatment of heart failure because of their ability to promote the reduction of preload through diuresis. Diuretics reduce the harmful effects of CHF (i.e., pulmonary edema, ascites, and increased cardiac work) by reducing plasma volume through various mechanisms.

Many different diuretics are available, and most work by inhibiting reabsorption of sodium and water in the loop of Henle or the distal tubules. If sodium ions remain in the tubules, they exert an increased osmotic "pull" on water molecules to cause them to remain in the tubules and be excreted as urine. The diuretics used most in veterinary medicine include furosemide, the thiazides, and spironolactone.

Furosemide

Furosemide is very powerful and is the most important and efficacious diuretic for removing edema from animals with heart failure (Hamlin, 2003). Furosemide may be administered intravenously, intramuscularly, subcutaneously, or orally and works rapidly to reduce pulmonary edema and other signs of CHF. It causes diuresis by reducing reabsorption of sodium and other electrolytes in the kidney tubules. Because much of the reabsorption occurs in the loop of Henle, furosemide is sometimes called a *loop diuretic*.

Clinical Uses. Furosemide is used for diuretic therapy (in CHF and other conditions) in all species.

Dosage Forms. Injectable and oral (solution, tablet, and bolus) products are used.

- **Furosemide tablets and injection** (Lasix)
- **Furosemide tablets and injection** (Salix), veterinary label
- **Furosemide tablets and injection**, generic

Adverse Side Effects. These include low blood potassium (hypokalemia), dehydration, low blood sodium (hyponatremia), ototoxicity (cats), weakness, and shock.

 TECHNICIAN NOTES

- Furosemide should be administered carefully to animals that are dehydrated or in shock.
- Furosemide should be used at the lowest effective dose to prevent hypokalemia, cardiorenal syndrome, and other potential adverse effects.
- Animals who are receiving diuretics such as furosemide should always have free access to water.
- Administer the dose at convenient times for the client because urination follows within 20 to 30 minutes.

Thiazides

Thiazide diuretics such as hydrochlorothiazide (HydroDiuril) and chlorothiazide (Diuril) act on the loop of Henle and distal tubules to inhibit reabsorption of sodium. Thiazides are seldom used in veterinary medicine. Adverse side effects are electrolyte imbalances.

Spironolactone

Spironolactone is a potassium-sparing diuretic (it does not normally cause hypokalemia) and an antagonist of aldosterone. By inhibiting aldosterone, it reduces the amount of sodium reabsorbed from the kidney tubules. Spironolactone (Aldactone) usually is not used alone but is combined with a loop diuretic to potentiate their effect (Plumb, 2015). Similar to the thiazides, it has limited use in veterinary medicine.

DIETARY MANAGEMENT OF HEART DISEASE

Dietary management is an important part of the overall treatment of patients with heart disease. Dietary measures often are instituted early in the pathogenesis of heart disease (before clinical signs are observed or drug therapy is begun). Two of the primary goals of dietary management of heart disease are sodium restriction and maintenance of good body weight and condition (reduction of obesity or cachexia). Specific nutrient deficiencies (taurine or carnitine), concurrent disease (chronic renal failure), and electrolyte disorders also may have to be addressed (Roudebush et al., 2000).

Sodium restriction has long been recognized as an important part of the management of CHF. As was previously mentioned, increased sodium levels in the body lead to water retention, increased plasma volume, and exacerbation of the clinical signs of heart failure. The primary source of sodium is food. However, water and treats also must be considered when dietary intake is limited. Prescription diets provide sodium-restricted nutrition for dogs and cats. These diets may also be restricted in chloride and phosphorus. They may have added taurine and/or carnitine, B-complex vitamins, and normal or added levels of potassium. Sometimes it is difficult to get an animal to accept a sodium-reduced diet because of palatability issues. These foods may be made more palatable by adding flavor enhancers or warming the food.

Cardiac diets should be highly digestible and easily metabolized because heart failure may impair other internal organs, such as the kidneys, gastrointestinal tract, and liver. They are balanced with adequate (but not excessive) levels of high-biologic-value protein to address potential renal failure. The energy level may need to decrease or increase on the basis of individual animal type and the cardiac condition of the animal. CHF in dogs with congestive failure have been seen with dietary supplementation of fish oils, which are high in omega-3 fatty acids (Ware, 2002).

TECHNICIAN NOTES

Clients should be instructed not to supplement their pet's diet with treats, human foods, or vitamin/mineral supplements when the animal is receiving a prescription sodium-restricted diet.

ANCILLARY TREATMENT OF HEART FAILURE

Various ancillary drugs and procedures are used in the treatment of heart failure. The following section provides a partial list of these therapies.

Bronchodilators

Bronchodilators such as aminophylline and theophylline are sometimes used in the treatment of heart failure. These agents increase the size of lung passageways to allow more efficient oxygenation of blood, to exert a mild positive inotropic effect on heart muscle, and to obtain a mild diuretic effect.

Oxygen Therapy

Oxygen therapy can be crucial in treating animals in the advanced stages of CHF. Animals with pulmonary edema benefit greatly from the administration of 40% to 50% oxygen via cage, mask, or nasal cannula.

Sedation

Animals with pulmonary edema caused by heart failure often experience a great deal of anxiety because of the dyspnea that they encounter. This anxiety often leads to hyperventilation and even greater oxygen demand and anxiety. To break the cycle and calm the animal, sedative drugs are often administered. The clinician may choose morphine, meperidine, diazepam, or other drugs.

Aspirin

Aspirin is known for its ability to reduce pain and inflammation, fever, and platelet aggregation. It is sometimes used in heart disease when clot formation may be a potential problem. It is used by some veterinarians to reduce the tendency for clot formation in heartworm treatment and for the same purpose in congestive cardiomyopathy in cats.

Thoracocentesis and Abdominocentesis

When heart failure is accompanied by excessive fluid (effusion) in the thoracic cavity, drawing fluid from the cavity may be lifesaving. Removal of ascitic fluid is controversial but may relieve pressure on the diaphragm and improve ventilation.

REVIEW QUESTIONS

1. Why is the heart considered to be two pumps functionally?
2. Cardiac cells are connected by intercalated disks and a fusion of cell membranes to form a _____.
3. Depolarization of cardiac cells is characterized by a rapid influx of _____ ions, a slower influx of _____ ions, and the outflow of _____ ions.
4. A relatively long _____ is important to cardiac cells to prevent a constant state of contraction from recycling impulses.
5. Define chronotropic and inotropic effects in relation to the heart.
6. Define preload and afterload in relation to the pumping mechanism of the heart.
7. List the four basic compensatory mechanisms of the cardiovascular system.
8. List five objectives of treatment for heart failure.
9. List four beneficial effects and one potential toxic effect of the use of the cardiac glycosides.
10. _____ is the preferred drug to be given during cardiac arrest because it provides stimulation for heart contractions and supports the circulatory system.
11. List five factors that may predispose the heart to arrhythmias.
12. List six categories of antiarrhythmic drugs and give an example of each.
13. List four vasodilator drugs and classify each as arteriolar dilator, venodilator, or mixed.
14. Why is Lasix sometimes called a loop diuretic?
15. List five ancillary methods of treatment for cardiovascular disease.
16. _____ is characterized by the rapid influx of sodium ions into the cell through channels, the slower influx of calcium ions, and the outflow of potassium ions.
17. _____ results when the pumping ability of the heart is impaired to the extent that sodium and water are retained in an effort to compensate for inadequate cardiac output.

18. ACE causes the conversion of _____ _____ to _____.
19. Nitroglycerin is supplied as an ointment. List the precautions that should be taken when applying.
20. What is hypokalemia?
21. What are the primary goals of the dietary management of heart disease?
22. List three effects of administration of catecholamines.
23. Gloves do not have to be worn when applying nitroglycerin.

a. True
b. False

24. A 50-lb dog with moderate heart failure will be treated with enalapril 0.5 mg/kg twice a day for 14 days and then reevaluated. Enacard tablets (10 mg) are available. How many will you dispense?
25. A 10-lb dog with advanced heart failure will be treated with furosemide at 8 mg/kg IV. Salix injection (50 mg/mL) will be used. How much will you draw up?

REFERENCES

Bill, R. (1994). Drugs affecting the cardiovascular system. In T. B. Barragry (Ed.), *Cardiac disease: Veterinary drug therapy*. Philadelphia: Lea and Febiger.

Boothe, D. M. (2012). *Therapy of cardiovascular diseases: Small animal clinical pharmacology and therapeutics*. Philadelphia: WB Saunders.

Christenson, D. E. (2020). *Veterinary medical terminology* (3rd ed.). St. Louis: Elsevier.

DeFrancesco, T. (2013). Can we delay progression of heart disease? In *Proceedings. Music City Veterinary Conference*, Murfreesboro, TN.

Ettinger, S. (2000). Therapy of heart failure. In S. Ettinger (Ed.), *Textbook of veterinary internal medicine* (5th ed.). Philadelphia: WB Saunders.

Ganong, W. (2003). Origin of the heartbeat and the electrical activity of the heart. In W. Ganong (Ed.), *Review of medical physiology* (21st ed.). New York: McGraw-Hill.

Hamlin, R. L. (2003). Cardiovascular system, introduction. In *Proceedings. Music City Veterinary Conference*, Nashville, TN.

Gordon SG, Saunders AB, P. Inotropes. Antiarrhythmics. In "The Merck Veterinary Manual" (online edition) http:merckveterinarymanual.com/; Accessed June 2019.

Papich, M. G. (2016). *Handbook of veterinary drugs* (4th ed.). St. Louis: Elsevier.

Plumb, D. C. (2015). *Veterinary drug handbook* (8th ed.). Ames, IA: Wiley-Blackwell.

Roudebush, P., Keene, B. W., & Mizelle, H. L. (2000). Cardiovascular disease. In M. S. Hand, C. D. Thatcher, & R. L. Remillard, et al. (Eds.), *Small animal clinical nutrition* (4th ed.). Topeka, KS: Mark Morris Institute.

Spinelli, J. S., & Enos, L. R. (1978). Drugs for treatment of cardiovascular disorders. In J. S. Spinelli, & L. R. Enos (Eds.), *Drugs in veterinary practice*. St. Louis: Mosby.

Upson, D. W. (1988). Cardiovascular system. In D. W. Upson (Ed.), *Handbook of clinical veterinary pharmacology* (3rd ed.). Manhattan, KS: Dan Upson Enterprises.

Ware, W. A. (2002). Problems in chronic heart failure management. In *Proceedings of the American Veterinary Medical Association*, Nashville, TN.

Williams, B. R., & Baer, C. (1990). Antiarrhythmic agents. In B. R. Williams, & C. Baer (Eds.), *Essentials of clinical pharmacology in nursing*. Springhouse, PA: Springhouse Publishing Co.

8

Drugs Used in Gastrointestinal System Disorders

OBJECTIVES

After studying this chapter, you should be able to

1. Exhibit a basic understanding of the anatomy and physiology of the gastrointestinal (GI) system.
2. Describe the various mechanisms of control of the GI system.
3. Explain the pathophysiology of vomiting and discuss drugs that induce vomiting and those that inhibit it.
4. List and describe antacid and antiulcer medications used in veterinary medicine.

5. Explain the pathophysiology of diarrhea and list the medications used to control this condition.
6. List the different categories of laxatives and explain their respective mechanisms of action.
7. List the two basic categories of GI prokinetics and stimulants.
8. Explain why digestive enzymes are used.
9. Discuss the use of antibiotics and antiinflammatory agents in GI disease.
10. List the categories of oral products and give an example from each category.

OUTLINE

KEY TERMS

Adsorbent
Anticholinergic
Chemoreceptor trigger zone
Cholinergic
Dentifrice
Emesis
Hematemesis

Melena
Motilin
Parietal cell
Peristalsis
Regurgitation
Segmentation
Vomiting center

INTRODUCTION

Problems of the gastrointestinal (GI) system are common reasons for visits to a veterinary practice. These problems include regurgitation, vomiting, diarrhea, weight loss, colic, bloating, flatulence, abnormal stools, and constipation. Veterinary technicians must be knowledgeable about this system because they are expected to answer clients' questions about the GI tract, administer therapeutic GI medications, and monitor the response to GI medications. They should have a basic knowledge of GI anatomy, physiology, pathophysiology, therapeutic principles, and medications.

ANATOMY AND PHYSIOLOGY

Anatomic and physiologic differences between the GI systems of different animal species are greater than for any other organ system. Despite these differences, the functions are basically the same in each species: (1) intake of food and fluid into the body, (2) absorption of nutrients and fluid, and (3) excretion of waste products. A discussion of the anatomy and physiology of the GI tract with an emphasis on similarities and differences between species follows.

The basic structures of the GI tract include (depending on the species) the mouth, teeth, tongue, salivary glands, esophagus, outpocketings of the esophagus (i.e., crop, reticulum, rumen, and omasum), stomach, liver, pancreas, duodenum, jejunum, ileum, cecum, colon, rectum, and anus.

Carnivorous or omnivorous species (e.g., cats, dogs, and primates) often are described as monogastric or simple-stomach animals because they have no outpocketings or forestomachs arising from the basic configuration (Fig. 8.1). The function of the stomach in these monogastric animals is primarily to store ingested material and to begin some enzymatic breakdown of protein. The salivary glands begin enzymatic digestion by producing enzymes that break down starch into simpler carbohydrates. Pancreatic enzymes delivered to the duodenum break down fats, carbohydrates, and proteins, and sodium bicarbonate from the pancreas neutralizes hydrochloric acid from the stomach. Bile salts, produced in the liver and delivered to the duodenum, aid in digestion by emulsifying fats. Bile is stored in the gallbladder, which is absent in some animals (e.g., horses and rats). Digestion and its control mechanisms are complex, and students should consult an appropriate text for further information.

Ruminant animals are herbivorous and have a GI system characterized by three forestomachs, the reticulum, rumen, omasum, and a "true" stomach—the abomasum (Fig. 8.2). The reticulum receives ingested material and passes it to the rumen, where it is mixed and acted on by microorganisms to digest cellulose and other coarse plant material (roughage). Some refer to the rumen as a "fermentation vat," where microorganisms break down coarse feeds into forms that can be used by the simple stomach portion of the GI system in ruminants. Partially digested material (cud) in the rumen is regurgitated and remasticated to further facilitate digestion. In an immature ruminant, an esophageal groove allows milk to bypass the rumen and

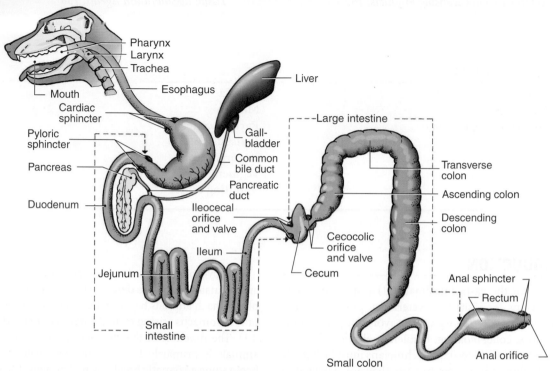

Fig. 8.1 The monogastric gastrointestinal system.

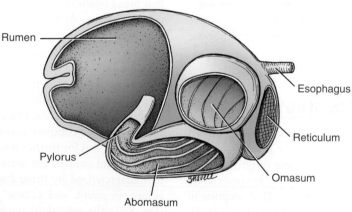

Fig. 8.2 Compartments of the ruminant forestomach.

flow directly into the abomasum, and the rumen gains full function only after several months.

Equines, rabbits, and some rodents are chiefly herbivorous animals that have a monogastric GI configuration. They possess, however, a large cecum, which is capable of limited roughage digestion (hindgut fermentation) (Fig. 8.3).

Birds have an outpocketing of the esophagus called the *crop,* which is used for food storage. They also have a ventriculus, or gizzard, which serves to grind coarse food material (Fig. 8.4).

The small intestine comprises three sections: the duodenum, which has a sharp bend and in which the pancreas is located; the long and highly coiled jejunum; and

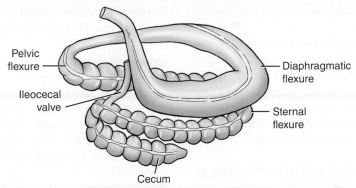

Fig. 8.3 The large intestine of a horse.

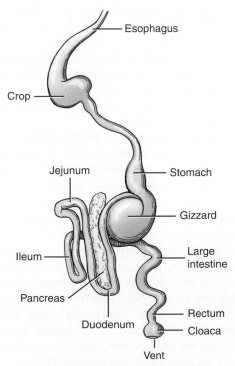

Fig. 8.4 The digestive system of a bird.

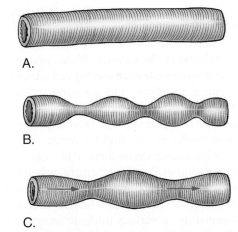

Fig. 8.5 Peristalsis and segmentation. (A) section of intestine exhibiting no activity; (B) Segmental contractions; (C) Peristaltic

Movements of the small intestine mix the intestinal contents, called *chyme,* and move them toward the large intestine. Normal intestinal motility includes two different patterns—peristalsis and segmentation (Fig. 8.5). Peristalsis is a wave of contractions that propels contents along the digestive tract. Segmentation is a periodic, repeating pattern of intestinal constrictions that serves to mix and churn the contents.

The colon has a considerably larger diameter than the small intestine. The colon is connected to the ileum and the cecum through the ileocecocolic valve. The surface of the colon may exhibit one or more longitudinal bands (depending on the species) called *teniae.* The wall of the colon may also form outpocketings, called *haustra.* The colon of monogastric animals has an ascending portion, a transverse portion, and a descending portion that leads into the rectum. Functions of the colon include

the short ileum, which connects to the large intestine. In the small intestine, contents passing from the stomach are mixed with intestinal secretions, pancreatic juice, and bile. The digestive process that began in the mouth and stomach is completed in the small intestine. Products of this process are absorbed together with most of the vitamins and a great deal of fluid. Villi and microvilli protrude from the mucosal surface into the lumen of the small intestine and greatly enhance the absorptive process.

absorption of water, synthesis of certain vitamins, and storage of waste material.

Movements of the colon include peristalsis and segmentation (as in the small intestine), as well as a third type called *mass action contraction* (Ganong, 2003). Mass action contraction is a result of simultaneous contraction of smooth muscle over a large area and serves to move fecal material from one portion of the colon to another and from the colon into the rectum.

REGULATION OF THE GASTROINTESTINAL SYSTEM

Regulation of GI system activity is complex but can be said to be under the influence of the following three basic control systems:

1. The autonomic nervous system (ANS).
   - Stimulation of the parasympathetic portion of the ANS increases intestinal motility and tone, increases intestinal secretions, and stimulates relaxation of sphincters. Drugs that mimic parasympathetic stimulation (i.e., cholinergic or parasympathomimetic) cause similar results. Anticholinergic, or parasympatholytic, drugs inhibit these ANS actions.
   - Stimulation of the sympathetic branch of the ANS decreases intestinal motility and tone, decreases intestinal secretions, and inhibits sphincters.
   - Stimulation of various intrinsic receptors in the GI tract, such as the myenteric plexus (stretch receptor), also may increase peristaltic activity. Some physiologists consider the intrinsic receptors (myenteric plexus and Meissner's plexus) to be a third portion of the ANS called the *enteric nervous system* (Ganong, 2003).
2. Gastrointestinal hormones such as gastrin, secretin, and cholecystokinin, when released from intestinal cells, exert control over many functions such as gastric secretion, emptying of the gallbladder, and gastric emptying.
3. Substances such as histamine, serotonin, and prostaglandin are released from specialized cells of the GI tract. Histamine attaches to H_2 receptors in gastric parietal cells to cause increased release of hydrochloric acid in the stomach. The influences of serotonin and prostaglandin are not as well defined.

Another factor that can have a major influence on GI activity is the presence of bacterial endotoxins. Endotoxins are components of the bacterial cell wall of certain bacteria (often gram-negative bacteria) that may increase the permeability of intestinal blood vessels and cause increased fluid loss and fever.

VOMITING

Vomiting is forceful ejection of the contents of the stomach, and sometimes the contents of the proximal small intestine, through the mouth. Vomiting is initiated by activation of the vomiting (emetic) center in the medulla of the brain. The vomiting center (emetic center) (Fig. 8.6) is connected by nerve pathways to the chemoreceptor trigger zone (CRTZ), the cerebral cortex, and peripheral receptors in the pharynx, GI tract, urinary system, and heart. Impulses from any of these areas activate the vomiting reflex; this requires a coordinated effort of the GI, musculoskeletal, respiratory, and nervous systems. Impulses may be generated by (1) pain, excitement, or fear (cortex), (2) disturbances of the inner ear (CRTZ), (3) drugs such as apomorphine and digoxin (CRTZ), (4) metabolic conditions such as uremia, ketonemia, or endotoxemia (CRTZ), and (5) irritation of peripheral receptors.

Multiple neurotransmitters are involved in the vomiting reflexes. Some of those include histamine (H_1), dopaminergic (D_2), serotonergic (5-HT_3), neurokinin (NK), acetylcholine (muscarinic, M_1), substance P, and other neurotransmitters. Agents that prevent emesis (antiemetics) exert their effects by blocking one or more of these neurotransmitters (Fig. 8.6A).

Occasional vomiting by a dog or cat is considered normal. However, persistent vomiting is not normal. Horses and rats do not normally vomit. Persistent vomiting can cause serious problems such as resultant dehydration, electrolyte disturbances, and acid–base imbalances. Sizable quantities of sodium, potassium, and chloride are lost in vomit. However, potassium loss is usually the most significant abnormality.

℞ Emetics

Emetics are drugs that induce vomiting. Emetics are administered to animals that have ingested toxins, but they must be used carefully to avoid serious complications. Emetics must be administered within 2 to 4 hours of the toxic ingestion to be effective. Emetics should not be used in animals that (1) are comatose or are having a seizure, (2) have depressed pharyngeal reflexes, (3) are in shock or have dyspnea, (4) bloat or esophageal damage, or (5) have ingested strong acid, alkali, or other caustic substances. Obviously,

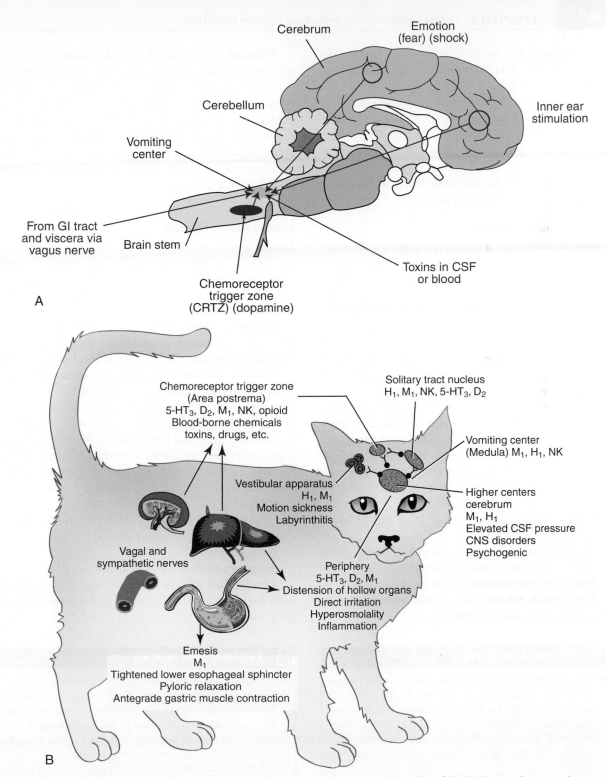

Fig. 8.6 (A) The vomiting center in the brainstem; (B) Sites that mediate the emetic reflex. Stimuli that mediate emesis at each site are listed below the neurotransmitter. *CNS,* Central nervous system; *CSF,* cerebrospinal fluid; *H₁,* histamine; *D₂,* dopaminergic; *5-HT₃,* serotonergic; *NK,* neurokinin; *M₁,* muscarinic (acetylcholine). (A, From Bill, R. L. [2006]. *Clinical pharmacology and therapeutics for veterinary technicians.* [3rd ed.]. St. Louis: Elsevier. B, From Boothe, D. M. [2012]. Gastrointestinal pharmacology. In *Small animal clinical pharmacology and therapeutics.* Philadelphia: WB Saunders, Fig. 19.2.)

emetics should not be given to animals that do not normally vomit, such as rabbits, some rodents, and horses. Emetics usually remove about 80% of the stomach contents. Therefore, the animal should be closely monitored for signs of toxicity after induced vomiting (Plumb, 2015).

Emetics are classified according to their site of action. Those acting on the CRTZ or emetic center are categorized as centrally acting, and those that act on peripheral receptors (GI tract) are locally acting.

Centrally Acting Emetics

Apomorphine. Apomorphine is a morphine derivative that stimulates dopamine receptors in the CRTZ, which then activates the vomiting center. This drug is poorly absorbed after oral administration and is therefore usually administered parenterally or topically in the conjunctival sac. Apomorphine tablets can be crushed and mixed with saline or water and placed in the eye. Vomiting follows rapidly after intravenous administration, 5 to 10 minutes after intramuscular injection, and variably (10 to 20 minutes) after conjunctival administration.

Clinical Uses. Apomorphine is used primarily for induction of vomiting in dogs. It is considered by many to be the emetic of choice for dogs. Its use in cats is controversial and generally not recommended because cats have fewer dopamine receptors and therefore is less effective. Xylazine, which is safer than apomorphine, is effective as an emetic in most cats.

Dosage Forms. Apomorphine is an opioid and a Class II controlled substance.

- **Apomorphine hydrogen chloride** (HCl) soluble tablets, from compounding pharmacies
- **Apomorphine injection** (Apokyn), human label
  Adverse Side Effects. These include protracted vomiting, restlessness, and depression.

Xylazine. Although xylazine (Rompun, Anased) is not classified as an emetic, the label indicates that it induces vomiting within 3 to 5 minutes in cats and occasionally in dogs. Some clinicians consider xylazine to be the agent of choice for inducing vomiting in cats. Normal precautions should be followed regarding administration of this product. Yohimbine or atipamezole can be used to reverse the emetic effects.

Locally Acting Emetics

Locally acting emetics act on peripheral receptors in the GI tract. Hydrogen peroxide is the primary agent. Other locally acting emetics that have been used but are rarely effective include mustard and water, and warm salt water.

Hydrogen Peroxide. A 3% solution of hydrogen peroxide can be used orally to induce vomiting. Vomiting is induced by a direct irritant effect on the oropharynx and stomach lining. Dogs usually vomit within 5 to 10 minutes after administration of the hydrogen peroxide. The dosage is 1 mL/lb (1 teaspoon (5 mL) per 5 pounds) of body weight or 2.2 mL/kg not to exceed 45 mL, and this dose can be repeated once if not successful on the first attempt (Plumb, 2015). Hydrogen peroxide should not be used in cats as they are at risk of developing esophagitis and hemorrhagic gastritis.

Clinical Uses. Hydrogen peroxide is used for the induction of vomiting in dogs, pigs, and ferrets.

Dosage Form
- **Hydrogen peroxide 3% solution**
  Adverse Side Effects. There are few adverse side effects, but they could include aspiration pneumonia or gastric ulceration.

 TECHNICIAN NOTES

- Whole or divided apomorphine tablets may be placed in the conjunctival sac of the eye. These tablets or portions can also be crushed or dissolved in saline and placed in the conjunctiva. Once vomiting has occurred, the remaining apomorphine should be rinsed from the conjunctiva to prevent protracted vomiting.
- Naloxone may be used to treat an overdose or toxicity.
- Intravenous cefazolin may cause vomiting.

TECHNICIAN NOTES

- Animals must be closely monitored to prevent aspiration of the material.
- Timing of administration of emetics is important; do not use hydrogen peroxide to induce emesis if the animal has already vomited, is lethargic, has respiratory distress, or poor swallowing reflex.
- Emetics must not be used in animals that do not normally vomit, such as rodents and rabbits, as intestinal blockage can occur.

℞ Antiemetics

Antiemetics are drugs that are used to prevent or control vomiting by blocking receptors centrally in the CRTZ, emetic center, and peripheral receptors. The use of antiemetics is a form of symptomatic treatment because these drugs do not necessarily correct the underlying cause of the vomiting. Many cases of vomiting in small animals are self-limiting or can be controlled by withholding food and water for 24 to 48 hours. Other cases are more difficult to control and necessitate the use of antiemetic agents and careful attention to determining the underlying cause. Antiemetics usually are given parenterally because vomiting precludes use of the oral route.

Phenothiazine Derivatives

Phenothiazine-derivative antiemetics act centrally by blocking dopamine receptors in the CRTZ and possibly by direct inhibition of the vomiting center. These agents are commonly used in veterinary medicine. They are very useful in preventing motion sickness in dogs and cats but may be less effective against irritant emetics (Upson, 1988). Common side effects include hypotension and sedation.

Acepromazine. Acepromazine is a phenothiazine tranquilizer that has multiple systemic effects. It is used as a sedative, tranquilizer, anesthetic adjunct, and has antiemetic effects.

Clinical Uses. Acepromazine is used to control vomiting caused by motion sickness and nausea.

Dosage Forms
- **Acepromazine maleate** injectable
- **PromAce injectable**, tablets
- **ACE** (Acepromazine)

Adverse Side Effects. Sedation, ataxia, and hypotension are common side effects. Penile prolapse has been reported in horses.

Chlorpromazine. Chlorpromazine is a phenothiazine-derivative tranquilizer that has little popularity as a tranquilizer in veterinary medicine and is more often used as an antiemetic.

Clinical Uses. Chlorpromazine is used as an antiemetic in dogs and cats. It is more effective in dogs than in cats.

Dosage Forms
- **Chlorpromazine tablets** (Thorazine)
- **Chlorpromazine capsules**
- **Chlorpromazine oral solution**
- **Chlorpromazine injection**

Adverse Side Effects. These are primarily limited to sedation, ataxia, and hypotension.

Prochlorperazine. Prochlorperazine is a phenothiazine derivative agent with moderate sedative effects and strong antiemetic effects. The approved form of this drug is a combination product that contains an anticholinergic agent (Darbazine). Prochlorperazine is available singly as Compazine (human label).

Clinical Uses. These include control of vomiting (prochlorperazine alone) in dogs and cats, and treatment of vomiting, gastroenteritis, diarrhea, spastic colitis, and motion sickness (combination product).

Dosage Forms
- **Prochlorperazine**—injection, oral syrup, sustained-release capsules (Compazine)
- **Prochlorperazine/isopropamide**—injectable and capsule (Darbazine)

Adverse Side Effects. These are similar to those of chlorpromazine but may also include dry mucous membranes, dilated pupils, and urinary retention caused by the effects of the anticholinergic in the combination product.

Procainamide Derivatives: Metoclopramide

Metoclopramide is a derivative of procainamide and has central and peripheral antiemetic activities. Centrally, it blocks dopamine receptors in the CRTZ, whereas peripherally, it increases gastric contraction, speeds gastric emptying, increases peristalsis of the small intestine, and causes relaxation of the pyloric sphincter. Metoclopramide has a limited influence on GI secretions. This drug has a short half-life and may have to be administered often or in a continuous drip in severe cases of vomiting (Plumb, 2015).

Clinical Uses. Metoclopramide is used as an antiemetic for parvoviral enteritis, uremic vomiting, and vomiting associated with chemotherapy. It is also used to treat gastric motility disorders.

Dosage Forms
- **Metoclopramide HCl tablets** (Reglan)
- **Metoclopramide HCl oral solution** (Reglan)

- **Metoclopramide HCl injection** (Reglan)
Adverse Side Effects. The most common side effects in horses, dogs, and cats are behavioral or other disorders associated with the central nervous system (CNS). Constipation also may occur.

> **TECHNICIAN NOTES**
>
> - Metoclopramide (reglan) is contraindicated if GI obstruction is suspected.
> - Atropine and the opioid analgesics may antagonize the actions of metoclopramide.

Antihistamines (H₁ Blockers)

Antihistamines are most effective as antiemetics in dogs and cats when vomiting is a result of motion sickness or inner ear abnormalities. Antihistamines inhibit vomiting at the level of the CRTZ through H_1 blockade. All antihistamines may cause sedation.

Dosage Forms

- **Trimethobenzamide HCL** (Tigan). Trimethobenzamide is an antiemetic for use in dogs only.
- **Dimenhydrinate** (Dramamine). Dimenhydrinate is an antihistamine labeled for treatment of motion sickness in dogs and cats. It is available in tablet, liquid, and injectable forms.
- **Diphenhydramine** (Benadryl). Diphenhydramine is used in veterinary medicine as an antiemetic and for the treatment of motion sickness, pruritus, and allergic reactions. It is available in tablet, capsule, oral elixir, and injectable forms.
- **Meclizine** (Antivert). Meclizine is used mainly in small animals for the treatment of motion sickness.

Serotonin Receptor (5-HT3) Antagonists

Serotonin receptors are found on vagal nerve terminals and in the CRTZ (Plumb, 2015). Blockade of these 5-HT3 receptors causes antiemetic activity.

Clinical Uses. They are used primarily for severe vomiting in dogs and cats. It is effective for treating chemotherapy associated vomiting.

Dosage Forms

- **Ondansetron** (Zofran). Zofran is used mainly as an antiemetic during chemotherapy and is noted for its special effectiveness during this application.
- **Dolasetron** (Anzemet)
- **Granisetron** (Kytril) is used primarily for its antiemetic effects during chemotherapy (Papich, 2016).

NK-1 Receptor Antagonists

NK-1 antagonists block the binding of substance P (a neurotransmitter peptide found in the emetic center) to NK-1 receptors in the CRTZ.

Clinical Uses. Uses include the prevention and treatment of vomiting in dogs resulting from motion sickness or other causes. Maropitant injectable is approved for vomiting in cats and acute vomiting in dogs.

Dosage Forms

- **Maropitant citrate** (Cerenia) tablets. Labeled for use in dogs.
- **Maropitant** (Cerenia) injectable is labeled for use in dogs and cats.

> **TECHNICIAN NOTES**
>
> - When using maropitant to prevent motion sickness in dogs it is best to have the owner feed a small meal approximately 3 hours prior to traveling, then administer maropitant an hour later.

Adverse Side Effects. Side effects included diarrhea, anorexia, and excessive salivation.

® Antacids and Antiulcer Medications

Gastric parietal cells produce hydrochloric acid when H_2 receptors (located in the stomach) are stimulated by histamine binding. Gastric ulcers may occur in animals for various reasons, including stress, metabolic disease, gastric hyperacidity, and drug therapy (e.g., corticosteroids or nonsteroidal antiinflammatory agents) (Hall, 2001). Anorexia, hematemesis, pain, and melena are common signs of gastric ulcer. Most cases of gastric ulceration involve increased gastric acid production and require treatment of the underlying cause and symptomatic therapy. Five classes of drugs are most commonly used to treat gastric ulcers: (1) H_2 receptor antagonists, (2) proton pump inhibitors, (3) antacids, (4) gastromucosal protectants, and (5) prostaglandin E1 analogues.

H₂ Receptor Antagonists

One of the primary stimuli for secretion of hydrochloric acid by gastric parietal cells is activation of H_2 receptors by histamine. By blocking H_2 receptors, H_2 receptor antagonists reduce the release of hydrochloric acid, thus decreasing irritation of the eroded mucosa and promoting healing (Fig. 8.7). H_2 blockers in current use include cimetidine, ranitidine, famotidine, and nizatidine. These are all available as over-the-counter products.

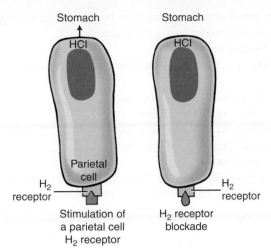

Fig. 8.7 H$_2$ receptor blockade (parietal cell). *HCl,* Hydrochloric acid.

Cimetidine. Cimetidine competitively inhibits histamine at H$_2$ receptors of gastric parietal cells, thereby reducing hydrochloric acid secretion by these cells. Cimetidine, the least potent of the H$_2$ receptors, must be given three to four times daily to be effective (DeNovo, 2002).

Clinical Uses. Cimetidine is used for the treatment or prevention of gastric, abomasal, or duodenal ulcers; hypersecretory conditions of the stomach; esophagitis; gastric reflux; and experimentally as an immunomodulator.

Dosage Forms. Products approved for use in humans are also used in animals.

- **Cimetidine tablets** (Tagamet)
- **Cimetidine oral solution** (Tagamet)
- **Cimetidine HCl for injection** (Tagamet)

Adverse Side Effects. These are rare in animals; however, cimetidine does inhibit microsomal enzymes in the liver and thus may alter the rate of metabolism of other drugs.

 TECHNICIAN NOTES

- Because of its inhibition of liver microsomal enzymes, cimetidine may prolong the effects of drugs that are highly metabolized by the liver (e.g., lidocaine, propranolol, metronidazole, diazepam, and others). References should be checked before cimetidine is used in combination with other drugs.
- If cimetidine is used with antacids, metoclopramide, digoxin, sucralfate, or ketoconazole, doses should be separated by at least 2 hours.

Ranitidine. Ranitidine is also an H$_2$ receptor antagonist that competitively inhibits histamine at parietal cell receptors and reduces hydrochloric acid secretion. Ranitidine has little effect on hepatic microenzymes and is unlikely to cause drug interactions. Ranitidine is the H$_2$ receptor antagonist preferred by many clinicians because of its greater potency (five times that of cimetidine) and greater duration of action. Ranitidine also has prokinetic activity in that it promotes gastric emptying (DeNovo, 2002).

Clinical Uses. Ranitidine is used for the treatment or prevention of gastric, abomasal, or duodenal ulcers; hypersecretory conditions of the stomach; esophagitis and gastric reflux.

Dosage Forms

- **Ranitidine HCl tablets** (Zantac)
- **Ranitidine HCl oral syrup** (Zantac)
- **Ranitidine injection** (Zantac)

Adverse Side Effects. Adverse side effects are rare in animals and are usually only seen with decreased renal clearance.

 TECHNICIAN NOTES

A practical advantage of ranitidine over cimetidine is its reduced frequency of dosing (twice a day rather than three or four times daily).

Famotidine. Famotidine is an H$_2$ receptor antagonist that is considerably more potent than cimetidine. It is administered once a day and may have fewer drug interactions than cimetidine or ranitidine.

Clinical Uses. Clinical uses are similar to those of cimetidine and ranitidine.

Dosage Forms

- **Famotidine film-coated tablets** (Pepcid or Pepcid AC)
- **Famotidine oral powder** (Pepcid)
- **Famotidine injection** (Pepcid IV)

Adverse Side Effects. Because of limited use, side effects have not been determined.

Nizatidine. Nizatidine is an H$_2$ receptor antagonist that also has prokinetic activity, similar to ranitidine.

Clinical Uses. Even though nizatidine is an H$_2$ receptor blocker, it is used primarily in small animal medicine as a prokinetic agent for the treatment of constipation, gastric ulcers, and delayed gastric emptying (Plumb, 2015).

Dosage Forms
- **Nizatidine** (Axid) tablets, capsules, and oral solution

Proton Pump Inhibitors

These agents bind irreversibly at the secretory surface of the parietal cell to the enzyme Na-K-ATPase. This enzyme is responsible for "pumping" hydrogen ions into the stomach against a concentration gradient. When bound in this way, the enzyme is inactivated and the cell is unable to secrete acid until a new enzyme is synthesized; therefore, the stomach has a less acidic environment.

Clinical Uses. These agents are used to treat gastric or duodenal ulcers and esophagitis and may be useful in treating parietal hypersecretion associated with gastrinoma and mastocytosis (DeNovo, 2002). Omeprazole has a veterinary-approved label for the treatment and prevention of recurrence of gastric ulcers in horses and foals (Foushee, 2000). Omeprazole binds to the proton

pump and stops acid formation by preventing hydrogen molecules from going to the stomach.

Dosage Forms
- **Omeprazole oral sustained-release capsules** (Prilosec)
- **Omeprazole** (Losec) (Canada)
- **Omeprazole Oral Paste**
- **GastroGard** (equine product)
- **UlcerGard** (equine product)
- **Pantoprazole**

Adverse Side Effects. These include constipation, sedation, ileus, pancreatitis, and CNS effects.

Antacids

Antacids used in veterinary medicine are (relatively) non-absorbable salts of aluminium, calcium, or magnesium. Antacids are used to decrease hydrochloric acid levels in the stomach as an aid in the treatment of gastric ulcers. In ruminants, antacids such as magnesium hydroxide are

---

BOX 8.1   Case Scenario Hemorrhagic Gastroenteritis

Bella, a 5-year-old female spayed Sheltie, presented with the chief complaint of profuse bloody vomiting and diarrhea.

History: The owner stated that she was acting normally up until this morning when she began vomiting and having diarrhea with blood. The owner thinks that she got into the garbage 2 days ago. Bella often goes to the park but no other travel history. She is up to date on vaccines.

Additional history: No other dietary indiscretions.

Physical examination findings: Bella was listless and depressed. Temperature: 103°F, pulse 150 bpm (tachycardia) with poor pulse quality, respirations panting with normal effort, and lung sounds clear, mucous membranes: dark red, CRT: 3 seconds, rectal exam revealed bloody stool and a sample was collected for analysis.

The veterinary technician prepared for IV catheter placement, fluids, blood tubes for complete blood count (CBC) and chemistry, ECG, blood pressure, abdominal radiographs, etc.

Diagnostic results: Sinus tachycardia with intermittent single premature ventricular contraction (PVC) revealed from ECG, blood pressure: 50 mm Hg and post IV fluid boluses 90 mm Hg, CBC revealed hemoconcentration with PCV of 68% and TP of 5 g/dL, normal platelet count, inflammatory leukogram, blood glucose: 70 mg/dL, chemistry was unremarkable. Abdominal

radiographs: unremarkable, fecal: no enteric pathogens seen, Parvo test: negative.

Diagnosis: Hemorrhagic Gastroenteritis

The patient was treated with multiple IV fluid boluses of crystalloids, maropitant as an antiemetic, and famotidine as a gastric protectant. Per doctor's orders the veterinary technician began IV fluids with crystalloids for the first hour, 2.5% dextrose solution was then started due to low blood glucose levels and she continued to monitor the blood glucose periodically and communicated the test results to the veterinarian. The patient was then put on 0.9% NaCl and were modified to match the ongoing losses.

Once the vomiting was controlled the patient was offered small amounts of canned food (highly digestible, low fat, and low fiber) so the gut could begin to repair itself.

The veterinary technician having knowledge of the disease was able to adequately prepare for diagnostic testing, as well as understand that aggressive fluid therapy is a primary goal to replace the fluid deficits from the vomiting and diarrhea and adjusting the rates to maintain proper hydration. She consistently monitored the fluid drip rate, urine output, PCV and TP, serum electrolytes, blood pressure, and body weight. This demonstrated diligent patient monitoring and excellent communication skills.

used to treat rumen acidosis (rumen overload syndrome) and are used as a laxative. Antacids also may be used in patients with renal failure to bind with (chelate) intestinal phosphorus and reduce hyperphosphatemia.

Clinical Uses. These include treatment of gastric ulcer, gastritis, esophagitis, constipation, and hyperphosphatemia in small animals. In ruminants, they are used to treat rumen overload (rumen acidosis).

Dosage Forms
- **Human label**
  - Aluminum/magnesium hydroxide (Maalox, Mylanta)
  - Aluminum carbonate (Basaljel)
  - Aluminum hydroxide (Amphojel)
  - Magnesium hydroxide (milk of magnesia)
- **Veterinary label**
  - Magnesium hydroxide (Magnalax)—for oral administration to ruminants

Adverse Side Effects. Adverse side effects in monogastric animals include constipation (with aluminium- and calcium-containing products) and diarrhea (with magnesium-containing products). Patients with renal disease should not be given aluminum and magnesium products on a long-term basis due to absorption and excretion by the kidneys.

TECHNICIAN NOTES

- Generally, do not give oral antacids within 1 to 2 hours of other oral medications because of their ability to decrease the absorption of drugs such as tetracycline, cimetidine, ranitidine, digoxin, captopril, corticosteroids, and ketoconazole.
- Magnesium-containing antacids are contraindicated in animals with renal disease.

Gastromucosal Protectants

Sucralfate is the only gastromucosal protectant in common use in veterinary medicine. This drug is a disaccharide that, when administered orally, forms a pastelike substance in the stomach that binds to the surfaces of gastric ulcers. This pastelike material forms a barrier over the ulcer to protect it from further damage and to promote healing. Because sucralfate binds better to ulcers in an acidic environment, it should be administered 30 minutes to 1 hour before H_2 receptor antagonists (antacids) are given. It also may reduce the availability of some other drugs.

Clinical Uses. Sucralfate is used in the treatment of oral, esophageal, gastric, and duodenal ulcers.

Dosage Form
- **Sucralfate** (Carafate)

Adverse Side Effects. These usually are limited to constipation. However, drug interactions may be notable.

TECHNICIAN NOTES

- Sucralfate should be given 2 hours before cimetidine, tetracycline, phenytoin, fluoroquinolones, or digoxin is administered.
- Sucralfate should be given a half hour before H_2 receptor antagonists or antacids are given because it requires an acid environment to be effective.

Prostaglandin E1 Analogues

Misoprostol is a synthetic prostaglandin E1 analogue that directly inhibits the parietal cell from secreting hydrogen ions into the stomach. It also protects the gastric mucosa by increasing the production of mucus and bicarbonate.

Clinical Uses. Prostaglandin E1 analogues are used primarily to prevent or treat gastric ulcers associated with the use of nonsteroidal antiinflammatory drugs (NSAIDs).

Dosage Form
- **Misoprostol oral tablets** (Cytotec)

Adverse Side Effects. Side effects include diarrhea, vomiting, flatulence, abdominal pain, and colic in horses.

TECHNICIAN NOTES

Misoprostol is a prostaglandin which will increase uterine contractions and can cause premature birth or abortion and therefore should not be used in pregnant animals.

DIARRHEA

Diarrhea is the passage of loose or liquid stools, often with increased frequency. Diarrhea can result from primary disease of the intestinal tract or may accompany non-GI disease. Explanation of the pathophysiology of diarrhea is beyond the scope of this text. However, categories of mechanisms described in veterinary references include hypersecretion, increased permeability, osmotic overload, and altered intestinal motility. Parasitism is a common cause of diarrhea in all domestic animal species; it results in diarrhea through a combination of previously described mechanisms. Parasitism always should be ruled out when a diagnosis is determined.

Increased secretion of fluid from the intestine may result from the actions of bacterial endotoxins from microorganisms such as *Escherichia coli*, *Clostridium perfringens*, *Clostridium difficile*, *Campylobacter jejuni*, and *Helicobacter*. Intestinal epithelium damaged by viruses or other organisms may lose fluid as the result of increased permeability. Osmotic overload may occur because of poorly digestible foods, a rapid change in diet, or maldigestion or malabsorption. Although diarrhea has often been associated with hypermotility of the GI tract, the current belief is that most patients with diarrhea actually have hypomotility.

Decreased segmental contractions (hypomotility) increase the diameter of the lumen and allow rapid passage of contents, resulting in diarrhea. Normal segmental constrictions narrow the diameter of the intestinal lumen and actually slow the passage of contents. Diarrhea, if not controlled, can result in substantial fluid and electrolyte (i.e., sodium, chloride, potassium, and bicarbonate) losses. Dehydration, acidosis, weakness, and anorexia may follow.

Acute diarrhea, similar to acute vomiting, in dogs and cats often responds to dietary management and conservative treatment, and in many cases are self-limiting. In cases that do not respond to conservative management, symptomatic and specific treatments are essential.

Ⓡ Antidiarrheal Medications
Narcotic Analgesics

Narcotic analgesics (opiates) are effective agents in the control of diarrhea because of their ability to (1) increase segmental contractions, (2) decrease intestinal secretions, and (3) enhance intestinal absorption. Many clinicians consider opiates to be the drugs of choice for the control of diarrhea in dogs. They also are used for the treatment of diarrhea in calves, but their use in cats and horses is controversial because of their tendency to cause CNS stimulation. Narcotic agents are sometimes prepared as combination products with other classes of antidiarrheals.

Clinical Uses. The opiates are used in GI therapy for the control of diarrhea.

Dosage Forms
• **Diphenoxylate** (Lomotil). Diphenoxylate is a synthetic narcotic agent (Class V) that is structurally similar to meperidine. Atropine sulfate is added to commercial preparations to discourage substance abuse.
• **Loperamide** (Imodium). Loperamide is a synthetic narcotic that is available in a nonprescription preparation. Loperamide poorly penetrates the CNS in cats and is acceptable in this species (Willard, 1998).
• **Paregoric/kaolin/pectin** (Parepectolin).

Adverse Side Effects. Adverse side effects of all the opiates include constipation, ileus, sedation, and CNS excitement (cats and horses).

Anticholinergics/Antispasmodics

Anticholinergics and antispasmodics have been widely used in veterinary medicine for the treatment of diarrhea. Anticholinergics and antispasmodics should be used with caution for the treatment of diarrhea because hypomotility rather than hypermotility is now considered to be associated with most cases of diarrhea. A few commercial antidiarrheal preparations contain an anticholinergic plus a CNS depressant.

Clinical Uses. Anticholinergics/antispasmodics are used for the treatment of diarrhea; they significantly decrease intestinal motility and secretions.

Dosage Forms
• **Hyoscyamine** (Levsin) may be used as an alternative to other anticholinergics for treating bradycardia or irritable bowel syndrome in dogs (Plumb, 2015).
• **Isopropamide**
• **Propantheline** (Pro-Banthine).

Adverse Side Effects. Adverse side effects include dry mucous membranes, constipation, urinary retention, tachycardia, and behavioral changes (Papich, 2016).

Protectants/Adsorbents

Products in this category may have protectant or adsorbent qualities in the GI tract. The coating action of these drugs protects inflamed mucosa from further irritation. Their adsorbent activity binds bacteria or their toxins to protect against the harmful effects of these organisms and are less likely to be further absorbed into the body. Kaolin and pectin are two ingredients often used in protectant compounds. The ability of protectants to control diarrhea has been questioned by some clinicians.

Bismuth subsalicylate is a compound found in products such as Corrective Suspension and Pepto-Bismol. Bismuth subsalicylate is converted to bismuth carbonate and salicylate in the small intestine. The bismuth has a coating and antibacterial effect, and the salicylate (an aspirin-like compound) has an antiinflammatory effect and reduces secretion by inhibiting prostaglandins (Boothe, 2012). Caution should be used when using salicylates in cats.

Activated charcoal is an adsorbent that is used primarily to treat poisoning to prevent further GI absorption.

Clinical Uses. These agents are used to control diarrhea and act as adsorbents to protect the intestinal wall.

Dosage Forms
- **Bismuth subsalicylate**
  - Corrective Suspension (veterinary approved)
  - BismuKote
  - Bismusal
  - GastroCote
  - Pepto-Bismol (human label)
- **Kaolin/pectin**
  - Kaopectolin
  - Kao-Pec
- **Activated charcoal**
  - ToxiBan Suspension and Granules
  - CharcoAid
  - Liqui-Char

Adverse Side Effects. Adverse side effects are rare and usually are limited to constipation.

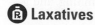

> **TECHNICIAN NOTES**
>
> - Bismuth subsalicylate compounds should be used with caution in cats because of the conversion to aspirin.
> - Bismuth may appear opaque on radiographs and may interfere with visualization of abdominal organs.
> - Administration of bismuth subsalicylate can result in black stools that resemble melena.

Laxatives

Laxatives are substances that loosen bowel contents and encourage their evacuation. Laxatives with a strong or harsh effect are called cathartics, or purgatives. Categories of laxatives include saline/hyperosmotic agents, bulk-producing agents, lubricants, surfactants/stool softeners, irritants, and miscellaneous agents.

Saline/Hyperosmotic Agents

Saline or hyperosmotic laxatives contain magnesium or phosphate anions that are very poorly absorbed from the GI tract. It generally is believed that these anions hold water in the tract osmotically. Increased water

in the GI tract then softens the stool and stimulates stretch receptors in the gut wall to enhance peristalsis.

Clinical Uses. These agents are used for the relief of constipation.

Dosage Forms. Dosage forms include suspensions, crystals, powders, and boluses.
- **Lactulose** (Cephulac, Constulose, Enulose). Lactulose also reduces blood ammonia levels in some hepatic diseases.
- **Magnesium hydroxide**
  - Milk of Magnesia is a suspension for use in dogs.
  - Carmilax Powder and Bolets is for use in cattle (laxative/antacid).
  - Magnalax Bolus and Powder is for use in cattle.
  - Polyox II Bolus is for use in cattle.
- **Magnesium sulfate**
  - Epsom salts has been used in horses and birds.

Adverse Side Effects. These are rare but may include cramping or nausea. Overdose or overuse may result in dehydration or electrolyte imbalances (especially in cats). Products containing high phosphates should not be used in cats.

Bulk-Producing Agents

Bulk-producing agents are often indigestible plant materials (e.g., fiber and celluloses derived from cereal grains and bran) that act by absorbing water (pulling water into the bowel lumen) and swelling to increase the bulk of intestinal contents, thereby stimulating peristalsis.

Clinical Uses. Bulk-producing agents are used for relief of constipation and for relief of some types of impaction (sand primarily) in horses.

Dosage Forms. Dosage forms primarily consist of psyllium preparations. Psyllium is obtained from the ripe seed of a species of *Plantago* (Plumb, 2015).
- **Metamucil**
- **Equine Enteric Colloid**
- **Equi-Phar Sweet Psyllium**
- **SandClear**
- **Bran**—a bulk-producing agent often used for horses (bran mash)
- **Vetasyl** Fiber for Cats and Dogs

Adverse Side Effects. Adverse side effects are rare.

> **TECHNICIAN NOTES**
>
> Animals should be well hydrated before bulk-producing agents or laxatives are administered.

Lubricants

Lubricants are typically oils or other hydrocarbon derivatives (petrolatum) that soften the fecal mass and make it easier to move through the GI tract.

Clinical Uses. These include treatment of constipation and fecal impaction.

Dosage Forms. Dosage forms include liquids (mineral oil) and a jellylike mass (petrolatum).

- **Mineral oil.** Mineral oil is used in horses for the treatment of constipation, colic, and impaction. This substance is also used as a laxative in other species. Heavy mineral oil is preferred over light mineral oil.
- **Petrolatum.** This is a jellylike mass that is insoluble in water and is only slightly soluble in alcohol. Petrolatum is the principal ingredient in many of the oral laxatives for hairball treatment in cats.
  - Laxatone
  - Felilax
  - Cat Lax

Adverse Side Effects. These are minimal when used appropriately. Aspiration may occur when administering mineral oil orally to patients.

TECHNICIAN NOTES

When mineral oil is administered orally to a patient, care should be taken to avoid aspiration. Mineral oil is very bland and may not readily stimulate a swallowing reflex.

Surfactants/Stool Softeners

Surfactants reduce surface tension and allow water to penetrate GI contents, thus softening the stool. They also may increase intestinal secretions.

Clinical Uses. Clinical uses include the treatment of hard, dry feces in small animals; impaction in horses; and occasionally digestive upset in cattle.

Dosage Forms. These products are available in liquid, syrup, capsule, tablet, and enema forms. Docusate sodium, also called dioctyl sodium sulfosuccinate, is the main ingredient.

- **Disposable Enema**
- **Pet-Enema**
- **Docusate Sodium Enema**
- **Docusate sodium oral liquid** (Veterinary Surfactant)
  Adverse Side Effects. Adverse side effects are rare.

Irritants

Irritants act by irritating the gut wall, causing stimulation of GI smooth muscle and increased peristalsis.

These drugs are seldom used in veterinary medicine. This category includes several agents that are sometimes used in the treatment of constipation in humans.

- **Bisacodyl** (Dulcolax) is an effective stimulant laxative in cats when given with fiber supplementation for long-term management of constipation.
- **Castor oil**

TECHNICIAN NOTES

- Docusate sodium given with mineral oil may result in some absorption of mineral oil.
- Phosphate enemas (human label) should not be used in cats or puppies because of the potential for causing electrolyte imbalances.

® Gastrointestinal Prokinetics/Stimulants

Prokinetic/stimulant drugs increase the motility of a part or parts of the GI tract and by doing this enhance the transit of material through the tract. Several classes of drugs, including dopaminergic antagonists, serotonergic drugs, motilin like drugs, direct cholinergics, and acetylcholinesterase inhibitors, have the ability to enhance GI motility. As was previously noted, some H_2 receptor antagonists exhibit prokinetic activity (see Ranitidine earlier).

Dopaminergic Antagonists

Dopaminergic antagonists used as prokinetics in veterinary medicine include metoclopramide and domperidone (Hall & Washabau, 1997). These agents stimulate motility of the gastroesophageal sphincter, stomach, and small intestine. Domperidone has had limited use as a prokinetic in the United States but is approved in Europe for the treatment of nausea, vomiting, and gastric reflux in humans (Parker, 2001).

Clinical Uses. Metoclopramide is used for treatment of gastroesophageal reflux and delayed gastric emptying, for stimulation of the GI tract in foals, and for GI motility disorders in dogs and cats. Metoclopramide has been shown to enhance gastric emptying. The use of metoclopramide as an antiemetic is discussed in a previous section.

Dosage Forms
- **Metoclopramide** (Reglan) tablets, syrup, and injection.
- **Domperidone** (Motilium, Equidone). Domperidone may have use in regulating GI motility in horses, cats, and dogs.

Adverse Side Effects. Side effects include behavioral changes in dogs, cats, and adult horses. Cats have shown frenzied behavior (Plumb, 2015), and adult horses have exhibited alternating periods of sedation and excitement.

Serotonergic Drugs

Cisapride is the serotonergic prokinetic that is used in veterinary medicine. Cisapride stimulates motility of the proximal and distal GI tract, including the gastroesophageal sphincter, stomach, small intestine, and colon (Boothe, 2012). Cisapride is not effective as an antiemetic but may be better than metoclopramide in treating some motility disorders and in promoting gastric emptying of solid material.

Clinical Uses. Uses include the treatment of constipation (along with dietary and/or surgical considerations) in cats and gastroesophageal reflux and GI stasis in dogs, cats, and horses.

Dosage Form
- **Cisapride.** This drug has been removed from the market but may be available from compounding pharmacies.

Adverse Side Effects. Side effects may include diarrhea and abdominal pain.

Motilin-Li3ke Drugs

Erythromycin has been used by veterinarians to treat bacterial and mycoplasmal infections for many years. This drug has been shown to stimulate GI motility by mimicking the effect of the hormone motilin (Hall & Washabau, 2000). Erythromycin stimulates motility in the esophageal sphincter, stomach, and small intestine at microbially ineffective doses.

Clinical Uses. Uses may include increasing lower esophageal sphincter pressure, accelerating gastric emptying by increasing stomach contractions, and facilitating intestinal transit time.

Dosage Form
- **Erythromycin** (Erythro)

Adverse Side Effects. Side effects may include anorexia, vomiting, diarrhea, and abdominal pain.

Direct Cholinergics

Clinical Uses. These include postoperative treatment of ileus—or retention of flatus or feces—and equine colic (without obstruction).

Dosage Forms
- **Dexpanthenol** (D-Panthenol Injectable, D-Panthenol Injection)—veterinary label

- **Dexpanthenol** (Ilopan injection)—human label

Adverse Side Effects. Adverse side effects are rare but may include cramping and diarrhea.

> ### TECHNICIAN NOTES
>
> Dexpanthenol should not be used within 12 hours of the use of neostigmine, parasympathomimetic agents, or succinylcholine.

Acetylcholinesterase Inhibitors

These drugs increase the amount of acetylcholine available to bind smooth muscle receptors.

Clinical Uses. These agents are used to treat rumen atony, to enhance gastric emptying (ranitidine), to stimulate peristalsis, to empty the bladder of large animals, and to aid in the diagnosis of myasthenia gravis (neostigmine) in dogs. They also may be used to treat curare overdose.

Dosage Forms
- **Neostigmine methylsulfate** (Prostigmine)
- **Ranitidine** (Zantac)

Adverse Side Effects. Adverse side effects are cholinergic and may include nausea, vomiting, diarrhea, drooling, sweating, lacrimation, bradycardia, and various others.

> ### TECHNICIAN NOTES
>
> Ranitidine and nizatidine, H_2 receptor antagonists, increase acetylcholine by inhibiting acetylcholinesterase. The increase in acetylcholine stimulates smooth muscle in the stomach and promotes gastric emptying to reduce vomiting in patients with gastritis and related disorders.

℞ Digestive Enzymes

Pancrelipase is a product that contains pancreatic enzymes that aid in the digestion of fats, proteins, and carbohydrates. The powder that contains the enzymes is mixed with the animal's food, which is allowed to stand for 15 to 20 minutes before feeding.

Clinical Uses. This product is used to treat exocrine pancreatic insufficiency (EPI) in which maldigestion and malabsorption of nutrients occurs.

Dosage Forms
- **Pancrelipase** (Viokase-V powder, Pancrezyme powder)

Adverse Side Effects. Adverse side effects of high doses include cramping, nausea, and diarrhea.

Miscellaneous Gastrointestinal Drugs

Antibiotics

Antibiotics are not routinely used in the treatment of GI tract disease in small animals because these agents may destroy normal inhabitants of the GI tract and allow pathogenic bacteria (e.g., *Salmonella* species, *C. jejuni, C. perfringens, C. difficile, Helicobacter,* and others) to grow on the mucosal surface. Bloody diarrhea or signs of sepsis may indicate the need for antibiotic therapy. Antibiotics that are often used for treating bacterial overgrowth and other GI conditions include metronidazole, amoxicillin, clavamox, and tylosin.

Metronidazole. Metronidazole is a synthetic antibacterial and antiprotozoal agent. This drug is prohibited from use in food-producing animals by the U.S. Food and Drug Administration (FDA).

Clinical Uses. Metronidazole is used for treatment of giardiasis, trichomoniasis, balantidiasis, plasmacytic/lymphocytic enteritis, ulcerative colitis, hepatic encephalopathy, and anaerobic infection in dogs. It is also used to treat giardiasis and anaerobic infections in cats and anaerobic infections in horses.

Dosage Form
- **Metronidazole** (Flagyl tablets, Flagyl capsules, Metronidazole Injection)

Adverse Side Effects. These include CNS signs (disoriented, head tilt, and seizures), anorexia, hepatotoxicity, neutropenia, vomiting, and diarrhea.

Antiinflammatory Agents

Antiinflammatory agents are used in the treatment of idiopathic inflammatory bowel disease in animals. Increased numbers of lymphocytes, macrophages, plasma cells, or eosinophils in the intestinal wall characterize these diseases. Treatment often involves the use of hypoallergenic diets and antiinflammatory agents.

Dosage Forms. Antiinflammatory agents used in the treatment of inflammatory bowel disease include prednisone, azathioprine, sulfasalazine, and olsalazine.
- **Prednisone/prednisolone.** Many generic and trade name products are available.
- **Azathioprine** (Imuran). A purine antagonist antimetabolite that may be used in the treatment of inflammatory bowel disease because of its immunosuppressive effects.
- **Sulfasalazine** (Azulfidine). An antibiotic drug that is converted by intestinal bacteria to a sulfa drug (sulfapyridine) and aspirin (salicylic acid). Aspirin is the active component that has an antiinflammatory effect and is useful in many cases of colitis in dogs and cats. It should be used with care in cats because of their poor ability to metabolize aspirin.
- **Olsalazine** (Dipentum). Olsalazine is used for the treatment of dogs with chronic colitis that cannot tolerate sulfasalazine or that respond poorly to the product.

Antifoaming Agents

Antifoaming agents are used to treat frothy bloat in ruminants. In this condition, gas bubbles form and become trapped in the rumen fluid as a result of consumption of wheat pasture or legumes, such as alfalfa or clover. The trapped bubbles cause a form of bloat that cannot be relieved by usual means.

Antifoaming agents act as surfactants (reduce surface tension) and cause bubbles to break down so that gas can be relieved by eructation (belching) or by the stomach tube. These products are given orally.

Clinical Uses. Antifoaming agents are used for the treatment of frothy bloat in ruminants by decreasing the surface tension of foam in the rumen.

Dosage Forms
- **Bloat Guard**
- **Bloat Treatment**
- **Bloat-Pac**
- **Therabloat**

Adverse Side Effects. These are rare if the products are given as directed.

Probiotics

In healthy animals a balance exists between beneficial and harmful bacteria in the GI tract. Beneficial bacteria contribute to the maintenance or restoration of good health by modulating the immune system, competitively inhibiting enteropathogens, processing nutrients, and producing vitamins and fatty acids. Probiotics are beneficial live microbes that are administered orally to animals to support intestinal and overall health. Commercial probiotic products typically contain strains of *Lactobacillus* species, *Bifidobacterium* species, and *Enterococcus* species. The number of microbes, bacteria, or yeast in a commercial product is usually quantified on the label and in promotional literature as colony-forming units (CFUs). One billion to 10 billion CFUs per day is a recommended dose (Loes, 2012). The composition of the microbe mixture and the number of microbes are both likely to be important in the effectiveness of the product (Tams, 2012).

Prebiotics are nondigestable food ingredients that are beneficial to the bacterial population. Synbiotics contain both prebiotics and probiotics.

Clinical Uses. Probiotics are used to treat stress-related GI upset, antibiotic-associated diarrhea, diarrhea associated with dietary change, inflammatory bowel disease, gingival disease, and some conditions associated with other body systems.

Dosage Forms
- **FortiFlora**
- **Proviable-Forte**
- **Proviable DC**
- **Proviable EQ**
- **Probios**
- **Bactaquin**
- **Visbiome**
- **Numerous others**

Appetite Stimulants

Stimulating an animal to eat can be an important component of a therapy regimen. Proper nutrition is essential for optimal functioning of the immune system as well as for proper organ function. Cats who do not eat adequately for a period of time may develop a "fatty liver" syndrome that can be life threatening. The following is a partial list of appetite stimulants:

- **Diazepam**—medication that produces a transient appetite stimulation when given intravenously
- **Oxazepam** (Serax)—oral use in dogs and cats
- **Cyproheptadine**—oral antihistamine used as an appetite stimulant primarily in cats
- **Mirtazapine** (Remeron)—oral use in dogs and cats
- **Capromorelin** (Entyce)—oral use in dogs only

℞ Oral Products

An increased emphasis on dentistry in veterinary practice in recent years has fueled a demand for products that promote and maintain oral health. Many of these products help to remove food particles and plaque, and assist in the maintenance of pleasant-smelling breath. Some are labeled as a dentifrice, and others may be applied as an oral rinse or with a toothbrush. They are prepared as solutions, gels, and premoistened gauze sponges. Various flavors are available, as are products with fluoride. These products should not be considered a substitute for veterinary dental treatment. Clients should be advised to look for products with the Veterinary Oral Health Council (www.vohc.org) seal when purchasing dental hygiene products.

Other oral products include grit impregnated in paste for polishing teeth and smoothing rough surfaces left by scaling, as well as disclosing solution used to help identify plaque.

Dentifrice and Cleansing Products
- C.E.T. Enzymatic Toothpaste
- Nolvadent oral cleansing solution—active ingredient: chlorhexidine acetate; also contains a peppermint flavor; may be used with a toothbrush or as a rinse
- OraVet Plaque Prevention Gel
- OraVet Barrier Sealant
- C.E.T. Oral Hygiene Rinse for dogs and cats
- C.E.T. HEXtra Premium Chews for Dogs
- C.E.T. Oral Hygiene Enzymatic Chews for Cats
- C.E.T Veggiedent tartar control chews for dogs
- C.E.T. Oral Tatar Control Toothpaste
- Hills t/d Diets
- Healthy Mouth products
- Canine Greenies
- Chlorhexidine oral rinse and gel
- Purina Pro Plan Veterinary Diets
- Sanos Dental Sealant
- Various others

Fluoride Products

- Fluoride Gel

Perioceutic Agents

Doxirobe. Doxirobe is placed in the periodontal pocket after dental cleansing with the use of a cannula. Upon contact with the aqueous environment, the product coagulates and releases doxycycline for several weeks.

Tissue Regeneration Agents

- Consil Dental—a substance used to promote the regeneration of bone lost as the result of periodontal disease or tooth extraction
- Enamel matrix protein (Emdogain)—a substance derived from fetal pig teeth that may be used to promote periodontal ligament growth and proliferation

Polishing Paste

Polishing paste is used as a part of the dental prophylaxis to remove irregularities on the tooth surface which may promote the accumulation of plaque.

- C.E.T. prophypaste
- iClean prophy paste
- Vetcare prophy paste

REVIEW QUESTIONS

1. List three general functions of the GI tract.
2. List three examples of monogastric animals.
3. What is the GI configuration of ruminant animals?
4. What is the difference between vomiting and regurgitation?
5. Ruminants are animals that use _____ to digest coarse plant material.
6. What are the three basic control mechanisms of the GI tract?
7. What is the significance of the presence of bacterial endotoxins in the GI tract?
8. The CRTZ stimulates vomiting when activated by _____.
9. List two examples of centrally acting emetics and two examples of peripherally acting emetics.
10. Drugs that inhibit vomiting are called _____.

11. List two H_2 receptor antagonists.
12. What are the two types of intestinal motility patterns?
13. Acute vomiting and diarrhea in dogs and cats often respond to conservative management such as _____.
14. List two species that do not vomit.
15. What is the mechanism of action of saline/hyperosmotic laxatives?
16. Direct cholinergic drugs stimulate the GI tract by what mechanism?
17. List four products used as dentifrice/oral cleansing agents.
18. What is the difference between peristalsis and segmentation?
19. Stimulation of the parasympathetic portion of the ANS decreases intestinal motility.
    a. True
    b. False
20. About what percent of the stomach's contents do emetics usually remove?
21. How does sucralfate work to treat/prevent gastric ulcers?
22. The crop in birds is used for _____.
    a. a stomach
    b. food storage
    c. feces storage
    d. a place where food goes to mix with hydrochloric acid to aid in the breakdown of foodstuffs
23. _____ are substances that loosen bowel contents and encourage their evacuation.
    a. Protectants
    b. Adsorbents
    c. Antispasmodics
    d. Laxatives
24. A 20-lb puppy will be given a continuous intravenous (IV) infusion of metoclopramide over 24 hours for vomiting. The dosage is 2 mg/kg and the Reglan solution contains 5 mg/mL. How many milliliters of Reglan will you draw up to add to the IV fluids?
25. A 1200-lb horse will be treated with omeprazole for gastric ulcers at 4 mg/kg once daily for 2 weeks. GastroGard oral paste is available in syringes containing 2.28 g. How many syringes will you dispense?

REFERENCES

Boothe, D. M. (2012). Gastrointestinal pharmacology. In *Small animal clinical pharmacology and therapeutics*. Philadelphia: WB Saunders.

DeNovo, R. C. (2002). Chronic vomiting in the cat and dog. In *Proceedings. Annual Meeting of the American Veterinary Medical Association*. Nashville, TN.

Foushee, L. L. (2000). Omeprazole. *Compendium on Continuing Education for the Practising Veterinarian*, *22*(8), 746–749.

Ganong, W. (2003). Regulation of gastrointestinal function. In W. Ganong (Ed.), *Review of medical physiology* (21st ed.). New York: McGraw-Hill.

Hall, J. A. (2001). Diseases of the stomach. In S. J. Ettinger (Ed.), *Pocket companion to textbook of veterinary internal medicine*. Philadelphia: WB Saunders.

Hall, J. A., & Washabau, R. J. (1997). Gastrointestinal prokinetic therapy: Dopaminergic antagonist drugs. *Compendium on Continuing Education for the Practising Veterinarian*, *19*(2), 214–219.

Hall, J. A., & Washabau, R. J. (2000). Gastrointestinal prokinetic agents. In *Kirk's current veterinary therapy XIII: Small animal practice*. Philadelphia: WB Saunders.

Loes, N. (2012). Probiotics: Healthy from the inside out. In *Proceedings. Annual Meeting Tennessee Veterinary Medical Association*. Nashville, TN.

Parker, A. R. (2001). Domperidone. *Compendium on Continuing Education for the Practising Veterinarian*, *23*(10), 906–908.

Papich, M. G. (2016). *Saunders handbook of veterinary drugs* (4th ed.). St. Louis: Elsevier.

Plumb, D. C. (2015). *Veterinary drug handbook* (8th ed.). Ames, IA: Wiley-Blackwell.

Tams, T. R. (2012). Gastrointestinal medicine—diarrhea. In *Proceedings. Annual Meeting Tennessee Veterinary Medical Association*. Nashville, TN.

Upson, D. W. (1988). Gastrointestinal system. In D. W. Upson (Ed.), *Handbook of clinical veterinary pharmacology* (3rd ed.). Manhattan, KS: Dan Upson Enterprises.

Willard, M. D. (1998). Gastrointestinal drugs. In D. M. Boothe (Ed.), *The veterinary clinics of North America, small animal practice*. Philadelphia: WB Saunders.

9

Drugs Used in Hormonal, Endocrine, and Reproductive Disorders

OBJECTIVES

After studying this chapter, you should be able to

1. Discuss the control mechanisms (physiology) of the endocrine system.
2. List the endocrine glands.
3. List the reasons why hormones are clinically used.
4. Describe the difference between an endogenous and an exogenous hormone.
5. Describe the location and functions of the pituitary gland.
6. Differentiate between a positive and a negative feedback control mechanism and describe a neurohormonal reflex.
7. Discuss control of the reproductive system in animals.
8. Discuss the uses and classes of gonadotropins, gonadal hormones, estrogens, androgens, progestins, and prostaglandins used in veterinary medicine.

9. Describe the uses and classes of drugs that affect uterine contractility. In addition, discuss miscellaneous reproductive drugs.
10. Define *pheromone* and give an example.
11. Describe the location, function, and hormonal products of the thyroid gland.
12. Describe the hormonal treatment of hypothyroidism and hyperthyroidism.
13. Describe Addison's disease and list the drugs used to treat Addison's disease.
14. List the two forms of spontaneous Cushing's syndrome and list two or more drugs used to treat Cushing's syndrome.
15. Describe diabetes mellitus and list the classes of insulin products used to treat diabetes mellitus.
16. Describe the method of action of the growth promoters.
17. List the clinical uses for the anabolic steroids.

OUTLINE

KEY TERMS

Addison's disease
Anabolism
Analogue
Cushing's syndrome
Dystocia
Diabetes mellitus
Endometrium
Euthyroid
Feed efficiency
Feedback
Gonadotropin

Hypophyseal portal system
Iatrogenic
Involution
Ketone bodies
Levo isomer
Myofibril
Nitrogen balance
Primary hypothyroidism
Releasing factor (releasing hormone)
Trophic hormone

INTRODUCTION

The traditional definition of the endocrine system states that it is composed of organs (glands) or groups of cells that secrete regulatory substances (hormones) directly into the bloodstream. This definition has now been extended to include regulatory substances that are distributed by diffusion across cell membranes.

The endocrine system and the nervous system constitute the two major control mechanisms of the body. These two control mechanisms are linked together through the complex integrating action of the hypothalamus (Fig. 9.1). Coordination of these two systems allows an individual to adapt its reproductive and survival strategies to changes in the environment.

Endocrine glands include the pituitary, adrenals, thyroid, ovaries, testicles, pancreas, and kidneys. These glands produce hormones that are carried to target organs, where they influence the physiologic activity of these structures.

Hormones generally are administered to animals for one of two reasons: (1) to correct a deficiency of that hormone or (2) to obtain a desired effect (e.g., to postpone estrus). Hormones that are administered to an animal are called *exogenous* hormones, whereas those produced naturally in the body are *endogenous* hormones.

ANATOMY AND PHYSIOLOGY

Pituitary Gland

The pituitary gland has been called the master gland of the endocrine system because of the control it exerts over the regulation of this system. It is located at the base of the brain just ventral to the hypothalamus and is connected to the brain by a stalk. It is divided into two main lobes—an anterior lobe (adenohypophysis), which arises from the embryologic pharynx, and a posterior lobe (neurohypophysis), which arises from the brain (Fig. 9.2).

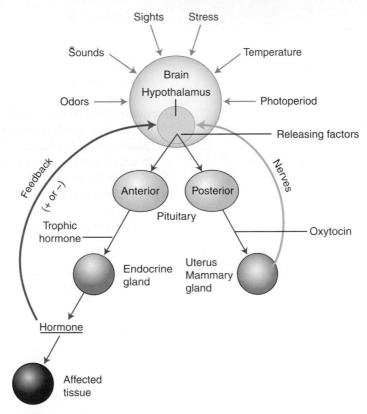

Fig. 9.1 Hypothalamic integration of endocrine and nervous systems.

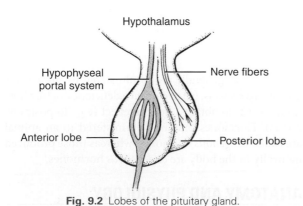

Fig. 9.2 Lobes of the pituitary gland.

The hypothalamus exerts control over the anterior pituitary through the transport of **releasing hormones,** or **factors,** down the **hypophyseal portal system.** In the anterior pituitary, these releasing factors cause the secretion of **trophic hormones** into the circulation. Trophic hormones produced by the anterior pituitary include thyroid-stimulating hormone (TSH), adrenocorticotropic hormone (ACTH), luteinizing hormone (LH), follicle-stimulating hormone (FSH), prolactin (LTH), and growth hormone (GH or somatotropin). These trophic hormones are sometimes called *indirect-acting hormones* because they cause their target organ to produce a second hormone, which in turn influences a second target organ or tissue (Table 9.1). For example, TSH stimulates the thyroid gland to produce triiodothyronine (T_3) and tetraiodothyronine (T_4), which are hormones that in turn influence the metabolic rate of all tissues in the body.

The two hormones of the posterior pituitary are vasopressin (antidiuretic hormone) and oxytocin. These hormones are produced in the hypothalamus and subsequently travel down nerve fibers to the posterior pituitary, where they are stored for release into the circulation. The hormones of the posterior pituitary are called *direct-acting hormones* because they produce the desired activity (e.g., contraction of the uterus) directly in the target organ.

TABLE 9.1	Pituitary Hormones.
Source and Name	**Target and Actions**
Anterior Lobe	
Thyroid-stimulating hormone (TSH)	Stimulates the thyroid to produce T_3/T_4
Follicle-stimulating hormone (FSH)	Stimulates ovarian follicle growth (female) and spermatogenesis (male)
Luteinizing hormone (LH)	Stimulates ovulation (female) and testosterone production (male)
Growth hormone (somatotropin)	Accelerates body growth and increases milk production
Adrenocorticotropic hormone (ACTH)	Stimulates production of corticosteroids by adrenal cortex
Posterior Lobe	
Oxytocin	Stimulates uterine contraction and milk letdown
Vasopressin (antidiuretic hormone, ADH)	Stimulates water retention

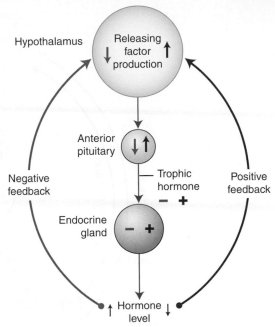

Fig. 9.3 Feedback control mechanisms. Positive and negative feedback mechanisms control the quantity of a particular hormone.

Control of the Endocrine System

Feedback Mechanism. The nervous system is sensitive to levels of hormones through a mechanism called **feedback.** By this mechanism, the plasma level of a particular hormone controls the activity of the gland that produces it. The feedback may be negative or positive (Fig. 9.3).

With negative feedback, high plasma levels of a hormone are sensed by the hypothalamus, which then reduces the amount of the appropriate releasing factor (or hormone). A decreased amount of releasing factor reduces the amount of trophic hormone released from the pituitary, causing less activity in the organ that is producing the hormone in question. The overall effect is to lower the amount of the hormone in the plasma.

In the positive feedback scheme, low levels of a hormone are sensed by the hypothalamus, and release of the appropriate releasing factor increases. Increased amounts of the corresponding trophic hormone are then secreted, causing increased activity in the target organ and a corresponding rise in the plasma levels of the hormone.

Neurohormonal Reflex. The neurohormonal reflex applies to the release of oxytocin by the posterior pituitary. The first step in this reflex can be initiated by (1) stimulation of the udder by a nursing calf or by preparation of the udder for milking, (2) stimulation of the uterus and vagina in parturition, or (3) stimulation of the cerebral cortex by sensory stimuli associated with nursing or milking.

Control of the Reproductive System

The reproductive (estrus) cycle in animals traditionally has been divided into four stages called *proestrus*, *estrus*, *diestrus*, and *anestrus*. The cycle also may be divided into a follicular phase and a luteal phase. In the follicular phase, the cycle is under the influence of estrogen produced by a developing follicle, and in the luteal phase, it is under the influence of progesterone made by the corpus luteum.

Control of the reproductive system is coordinated in the hypothalamus, where the gonadotropin-releasing hormone (GnRH) is produced in response to various stimuli (Fig. 9.4). These stimuli can include day–night length (photoperiod), pheromones, and positive and negative internal feedback mechanisms. GnRH causes the release of FSH and LH from the anterior pituitary.

FSH causes the growth and maturation of a follicle, which begins to produce increasing amounts of estrogen as it matures. Estrogen causes the changes that occur in proestrus and estrus, including the behavioral characteristics associated with estrus (e.g., standing to be mounted). The follicle also produces inhibin,

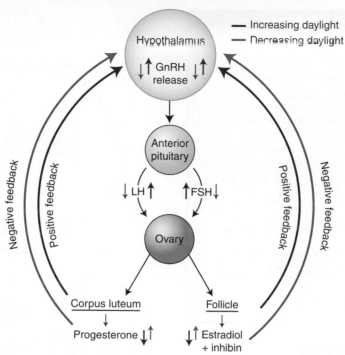

Fig. 9.4 Control of the reproductive system is achieved through feedback mechanisms responding to increased or decreased levels of estradiol and progesterone in the bloodstream and increasing or decreasing daylight. *FSH*, Follicle-stimulating hormone; *GnRH*, gonadotropin-releasing hormone; *LH*, luteinizing hormone.

which—along with estrogen—serves as negative feedback to the hypothalamus to inhibit the release of GnRH.

LH release causes ovulation of the mature follicle and the formation of a corpus luteum in its place. This event signals the beginning of diestrus and the beginning of the luteal phase of the cycle. The corpus luteum produces progesterone, which prepares the uterus for pregnancy. Once pregnancy occurs, the corpus luteum maintains a uterine environment conducive to normal progression of the pregnancy. Progesterone levels in the blood serve as negative feedback to prevent the release of GnRH and the development of new follicles during pregnancy.

When the gestation period nears its end, the fetus begins to produce increasing amounts of ACTH. ACTH causes increased amounts of cortisol to be produced by the adrenal glands. The increased cortisol levels result in increased production of estrogen and prostaglandin by the uterus. These two substances sensitize the uterus to the contraction-producing effects of oxytocin and allow parturition to begin. Prostaglandin also causes the breakdown (lysis) of the corpus luteum at the end of pregnancy and at the end of diestrus if pregnancy does not occur.

HORMONAL DRUGS ASSOCIATED WITH REPRODUCTION

Ⓡ Gonadotropins and Gonadal Hormones

Products in this category are used in veterinary medicine for various reasons. Some of these include synchronization of estrus, suppression of estrus, induction of estrus, treatment of cystic ovaries, and termination of pregnancy.

Gonadotropins

Gonadotropins are drugs that act similarly to GnRH, LH, or FSH. Gonadotropins cause the release of LH and FSH or cause activity similar to that of LH or FSH. LH may be prepared from the pituitary glands of slaughtered animals, from the urine of pregnant women in the form of human chorionic gonadotropin (hCG), or in pure form through recombinant techniques. FSH may be obtained from pituitary glands (FSH-P), from the serum of pregnant mares (PMS) between the 40th and 140th days of pregnancy, or from recombinant sources. GnRH is prepared synthetically.

FSH that is released endogenously by the anterior pituitary causes growth and maturation of the ovarian follicle in females and spermatogenesis in males. LH, also released by the anterior pituitary, causes ovulation in females and production of testosterone in males.

Gonadorelin. Gonadorelin (GnRH) is produced endogenously by the hypothalamus. Gonadorelin causes the release of FSH and LH by the anterior pituitary.

Clinical Uses. Gonadorelin is used to treat cystic (follicular) ovaries in dairy cattle. It has also been used in cats and horses (with limited success) to induce estrus.

Dosage Forms

- **Gonadorelin** (Cystorelin) for injection; used in dairy cattle for cystic ovaries.
- **Gonadorelin** (Factrel) for injection; used in cattle for the treatment of ovarian follicular cysts; it is also approved for use with Lutalyse to synchronize estrous cycles in beef or dairy heifers and cows.
- **Gonadorelin** (Fertagyl) for injection; used in dairy cattle for cystic ovaries.
- **Gonadorelin** (Gonabreed) for injection; used in beef and diary cattle. Used in dairy cattle for cystic ovaries. Used with cloprostenol sodium to synchronize estrous cycles in beef and dairy cows.
- **Deslorelin** (SucroMate, Ovuplant). Deslorelin is used to induce and time ovulation in mares and may have some potential as a contraceptive agent in dogs (extralabel).

Adverse Side Effects. These are minimal with the use of this product. May cause local swelling at the site of injection, which usually subsides within 5 days (Plumb, 2015).

Chorionic Gonadotropin. hCG is a hormone secreted by the uterus and obtained from the urine of pregnant women. It mimics the effects of LH, although it has limited FSH activity. In males, it stimulates the production of male hormones by the testicles and may facilitate descent of the testicles.

Clinical Uses. Chorionic gonadotropin is used to treat cystic ovaries (nymphomania) in dairy cattle. In males, it has been used to treat cryptorchidism and infertility caused by low testosterone levels.

Dosage Forms

- **hCG injection** (Follutein)
- **Combination hCG and PMS** (P.G. 600); contains both LH and FSH activity
- **hCG injection** (Chorulon)
- **Chorionic gonadotropin injection** (generic)

Adverse Side Effects. These are limited but may include hypersensitivity reaction and abortion in mares if given before the 35th day of pregnancy (Plumb, 2015).

Follicle-Stimulating Hormone. FSH causes growth and maturation of the ovarian follicle. FSH-P, prepared from the pituitary glands from slaughtered animals, is no longer available. Purified recombinant human FSH may be obtained, but it is expensive. Chorionic gonadotropin is readily available and causes FSH-like activity (and LH activity) and is more likely to be used in reproductive cases.

Clinical Uses. FSH has been used in veterinary medicine to induce superovulation and for out-of-season breeding.

Dosage Form

- **FSH** (Follitropin alpha), human label

Adverse Side Effects. These include endometrial hyperplasia, superovulation, and follicular cysts.

Estrogens

Estrogens are a group of hormones synthesized by the ovaries and—to a lesser extent—by the testicles, adrenal cortex, and placenta. Estrogens are classified as sex steroids and are synthesized from a cholesterol precursor. Estrogens are necessary for normal growth and development of the female gonads. They cause secondary female characteristics and are responsible for female sex drive. These hormones inhibit ovulation, increase uterine tone, and cause proliferation of the endometrium.

Clinical Uses. In cattle, estrogens are used to treat persistent corpus luteum, to expel purulent material from the uterus, to expel retained placentas and mummified fetuses, and to promote weight gain. In dogs, estrogens may be used to control urinary incontinence. In horses, they may be used for induction of estrus in the nonbreeding season.

Dosage Forms

- **Estradiol cypionate** (ECP) injection
- **Estradiol cypionate for injection** (Depo-Estradiol), human label
- **Estradiol valerate for injection** (Delestrogen), human label
- **Diethylstilbestrol** (DES) compounded capsules and tablets
- **Estriol** (Incurin), for control of urinary incontinence in spayed dogs

Adverse Side Effects. These include severe anemia, prolonged estrus, genital irritation, and follicular cysts.

📋 TECHNICIAN NOTES

- Estrogens should not be given during pregnancy.
- Estrogens can cause infection in the uterus and pyometra.
- Estrogen administration can cause severe anemia (aplastic anemia).
- Synthetic DES has been banned from use in food-producing animals because of its possible link with cervical cancer in women.

Androgens

Androgens are male sex hormones produced in the testicles, the ovaries, and the adrenal cortex. Similar to the other gonadal hormones, they have a steroidal parent molecule. These hormones are necessary for growth and development of the male sex organs. They cause secondary male sex characteristics and produce male libido. The androgens promote tissue **anabolism,** weight gain, and red blood cell formation.

Methyltestosterone, Testosterone Cypionate, Testosterone Enanthate, and Testosterone Propionate. These injectable testosterone products are available under a human label. Because of expense and unpredictable efficacy, these drugs are not commonly used in veterinary medicine.

Clinical Uses. These androgens are rarely used to treat urinary incontinence in male dogs and to increase libido and fertility in domestic animals (with generally poor results).

Dosage Forms
- **Methyltestosterone** (Android), human label
- **Danazol** (Danocrine), synthetic androgen (human label)
- **Testosterone cypionate injection** (generic)
- **Testosterone enanthate** (generic)
- **Testosterone propionate injection** (generic)

Adverse Side Effects. Adverse effects include edema, testicular atrophy, prostatic disorders, hepatotoxicity, and behavior changes.

 TECHNICIAN NOTES

Testosterone products are Class III controlled substances.

Mibolerone. Mibolerone is an androgen used for prevention of estrus in dogs. Mibolerone blocks the release of LH by the pituitary and prevents complete development of the follicle. Ovulation does not occur. This drug is an anabolic steroid and has been abused by people for use as a body-building drug. Mibolerone has been discontinued by the manufacturer (Papich, 2016).

Clinical Uses. This product is used for prevention of estrus in adult female dogs and for treatment of pseudocyesis.

Dosage Forms
- It may be available through compounding pharmacies.

Adverse Side Effects. Adverse side effects reported in the product insert include premature epiphyseal closure and vaginitis in immature females. In mature females, vulvovaginitis, clitoral hypertrophy, riding behavior, increased body odor, and various other side effects have been reported. It is further reported that side effects usually resolve with discontinuation of therapy.

 TECHNICIAN NOTES

Mibolerone should not be used in cats because of a very low margin of safety in this species.

Progestins

Progestins are a group of compounds that are similar in effect to progesterone. Endogenous progestins are produced by the corpus luteum. They cause increased secretions by the endometrium, decreased motility in the uterus, and increased secretory development in the mammary glands. They also inhibit the release of gonadotropins by the pituitary to produce an inactive ovary. In some situations, they can cause elevated blood glucose levels (antiinsulin effect) or serious suppression of the adrenal glands. These hormones are used clinically to suppress estrus and to treat false pregnancy, behavioral disorders, and progestin-responsive dermatitis. The root "gest" often allows name recognition of the progestins.

Megestrol Acetate. Megestrol acetate is a synthetic progestin labeled for use in dogs. It is used, however, in cats for some behavioral and dermatologic conditions.

Clinical Uses. Megestrol acetate is labeled for use in dogs to control estrus, treat false pregnancy, prevent vaginal hyperplasia, treat severe galactorrhea, and control unacceptable male behavior. Megestrol acetate has been used in cats for various dermatologic (alopecia) and behavioral problems (urine spraying in cats) and for suppression of estrus.

Dosage Forms
- **Megestrol acetate** (Ovaban) tablets in bottles or foil strips

Adverse Side Effects. These can include hyperglycemia, adrenal suppression (cats), endometrial hyperplasia, and increased appetite.

 TECHNICIAN NOTES

Clients should be made aware of the potential dangers associated with the use of megestrol acetate and should be asked to report any changes in their pet's health status that occur after initiation of therapy.

Medroxyprogesterone Acetate. Medroxyprogesterone acetate (MPA) is a human-label progestin that has been used to treat certain behavioral and dermatologic problems and to suppress estrus in dogs and cats.

Clinical Uses. Medroxyprogesterone acetate is used for (1) treatment of behavioral problems, such as aggression, roaming, spraying, or mounting in males; and (2) treatment of certain dermatologic conditions.

Dosage Forms
- **MPA for injection** (Depo-Provera)
- **MPA tablets** (Provera)

Adverse Side Effects. These are potentially numerous and include pyometra, personality changes, depression, lethargy, mammary changes, and increased appetite.

 TECHNICIAN NOTES

Progestins should be administered with strict adherence to an accepted protocol to minimize side effects such as pyometra.

Altrenogest. Altrenogest is an oral progestin labeled for use in horses and swine. This drug is used to suppress estrus in mares and sexually mature gilts. Mares stop cycling within 3 days of treatment and begin cycling again 4 to 5 days after treatment is stopped. It is also used to manage other reproductive conditions that are listed later.

Clinical Uses. Altrenogest is used to suppress estrus for synchronization, to suppress estrus for long periods, or to maintain pregnancy in mares with low levels of progesterone.

Dosage Form
- **Altrenogest in oil oral solution (Regu-Mate)** for use in horses
- **For use in sexually mature gilts (Matrix);** for use in swine; extralabel use is prohibited

Adverse Side Effects. These have been reported as minimal when altrenogest is used correctly.

 TECHNICIAN NOTES

Altrenogest can be absorbed through the skin and should be used with great caution by pregnant women or anyone with vascular disorders. Read the label carefully before using.

Norgestomet. Norgestomet is a synthetic progestin that is used in combination with an estrogen (estradiol valerate) for synchronization of estrus in beef cows and nonlactating dairy cows. A treatment consists of one implant and an injection at the time of implantation.

Clinical Uses. Norgestomet is used for synchronization of estrus and/or ovulation in cattle.

Dosage Form
- **Syncro-Mate-B**

Adverse Side Effects. Adverse side effects are not reported in the insert.

Melengestrol Acetate (MGA). Melengestrol acetate is an approved progestogen that is used as a feed additive in cattle to promote growth and to suppress the estrous cycle in heifers.

Ⓡ Prostaglandins

Prostaglandins consist of a group of naturally occurring, long-chain fatty acids that mediate various physiologic events in the body. The primary use of prostaglandins in veterinary medicine is for regulation of activity in and treatment of conditions of the female reproductive tract. Of the six classes (A, B, C, D, E, and F), only prostaglandin F_{2alpha} has significant clinical application in the reproductive system.

Prostaglandin F_{2alpha} causes lysis of the corpus luteum, contraction of uterine muscle, and relaxation of the cervix. Lysis of the corpus luteum results in a decline in plasma levels of progesterone and, through the negative feedback mechanism, initiation of a new estrus cycle. Contraction of uterine muscle can facilitate evacuation of uterine contents (pus or a mummified fetus) or produce an abortion.

Bronchoconstriction, increased blood pressure, and smooth muscle contraction have been reported in other species, including humans. For these reasons, pregnant women and asthmatic individuals should handle prostaglandin products with extreme caution; exposure (through injection or skin contact) can cause abortion or an asthma attack.

Name recognition of the prostaglandins is made easier by looking for "prost" in the drug name.

Dinoprost Tromethamine

Dinoprost tromethamine is a salt of the naturally occurring prostaglandin F_{2alpha} and is labeled for use in cattle, horses, and swine. It also has accepted clinical uses in dogs, cats, sheep, and goats. It is effective only in animals with a corpus luteum.

Clinical Uses. Labeled clinical uses include estrus synchronization, treatment of silent estrus, and pyometra in cattle. It is also used for abortion of feedlot and other non-lactating cattle. In swine, dinoprost tromethamine induces parturition. It can be used for controlling the timing of estrus in cycling mares and in anestrous mares that have a corpus luteum. In dogs and cats, dinoprost tromethamine is used to treat pyometra and endometrial hyperplasia and as an abortion-producing agent. In sheep and goats, the uses are similar to those for cattle.

Dosage Forms
- **Dinoprost tromethamine for injection** (Lutalyse)
- **In Synch**
- **ProstaMate**

Adverse Side Effects. These can include sweating (horses), abdominal pain (horses, dogs, cats, and swine), urination/defecation (dogs, cats, and swine), dyspnea and panting (dogs and cats), tachycardia (dogs), and increased vocalization (cats and swine) (Plumb, 2015). Most of the side effects are self-limiting and disappear within a short time.

Cloprostenol Sodium

Cloprostenol sodium is an analogue of prostaglandin F_{2alpha} for use in cattle. This product is chemically very similar to dinoprost and fenprostalene and is labeled for uses that are very similar to those of dinoprost and fenprostalene in cattle. The same precautions should be taken when this drug is used as are taken with the other prostaglandins.

Clinical Uses. This drug is used for treatment of luteal cysts and mummified fetuses, termination of pregnancy, and estrus synchronization.

Dosage Forms
- **Cloprostenol** (Estrumate) for injection
- **estroPLAN**

Adverse Side Effects. At high doses, adverse side effects may include uneasiness, frothing at the mouth, and milk letdown.

 TECHNICIAN NOTES

- When administering any of the prostaglandins do not administer by intravenous injection.
- Skin that is accidentally exposed during administration should be washed off immediately.
- Pregnant women and individuals with asthma or bronchial disease should handle this product with great caution.

Drugs That Affect Uterine Contractility

Several drugs have the ability to increase the contractility of uterine muscle. Some are used during pregnancy to cause abortion, and others are used at term to induce parturition, to aid in delivery of the fetus or the placenta, and to cause involution of the uterus after delivery. Great care should be taken to ensure that the cervix is dilated before these drugs are administered.

One of these drugs, oxytocin, also causes contraction of the myoepithelial cells in the mammary glands to facilitate milk letdown.

Oxytocin

Oxytocin is a polypeptide made in the hypothalamus and stored in the posterior pituitary for release in response to appropriate stimuli from the reproductive tract or mammary glands. This hormone causes stronger uterine contractions by increasing the contractility of uterine myofibrils. The uterus must be primed for a period by progesterone and estrogen before oxytocin is effective in stimulating the uterus.

Oxytocin is used clinically to cause more forceful uterine contractions as an aid in delivery of a fetus. It is also used to assist delivery of the placenta, to cause uterine involution, and to reduce bleeding of the uterus after delivery. It should be used only when the cervix is sufficiently dilated and when it can be determined that the fetus can be delivered normally through the pelvic canal.

This hormone is responsible for milk letdown from the mammary glands through its stimulation of myoepithelial cells in the alveolar wall of the glands. It is released endogenously after stimulation of the udder or in response to environmental stimuli, such as the sound of milking machines or other sights, sounds, or smells associated with nursing/milking.

Clinical Uses. Oxytocin is used to augment the force of uterine contractions during delivery, aid in delivery of the placenta, facilitate involution of the uterus (for reduction of bleeding or replacement of a prolapse), induce milk letdown, and assist in the treatment of agalactia in sows.

Dosage Form
- **Oxytocin injection;** generic form from many sources

Adverse Side Effects. These are minimal when used according to recommendations.

 TECHNICIAN NOTES

- Oxytocin should be used in dystocia (difficult labor) only when the reproductive tract has been adequately examined. Inappropriate use can result in uterine torsion or rupture and can lead to death.
- A single dose of oxytocin lasts approximately 15 minutes.

Prostaglandins

Prostaglandins, as mentioned in a previous section, stimulate uterine smooth muscle and can be used to induce parturition or abortion.

Corticosteroids

Corticosteroids comprise a group of hormones produced by the adrenal cortex that are used primarily for their antiinflammatory effect but can cause induction of parturition in the last trimester of pregnancy. This effect occurs because exogenous administration of the drug mimics the natural rise in production of corticosteroids by the fetus as the time for delivery draws near. Induction of parturition or abortion is not a labeled use for the corticosteroids, but they have been applied clinically for this purpose.

Ⓡ Miscellaneous Reproductive Drugs
Bromocriptine

Bromocriptine is a dopamine agonist and prolactin inhibitor that has been used mainly in dogs for pregnancy termination after mis-mating or for the treatment of pseudopregnancy.

Cabergoline

Cabergoline is an ergot derivative used in dogs and cats for reduction of milk production, for pregnancy termination, and for estrus induction (dogs).

Leuprolide

Leuprolide is a synthetic analogue of GnRH that is used for the treatment of adrenal endocrinopathy in ferrets and for the treatment of inappropriate egg laying in cockatiels.

Melatonin

Melatonin is a naturally occurring hormone that is produced in the pineal gland. In addition to its use in the treatment of alopecia in dogs and sleep disorders in cats and dogs, melatonin has been used to improve early breeding and ovulation in sheep and goats.

Metergoline

Metergoline is a serotonin antagonist that may be used for treating pseudopregnancy in dogs.

Ⓡ Pheromones

Pheromones are odors released by animals that influence the behavior of other animals of the same species. Although pheromones do not fit exactly into the endocrine category, they are considered in this section.

The first pheromone made commercially available was a boar odor aerosol called SOA/Sex. This product is a synthetic version of the natural pheromone that causes the typical boar odor and is used for heat detection in sows and gilts. Label instructions call for spraying the pheromone directly at the nostrils of the sow or gilt for 2 seconds. If the sow or gilt is in heat, she will demonstrate mating reflexes, such as rigid posture, deviations of the tail, and erect ears.

Other products (Feliway, Comfort Zone-Feline) are analogues of the feline facial pheromone. They are labeled for use in stopping or preventing urinary marking by the cat and to comfort the cat in an unknown or stressful environment. Cats deposit facial pheromones by rubbing an object with the side of the face. The manufacturers recommend spraying this product directly onto the places soiled by the cat and also on prominent objects that could be attractive to the cat. The products should be applied daily at a height of 8 inches from the floor until the cat is seen rubbing the area with its head. Pheromones can also be used to familiarize cats with new environments, such as carriers and cages. They may be dispensed over a large area with the use of a plug-in diffuser.

Another pheromone available in the veterinary market is called dog-appeasing hormone (D.A.P. and Comfort Zone-Canine). The manufacturers indicate that this product mimics the appeasement pheromones, which female dogs secrete to comfort and reassure their nursing puppies. Label indications for use include calming dogs during stressful situations, such as thunderstorms, fireworks, visits by strangers, or moving the dog to a new environment. It is available as a spray, collar, or room diffuser.

THYROID HORMONES

The thyroid gland is made up of two lobes (one on each side of the trachea) and is located near the thyroid cartilage of the larynx (Fig. 9.5). Microscopically, the thyroid is composed of follicles that, on stimulation by TSH from the anterior pituitary, produce two metabolically active hormones. The thyroid synthesizes these hormones by first trapping iodide from the blood and then oxidizing the iodide to iodine. The iodine is combined with the amino acid tyrosine to form (through several intermediary steps) T_3 and T_4. T_3 is considered to be the active form at the cellular level. Although both T_3 and T_4 are released from the thyroid gland, some of the T_4

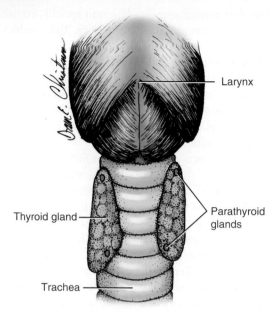

Larynx

Thyroid gland

Parathyroid glands

Trachea

Fig. 9.5 Canine thyroid and parathyroid glands. (From Christenson, D. E. [2008]. *Veterinary medical terminology* [2nd ed.]. St. Louis: Elsevier.)

is converted to T_3 after release. T_4, also called *thyroxine,* is found in higher levels than T_3 in **euthyroid** animals.

Thyroid hormones control many events in the body, including metabolic rate, growth and development, body temperature, heart rate, metabolism of nutrients, skin condition, resistance to infection, and others. Two abnormalities of thyroid function that are encountered in veterinary medicine are hypothyroidism (low production of thyroid hormone) and hyperthyroidism (overproduction of thyroid hormone).

Hypothyroidism is noted most often in dogs and is characterized by lethargy, weight gain, cold intolerance, dry and scaly haircoat, decreased function of the estrous cycle, and bradycardia. Hyperthyroidism is encountered more often in older cats and is accompanied by weight loss despite increased appetite, heat intolerance, restlessness, hyperexcitability, polyuria, polydipsia and tachycardia. Diagnosis of thyroid conditions is made by observing clinical signs and by measuring serum levels of T_3 and T_4 before and after TSH administration.

Goiter is a hypothyroid condition that is caused by inadequate levels of iodide in the diet. Lack of iodide causes the thyroid to be unable to produce T_3 or T_4. The thyroid attempts to increase its output by enlarging, often to a size that can be palpated and visualized. Goiter is almost nonexistent in animals receiving a commercial diet.

℞ Drugs Used to Treat Hypothyroidism

Treatment of hypothyroidism consists of supplementation of thyroid hormones on a daily basis. Clinical signs usually resolve within a short time of treatment initiation, but lifelong therapy is required.

Thyroid hormones can be extracted from thyroid glands or can be prepared synthetically. Purification of the animal source hormones is difficult and has led to the common use of synthetic products. Synthetic thyroxine (T_4) is considered to be the compound of choice in the treatment of hypothyroidism. T_3 products are recommended only when a poor response to T_4 occurs.

Levothyroxine Sodium (T_4)

Levothyroxine is a synthetic **levo isomer** of T_4. It is the compound of choice for the treatment of hypothyroidism in all species.

Clinical Uses. Levothyroxine is used for the treatment of hypothyroid conditions.

Dosage Forms
- **Levothyroxine tablets** (Thyro-Tabs) for dogs
- **Levothyroxine powder** (Thyro-L), for horses
- **Equine Thyroid Supplement**

Adverse Side Effects. These are rare when used according to recommendations.

Liothyronine Sodium

Liothyronine sodium (T_3) is a synthetic salt of endogenous T_3. T_3 is not recommended as the compound of choice for the treatment of hypothyroidism because it has a shorter half-life, requires administration three times daily, and is more likely to cause iatrogenic hyperthyroidism (Scott-Moncrieff, 2014). It may be useful, however, in cases that do not respond well to T_4.

Clinical Uses. T_3 is used for the treatment of hypothyroidism in cases that respond poorly to T_4.

Dosage Forms
- **Triostat,** human label
- **Cytomel,** human label

Adverse Side Effects. These are probably minimal with careful use.

Thyroid-Stimulating Hormone

Thyrotropin alpha is a recombinant TSH. It is used as an aid in the diagnosis of hypothyroidism. The bovine source of TSH is no longer available.

Clinical Uses. In veterinary medicine, thyrotropin is used for diagnosis of **primary hypothyroidism** in the TSH stimulation test.

Dosage Form

- **Thyrogen powder for injection**
    Adverse Side Effects. Allergic reactions may occur in animals sensitive to human protein.

℞ Drugs Used to Treat Hyperthyroidism

Treatment of hyperthyroidism is directed at lowering blood levels of T_3 and T_4. This can be accomplished by destruction or removal of the overproducing thyroid or by blocking of hormone production. The thyroid can be removed surgically or destroyed with radioactive iodine. Drug therapy to block hormone production can be effective but is continuous and is not curative (Boothe, 2012).

The two antithyroid drugs used most often are methimazole and carbimazole. These compounds are used for long-term therapy and for presurgical preparation of patients. Cats with hyperthyroidism are often high surgical risks, primarily because of tachycardia and other potential cardiac abnormalities.

Methimazole

Methimazole is a compound that interferes with incorporation of iodine into the precursor molecules of T_3 and T_4. It does not alter thyroid hormones already released into the bloodstream.

Clinical Uses. Methimazole is used for the treatment of feline hyperthyroidism.

Dosage Form

- **Methimazole tablets** (Felimazole), approved for cats
- **Methimazole can be compounded as an oral liquid or in the form of a transdermal gel** that is applied to a hairless area of skin, usually on the inside of the ear.
- **Methimazole tablets** (Tapazole), human approved

TECHNICIAN NOTES

- Veterinary staff and owners should wash hands with soap and water after administration of Felimazole to avoid exposure to drug.

Adverse Side Effects. These include anorexia, vomiting, and skin eruptions. Kittens should receive a milk replacement after receiving colostrum from mothers given methimazole.

Carbimazole

Carbimazole is a product similar to methimazole that is used in Canada and other countries. Most of this drug is converted to methimazole after administration to the cat. It inhibits the synthesis of thyroid hormones.

Clinical Uses. Carbimazole is used for the treatment of feline hyperthyroidism.

Dosage Forms

- **Carbimazole** (Carbizole), human label
    Adverse Side Effects. Side effects are similar to those of methimazole.

Radioactive Iodine

Radioactive iodine (I-131) may be given intravenously to destroy overproductive thyroid tissue. I-131 concentrates in the thyroid, where it remains and destroys thyroid tissue. This method has appeal because it is performed only once and is not especially stressful to patients. However, it must be done at facilities that can handle radioactive materials.

Propranolol

Propranolol (Inderal) may be used preoperatively to treat the tachycardia associated with hyperthyroidism in cats.

℞ Drugs Used to Treat Hypoadrenocorticism (Addison's Disease)

Hypoadrenocorticism or Addison's disease primarily affects dogs and results in inadequate secretions of glucocorticoids (cortisol) and/or mineralocorticoids (aldosterone) by the adrenal glands. The adrenal glands are located near the kidneys (Fig. 9.6). Adrenal hormones are necessary to control sodium, potassium, and water balance. Production of cortisol is regulated by hormones produced in the brain from the pituitary gland. Production of aldosterone is regulated by the renin-angiotensin system (Fig. 9.7) and helps maintain sodium and water balance as well as regulating blood pressure in the body. Addison's disease is seen mostly in young to middle-aged, female dogs. The clinical signs associated with this disease include hypotension, dehydration, hypoglycemia, hyponatremia (decreased sodium), azotemia, and hyperkalemia (increased potassium).

Mineralocorticoids

Desoxycorticosterone pivalate. Desoxycorticosterone pivalate (DOCP) is a drug that mimics the effects of aldosterone.

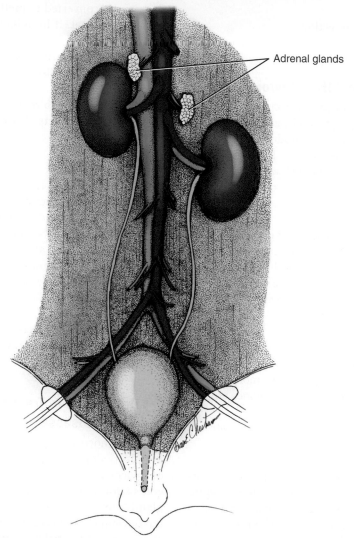

Fig. 9.6 Adrenal glands. (From Christenson, D. E. [2008]. *Veterinary medical terminology* [2nd ed.]. St. Louis: Elsevier.)

Dosage Form

• **Desoxycorticosterone pivalate** (Percorten-V)

Adverse Side Effects. Side effects include depression, vomiting, anorexia, polyuria, polydipsia, and anemia (Plumb, 2015).

Fludrocortisone

Fludrocortisone is a mineralocorticoid alternative to DOCP and can also be used as adjunctive therapy in hyperkalemia (Plumb, 2015).

Dosage Form

• **Florinef**

Adverse Side Effects. Side effects include polyuria, polydipsia, hypertension, and hypokalemia are possible.

Glucocorticoids

Dexamethasone sodium phosphate. Dexamethasone is a glucocorticoid used to treat antiinflammatory, immune-mediated, and many other conditions. Dexamethasone is used in the treatment of adrenal insufficiency to replace glucocorticoid activity. It will not interfere with cortisol assays.

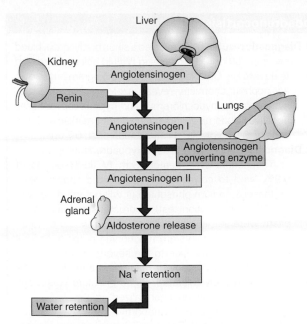

Fig. 9.7 Renin-angiotensin system. (From Summers, A. [2020]. *Common diseases of companion animals* [4th ed.]. St. Louis: Elsevier.)

Dosage Form
- **Azium**
- **Dexasone**
- **DexaJect**
- Many other generic brands

Adverse Side Effects. Side effects from corticosteroids are many and include polyphagia, polydipsia, polyuria, gastrointestinal ulceration, delayed wound healing, immunosuppression, and many other effects.

Prednisone

Prednisone is a glucocorticoid used to treat various conditions such as adrenal insufficiency, inflammatory conditions, and certain autoimmune diseases. Prednisone will interfere with cortisol assays.

Dosage Form
- **Deltasone**
- Other generic brands

Adverse Side Effects. Side effects are very similar to dexamethasone.

Refer to Chapter 14 for more information on corticosteroids.

℞ Drugs Used to Treat Hyperadrenocorticism (Cushing's Syndrome)

Hyperadrenocorticism or **Cushing's syndrome** is one of the most commonly diagnosed endocrine disorders in dogs and horses. Most cats diagnosed with Cushing's syndrome also have concurrent diabetes mellitus. Cushing's syndrome is usually seen in older dogs and can be spontaneous or **iatrogenic.** The signs associated with this syndrome occur because of an excess of circulating glucocorticoids, especially cortisol. Cortisol (see Chapter 14) is a hormone produced in the cortex of the adrenal gland on stimulation by ACTH from the pituitary. Its function is to help the body respond to stress and to prepare the body for the flight-or-fight response. It does this by mobilizing nutrients, modifying the response to inflammation, raising the blood glucose level, and controlling the amount of water in the body.

There are two forms of spontaneous Cushing's syndrome:
- **Pituitary-dependent hyperadrenocorticism** (PDH). This is the most common of spontaneous cases and often occurs due to a benign tumor of the pituitary gland. This tumor causes the pituitary to produce large amounts of ACTH, which stimulates the adrenal to make large amounts of cortisol.
- **Adrenal-dependent hyperadrenocorticism** (ADH). This is a less common form of the spontaneous disease. It occurs due to a tumor of one or both of the adrenal glands and results in the production of a large amount of cortisol independent of ACTH.

Differentiating between these two forms of disease in the dog can be difficult.

In the equine patient, Cushing's syndrome is a disease of older horses that is the result of pituitary pars intermedia dysfunction (PPID), which makes it different from Cushing's syndrome in the dog. Adrenal gland tumors are apparently rare in the horse.

Ketoconazole

Ketoconazole is an antifungal agent that can be used in the treatment of hyperadrenocorticism if other agents like mitotane are not effective. Ketoconazole inhibits the synthesis of glucocorticoids and androgens.

Dosage Form
- **Ketoconazole tablets,** human label

Adverse Side Effects. Side effects include vomiting, diarrhea, and anorexia.

BOX 9.1   Case Scenario Addisonian Crisis (Hypoadrenocortisism)

A 4-year-old spayed female Standard Poodle as presented for severe vomiting and bloody diarrhea, collapsed, and unable to stand.

History: The owner started that she had intermittent vomiting and diarrhea whenever she is boarded or there are guests that come over to her home. She has always been a picky eater and there was no way that she could have gotten into anything. She went to the groomer 3 days ago and since then she seemed more lethargic and has not been feeling well. She started vomiting and having diarrhea 2 days ago. Today was the first day that she noticed bloody diarrhea. She vomited a large amount and then collapsed this morning (about 15 minutes ago).

Additional history: She is not on any medications and is up to date on vaccinations. No travel history but frequently goes to the dog park for exercise.

Physical examination findings: Obtunded, Temperature: 99°F, pulses: 70 bpm with poor femoral pulse quality, respirations: 20 bpm with normal effort, mucous membranes: pink but tacky, CRT (capillary refill time): 2–3 seconds. Patient is showing signs of hypovolemic shock but interestingly is not tachycardic.

The veterinary technician placed an intravenous (IV) catheter and started the patient on IV fluids (0.9% sodium chloride [NaCl]) for the hypovolemic shock per doctor's orders. The 0.9% NaCl was chosen because it offers a higher amount of sodium and lower amount of potassium. Additional veterinary technicians prepared for the diagnostic tests.

Diagnostic tests: The veterinarian ordered an ECG, blood pressure, complete blood count (CBC) and chemistry, abdominal radiographs, cortisol and ACTH stimulation tests.

The veterinary technician prepared synthetic ACTH (cosyntropin) to run the ACTH stimulation test. ACTH is a hormone produced in the pituitary gland that stimulates the adrenal glands to release cortisol and aldosterone.

All technicians worked quickly and systematically implementing the treatment plan.

Diagnostic results: ECG revealed a sinus bradycardia, blood pressure: 50 mm Hg, following IV fluid bolus it increased to 90 mm Hg; CBC: lack of a stress leukogram but also an eosinophilia; chemistry reveals azotemia, hyperkalemia, hyponatremia, hypochloremia, and hypoglycemia. Fecal: negative, abdominal radiographs: unremarkable, basal cortisol: 0.5 ug/dL, ACTH stimulation post: 0.7 ug/dL.

Diagnosis: Addison's disease (Hypoadrenocortisism)

The patient was treated with IV fluid boluses of 0.9% NaCl to correct the hypovolemic shock. Dexamethasone sodium phosphate (it will not interfere with the ACTH stimulation test), fludrocortisone, and maropitant were administered. Urine output was monitored to ensure the kidneys are functioning properly as well as for fluid therapy. Due to the severity of dehydration urine output may be lower than volume input until the pet is adequately hydrated. Blood pressure was monitored every 2 hours until normalized.

After 24 hours, with supportive care, the patient's vital signs stabilized. She was bright, alert, and responsive. The veterinary technician understood the importance of appropriate nutrition for these patients and tempted the patient to eat. The patient starting eating and drinking on her own. She was discharged with prednisone and fludrocortisone.

A follow-up was scheduled in 7 days to monitor her electrolytes closely and transition to DOCP (desoxycorticosterone pivalate) injections, to replace fludrocortisone, for long-term mineralocorticoid supplementation. DOCP requires the pet to have an injection every 21–30 days.

An adrenal crisis is an acute medical emergency and requires the staff to work quickly in order for the patient to have the best chance of survival. Dealing with an Addisonian crisis requires treating the patient's shock and focus should be on treating the hypotension and hypovolemia. This scenario depicts teamwork, communication, accurate monitoring, and an understanding of the disease so that preparation of drugs can be ready for administration when needed.

Courtesy of Tara J. Fetzer, DVM, DACVECC

Metyrapone

Metyrapone is an agent used to treat cats with hyperadrenocorticism, especially for stabilization of patients before adrenalectomy.

Dosage Form

- **Metyrapone** (Metopirone), oral capsule, human label

    Adverse Side Effects. Metyrapone is relatively well tolerated in cats.

Mitotane

Mitotane is used for the treatment of PDH. This agent is an adrenal cytotoxic agent that inhibits or destroys the cortisol-producing layers of the adrenal gland.

Dosage Form

- **Mitotane tablets** (Lysodren) human label

    Adverse Side Effects. Side effects include lethargy, ataxia, weakness, vomiting, diarrhea, and others.

Long-term glucocorticoid and possibly mineralocorticoid replacement therapy may be needed in some patients treated with mitotane.

Selegiline

Selegiline is a monoamine oxidase B (MAO-B) inhibitor that is used for cognitive dysfunction and PDH in dogs. Its use for Cushing's syndrome is controversial because of disappointing clinical studies (Plumb, 2015).

Dosage Form
- **Selegiline tablets** (Anipryl)

Adverse Side Effects. Side effects may include vomiting, diarrhea, restlessness, salivation, and others.

Trilostane

Trilostane is an adrenal steroid synthesis inhibitor that is used to treat PDH or hyperadrenocorticism due to adrenal tumors in dogs. Trilostane is considered the treatment of choice for dogs.

Dosage Form
- **Trilostane capsules** (Vetoryl)

Adverse Side Effects. Side effects may include loss of appetite, lethargy, weakness, diarrhea, or vomiting.

Ⓡ Agents for the Treatment of Diabetes Mellitus

Insulin

The pancreas produces two principal hormones in special cells of the islets of Langerhans: insulin and glucagon. Insulin is produced by beta cells, and glucagon is produced by alpha cells. Insulin causes a decrease in blood glucose levels, and glucagon promotes an increase. Only insulin is used clinically.

Insulin facilitates cellular uptake of glucose and its storage in the form of glycogen and fat. It inhibits the breakdown of fat, protein, and glycogen into forms that may be used as energy sources. Further, it promotes synthesis of protein, fatty acids, and glycogen. In the absence of insulin, the body cannot use glucose and must break down its own fat and protein that can be used for energy.

Diabetes mellitus is a complex disease that results from the inability of the beta cells of the pancreas to produce enough insulin or from altered insulin action within cells. Diabetes mellitus that results from inadequate secretion of insulin is called *type I*, or *insulin-dependent, diabetes mellitus*. This is the most common type of diabetes mellitus in dogs and cats. Diabetes mellitus that results from resistance of tissue to the action of insulin is called *type II*, or noninsulin-dependent, diabetes mellitus (NIDDM). NIDDM is rare in dogs but is occasionally encountered in cats.

Both forms of diabetes mellitus eventually cause polydipsia, polyuria, polyphagia, and weight loss. Untreated diabetes mellitus proceeds to the condition called *diabetic ketoacidosis,* in which body fat is metabolized as a substitute energy source. Metabolism of body fat results in accumulation of by-products of this process called *ketone bodies,* which promote a metabolic acidosis that can lead to death.

Corticosteroids, epinephrine, and progesterone should be given with caution to diabetic animals because they can increase blood glucose levels. Sudden changes in diet and exercise level should also be avoided because they can alter blood glucose levels and cause an imbalance in the ratio of insulin to glucose.

Insulin is not effective when given orally because the digestive tract breaks down the protein molecule before it can be absorbed. Insulin usually is administered by subcutaneous injection. However, some forms may be given intravenously or intramuscularly.

Sources of insulin have traditionally included beef or pork pancreas and preparations consisting of a purified (pure beef source or pure pork source) form or a combination beef/pork form. The beef/pork form is best suited to the treatment of diabetes mellitus in dogs and cats. Pork insulin is very close in structure to dog and human types of insulin, whereas beef insulin is very similar to cat insulin.

Most human insulin products are now prepared through recombinant DNA or synthetic processes. Only two animal-labeled products (ProZinc and Vetsulin) are currently approved for use in the United States. The availability of insulin products is subject to change, and technicians should always consult current information when dealing with products for diabetic patients.

Insulin concentration is measured in units of insulin per milliliter. It is available in concentrations of 40 (U-40) and 100 (U-100). Animal-approved products are U-40. Both animal-approved and human-approved insulin preparations are used in animals.

U-40 syringes must be used with U-40 insulin, and U-100 syringes must be used with U-100 insulin. U-40 syringes have a red top, and U-100 syringes have an orange top (Fig. 9.8). U-100 syringes are available in 0.3 mL (30 units), 0.5 mL (50 units), and 1.0 mL (100 units) sizes (Fig. 9.9). U-40 syringes are also produced in 0.3 mL (12 units), 0.5 mL (20 units), and 1.0 mL (40 units) sizes. Table 9.2 lists insulin syringe manufacturers.

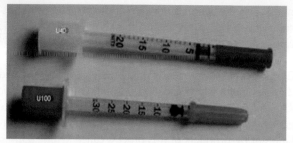

Fig. 9.8 U-40 syringe (red top) and U-100 syringe (orange top).

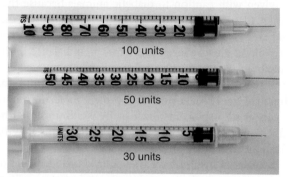

Fig. 9.9 U-100 insulin syringes: 30 unit, 50 unit, and 100 unit. (From Mulholland, J. [2011]. *The nurse, the math, the meds.* St. Louis: Elsevier.)

TABLE 9.2	Insulin Syringe Manufacturers.
U-100	**U-40**
BD (Becton Dickinson)	Ulti Care
Turemo	Ulti Guard
Monoject	MVP
Ulti Med	Vetsulin
Aimsco	BD
ReliOn (Walmart)	
Abbott Laboratories	
Can-Am Care	
Inviro Medical Devices	
Excel International	

When U-40 insulin is drawn into a U-40 syringe, each mark on the syringe barrel denotes 1 unit of insulin. A 100-unit, 1-mL syringe may be marked in 2-unit increments (e.g., 2, 4, 6, 8) or in 1-unit increments (e.g., 1, 2, 3, 4, 5); care should be taken to note which is being used. Small volume 100-unit (0.3 mL and 0.5 mL) syringes are marked in 1-unit increments.

U-100 syringes can be used to administer U-40 insulin by multiplying the required units of U-40 insulin by 2.5 (Plumb, 2015).

Needles for insulin syringes are either 1/2 or 5/16 inches in length and standard gauges are 28, 29, and 31.

Insulin Classifications. Insulin is usually classified according to its duration of action, that is, short acting, intermediate acting, or long acting. Short-acting insulin is regular insulin. Neutral protamine Hagedorn (NPH), and Lente (porcine insulin zinc suspension) are intermediate-acting insulins. Glargine, detemir, and protamine zinc insulin (PZI) are long-acting products. Two different forms are sometimes combined in the same preparation. See Table 9.3 for a partial listing of insulin products in each category. The technician involved in treating diabetic animals should remain current with the literature on this topic because insulin products and classifications tend to change periodically.

The onset of effect and route of administration are other important characteristics of insulin preparations to be considered. For an in-depth discussion of insulin forms and characteristics, other references should be consulted.

Short-Acting Insulin. *Regular crystalline insulin.* Regular insulin is a fast-acting insulin that is made from zinc insulin crystals; it is a clear solution that may be administered intravenously, intramuscularly, or subcutaneously. It is used mainly to treat diabetic ketoacidosis until blood glucose levels are reduced and the animal is metabolically stable. At that time, the animal is usually switched to a longer-acting form.

Clinical Uses. Regular crystalline insulin is used primarily for the treatment of diabetic ketoacidosis.

Dosage Forms. Many products approved for humans are available.

- **Humulin R (U-100)**
- **Novolin R (U-100)**

Adverse Side Effects. These usually are related to overdose and may include weakness, ataxia, shaking, and seizures.

📋 **TECHNICIAN NOTES**

- Although not required by label on the newer products, refrigeration probably enhances storage life. Do not freeze.
- Do not use regular insulin preparations if discoloration or precipitates are present.

TABLE 9.3	Insulin Products Commonly Used in Dogs and Cats.			
Brand Name	**Generic Name**	**Source**	**Duration**	**Concentration**
Humulin R	Regular crystalline insulin	Human recombinant	Short-acting	U-100
Humulin N Novolin N	Neutral protamine Hagedorn	Human recombinant	Intermediate-acting	U-100
Vetsulin	Lente	Porcine	Intermediate-acting	U-40
ProZinc	Protamine zinc	Human recombinant	Long-acting	U-40
Lantus	Glargine	Human recombinant	Long-acting	U-100
Levemir	Detemir	Human recombinant	Long-acting	U-100

Intermediate-Acting Insulin. *NPH and Lente.* NPH insulin is a cloudy suspension of zinc insulin crystals and protamine zinc. Protamine (a fish protein) and zinc prolong the absorption and activity of the product. These insulin types are longer acting than regular insulin. They are commonly used for the control of uncomplicated diabetes in dogs and cats. Lente insulin is similar in activity to NPH insulin but is made without the use of protamine.

Clinical Uses. NPH insulin is used in the treatment of uncomplicated diabetes mellitus.

Dosage Forms
- **Humulin N (U-100)**
- **Novolin N (U-100)**
- **Lente (U-40),** porcine insulin zinc suspension (Vetsulin); U.S Food and Drug Administration (FDA) approved for use in cats and dogs

Adverse Side Effects. These are similar to those of regular insulin.

TECHNICIAN NOTES

- Resuspension, by gently rolling the bottle, is required before the product is withdrawn from the bottle. An exception to this rule is Vetsulin, whose label reads: "Shake the vial thoroughly until a homogenous, uniformly milky suspension is obtained."
- Store in the manner of regular insulin. Do not freeze.
- Neutral protamine Hagedorn insulin is usually administered once a day although maintenance doses of insulin in dogs and cats can be highly individualized.

Long-Acting Insulin. Protamine zinc (PZI; ProZinc), Glargine (Lantus), and detemir (Levemir) insulin are long-acting insulins. Lantus is marketed as a peakless insulin. Care should be taken to avoid confusing Lantus and Levemir with other clear insulins.

Clinical Uses. Glargine is used for the treatment of uncomplicated diabetes mellitus. ProZinc insulin is used to reduce hyperglycemia in cats with diabetes mellitus.

Dosage Forms
- **Protamine zinc insulin (U-40)** (PZI; ProZinc), FDA approved for use in cats
- **Clear, long-acting glargine insulin (U-100)** (Lantus)
- **Clear, detemir insulin (U-100)** (Levemir)

Adverse Side Effects. These are similar to those of regular and intermediate-acting insulins.

Use of Insulin Products. Technicians who are counseling clients about the use of insulin products should take great care to become thoroughly familiar with the products they are using. The onset of action of various insulin products can vary from a few minutes to a few hours. Peak activity time and duration of activity can also vary greatly between products. Exercise levels and eating patterns may influence insulin activity. An overdose of insulin can lead to various degrees of hypoglycemia that produce clinical signs ranging from mild weakness to coma. Clients should be shown how to give subcutaneous injections of insulin, and they should be given written instructions about monitoring the insulin response and making appropriate adjustments. Tips regarding the use of insulin products follow as technician's notes.

One of the issues involved in treating animals with human insulin products is the high cost. To reduce the cost of these products many veterinarians are choosing the ReliOn (Walmart) line of products, which may reduce the cost of some products by half or more (Jordan, 2013).

TECHNICIAN NOTES

- It is usually best to feed the animal 30 minutes before giving the insulin injection.
- Roll "cloudy" insulins between your palms; do not shake (except Vetsulin).
- Neutral protamine Hagedorn insulin should not be mixed with any Lente insulin.
- It is the opinion of some people that insulin should be disposed of after 30 days or 100 injections.
- Injection sites should be rotated (Fig. 9.10).
- Clients should be advised to use insulin syringes only once.
- Mild to moderate hypoglycemia resulting from an overdose can be treated by feeding the animal or administering corn (Karo) syrup.

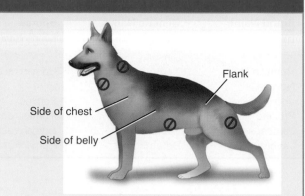

Fig. 9.10 Insulin injection sites include the side of the chest, belly or at the flank. The red circle indicates an area where injections should not be made. (From Civco T. [2010]. *Diabetic treatment & management protocols* [website]. http://abbottanimalhealthce.com. Accessed March, 28, 2013.)

Oral Hypoglycemic Agents

Sulfonylurea (glipizide) is an oral hypoglycemic agent used to promote insulin secretion from the pancreas and is sometimes used in cats with diabetes. It is only recommended for use in cats with owners who refuse insulin therapy, and only with concurrent dietary therapy (Behrend, 2018). Although oral glipizide therapy can be considered, insulin continues to be the treatment of choice.

℞ Hyperglycemic Agents

Several drugs such as corticosteroids, epinephrine, and progesterone incidentally elevate blood glucose levels. Two products that are marketed for this purpose, however, are diazoxide (Proglycem) and octreotide (Sandostatin). These are used to treat the low blood glucose levels associated with hypersecretion of insulin that occurs in tumors of the beta cells of the pancreas (insulinoma) in dogs and ferrets (Plumb, 2015). These products act by inhibiting the release of insulin from beta cells of the pancreas and raise blood glucose levels.

HORMONES THAT ACT AS GROWTH PROMOTERS

℞ Sex Steroids, Synthetic Steroid Analogues, and Nonsteroidal Analogues

The factors that control growth, feed efficiency, and carcass composition in animals involve a complex interrelationship between genetic, metabolic, and hormonal mechanisms that are not always totally understood. It is possible, however, to increase growth (weight gain) in ruminants by administering sex steroid hormones (estrogen, testosterone, or progesterone), synthetic steroid hormone analogues (trenbolone), or certain nonsteroidal hormone analogs (zeranol).

The primary sex steroid used to promote weight gain is estrogen (estradiol). The mechanisms by which estradiol promotes weight gain include (1) increased water retention, (2) increased protein synthesis, (3) increased fat deposition, and (4) possible increased release of growth hormone (bovine somatotropin [BST]).

Testosterone is used as an adjunct to estradiol in some growth-promotion products because it is an anabolic agent in itself and because a second component in the compound slows down the release of estradiol and prolongs its effective life span.

Progesterone is also added to growth promoters to slow the release of estradiol. It apparently has little anabolic effect of its own.

Trenbolone is a synthetic anabolic agent that improves feed efficiency and promotes weight gain in steers. It is used as the sole agent in some growth-promoting preparations.

Zeranol is an analogue of a naturally occurring plant estrogen that increases feed efficiency, protein synthesis, and growth rate.

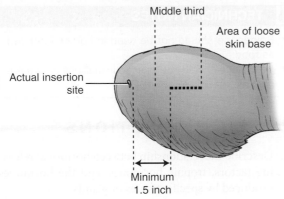

Fig. 9.11 Implantation site for growth-promoting pellets (posterior view of the ear).

All of the growth-promoting products for use in cattle and sheep are prepared as compressed pellets that are implanted in the subcutaneous tissue of the dorsal, middle third of the ear (Fig. 9.11). These pellets are designed for use with corresponding needle devices and should be implanted with close adherence to product instructions (failure to do so is a violation of federal law in some cases).

The growth-promotion products are considered here as a group, and minimal information is provided about each product.

Clinical Uses. These drugs are used to promote feed efficiency and weight gain in calves, steers, heifers, or sheep (depending on the product).

Dosage Forms

- **Estradiol/progesterone implant** for use in calves older than 45 days (Synovex C)
- **Estradiol/testosterone implant** for use in heifers (Synovex H, Implus-H)
- **Estradiol/testosterone implant** for use in steers (Synovex S)
- **Estradiol implant** for use in steers (Compudose)
- **Trenbolone implant** for use in feedlot heifers (Finaplix-H)
- **Trenbolone and estradiol implant** for use in feedlot steers (Revalor-S)
- **Zeranol implant** for use in growing cattle, feedlot heifers, feedlot steers, and suckling and weaned calves (Ralgro beef cattle implant)

Adverse Side Effects. These may include mounting, elevated tail heads, rectal prolapse, and udder development.

℞ Growth Hormone: Bovine Somatotropin, Bovine Growth Hormone

Growth hormone, also called *somatotropin,* is a hormone produced by the anterior pituitary. Its function before the onset of puberty is to stimulate growth. It is released throughout life to promote anabolic activity (e.g., to increase protein synthesis). It has been shown to increase growth rate and feed efficiency in farm animals. Many of the growth-promoting agents listed in the previous section may work by stimulating the release of somatotropin. Somatotropin is also a potent stimulator of milk production. Claims of a 20% boost in milk production in dairy cows have been made after administration of somatotropin.

The FDA approved a recombinant (genetically engineered) BST for commercial production in 1993. This product, Posilac, was manufactured originally by Monsanto and was later acquired by Elanco. Its market availability has sparked intense debate among certain groups. Some dairy producers have opposed its use because of their fear that increased production would drive milk prices down and reduce their overall income. Other groups have resisted the use of BST because of their concerns about residues of the hormone in milk products, even though the FDA has stated that milk from cows receiving BST is completely safe. People who advocate the use of "organic" food products may oppose the use of this product.

ANABOLIC STEROIDS

Anabolic steroids are steroids that produce a tissue-building (anabolic) effect. Testosterone is a naturally occurring anabolic steroid that produces masculinization in addition to its anabolic effects. Synthetic anabolic steroids are designed to prevent most masculinizing effects.

Anabolic steroid administration causes positive nitrogen balance and reverses processes that break down tissue. An increase in appetite, weight gain, improved overall condition, and recovery are promoted.

These products are labeled for clinical use in dogs, cats, and horses for anorexia, weight loss, and debilitation. In working animals, they may be used in cases of overwork or overtraining. Anabolic steroids also promote red blood cell formation and are used to treat some forms of anemia. The product insert for a commonly used anabolic steroid states that "anabolic therapy is intended primarily as an adjunct to other specific and supportive therapy, including nutritional therapy."

The DEA has now classified anabolic steroids as Class III controlled substances because of the potential for abuse by bodybuilders and other athletes.

Stanozolol

Stanozolol is an anabolic steroid that has been found to have an unusual pattern of biologic activity in that its anabolic effect far outweighs its weak androgenic influence.

Clinical Uses. Stanozolol is used for the treatment of anorexia, debilitation, weight loss, overwork, and anemia.

Dosage Forms
- **Stanozolol sterile suspension** for injection in dogs, cats, and horses (Winstrol-V)
- **Stanozolol tablets** for use in dogs and cats (Winstrol-V)

Adverse Side Effects. These may include mild androgenic effects after prolonged use or overdose.

TECHNICIAN NOTES

- Winstrol-V should not be used in pregnant dogs, mares, or stallions.
- Winstrol-V should not be given to horses intended for food uses.

Boldenone Undecylenate

Boldenone undecylenate is a steroid ester that possesses marked anabolic activity and a minimal amount of androgenic activity. It is labeled for use in horses.

Clinical Uses. Boldenone undecylenate acts as an aid in the treatment of debilitated horses.

Dosage Form
- **Boldenone injection** for horses (Equipoise)

Adverse Side Effects. These include androgenic effects such as over aggressiveness.

TECHNICIAN NOTES

- Boldenone should not be used in horses intended as food.
- Boldenone should not be used in stallions or in pregnant mares.

REVIEW QUESTIONS

1. Describe the relationship between hormonal releasing factors, trophic hormones, and the hormones produced by specific tissues or glands.
2. List the major endocrine glands.
3. What are the reasons for using hormonal therapy in veterinary medicine?
4. Endogenous hormones are those that are produced _____, whereas exogenous hormones come from _____ sources.
5. Describe the difference between a negative and a positive feedback control mechanism in the endocrine system.
6. Hormonal products with "gest" in their name are classified as _____.
7. List three potential uses of the prostaglandins in veterinary medicine.
8. Human skin contact or injection with prostaglandins can be a serious health risk to _____ women and individuals with _____.
9. What precautions should be taken before oxytocin is administered?
10. What two active hormones are produced by the thyroid gland?
11. List two drugs used in the treatment of hypothyroidism.
12. List the three major classes of insulin.
13. Which form of insulin is used in the treatment of diabetic ketoacidosis?
14. What are some signs of insulin overdose?
15. Growth promoters generally should not be used in animals intended for _____.
16. Why are anabolic steroids classified as controlled substances?
17. Which insulin product should be shaken thoroughly prior to use?
18. What precautions should be taken by pregnant women when Regu-Mate is administered?

19. Why was synthetic DES banned from use in food-producing animals?

20. A _____ hormone is one that results in the production of a second hormone within a target gland.
    a. gonadotropin
    b. euthyroid
    c. trophic
    d. myofibril

21. Androgens are female sex hormones produced in the ovaries, adrenal cortex, and testicles.
    a. True
    b. False

22. Corticosteroids are produced by the _____.
    a. thyroid gland
    b. adrenal cortex

c. kidneys
d. hypothalamus

23. Pituitary-dependent hyperadrenocorticism in dogs may be treated with _____.
    a. Lysodren
    b. Vetoryl
    c. Captopril
    d. both a and b

24. A 1100-lb mare will be given altrenogest at 0.044 mg/kg daily to maintain pregnancy. The concentration of altrenogest (Regu-Mate) is 0.22%. What quantity will you give daily?

25. A 13-lb diabetic cat with a blood glucose of 450 mg/dL will be treated with ProZinc (U-40) at a dosage of 0.5 U/kg twice a day. How many units will you give with each dose?

REFERENCES

Behrend, E., Holford, A., Lathan, P., Rucinsky, R., & Schulman, R. (2018). Diabetes management guidelines for dogs and cats. *Journal of the American Animal Hospital Association, 54*, 1–21.

Boothe, D. M. (2012). Drug therapy for endocrinopathies. In D. M. Boothe (Ed.), *Small animal clinical pharmacology*. Philadelphia: WB Saunders.

Jordan, D. G. (2013). Trends in veterinary therapeutics. In *Proceedings Music City Veterinary Conference*. Murfreesboro, TN.

Papich, M. G. (2016). *Handbook of veterinary drugs* (4th ed.). St. Louis: Elsevier.

Plumb, D. C. (2015). *Veterinary drug handbook* (8th ed.). Ames, IA: Wiley-Blackwell.

Scott-Moncrieff., et al. (2014). *Canine hypothyroidism. Kirk's current veterinary therapy XV*. St. Louis: Elsevier.

Drugs Used in Ophthalmic and Otic Disorders

KEY TERMS

Blepharospasm
Cerumen
Conjunctivitis
Cycloplegia
Distichia (distichiasis)
Ectropion
Entropion
Glaucoma
Horner's syndrome
Hyphema

Intracameral injection
Keratitis
Miotics
MRSA
Mydriasis
Open-angle glaucoma
Otoacariasis
Uvea
Uveitis

INTRODUCTION

The sense of smell is highly developed in animals, but the sense of sight also plays an important role in an animal's health and well-being. Cats rely on excellent eyesight because they are animals of prey. This prey trait can provide cat owners with much laughter as a string or a feather toy is pulled around the house. Horses rely on good eyesight to perform their best in equestrian events. Police dogs, hunting dogs, seeing-eye dogs, and herd dogs rely on their eyesight to interpret hand signals when working in the field.

An ophthalmic examination includes the use of diagnostic agents to determine any ocular problems that may be present in the patient. Additionally, an examination of the ocular features (eyelids, eyelashes, sclera, cornea, third eyelid [i.e., nictitating membrane], pupil, anterior chamber, iris, and lens), all of which can be seen without highly specialized equipment (Bassert, 2018), are also important to evaluate. Some dog breeds (shar-pei, cocker spaniels, English bulldogs, and others) are genetically predisposed to conditions that may

require cosmetic surgery to correct faults. Three of these conditions are known as entropion, ectropion, and distichiasis.

Topical administration of eye drops or ointment is the most common method of treatment involving disorders of the eye. It is the veterinary technician's duty to educate the client by demonstrating the proper way to administer eye medication. Products for ocular treatment are usually available as solutions or ointments. Drug penetration is one factor that veterinarians must consider when choosing a topical ophthalmic agent. Topical agents are more readily absorbed into the anterior chamber than the posterior chamber. For this reason, these agents have limited use in posterior eye disorders. Systemic agents may be more effective. Lipid-soluble agents readily penetrate the corneal epithelium and endothelium layers. Water-soluble agents readily penetrate the corneal stroma layer (Figs. 10.1 and 10.2). Most topical ophthalmic medications require several applications per day because the eye continuously secretes tears that wash away the medication. Ointments tend to necessitate less frequent applications than drops. However,

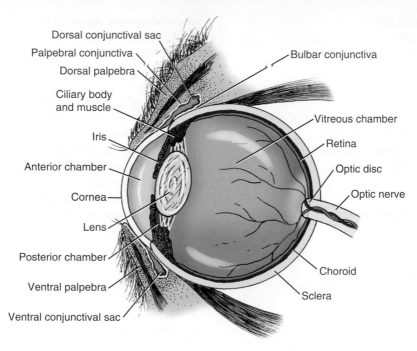

Fig. 10.1 Internal structures of the eye. (From Christenson, D. E. [2008]. *Veterinary medical terminology* (2nd ed.). St. Louis: Elsevier.)

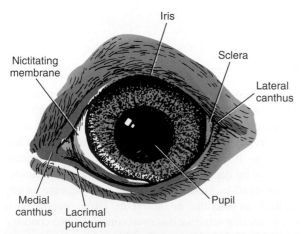

Fig. 10.2 External structures of the eye. (From Summers, A. [2020]. *Common diseases of companion animals* (4th ed.). St. Louis: Elsevier.)

ointments may blur an animal's vision for a short period after application. Recently, some clinicians believe that ophthalmic drops may be more effective than ointments.

Client education is invaluable for proper treatment of an eye disorder. It is important that clients understand that the applicator tip of the drug's container should not touch the eye's surface or the conjunctiva because bacteria from the patient's eye may contaminate the remaining drug contents inside the container. This is also important to remember when veterinary personnel are treating several patients in a veterinary hospital with the same drug container.

Clients placing telephone calls to the veterinary hospital to discuss a potential eye problem in a companion animal should be made to realize that these situations may be considered an emergency. Unfortunately, some clients tend to let an ocular problem progress to severe stages before treatment is sought. Veterinary technicians should remind clients that animals have only two eyes and the importance of vision should not be minimized.

DIAGNOSTIC AGENTS

The use of diagnostic agents to determine what problems may exist with the eyes is an important part of the ophthalmic examination. Some diagnostic agents should be used before others so that results are not misinterpreted.

TECHNICIAN NOTES

The Schirmer tear test is one of the first diagnostic procedures to be employed so that tear evaluation is calculated correctly.

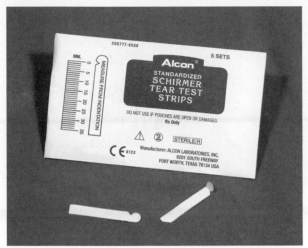

Fig. 10.3 Schirmer Tear Test. (From Taylor, S. M. [2010]. *Small animal clinical procedures* (1st ed.). St. Louis: Elsevier.)

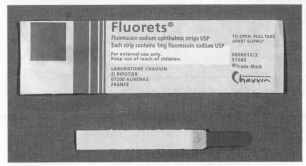

Fig. 10.4 Fluorescein test strips. (From Taylor, S. M. [2010]. *Small animal clinical procedures* (1st ed.). St. Louis: Elsevier.)

- **Fluor-I-Strip**
- **Bio-Glo**

📋 **TECHNICIAN NOTES**

If a bacterial culture is indicated, the culture should be obtained before cleaning the eye or administering other ophthalmic drugs. Therefore, an eye examination should be carried out in a methodical manner in order for a proper diagnosis to be made.

📋 **TECHNICIAN NOTES**

- Moisten the fluorescein strip with a few drops of eye wash. Then, hold the eye open and place the strip over the eye, allowing a drop of dye to fall onto the corneal surface or you can touch the moistened strip to the bulbar conjunctiva. Irrigate the eye with liberal amounts of sterile eyewash (irrigating solution) to remove excess stain.
- Do not allow the fluorescein strip to touch the cornea.
- Horses have strong palpebral muscles. If stain is to be used in this species, it may be necessary to have another person keep the eyelids spread apart while the stain is introduced into the eye.
- Fluorescein stains the hair if allowed to drain on the face. Use cotton or gauze to wipe away excess fluorescein stain because it is softer than a paper towel.
- Use care to prevent the stain from causing temporary staining of the patient's fur, as this may make some owners unhappy (especially on white-coated breeds that have just been groomed).

Schirmer Tear Test

Clinical Uses. The Schirmer tear test (Fig. 10.3) is used clinically to measure tear production.

Dosage Forms. Paper strips are placed in the animal's lower eyelid (conjunctival sac) making contact with the cornea.

- **Schirmer Tear Test**

Adverse Side Effects. These are uncommon.

Fluorescein Sodium

Clinical Uses. Fluorescein stain is commonly used to stain the patient's cornea in cases in which a corneal ulcer is suspected. The stain fluoresces, and if a corneal ulcer is present it can be observed with the use of a cobalt blue filter and a light source. The corneal epithelium will not stain because the corneal stroma, which is a lipid membrane, repels the stain. Fluorescein stain is also used to diagnose patency of the nasolacrimal outflow duct.

Dosage Forms. Fluorescein stain (Fig. 10.4) is manufactured on paper strips and are preferred to fluorescein solution to ensure sterility.

- **Ful-Glo**

Lissamine Green

Clinical Uses. Lissamine green is used to diagnose corneal damage and to quantify tear production. This product does not sting like Rose Bengal, but interpretation requires more experience. Fluorescein stain is a more reliable indicator of corneal damage.

Dosage Form

- Manufactured on paper strips

Adverse Side Effects. Side effects are uncommon.

Phenol Red Thread

Clinical Uses. This product is used to evaluate tear production. Phenol red thread is a new accurate way to measure tear production as compared with the Schirmer tear test.

Dosage Form
- A long (75-mm) yellow-colored thread impregnated with phenol red, which is a sensitive pH indicator (Zone-Quick Diagnostic Threads)

Adverse Side Effects. Side effects are uncommon.

Rose Bengal

Clinical Uses. Rose bengal is used most commonly to detect the presence of canine and feline herpesvirus keratitis. It can also be used to evaluate corneal epithelium that may be damaged due to keratoconjunctivitis sicca (KCS).

Dosage Forms
- Manufactured by Akorn as a solution or an impregnated strip (Rosets).

Adverse Side Effects. This product may be toxic to the cornea and should be thoroughly flushed from the eye to prevent irritation. Hypersensitivity reactions may occur. It may also stain clothing.

OCULAR ANESTHETICS

Ocular anesthetics are used during tonometry or for relief of corneal pain during performance of an ocular examination.

Proparacaine Hydrogen Chloride

Clinical Uses. Proparacaine hydrogen chloride (HCl) is a topical anesthetic used for a variety of ophthalmic procedures. Proparacaine should be protected from light and should be refrigerated.

Dosage Forms. Drops placed in the eye (Fig. 10.5)
- **Proparacaine HCL**
- **Parcaine**
- **Alcaine**

Adverse Side Effects. Side effects are uncommon.

Tetracaine HCl

Clinical Uses. Tetracaine HCl is used to produce local anesthesia of short duration for ophthalmic procedures.

Dosage Forms. Drops placed in the eye
- **Tetracaine HCL**
- **Altacaine**

Adverse Side Effects. Tetracaine may be more irritating than proparacaine; it is only sometimes used in veterinary medicine. Prolonged use may cause delayed wound healing and corneal ulcers and may retard the blink reflex. Repeated use may cause development of tolerance to the drug.

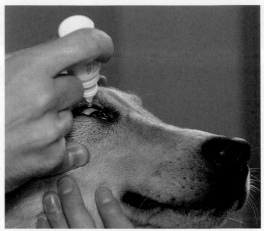

Fig. 10.5 Instilling ocular medication. (From Taylor, S. M. [2010]. *Small animal clinical procedures* [1st ed.]. St. Louis: Elsevier.)

PARASYMPATHOMIMETICS

These are also known as *miotics.* Parasympathomimetics are used to induce contraction of the intraocular smooth muscle (miosis), which helps to reduce intraocular pressure (IOP). Miotics are drugs that constrict the pupil.

Carbachol

Clinical Uses. Carbachol may be used to cause miosis in the treatment of glaucoma. Veterinary ophthalmologists may also use it at the conclusion of cataract removal to prevent cases of postoperative increased IOP.

Dosage Forms. Intracameral injection
- **Miostat Intraocular**

Adverse Side Effects. In humans, the following have been reported: headaches, muscle spasms of accommodation, retinal detachment, and iritis (postoperatively).

Pilocarpine HCl

Clinical Uses. Pilocarpine is a cholinergic agonist (miotic) that is sometimes used in the treatment of canine primary glaucoma, but has been replaced by beta-blockers and prostaglandin agents. It was used orally as a primary treatment of neurogenic KCS in dogs, prior to the approval of cyclosporine (Plumb, 2015).

Dosage Forms. Various solutions and gels
- **Isopto Carpine**
- **Piloptic**

Adverse Side Effects. This drug should not be used in secondary glaucoma (uveitis) cases. With repeated use, it may cause vomiting, diarrhea, increased salivation, bronchiolar spasm, and pulmonary edema (Plumb, 2015).

Demecarium Bromide

Clinical Uses. Used to reduce IOPs for up to 48 hours in dogs. Causes miosis. Generally, this drug is used to manage potential glaucoma in the eye opposite from which a diagnosis of an acute congestive crisis of primary glaucoma is made. It is not available from a veterinary pharmaceutical manufacturer and can be compounded by a specialty pharmacy.

Dosage Form
• **Ophthalmic drops**

Adverse Side Effects. Do not use in pregnant animals. Use with caution when other cholinesterase inhibitors are used. May cause ciliary muscle spasm, headache, blurred vision, local inflammation, vomiting, diarrhea, increased salivation, and cardiac effect especially when used in high doses in small-breed dogs.

SYMPATHOMIMETICS

These are also known as *alpha₂-agonists*. Sympathomimetic drugs decrease IOP. Long-term use may result in an increase in uveoscleral outflow.

Apraclonidine

Clinical Uses. Apraclonidine is used to reduce aqueous humor formation. Effects are usually noted 3 to 5 hours after a single dose.

Dosage Forms
• **Ophthalmic solution** (Iopidine)

TECHNICIAN NOTES

Do not use apraclonidine in cats.

Adverse Side Effects. Adverse effects include conjunctival blanching and mydriasis. Do not use in cats; they can experience vomiting, diarrhea, hypersalivation, and bradycardia (Plumb, 2015).

Brimonidine

Clinical Uses. Brimonidine has a longer duration of action than does apraclonidine. It is used to treat elevated IOP, reduces aqueous humor formation, and increases uveoscleral outflow.

Dosage Forms. Ophthalmic solution
• **Alphagan P**
• **Combigan**

Adverse Side Effects. Animals seem to better tolerate side effects from brimonidine than from apraclonidine.

Side effects include allergic conjunctivitis, eye itching, and eye irritation.

Epinephrine

Clinical Uses. Epinephrine is used clinically as an intracameral injection to cause mydriasis and to prevent bleeding after intraocular surgical procedures.

Dosage Forms. Topical ophthalmic solution
• **Epifrin**
• **Glaucon**

Adverse Side Effects. These include possible eye irritation at administration.

BETA-ADRENERGIC ANTAGONISTS

These drugs aid in reducing IOP.

Timolol

Clinical Uses. Timolol is primarily used to prevent glaucoma from developing in the contralateral eye of a dog that has primary glaucoma in one eye. The drug reduces IOP.

Dosage Forms. Ophthalmic solution; no veterinary product is available.
• **Timoptic**

Adverse Side Effects. These include miosis in dogs and cats to a slight degree. It may also trigger bronchospasms in cats with asthma.

TECHNICIAN NOTES

Caution should be used if timolol is prescribed for cats with asthma.

CARBONIC ANHYDRASE INHIBITORS

These drugs are most useful in treating primary open-angle glaucoma and secondary glaucoma in humans.

Brinzolamide HCl

Clinical Uses. Brinzolamide reduces aqueous humor production (decrease IOP) in animals with glaucoma.

Dosage Forms
• **Ophthalmic topical solution** (Azopt)

Adverse Side Effects. Side effects include burning and irritation; cats are more susceptible to irritation from brinzolamide than other species (Plumb, 2015).

Dorzolamide HCl

Clinical Uses. This drug is often used in the contralateral eye of a dog with primary glaucoma to prevent development of bilateral disease. It is also used for secondary glaucoma in dogs and cats because it does not affect pupil size; it is used to decrease IOP.

Dosage Forms. Ophthalmic topical solution
- **Trusopt**
- **Cosopt**

Adverse Side Effects. These may include a stinging sensation in cats. Hypersensitivity may also occur.

Other carbonic anhydrase inhibitors include (Whelan, 2019):
- **Acetazolamide** (Diamox)
- **Dichlorphenamide** (Daranide)
- **Methazolamide** (Neptazane)

PROSTAGLANDINS

These drugs act on prostanoid receptors to lower IOP.

Latanoprost

Clinical Uses. Latanoprost reduces IOP, especially in canine primary glaucoma cases; results are even better when this drug is combined with carbonic anhydrase inhibitors. It is not effective for feline glaucoma.

Dosage Form
- **Latanoprost ophthalmic solution** (Xalatan)

Adverse Side Effects. Topical irritation and hyperemia of the conjunctiva may be noted. Various other effects may also occur.

> **TECHNICIAN NOTES**
>
> - Do not use latanoprost in horses because of adverse side effects.
> - Refrigerate until use; store at room temperature for 6 weeks after opening.

Bimatoprost

Clinical Uses. Bimatoprost is used to lower IOP in patients with glaucoma. It is not effective for feline glaucoma.

Dosage Forms. Ophthalmic drops
- **Lumigan**

Adverse Side Effects. Topical irritation and hyperemia of the conjunctiva may be noted. Various other effects may also occur.

OSMOTIC AGENTS FOR THE TREATMENT OF GLAUCOMA

Osmotic agents increase osmotic pressure of plasma and create a concentration gradient that will draw fluid out of the intraocular environment. These agents are systemically administered with concurrent water deprivation (4–6 hours) and are indicated only for acute episodes of glaucoma not maintenance (Plumb, 2015).

MYDRIATIC CYCLOPLEGIC VASOCONSTRICTORS

Cyclopentolate

Clinical Uses. This drug is an anticholinergic agent that causes the sphincter of the iris and ciliary muscles to relax. This drug is mainly used to induce mydriasis (dilates pupil) and cycloplegia (paralysis of the ciliary muscle) for diagnostic purposes.

Dosage Forms. Ophthalmic solution
- **Cyclogyl**

> **TECHNICIAN NOTES**
>
> Cyclopentolate increases IOP and should never be used in animals with glaucoma.

Adverse Side Effects. These may include stinging sensations and irritation. It is contraindicated in animals with glaucoma as it causes increased IOP.

Phenylephrine HCl

Clinical Uses. Phenylephrine is a direct acting, alpha$_1$-agonist vasoconstrictor drug that is commonly used in veterinary medicine to induce mydriasis before cataract removal. This drug can also be used to control bleeding for minor surface procedures. On administration, phenylephrine HCl lasts approximately 2 to 18 hours. It can be used in the treatment of Horner's syndrome (Plumb, 2015).

Dosage Form
- **Ophthalmic solution** (Altafrin, Neofrin)

Adverse Side Effects. Local irritation may occur. In cats and rabbits, stromal clouding may occur if the corneal epithelium is damaged.

Atropine Sulfate

Clinical Uses. Atropine controls pain caused by corneal and/or uveal disease. It may be used to dilate the pupil for an ophthalmic examination or before ophthalmic surgery. Do not use in patients with primary glaucoma.

Dosage Forms
- Manufactured as an **ophthalmic solution or ophthalmic ointment** (Atrophate)

Adverse Side Effects. This drug causes mydriasis and accommodation paralysis. Hypersalivation may occur in cats when atropine drops are administered. Atropine can cause a decrease in tear production in small animals. In horses, repeated treatment with atropine may cause colic, although this is rare.

TECHNICIAN NOTES

- In the dog, dilation may persist for up to 120 hours. Dogs and cats should be placed in darkened quarters until the pupil is at its normal size.
- Ointments or drops may be used in dogs.
- Atropine is very long lasting when used in horses, and dilation may last for days to weeks.
- Do not use in patients with primary glaucoma.
- Atropine ointment should be used in cats to prevent hypersalivation caused by the bitter taste of atropine drops.

Tropicamide

Clinical Uses. Tropicamide has a more rapid onset of action and a shorter duration of action than atropine. This drug causes mydriasis which makes it useful for funduscopic examinations. In dogs, IOP does not seem to be affected by the action of tropicamide.

Dosage Forms. Ophthalmic solution
- **Mydriacyl**

Adverse Side Effects. Side effects include less effective pain control than atropine; hypersalivation, especially in cats; stinging of the eye on administration; and may decrease tear production for several hours after administration (Plumb, 2015).

ANTIINFLAMMATORY/ANALGESIC OPHTHALMIC AGENTS

Cromolyn Sodium

Clinical Uses. Cromolyn sodium is a mast cell stabilizing agent. This drug blocks the release of histamine from mast cells after antigen recognition. This drug is particularly useful in treating patients with allergic conjunctivitis and may help alleviate seasonal allergies affecting the eyes.

Dosage Form
- **Ophthalmic solution** (Crolom, Opticrom)

Adverse Side Effects. A stinging sensation has been reported at administration.

Olopatadine HCl

Clinical Uses. This drug is used to relieve the symptoms of ocular allergies (pruritis).

Dosage Form
- **Ophthalmic solution** (Patanol)

NONSTEROIDAL ANTIINFLAMMATORY AGENTS

Nonsteroidal antiinflammatory drugs (NSAIDs) are used in veterinary medicine to control inflammation and to provide pain relief. They may be used postoperatively to help the cornea to heal. Additionally, they may also be used to treat allergic conjunctivitis.

Clinical Uses. Bromfenac is used after cataract removal to minimize inflammation. Diclofenac sodium is used for the treatment of uveitis. Flurbiprofen sodium may be useful in the management of uveal inflammation, especially if topical steroids are also used. Ketorolac tromethamine is most commonly used to control surgical or nonsurgical uveitis, especially in cases with corneal bacterial infection or ulceration. Nepafenac is used in veterinary medicine to control the pain and inflammation that accompanies cataract surgery. Suprofen may be useful in the management of uveal inflammation.

Dosage Forms. Ophthalmic solution
- **Bromfenac** (Xibrom)
- **Diclofenac sodium** - this product is not commercially available and can be prepared through a compounding pharmacy.
- **Flurbiprofen sodium** (Ocufen)
- **Ketorolac tromethamine** (Acular)
- **Nepafenac** (Nevanac)
- **Suprofen** (Profenal)

Adverse Side Effects. Bromfenac is not to be used in patients with known hypersensitivity to any ingredient found in bromfenac. Do not use flurbiprofen in patients with infected corneal ulcers because this drug can be as immunosuppressive as topical corticosteroids. Nepafenac may cause bleeding of ocular tissues. All topical NSAIDs may slow healing time. Other adverse reactions also exist.

STEROIDAL ANTIINFLAMMATORY AGENTS

This group of drugs is used to treat diseases of the eye that may include the conjunctiva, the sclera, the cornea, and the anterior chamber. For maximum results from these agents, the frequency of administration should be increased instead of increasing the drug's concentration. Some side effects may occur when steroidal antiinflammatory agents are used. These are more common in humans than in animals but may include the development of cataracts, increased IOP, infection, decreased wound healing, mydriasis, and calcific keratopathy. These drugs should not be used to treat conjunctivitis in cats.

Prednisolone

Clinical Uses. This drug is typically used in the treatment of anterior uveitis and is also used to treat uveitis in horses.

Dosage Forms. Suspension drops can be prepared through a compounding pharmacy.
- **Pred Forte**
- **Omnipred**

Adverse Side Effects. These are uncommon.

Dexamethasone

Clinical Uses. This drug is used for antiinflammatory purposes.

Dosage Forms. Manufactured as an ophthalmic solution and ophthalmic ointment.

Betamethasone

Clinical Uses. Antimicrobial-steroid combination used for inflammatory conditions of the eye.

Dosage Form
- Ophthalmic drops are no longer commercially available but can be prepared through a compounding pharmacy.

 TECHNICIAN NOTES

- Never use this product if corneal ulceration or abrasion is suspected.
- Do not use to treat herpes keratitis in cats.

Fluorometholone

Clinical Uses. This drug is used for antiinflammatory purposes.

Dosage Form. Manufactured as an ophthalmic ointment and suspension.
- **FML**
- **Flarex**

Adverse Side Effects. High concentrations of this drug may raise IOP.

Loteprednol

Clinical Uses. Loteprednol is used for antiinflammatory purposes. It is not suitable to raise IOP.

Dosage Forms. Ophthalmic suspension
- **Lotemax**
- **Alrex**

Adverse Side Effects. Do not use this product to treat herpes keratitis or if corneal ulceration or abrasion are suspected (Plumb, 2015).

Rimexolone

Rimexolone is used for antiinflammatory purposes.

Dosage Form
- **Ophthalmic suspension** (Vexol)

OPHTHALMIC ANALGESICS

These agents are for eye pain relief.

Morphine Sulfate

Clinical Use. Morphine sulfate is used for corneal ulcer pain relief and may also be used to lessen blepharospasms. Morphine sulfate is a Class II controlled substance.

Dosage Forms
- No veterinary- or human-label products available
- May be compounded as a solution by a compounding pharmacy

ANTIMICROBIAL OPHTHALMIC THERAPY

Antimicrobials aid in the treatment and management of ocular disease.

Amikacin Sulfate

Clinical Uses. This drug is useful in the treatment of corneal infections, as well as in treating bacterial endophthalmitis. It does not cause retinal toxic effects.

Dosage Forms
- Not available as a veterinary- or human-label drug
- Must be compounded into a topical preparation (Plumb, 2015)

Neomycin Sulfate

Clinical Uses. This drug is useful in treating superficial corneal ulcers or infections of the ocular surface.

Dosage Forms. This drug is manufactured as an ophthalmic ointment or ophthalmic solution. Most are a combination of bacitracin/neomycin/polymyxin B (triple antibiotic).

- TriOptic
- Vetropolycin
- Optiprime

Adverse Side Effects. The neomycin in this product may cause contact sensitivity and should not be used in patients with a history of this problem.

Gentamicin Sulfate

Clinical Use. This drug is most commonly used for keratitis caused by *Pseudomonas aeruginosa*.

Dosage Forms
- **Ophthalmic ointment and ophthalmic solution** available (Gentocin)

 TECHNICIAN NOTES

- Do not use if there is corneal penetration as gentamicin is toxic to the interior of the eye.

Tobramycin Sulfate

Clinical Uses. This is an antimicrobial product used in animals with ocular infections of *Pseudomonas aeruginosa*.

Dosage Forms. Manufactured as an ophthalmic ointment and ophthalmic solution
- No veterinary-label products available
- **Tobrex**—human label

Adverse Side Effects. Systemic use of this drug is not beneficial in ocular infections.

MISCELLANEOUS OCULAR ANTIBIOTICS

Chloramphenicol

Clinical Uses. This is a broad-spectrum antibiotic that is able to cross the corneal barrier and gain entrance into the anterior chamber. (Very few infections, however, happen in the anterior chamber.) Generally speaking, *Staphylococcus* spp. and *Streptococcus* spp. are destroyed by chloramphenicol, but *Pseudomonas* spp. are resistant to it. It is used in dogs and cats for the topical treatment of bacterial conjunctivitis caused by pathogens susceptible to chloramphenicol.

Dosage Forms
- **Chloramphenicol ophthalmic solutions** are no longer commercially available but can be prepared through a compounding pharmacy.

Polymyxin B

Clinical Uses. This drug is a surface detergent (cationic). Its efficacy is against gram-negative organisms and can be combined with other antimicrobials with gram-positive activity. Terramycin is used in dogs, cats, horses, and cattle with superficial ocular infections, such as conjunctivitis, pink eye, corneal ulcer, and bacterial inflammatory conditions.

Dosage Form
- **Terramycin Ophthalmic Ointment**

Sulfacetamide

Clinical Uses. This drug is useful in the treatment of conjunctivitis and superficial eye infections.

Dosage Forms. No veterinary products are available.
- **Bleph-10**

Adverse Side Effects. Side effects include gastrointestinal (GI) disturbances, allergies, renal damage, and damage to lacrimal acinar cells (KCS).

Vancomycin

Clinical Uses. This drug is used in rabbits to treat methicillin-resistant *Staphylococcus aureus* (MRSA).

Dosage Forms
- Must be prepared through a compounding pharmacy
- Not approved in an ophthalmic dosage form in the United States (Plumb, 2015)

 TECHNICIAN NOTES

This should be the last drug of choice because it has a high potential for ototoxicity (leading to deafness) and nephrotoxicity that can lead to death.

OCULAR ANTIFUNGALS

Aspergillus is a common pathogen causing fungal keratitis in horses. These drugs are used to treat fungal infections in animals.

Amphotericin B

Clinical Uses. This is a broad-spectrum antifungal agent (derived from *Streptomyces nodosus*) used to treat fungal infections and fungal keratitis (Plumb, 2015).

Dosage Forms
- No veterinary-label products; it is not commercially available and can be prepared through a compounding pharmacy.

TECHNICIAN NOTES

Amphotericin B cannot be reconstituted with sodium chloride because it may cause degradation of the drug; it can only be reconstituted with sterile water.

Natamycin

Clinical Uses. This drug is used to treat superficial equine fungal keratitis (Plumb, 2015).

Dosage Form
• **Ophthalmic suspension** (Natacyn)

Adverse Side Effects. Natamycin may cause worsening of corneal edema.

Povidone Iodine

Clinical Uses. This drug can be used for chemical débridement of loose epithelium in canine ulcers.

Dosage Forms
• Must be compounded and diluted from commercially available povidone iodine solutions (Betadine)

Adverse Side Effects. These solutions need to be lavaged from the eye after no more than 5 minutes to prevent corneal epithelial damage.

Itraconazole

Clinical Uses. This is a broad-spectrum antifungal agent. Itraconazole is insoluble in water and must be diluted in dimethyl sulfoxide (DMSO) in order to form a solution for instillation into the eyes. This drug may be used in horses to treat fungal keratitis.

Dosage Forms
• Not commercially available and can be prepared through a compounding pharmacy.

Adverse Side Effects. Personnel treating horses with this drug should wear gloves to avoid having their skin absorb the DMSO.

Miconazole

Clinical Uses. This drug is used in horses to treat fungal keratitis.

Dosage Forms. Not commercially available and can be prepared through a compounding pharmacy.

OCULAR ANTIVIRALS

These drugs are most commonly used to treat feline ocular herpes virus infections.

Trifluridine

Clinical Uses. This drug is used occasionally to treat feline herpes virus infections of the eye. This agent may also be used to treat superficial punctate keratitis in equines, which is thought to occur due to equine herpes virus (EHV-2), which may cause problems with the cornea.

Dosage Forms. Ophthalmic solution
• **Trifluorothymidine** (Viroptic) – may be prepared through a compounding pharmacy.

Adverse Side Effects. Trifluridine must be administered quite frequently to obtain acceptable results. If cats do not respond well within a 3-week period, they are not likely to respond to this drug at all. Therefore, use should be discontinued. The conjunctiva and eyelid margins may be irritated in cats during therapy with this drug.

Idoxuridine

Clinical Uses. This drug may be used to treat herpes virus infections of the eye in cats.

Dosage Forms
• No veterinary products exist; this product is not commercially available but can be prepared through a compounding pharmacy.

Acyclovir, Valacyclovir, Famciclovir, Ganciclovir, Cidofovir, and Penciclovir

These drugs are used in the treatment of feline herpes ocular virus. Cats are sensitive to acyclovir and valacyclovir; these drugs may cause fatal myeloid dysplasia in the species. Famciclovir may be safely used in cats to reduce herpetic symptoms.

DRUGS FOR KERATOCONJUNCTIVITIS SICCA

Keratoconjunctivitis sicca, also called dry eye, is a disease in which tear production is decreased and causes changes in the cornea (ulcerations and corneal scarring) and conjunctiva (mucopurulent conjunctivitis). It is a common disorder in dogs, and it is believed from recent research that the disease may be due to an immune-mediated disease process.

Cyclosporine

Clinical Uses. Cyclosporine is used in the treatment of KCS. Cyclosporine is also used in the treatment of pannus.

Dosage Forms. Ophthalmic ointment
• **Optimmune**

Adverse Side Effects. Patients are usually given this drug for life to keep KCS symptoms under control. If the therapy is stopped, the clinical signs often return.

Tacrolimus

Clinical Uses. Tacrolimus was originally studied at the University of Tennessee College of Veterinary Medicine. Investigators there found this drug to be as equally effective as cyclosporine and effective for cyclosporine-resistant cases of KCS.

Dosage Form
- Not commercially available but can be prepared through a compounding pharmacy.

Pimecrolimus

This drug is also used in dogs with KCS.

Dosage Form
- Not commercially available but can be prepared through a compounding pharmacy.

 TECHNICIAN NOTES

Avoid contact with the skin as it has been associated with cancer; gloves must be worn when handling this drug (Plumb, 2015).

OCULAR LUBRICANTS/ARTIFICIAL TEAR PRODUCTS

These agents are used as a lubricant for dry eyes, to relieve eye irritation, and are also used during anesthetic periods when the patient's eyes remain open and tear production is reduced.

Artificial Tears
- **Adsorbotear**
- **Comfort Tears**
- **Tears Naturale**
- Various others

Ophthalmic Irrigants

The main purpose of these agents is to maintain the shape of the anterior chamber during cataract surgery.

ANTICOLLAGENASE AGENTS

These agents are used to treat corneal ulcers by stopping the melting effect of colla genases and proteases on the cornea.

Acetylcysteine

Dosage Form
- No veterinary product is available and must be prepared through a compounding pharmacy.

Edetate Disodium

Clinical Uses. This drug is used to stop the melting effect of collagenases and proteases on the cornea but are not useful for melting caused by infectious agents. It is used to remove superficial calcium deposits (Plumb, 2015).

Dosage Form
- No longer commercially available and must be prepared through a compounding pharmacy.

OTIC DRUGS

The ear consists of three major parts; the outer, middle, and inner ear (Fig. 10.6). The outer ear includes the pinna and the ear canal. The ear canal carries sound to the tympanic membrane (ear drum). The shape of the ear canal is "L" shaped and where cerumen and other secretions accumulate. The middle ear includes the tympanic membrane, auditory ossicles (bones that transmit and amplify air vibrations), and eustachian tube. The inner ear includes the cochlea (hearing) and vestibular apparatus (balance).

When a client obtains a new puppy, the veterinary technician should demonstrate the proper way to clean the pup's ears. Performance of the ear cleaning process at an early age will allow the puppy to submit more readily to the task as an adult dog. Unfortunately, those breeds with pendulous ears may tend to have otic problems. Long ear flaps (i.e., pinnae) tend to keep air from circulating into the external ear canal; consequently, the ear canal remains moist, which creates a perfect environment for yeast formation. Yeast is not the only problem that veterinarians encounter in dogs and cats. External parasites such as *Otodectes cynotis* (i.e., ear mites) can cause extreme discomfort in animals that are infested by these creatures. Patients whose ears remain untreated often experience aural hematomas caused by extreme shaking of the head and scratching of the ears (Hendrix, 2017).

Generally, ear problems are treated with topical medications. Sometimes, ear infections also must be treated with systemic medications. Topical preparations used to treat ear infections are often a combination of different types of drugs, such as antibacterial, antifungal, antipruritic, and antiinflammatory agents. Still other preparations are cleansers, drying agents, and parasiticides.

Cleansing agents are used to remove discharge and debris from the ear canal to prevent infections. Drying

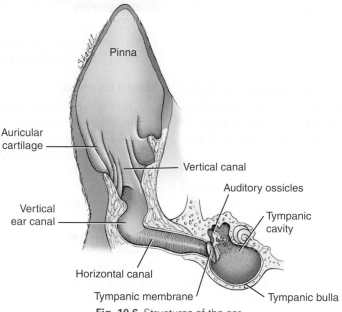

Fig. 10.6 Structures of the ear.

agents are used to decrease the amount of moisture in the ear canal.

 TECHNICIAN NOTES

- When a ruptured eardrum is suspected or confirmed, oil-based or irritating external ear preparations (e.g., chlorhexidine) and aminoglycosides should be avoided.
- Technicians play an important role in educating and demonstrating proper ear cleaning techniques to clients.

Ceruminolytic Agents

Clinical Uses. These products emulsify **cerumen** and purulent exudate. They work by providing a surfactant, detergent, and bubbling action. Do not use these products in patients with ruptured ear drum(s).

Dosage Forms
- **Cerumene**
- **Corium-20**
- **KlearOtic Ear Cleanser**
- **Douxo Micellar Solution**
- **Ear Cleansing Solution**
- **Earoxide Ear Cleanser**
- **Epiklean Ear Cleanser**

Cleaning/Drying Agents

Clinical Uses. These products are used after cleaning of the ears has occurred. These agents can be used as maintenance agents to prevent ear infections after swimming or bathing.

Dosage Forms
- **Corium-20**
- **Epi-Otic Cleanser with Spherulites**
- **Epi-Otic Advanced**
- **Euclens Otic Cleanser**
- **Gent-L-Clens**
- **MalAcetic Otic**
- **Nolva-Cleanse**
- **Nolvasan Otic**
- **Otic clear**
- **Oti-Clens**
- **Oti-Soothe**
- **OtiRinse solution**
- **Vetoquinol ear cleansing solution**
- **Zymox ear cleanser**
- **Various others**

Antiseptic Agents

Clinical Uses. These products are commonly used with other products to help heal ear infections. Chlorhexidine-containing products should be used carefully in animals with ruptured tympanic membranes.

Dosage Forms
- **MalAcetic Otic**
- **MalAcetic Ultra Otic**

BOX 10.1 Case Scenario Acute Otitis Externa

Lily, a 2-year-old Labrador, was presented by the owner stating that she has been scratching at her ears, shaking her head, and rubbing her head on the floor for the past week. The owner noted that her ears have an odor.

Additional history: Up to date on vaccinations. The owner noted that Lily likes to swim in the lake on their farm.

Physical examination findings: Lily was bright, alert, and responsive. Temperature: 101.5°F, pulses: 80 bpm, no pulse deficits, respirations: panting. The ear canal was palpated and pliable, not firm. No areas of alopecia or excoriation on the pinna. The otoscope examination of both ears revealed purulent (yellow-tan color) and thick exudate. The ear canal was red and inflamed but not painful; the tympanic membrane was intact.

A sample for ear cytology was taken from both ears and revealed occasional bacteria, moderate amount of yeast, and occasional epithelial cells.

Diagnosis: Acute otitis externa

The ear canal was cleaned with MalAcetic Ultra Otic and medicated with Animax.

A follow-up examination was scheduled to ensure that the ear canal is clean and also another ear cytology to ensure that the infection has resolved.

The veterinary technician discharged the patient with ear cleaning solution and Animax. She explained that routine ear cleaning should be done once daily until no debris is visible (usually 3–7 days), then clean the ears once weekly. The Animax is to be administered after cleaning the ear. She went on to say that if Lily should go swimming in the lake, that she will need to clean her ears afterward. She demonstrated to the owner how to properly clean the ears. It was emphasized that continued ear cleaning will be necessary to help prevent recurrence even if the ear looks good and there is no obvious odor or discharge. She also explained that if Lily starts scratching at her ears and shaking her head a hematoma can develop in which the blood vessels in the ear flap break, causing a painful swelling that requires surgical treatment. The veterinary technician explained how important it is to get the medication into the horizontal part of the ear canal. She further explained that unlike our ear canal, the dog's external ear canal is L-shaped and showed her a picture. The goal is to administer the medication into the lower part of the "L"—the horizontal ear canal.

The veterinary technician demonstrated to the owner how to properly clean the ears using the following steps:

- Gently pull the earflap up and slightly back with one hand.
- Using the other hand, apply a small amount of medication into the vertical part of the ear canal and wait a few seconds for the medication to run down into the ear canal.
- Put one finger in back of and at the base of the ear and your thumb in front.
- Gently massage the ear canal between your finger and thumb. You may hear a squishing sound; this tells you that the medication went into the horizontal ear canal.
- Release the ear and let your dog shake its head.
- You should then clean the outer part of the ear canal and the inside of the earflap with a cotton ball.
- **Do not** use cotton tipped applicators (Q-Tips) to do this, as they tend to push debris back into the vertical ear canal and you may cause damage to the ear.

- **Mal-A-Ket Plus TrizEDTA Flush**
- **OtoCetic Solution**

Antibiotic Potentiating Agents

Clinical Uses. Tromethamine-ethylenediaminetetraacetic acid (tris-EDTA) has antimicrobial and antibiotic potentiating activity. It is nonototoxic and safe to use in the middle ear. These products work better when used 15 to 30 minutes before a topical antibiotic (Plumb, 2015).

Dosage Forms
- **KetoTRIS Flush**
- **Mal-A-Ket Plus TrizEDTA Flush**
- **TrizEDTA Aqueous Flush or Crystals**
- **TrizULTRA + Keto**
- **TrizChlor**

Corticosteroid Preparations

Clinical Uses. These products are used in cases of acute or chronic otitis. They help to reduce the build-up of sebaceous and apocrine gland secretion.

Dosage Forms
- **Cort/Astrin Solution**
- **MalAcetic Ultra Otic**
- **Synotic Otic Solution**
- **Zymox Plus Otic-HC**

Antibacterials

Clinical Uses. Many antibacterial agents used in the ears are designed to treat infections caused by *Staphylococcus* spp. or *Pseudomonas* spp. Very few products contain an antibiotic to treat bacterial otitis; therefore, the veterinarian may resort to using ophthalmic products or injectable antibiotics directly into the ear canal to treat such infections. Some of the dosage forms below also contain other drugs

Dosage Forms
- **Enrofloxacin** (Baytril Otic)
- **Gentamicin** (Otomax, Gentocin otic)
- **Tobramycin** (Tobrex Ophthalmic Solution)
- **Neomycin** (Tresaderm, Panalog)

Antifungals

Clinical Uses. These are mainly used to treat *Malassezia* otitis and sometimes otic candidiasis.

Dosage Forms
- **Clotrimazole solution** (Otomax and various others)
- **Miconazole** (Conofite and various others)
- **Nystatin** (Panalog, Dema-vet)
- **Thiabendazole** (Tresaderm)
- Various others

Corticosteroid Plus Antimicrobial Preparations

Clinical Uses. These products are used in cases of acute and chronic otitis. They help reduce inflammation, decrease edema, tissue hyperplasia, pain, and pruritis, and to help eliminate any infectious organisms that may be present.

Dosage Forms
- **Ciprofloxicin** (Ciprodex)
- **Clotrimazole** (Otibiotic, Otomax, Vetromax)
- **Gentamicin** (GenOne Otic, GentaVed otic, Mometamax otic)
- **Nystatin** (Animax Ointment, DermaVet, Dermalog, Quadritop, Panalog)
- **Neomycin** (Tresaderm, Tritop)
- **Orbifloxacin** (Posatex)
- Various others

Antiparasitic Preparations

Clinical Uses. The following preparations are designed for use inside the ears to stop otoacariasis. Products such as selamectin or fipronil are preferred because *O. cynotis* are known to live outside the ears and can re-infest the ears (Plumb, 2015).

Dosage Forms
- **Ivermectin** (Acarexx Otic, Ivomec)
- **Adams Ear Mite**
- **Pyrethrins** (Cerumite 3x, Mita-clear, Eradimite, Otimite Plus)
- **Milbemycin** (MilbeMite Otic)
- **Thiabendazole** (Tresaderm)

- **QuadraClear Ear Drops**
- Various others

REVIEW QUESTIONS

1. Mydriatic agents are used to _____ the pupils.
2. Atropine is contraindicated in_____ and _____.
3. Miotic agents produce _____ _____ constriction.
4. Why are ophthalmic stains used?
5. _____ stain is the most commonly used dye for the detection of corneal epithelial defects.
6. Patients with ear mites, whose ears are left untreated, often experience _____ hematomas caused by excessive shaking of the head.
7. What type of administration is the most common method of treating disorders of the eye?
8. Why do most topical ophthalmic medications require several applications per day?
9. What is Proparacaine used for?
10. The appearance of fluorescein stain at the nostril opening is an abnormal finding when a fluorescein stain test is performed.
    a. True
    b. False
11. The nictitating membrane is also known as _____.
    a. sclera
    b. cornea
    c. third eyelid
    d. ciliary body
12. Mydriatic agents are used to _____ the pupils.
    a. dilate
    b. constrict
    c. hydrate
    d. teach
13. Atropine ophthalmic agents are used to produce _____.
    a. miosis
    b. mydriasis
14. Carbonic anhydrase inhibitors are useful in treating _____-angle glaucoma.
    a. closed
    b. open

15. Sympathomimetic drugs are used to _____ (increase, decrease) intraocular pressure.
16. Which one of the following is an ocular fluoro-quinolone used to treat gram-negative corneal infections?
    a. Ciprofloxacin
    b. Amphotericin B
    c. Itraconazole
    d. Neomycin
17. Fluorescein stain is used commonly to diagnose _____.
    a. glaucoma
    b. corneal ulcers
    c. entropion
    d. ectropion
18. _____ have very strong palpebral muscles, and it may be necessary to have another person assist when one is applying ophthalmic drugs.
    a. Canines
    b. Felines
    c. Equines
    d. Caprines
19. It is acceptable to use corticosteroid-type ointments in patients with corneal ulcers.
    a. True
    b. False
20. _____ has been developed for the treatment of *Otodectes* spp.
    a. Chloramphenicol
    b. Enrofloxacin
    c. Optimmune
    d. Acarexx
21. Clotrimazole and miconazole are _____ drugs used to treat Malassezia infections in the ear.
22. Ceruminolytic agents should not be used in patients with _____.
23. How many milligrams of tropicamide are in a 0.5% solution?
    a. 50 mg
    b. 500 mg
    c. 5 mg
    d. 0.5 mg
24. If the veterinarian prescribes amphotericin B in a 0.15% solution for ocular administration at a rate of 0.2 mL in the eye every 4 hours for 14 days, how much solution should be prepared for the patient?
    a. 8.4 mL
    b. 4.2 mL
    c. 16.8 mL
    d. 32.16 mL
25. A veterinary ophthalmologist must perform fluorescein staining on 21 dogs in a 1-week period. How many fluorescein strips need to be on hand to accomplish this task for a month?
    a. 64 strips
    b. 66 strips
    c. 94 strips
    d. 84 strips

REFERENCES

Bassert, J. M., Samples, O., & Beal, A. (Eds.). (2018). *McCurnin's clinical textbook for veterinary technicians* (9th ed.). Philadelphia: Elsevier.

Hendrix, C. M., & Robinson, E. (Eds.). (2017). *Diagnostic veterinary parasitology* (5th ed.). St. Louis: Mosby.

Plumb, D. C. (2015). *Veterinary drug handbook* (8th ed.). Ames, IA: Wiley-Blackwell.

Whelan N. Treatment of glaucoma. In: *The Merck veterinary manual* (online edition) http:merckveterinarymanual.com/; Accessed August 2019.

Drugs Used in Skin Disorders

After studying this chapter, you should be able to

1. List and describe the diagnostic procedures used to help determine the cause of skin problems (disease).
2. Exhibit a basic understanding of the anatomy and physiology of the skin.
3. Exhibit a basic understanding of wound healing, including describing the difference between primary and secondary intention healing.

4. Describe the use of topical antipruritics and antiinflammatories.
5. Describe the use of topical antimicrobials and antiseptics.
6. Explain the use of antifungals and topical retinoids.
7. Discuss the use of topical and oral antiparasitic agents.

OUTLINE

KEY TERMS

Antiseptic

Astringent

Collagen

Comedo (pl. comedones)

Dermatitis

Dermatophyte

Dermatophytosis

Erythema

Fatty acid

Furuncle (furunculosis)

Granulation tissue

Integumentary system

Keratolytic

Keratoplastic

Primary intention healing

Pruritus

Pseudomembranous colitis

Pyoderma

Seborrhea

Seborrhea oleosa

Seborrhea sicca

Secondary intention healing

INTRODUCTION

Dermatologic conditions are frequently seen in veterinary practice. From ectoparasitic problems to allergies, veterinarians are continually combating companion animal skin problems. As a veterinary technician, this is one area in which your expertise will be used because clients will ask many questions about shampoos, dips, conditioners, soaks, lotions, creams, ointments, sprays, powders, and topical products designed to have activity against fleas, ticks, and mosquitoes. Each of these products may be used to treat a full spectrum of dermatologic problems from parasites to **pyoderma**. Patients are often presented for examination of a skin disease when in reality they have an underlying systemic illness. Veterinarians use various diagnostic procedures (e.g., skin scrapings, allergy testing, and **dermatophyte** tests) to determine the cause of skin disease. Skin scraping is commonly used to identify mites such as *Sarcoptes*, *Demodex*, and *Cheyletiella*. Allergy testing is most commonly performed to determine atopic dermatitis or allergic inhalant dermatitis to help identify the specific allergens causing the problem. Dermatophyte tests include fungal cultures (DTM—Dermatophyte Test Medium), examination with a Wood's lamp, and direct microscopic examination of hair or skin scale. Technicians play a vital role by obtaining a complete history, knowing how to perform the diagnostic procedures used in a dermatologic workup, and providing client education. Client education is essential when skin disease is treated because clients must understand the purpose of medications and how they should be properly used.

ANATOMY AND PHYSIOLOGY

The skin is a part of the **integumentary system** and constitutes the largest organ in the body. It is made up of three layers (Fig. 11.1) and serves multiple functions. It provides a barrier against the outside world by preventing entry of pathogenic microorganisms and by protecting against physical and chemical insults. It senses heat, cold, pain, touch, pressure, and other sensations like **pruritus** (itching) and helps to regulate body temperature through mechanisms related to cutaneous blood

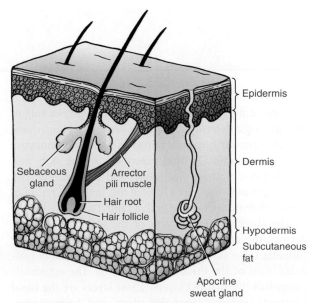

Epidermis

Dermis

Sebaceous gland

Arrector pili muscle

Hair root

Hair follicle

Hypodermis

Subcutaneous fat

Apocrine sweat gland

Fig. 11.1 Schematic representation of the skin layers of normal canine skin.

TABLE 11.1 Common Skin Disorders With Suggested Treatments and Various Products Available.

Disease	Sulfur	Salicylic Acid	Coal Tar	Benzoyl Peroxide	Chlorhexidine	Hydrocortisone	Therapeutic Products
Seborrhea sicca	✓	✓					SebaLyt Shampoo Sebolux Shampoo Allerseb-T Shampoo
Seborrhea oleosa	✓	✓	✓	✓			LyTar Shampoo Pyoben Shampoo SulfOxyDex Shampoo
Hot spots				✓	✓	✓	ChlorHex Shampoo Pyoben Gel Gentocin Topical Spray
Skinfold dermatitis				✓			OxyDex Gel Pyoben Gel
Deep pyoderma				✓			Pyoben Shampoo SulfOxyDex Shampoo Systemic antibiotics
Superficial pustular dermatitis				✓			Pyoben Shampoo OxyDex Shampoo SulfOxyDex Shampoo
Superficial folliculitis				✓	✓		ChlorHex Shampoo Pyoben Shampoo SulfOxyDex Shampoo
Atopy/ allergic contact dermatitis	✓	✓	✓			✓	Micro Pearls Advantage Seba-Moist Shampoo DermaCool-HC Spray
Schnauzer comedo syndrome				✓			Micro Pearls Advantage Benzoyl Plus Shampoo OxyDex Shampoo

flow, sweating, and the haircoat. The skin plays a role in immunologic defense through the actions of Langerhans (dendritic or antigen-presenting) cells and keratinocytes, produces vitamin D_3 from precursors in the skin, and acts as a reservoir for electrolytes and other substances. This organ may also play a limited role in the excretion of some substances from the body (Table 11.1).

The three primary layers of the skin are the epidermis, the dermis or corium, and the hypodermis or subcutis (also called the *panniculus*). The dermis provides most of the thickness of the skin. The epidermis comprises five distinct layers. These layers are the basal (deepest), spinous, granular, clear, and horny/cornified (superficial) layers. Epidermal cells are replenished in the basal layer and are pushed outward by newly forming layers. As these cells reach the surface, they are flattened and hardened to form a protective barrier. It normally takes 21 to 22 days for cells to reach the outer layer; this process is called the *epidermal turnover rate*. The epidermal turnover rate may be sped up in some disease processes. Continual shedding of these cells is called *desquamation*. When the process becomes excessive, scale or dandruff is seen. The epidermis includes a population of normal microorganisms that help to prevent overgrowth of pathogenic microorganisms.

The dermis or corium is located directly beneath the epidermis and is separated from and attached to it by the basement membrane. The dermis is a thick layer that comprises collagen fibers, blood vessels, nerves, lymphatics, and other structures such as hair follicles, sebaceous glands, and sweat glands. Sebaceous glands are found throughout haired skin, and their ducts empty into hair shafts. One type of sweat gland (eccrine) is found only in footpads and may play a role in body temperature regulation. The dermis gives stability and flexibility to the skin and acts to maintain and repair the skin.

The hypodermis is the deepest layer of the skin. It is made up of fat and connective tissue. Its functions are to provide padding and insulation and to serve as an energy store.

The skin produces hair and other keratinized structures like nail, horn, nasal pads, and footpads. Hair grows from follicles found in the dermis. In contrast to humans, who have one hair per follicle, dogs and cats have multiple hairs per follicle. Individual hair follicles have associated glandular structures (see earlier) and arrector pili muscles that are responsible for piloerection (hair standing on end). The hair follicle is frequently involved in bacterial, fungal, and demodectic infections. If a hair follicle loses the hair and becomes plugged with sebaceous secretions and keratin, a comedo (blackhead) results. There are three stages or phases of hair growth called *anagen* (growth), *telogen* (rest), and *catagen* (intermediate). Hair grows until it reaches a predetermined length, enters a resting phase, and then is shed. The hair cycle is controlled by day–night length (photoperiod), environmental temperature, hormones, and nutritional status. General illness, skin disorders, poor nutrition, overbathing, and stress are conditions that may result in excessive shedding.

WOUND HEALING

A wound is a type of injury to living tissue: lacerations, burns, punctures, abrasions, and incisions (surgical procedures).

> **TECHNICIAN NOTES**
>
> Normal wound healing can be divided into four stages: inflammation, débridement, repair, and maturation.

Wound healing is divided into four stages. The inflammatory phase usually begins with hemorrhage and is limited by vessel contraction and constriction. Serum leakage into the wound deposits fibrinogen and other clotting elements and blood vessels constrict to limit the blood loss. Later, this serum provides enzymes, proteins, antibodies, and complement. The débridement phase begins about

6 hours after injury and is facilitated by the appearance of neutrophils and monocytes that migrate to the wound. Neutrophils phagocytize bacteria and then die. Monocytes become macrophages and phagocytize necrotic debris. The repair phase is marked by the formation of a blood clot and is usually active by 3 to 5 days post injury. During the repair phase, fibroblasts produce collagen and other connective tissue proteins and begin to fill in the wound in order to bind the tissues. Capillaries infiltrate the wound to provide blood supply and oxygen. This process forms granulation tissue. Epithelial cells proliferate beneath the scab, and the wound begins to contract so that new skin can form and cover it. The maturation phase is the end of wound healing and is a period of remodeling which can take several months to years to heal. During this time, the wound consolidates and strengthens. Many important factors contribute to proper wound healing. These include patient factors (e.g., the age of the patient, nutritional status, rest, environment, and general health); wound factors, including wound characteristics (i.e., contaminated wounds versus noncontaminated wounds); external factors (e.g., temperature regulation [i.e., bandage]); whether lavage is performed; and how the wound is closed (e.g., primary or secondary closure). Primary intention healing occurs when there is no area for the body to fill in with granulation tissue. Healing of a clean, uninfected, surgical incision that is approximated by sutures is an example. Secondary intention healing occurs when there is a larger wound that cannot be opposed by sutures, therefore granulation tissue must form to fill in the opening. Once granulation tissue forms, contraction and epithelization occur to achieve structural integrity. A veterinarian must consider all these factors when determining how to treat a wound and when anticipating how well it will heal.

℞ Topical Antipruritics and Antiinflammatories

Noncorticosteroids

Aluminum Acetate Solution. This is also known as Burow's solution.

Clinical Uses. This is an astringent solution and an antipruritic agent that is useful for the treatment of superficial skin problems. It can be used to help with acute moist dermatitis, fold dermatitis, and contact dermatitis. Some doctors may use it to treat otitis externa. The exact manner in which this agent works is not fully known at this time.

Dosage Forms
- **Cort/Astrin Solution**
- **Corti-Derm Solution**

- Buro-O-Cort 2:1
- Hydro-B 1020

Adverse Side Effects. Do not use anything that prevents the evaporation of this solution from the skin. Avoid contact with the eyes. Gloves should be worn when applying the solution.

Colloidal Oatmeal

Clinical Uses. Colloidal oatmeal has unique properties in that it can be used topically as both an antiinflammatory and antipruritic agent. At this time, however, scientists are concerned about its mechanism of action. It is thought that perhaps it inhibits prostaglandin production.

Dosage Forms
- **DermAllay Oatmeal Spray, Shampoo, Conditioner**
- **Epi-Soothe Cream Rinse**
- **ResiSoothe Leave-On Lotion**
- **Aloe & Oatmeal Shampoo**
- **Aloe & Oatmeal Skin & Coat Conditioner**
- **Epi-Soothe Shampoo**
- **Cortisoothe Shampoo**

Adverse Side Effects. Colloidal oatmeal is very safe.

Topical Essential Fatty Acids

Clinical Uses. These products are commonly used for their antipruritic and antiinflammatory properties. They tend to help skin problems such as atopic dermatitis, sebaceous adenitis, and seborrhea. Some of these products have natural oils in them, which also may help skin problems. Essential fatty acids affect arachidonic acid levels and also affect the production of prostaglandins in the body, which can reduce inflammation and pruritus. Essential oils also help to create healthy skin.

Dosage Forms
- **Dermoscent ATOP 7**
- **Dermoscent Essential 6 Spot-On**
- **HyLyt EFA Shampoo, Cream Rinse**
- **Dermoscent EFA Treatment Shampoo**
- **DermaLyte Shampoo**
- **Allermyl Shampoo**
- **Allerderm Spot-On**
- Various others

Adverse Side Effects. These are uncommon.

Topical Diphenhydramine Hydrogen Chloride

Clinical Uses. Diphenhydramine is a first-generation antihistamine that has some local anesthetic properties. This drug can be absorbed transdermally but not enough to cause systemic effects.

Dosage Forms
- ResiHist Leave-On Lotion
- **Benadryl (human label)**
- **Benasoothe**
- **AtopiCream**

Adverse Side Effects. Avoid contact with eyes or mucous membranes. Diphenhydramine should not be applied to skin that is oozing. Gloves should be worn when applying these products.

 TECHNICIAN NOTES

Topical diphenhydramine should not be used 2 weeks before allergy testing.

Topical Lidocaine and Lidocaine/Prilocaine

Clinical Uses. This product can be applied topically as a skin anesthetic and also helps with pruritus. It may be used to treat acute moist dermatitis, pruritic lesions, or painful skin conditions.

Dosage Forms
- **Allercaine**
- **Allerspray**
- **DermaCool with Lidocaine Spray**
- **Hexa-Caine**
- **Biocaine**
- **EMLA Cream**

TECHNICIAN NOTES

EMLA cream may be used before intravenous catheter placement to ease the minor discomfort of the procedure.

Adverse Side Effects. Avoid contact with the eyes and do not use in ears. Gloves should be worn when applying these products.

Phytosphingosine

Clinical Uses. Phytosphingosine is useful in treating localized inflammatory and pruritic cases such as atopic dermatitis. It can also be sprayed on sutures postoperatively to aid in the wound healing process.

Dosage Forms
- **Douxo Calm Gel**
- **Douxo Calm Micro-emulsion Spray**
- **Douxo Calm Shampoo**
- **Douxo Seborrhea Shampoo**
- **Douxo Chlorhexidine PS**

- Douxo Seborrhea Micro-emulsion Spray
- Douxo Seborrhea Spot-on
  Adverse Side Effects. This product may cause skin redness or irritation.

Pramoxine Hydrogen Chloride

Clinical Uses. This agent has the ability to cause surface and local anesthetic characteristics, which can affect the peripheral nerves. It may be combined with other products to reduce pain or itching. At this time, scientists are unclear of this drug's mechanism of action.

Dosage Forms. The following are all veterinary-label products.
- Micro Pearls Advantage Dermal-Soothe Antiitch Spray
- Relief Shampoo, Relief Spray
- Pramosoothe HCl Spray
- Resiprox Leave-On Lotion
- Micro Pearls Advantage Dermal-Soothe Antiitch Shampoo, Cream Rinse
- Pramoxine Antiitch Shampoo, Cream Rinse, Spray
  Adverse Side Effects. Avoid contact with the eyes. This agent is not for ophthalmic use. Gloves should be worn when applying these products.

Phenol/Menthol/Camphor

Clinical Uses. These agents are used in equines for overexertion, soreness, or stiffness.

Dosage Forms
- White Liniment
- Choate's Liniment
- Cool Gel
- Ice-O-Gel
- Shin-O-Gel
- Scarlet Oil Pump Spray
  Adverse Side Effects. These products may cause local irritation. Do not use near the eyes. Do not use these products on cats.

Topical Neutralized Zinc Gluconate

Clinical Uses. This product can be used for mild itching, mild bacterial infections, and dry skin. It works well for relief from insect bites, acute moist dermatitis, acral lick dermatitis, fold dermatitis, feline acne, and postsurgical wounds. The exact mechanism of action is unclear at this time. Zinc has **antiseptic** and astringent ability.

Dosage Form
- Maxi/Guard Zn7 Derm Solution, Spray

Topical Corticosteroids

Clinical Uses. Topical corticosteroids are used in conjunction with other treatments for localized itching or inflammatory conditions. Products containing betamethasone should be used after other products have been tried because the risks associated with betamethasone use are greater than the risks involved with hydrocortisone use (Plumb, 2015).

Dosage Forms
- Gentocin Topical Spray
- GentaSpray
- Betagen Topical Spray
- Gentamicin Topical Spray
- GentaVed Topical Spray
- Otomax Ointment
- Vetromax Ointment
- MalOtic Ointment
- Icaderm Gel
- Betamethasone Dipropionate Ointment, Cream, Lotion
- Clotrimazole and Betamethasone Dipropionate
- Lotrisone
  Adverse Side Effects. Do not use in pregnant animals. Avoid contact with the eyes. The animal should not be allowed to lick or chew at the affected sites for at least 20 to 30 minutes after application (Plumb, 2015).

Topical Hydrocortisone

Clinical Uses. Topical hydrocortisone is useful in the treatment of localized pruritus and/or inflammatory conditions. Because topically applied corticosteroids reduce the ability of leukocytes and macrophages to attack infected skin, the area to which such agents are applied will have less redness, itching, and swelling.

Dosage Forms
- CortiCalm Lotion
- Sulfodene HC Antiitch Lotion
- Zymox Topical Cream, Spray, Wipes
- Relief HC Spray
- Pramosoothe HC Spray
- Cortispray
- DermaCool HC Spray
- Malacetic Ultra Shampoo, Spray
- Malacetic HC Wipes
- Cort/Astrin Solution
- Corti-Derm Solution
- Hydro-Plus
- Buro-O-Cort 2:1
- Hydro-B 1020
- Cortisoothe Shampoo

- **Chlorhexidine 4% HC Shampoo**
- **ResiCORT Leave-on Lotion**

Adverse Side Effects. These products may cause tuberculosis of the skin. Do not use in pregnant animals. Gloves should be worn when applying these products. Keep out of the eyes. Do not allow the animal to lick or chew the application site for at least 30 minutes. Stop using 2 weeks before allergy testing.

Topical Isoflupredone Acetate

Clinical Uses. This is a high-potency topical corticosteroid. It is used in the treatment of otic or skin itching or inflammation that may be associated with bacterial infections. These products should be used as a last resort because the risks associated with them are greater than those with hydrocortisone.

Dosage Forms
- **Tritop**
- **Neo-Predef with Tetracaine Powder**

Adverse Side Effects. These products may cause tuberculosis of the skin. Do not use in pregnant animals. Gloves should be worn when applying these agents. Do not allow the animal to lick or chew the affected site for 30 minutes after application. Allergic reaction to neomycin and/or tetracaine may happen.

Mometasone Furoate

Clinical Uses. Mometasone furoate is useful in the treatment of itching and inflamed skin that may be associated with bacterial or yeast infections. When hydrocortisone products do not produce desirable results, this may be used.

Dosage Forms
- **Mometamax** Otic Suspension

Adverse Side Effects. These products may cause tuberculosis of the skin. Do not use these products in pregnant animals. Use caution when treating a large area of skin or when the drug is used on small patients. Mometasone may delay wound healing when used for more than 7 days (Plumb, 2015).

Topical Triamcinolone Acetonide

Clinical Uses. This agent is useful as an adjunct in the treatment of pruritus. It is best suited for small lesions that only need to be treated for a short duration.

Dosage Forms. The following are all veterinary-label products.

- **Medalone Cream**
- **Cortalone Cream**
- **Genesis Spray**
- **Derma-Vet Cream, Ointment**
- **Panalog Ointment**
- **Animax Ointment**
- **Quadritop Ointment**
- **Dermalog Ointment**
- **Dermalone Ointment**
- **Resortin Ointment**

Adverse Side Effects. Do not use on pregnant animals. Keep out of the eyes. Do not allow the animal to lick or chew for 30 minutes after application. Stop using 2 weeks before allergy testing is to be done.

℞ Topical Antimicrobials
Benzoyl Peroxide

Clinical Uses. Benzoyl peroxide products are used topically as gels or shampoos. The shampoo products are usually used in cases involving oily skin, pyodermas, furunculosis, generalized demodicosis, and Schnauzer comedo syndrome (Plumb, 2015). Gels are used for treating pyodermas, chin acne, and localized demodex lesions. Benzoyl peroxide has antimicrobial actions. Gels can be used up to twice daily, but shampoos should only be used once a day.

Dosage Forms. The following are all veterinary-label products.
- **Pyoben Gel**
- **OxyDex Shampoo, Gel**
- **Micro Pearls Advantage Benzoyl Plus**
- **Benzoyl Peroxide Shampoo**
- **BPO-3 Shampoo**
- **SulfOxyDex Shampoo**
- **Oxiderm Shampoo**
- **OxyDex Shampoo**
- **DermaBenSs Shampoo**
- **PhytoVet PSS Shampoo**

> 📋 **TECHNICIAN NOTES**
>
> All shampoos should remain lathered on the skin for a minimum of 10 minutes before rinsing.

Adverse Side Effects. Do not use around eyes or mucous membranes. Gloves should be worn when applying these products. Benzoyl peroxide will bleach fabrics, jewelry, carpet, and the pet's fur.

Topical Clindamycin

Clinical Uses. This is used in the treatment of feline acne. ClinzGard may be used in the treatment of anal sac abscesses, other abscesses, and puncture wounds.

Dosage Forms. Most products are human label unless otherwise specified.
- **ClinzGard—veterinary label**
- **Clindamycin Phosphate**
- **Cleocin T**
- **Clindamax**
- **Clindagel**
- **Clindets**
- **Evoclin**

Adverse Side Effects. Avoid use in individuals allergic to clindamycin. Gloves should be worn when applying this product. Rarely, pseudomembranous colitis (caused by *Clostridium difficile*) may occur in some patients.

Topical Gentamicin Sulfate

Clinical Uses. This is used to treat primary and secondary bacterial infections. Topical gentamicin can be used to treat "hot spots." Products that contain betamethasone, mometasone, or clotrimazole can be used as otic treatments.

Dosage Forms
- **Gentocin Topical Spray**
- **GentaSpray**
- **Betagen Topical Spray**
- **Gentamicin Topical Spray**
- **GentaVed Topical Spray**
- **GenOne Spray**
- **Otomax Ointment**
- **DVMax Ointment**
- **Vetromax Ointment**
- **Mometamax Otic Suspension**

Adverse Side Effects. This agent may be absorbed systemically if used on ulcers or burned or denuded skin.

Mupirocin (Pseudomonic Acid A)

Clinical Uses. This agent is Food and Drug Administration (FDA)-approved for treating pyoderma, interdigital cysts and draining tracts, acne, and pressure point pyodermas (Plumb, 2015).

Dosage Forms. The following are human-label products unless otherwise specified.
- **Muricin—veterinary label**
- **Mupirocin**
- **Bactroban Cream, Ointment**
- **Centany**

Adverse Side Effects. Do not use in patients who are allergic to mupirocin or products containing polyethylene glycol.

Salicylic Acid

Clinical Uses. Salicylic acid is used to treat seborrheic disorders. It has some antipruritic activity, as well as antibacterial, keratoplastic, and keratolytic actions.

Dosage Forms. The following are all veterinary-label products.
- **KeraSolv Gel**
- **Derma-Clens cream**
- **Dermazole Shampoo**
- **SebaLyt Shampoo**
- **Nova Pearls Medicated Dandruff Shampoo**
- **Keratolux Shampoo**
- **Sebolux Shampoo**
- **Oxiderm Shampoo**
- **Oxiderm Shampoo + PS**
- **Micro Pearls Advantage Seba-Hex Shampoo**
- **NuSal-T**
- **Solva-Ker Gel**

Adverse Side Effects. Skin irritation is possible.

Topical Nitrofurazone

Clinical Uses. This can be used to treat or prevent superficial infections.

Dosage Form
- **Nitrofurazone Soluble Dressing**

 TECHNICIAN NOTES

United States federal law prohibits the use of nitrofurazone products in (or on) food animals, including horses to be used for food.

Silver Sulfadiazine (SSD)

Clinical Uses. This is used for second- and third-degree burns. It can also be used to treat skin infections caused by *Pseudomonas* spp. (Plumb, 2015).

Dosage Forms. No veterinary-labeled products are available for use.
- **Silvadene cream**
- **Thermazene**
- **SSD cream**

Adverse Side Effects. Patients that are hypersensitive to sulfonamides may react to SSD. Silver sulfadiazine may reduce granulation, so it should not be used in non-granulated wounds.

Ⓡ Antiseptics
Acetic Acid/Boric Acid

Clinical Uses. These products are used to treat skin infections caused by *Staphylococcus* spp., *Pseudomonas* spp., and *Malassezia* spp.

Dosage Forms. All of the following are veterinary-label products.
- **MalAcetic Ultra Spray**
- **Mal-A-Ket Shampoo, Wipes**
- **MalAcetic HC Wipes**
- **MalAcetic Shampoo, Spray Conditioner, Wet Wipes**

Adverse Side Effects. These include skin redness and irritation.

Chlorhexidine

Chlorhexidine may be easier on patients who are unable to tolerate benzoyl peroxide. It may have residual effects and can remain active on the skin after rinsing.

Clinical Uses. Chlorhexidine is used as a topical antiseptic for disinfection of wounds, to manage skin infections and used as a surgical scrub. It does not seem to have much efficacy against *Pseudomonas* or *Serratia* spp. (Plumb, 2015).

Dosage Forms. Chlorhexidine is available as a solution, scrub, shampoo, ointment, and spray. All of the following are veterinary-label products.
- **Chlorhexidine Spray, Flush (0.2%), Ointment**
- **Chlorhexidine Solution, Concentrate, Scrub**
- **Chlorhexidine Shampoo 2%, 4%**
- **Malaseb Shampoo, Concentrate rinse, Spray, Flush**
- **Douxo Chlorhexidine PS Micro-emulsion Spray**
- **Chlorhex 2X 4% Spray**
- **ChlorhexiDerm Spray, Flush**
- **ChlorhexiDerm Plus Scrub**
- **Ketoseb-D Spray, Flush, Wipes**
- **Mal-A-Ket Plus TrizEDTA Spray, Flush, Wipes**
- **TrizChlor 4 Shampoo, Spray, Flush, Wipes**
- **Douxo Chlorhexidine 3% PS Pads**
- **Dermachlor Flush Plus**
- **Hexadene Flush**
- **Nolvasan Shampoo**
- **KetoChlor Shampoo**
- **ResiKetoChlor Leave-On Conditioner**

Adverse Side Effects. This agent may damage the eyes. Chlorhexidine is safe to use on cats, although irritation and corneal ulcer have been reported (Plumb, 2015).

Chloroxylenol (PCMX)

Clinical Uses. Chloroxylenol is also known as *p*-chloro-*m*-xylenol (PCMX). It is an antimicrobial disinfectant that is effective against gram-negative and gram-positive bacteria. It is also effective against RNA and DNA viruses (Plumb, 2015). It may be used as a preoperative scrub of the skin, for cleaning wounds, for the treatment of bacteria and fungi, and for the treatment of yeast infections.

Dosage Forms. All of the following are veterinary-label products.
- **Medicated Shampoo**
- **Vet Solutions Sebozole Shampoo**
- **Vet Solutions Universal Medicated Shampoo**

Adverse Side Effects. Chloroxylenol may cause skin irritation.

Topical Enzymes

These include lactoperoxidase, lysozyme, and lactoferrin.

Clinical Uses. These are effective against *Staphylococcus* spp., *Pseudomonas* spp., *Malassezia* spp., *Candida albicans,* and *Microsporum* spp. and can be used on the skin (Plumb, 2015).

Dosage Forms. All of the following are veterinary-label products.
- **Zymox Topical Spray**
- **Zymox Topical Cream**
- **Zymox Enzymatic Shampoo**
- **Zymox Rinse**

Adverse Side Effects. These are uncommon.

Ethyl Lactate

Clinical Uses. This is useful in treating bacterial skin infections and superficial pyodermas.

Dosage Form
- **Etiderm Shampoo**

Adverse Side Effects. Erythema, pain, and itching are possible. Avoid contact in eyes. Gloves should be worn when using this product.

Ⓡ Antifungals
Enilconazole

Clinical Uses. No dosage forms are available for topical use in the United States. This drug has been used in the treatment of dermatophytosis in small animals and in horses. Not commercially available but can be prepared through a compounding pharmacy.

Adverse Effects. When used topically in felines, hypersalivation, vomiting, anorexia, weight loss, muscle weakness, and increased alanine aminotransferase (ALT) levels have been reported (Plumb, 2015).

> **TECHNICIAN NOTES**
>
> When using antifungals, gloves should be worn to protect the skin. Avoid contact with eyes.

Topical Ketoconazole

Clinical Uses. Ketoconazole is used against dermatophytes and yeasts. Patients with severe infections may need systemic therapy.

Dosage Forms. The following are all veterinary-label products.

- **Ketoseb-D Spray, Flush, Wipes**
- **Dermachlor Flush**
- **Mal-A-Ket Plus TrizEDTA Spray, Flush**
- **MalAcetic Ultra Spray**
- **Mal-A-Ket Shampoo, Wipes**
- **Ketochlor Shampoo**
- **ResiKetoChlor Leave-On Conditioner**

Adverse Side Effects. Skin irritation is possible.

Lime Sulfur

This is also known as sulfurated lime solution.

Clinical Uses. Lime sulfur is used in the treatment of dermatophytosis and for the treatment of *Malassezia*, *Cheyletiellosis*, chiggers, and mange. It is also used in the treatment of demodex in cats (Plumb, 2015).

Dosage Forms. The following are all veterinary-label products.

- **LimePlus Dip**
- **Vet Solutions Lime Sulfur Dip**
- **Vet Basics Lime Sulfur Dip**
- **Various others**

Adverse Side Effects. Lime sulfur may stain porous surfaces and discolor jewelry, and it may stain light-colored fur. Lime sulfur may cause skin irritation. Oral ingestion may cause nausea and oral ulcers, especially in cats; so, it is best to use an Elizabethan collar (i.e., E-collar) to prevent this.

Topical Miconazole

Clinical Uses. It is used in the treatment of dermatophytes and yeast.

Dosage Forms. The following are all veterinary-label products.

- **Micro Pearls Advantage Miconazole 1% Spray**
- **Conofite Spray 1%, Conofite Cream 2%**
- **MicaVed Spray 1%**

- **Malaseb Shampoo, Concentrated Rinse, Spray, Flush**
- **Micazole Spray, Lotion 1%**
- **MicaVed Lotion 1%**
- **Sebazole Shampoo**

Adverse Side Effects. Avoid contact with the eyes. Skin irritation may occur. Do not apply to eroded or ulcerated skin.

Nystatin

Clinical Uses. Nystatin is useful for treating topical lesions caused by yeast or yeast-like organisms.

Dosage Forms. The following are all veterinary-label products.

- **Derma-Vet Cream, Ointment**
- **Panalog Ointment**
- **Animax Ointment**
- **Quadritop Ointment**
- **Dermalog Ointment**
- **Resortin Ointment**

Adverse Side Effects. Avoid contact with eyes. Allergic reactions may occur.

Selenium Sulfide

Clinical Uses. Selenium sulfide is used for treating seborrheic disorders and *Malassezia*.

Dosage Forms. The following are all human-label topical products.

- **Selenium Sulfide**
- **Selsun Blue Medicated Treatment**
- **Head & Shoulders Intensive Treatment**
- **Selsun**

Adverse Side Effects. Do not use on cats. This agent may discolor jewelry and may stain hair coats. Mucous membranes and scrotal areas may become irritated.

Topical Terbinafine Hydrogen Chloride

Clinical Uses. Terbinafine is useful for treating local lesions caused by *Malassezia*.

Dosage Forms. No veterinary products are available. The following are all human-label products.

- **Lamisil AT**
- **Lamisil**
- **Lamisil Advanced**

Adverse Side Effects. Skin irritation is possible but usually is rare.

Precipitated Sulfur

Clinical Uses. Precipitated sulfur is used to treat seborrhea.

Dosage Forms. The following are all veterinary-label products.

- SebaLyt Shampoo
- **Micro Pearls Advantage Seba-Hex Shampoo**
- **Sebolux Shampoo**
- **Oxiderm Shampoo + PS**
- **Keratolux Shampoo**
- **DermaPet DermaSebS Shampoo**
- **Paraguard Shampoo**
- **SulfOxyDex Shampoo**

Adverse Side Effects. Skin irritation is possible. Sulfur may cause drying, itching, and irritation. The residual odor of this product may be offensive to clients.

Coal Tar

Clinical Uses. The use of coal tar shampoos has been somewhat controversial in veterinary medicine (Plumb, 2015). Manufacturing of almost all veterinary-label products has been discontinued. Coal tar has been used in treating seborrhea oleosa (oily) for many years.

Dosage Form
- **NuSal T Shampoo**
- **Sulfodene Shampoo**
- **Sulfur and Tar Shampoo**

Adverse Side Effects. The FDA believes that coal tar products with concentrations of 5% or less are safe for human use (Plumb, 2015). Carcinogenic risks may be associated with these products.

® Topical Retinoids

Tretinoin

Types of tretinoin include transretinoic acid and vitamin A acid. Tretinoin stimulates cellular division and increases cell turnover.

Clinical Uses. These products are useful in treating acanthosis nigricans, idiopathic nasal and footpad hyperkeratosis, callous pyodermas, and chin acne (Plumb, 2015).

Dosage Forms. No veterinary products are available. All of the following are human-label products.
- **Renova**
- **Retin-A Cream, Gel**
- **Avita Cream, Gel**
- **Altinac**

Adverse Side Effects. Avoid sun exposure. Avoid contact with eyes and mouth. Products may cause allergic reactions or local irritation.

® Topical and Oral Antiparasitic Agents

Amitraz

Clinical Uses. Amitraz is used in the treatment of generalized demodicosis. It is also used for flea and tick infestation prevention as a collar (Preventic).

Dosage Forms
- **Mitaban; no longer available**
- **Preventic collar**

Adverse Side Effects. These products are not for use in dogs younger than 4 months. If the skin around the eyes needs to be treated, use a petrolatum-based ophthalmic ointment. Amitraz may be toxic to rabbits and cats. Yohimbine may be used if an overdose occurs. Amitraz is contraindicated if an animal is taking monoamine oxidase inhibitors.

Crotamiton

Clinical Uses. This is a topical miticide and scabicide. It is used mainly for treating scaly leg mites in birds (*Knemidokoptes*) (Plumb, 2015).

Dosage Form
- **Eurax**—human label

Adverse Side Effects. Little is known about this product's safety. Irritation and allergic reactions are possible.

Deltamethrin

Clinical Uses. In the United States, deltamethrin-impregnated collars are labeled for killing fleas and ticks on dogs for up to 6 months. In countries in which leishmaniasis is a problem, deltamethrin-impregnated collars may be used for repelling and killing sand fly vectors (Plumb, 2015).

Dosage Form
- **Scalibor Protector Band for Dogs**

Adverse Side Effects. Do not use on dogs younger than 12 weeks. This product should be used very carefully around water because it is toxic to fish.

Dinotefuran Plus Pyriproxyfen (Plus Permethrin)

Clinical Uses. This is used for the control of adult and all immature flea stages. Vectra 3D also contains permethrin to help kill and repel adult and immature fleas, ticks, mosquitoes, biting and sand flies, lice, and mites (excluding mange mites). Vectra does not contain permethrin and is used to kill fleas only.

Dosage Forms
- **Vectra for Cats and Kittens**
- **Vectra for Cats**
- **Vectra for Dogs and Puppies**
- **Vectra 3D**

TECHNICIAN NOTES

- Do not use the dog product, which contains permethrin (i.e., Vectra 3D) on cats. Do not use this product on dogs that live in the same household as a cat.
- This product should not be used on geriatric animals, animals that are debilitated, or nursing animals.

Fipronil or Fipronil/(S)-Methoprene

Clinical Uses. Fipronil is approved for the treatment of fleas, ticks, and chewing lice, which infest dogs and cats. It has also been used to treat chigger infestation and aids in the control of sarcoptic mange. Frontline Plus also has an insect growth regulator (IGR) that kills flea eggs and flea larvae. Frontline Gold contains fipronil to kill adult fleas and ticks and (S)-methoprene and pyriproxyfen to kill flea eggs and larvae before they can develop into adult fleas. The only difference between the two products is that Frontline Gold kills fleas faster than Frontline Plus.

Dosage Forms
- **Frontline Spray Treatment**
- **Frontline Plus for Cats and Kittens**
- **Frontline Gold for Cats and Kittens**
- **Frontline Plus for Dogs and Puppies**
- **Frontline Gold for Dogs and Puppies**
- **Effipro Plus for Dogs contains fipronil and pyriproxyfen**
- **Effitix Plus for Dogs contains fipronil, permethrin, and pyriproxyfen**

Adverse Side Effects. These products are not to be used on puppies younger than 8 weeks. Do not use in rabbits. The product label states that the product is effective after bathing, but animals should not be bathed within 48 hours of application for best results. The product label also states that the product is effective after water immersion and exposure to sunlight. Areas of the skin to which the product has been applied may remain oily for up to 24 hours after application.

Imidacloprid, Imidacloprid With Permethrin, and Imidacloprid With Moxidectin

Clinical Uses. Imidacloprid topical solution is used for the treatment of adult and larval flea stages in dogs and cats. The combination product with permethrin (K9 Advantix II) kills adult and larval forms of fleas, repels and kills ticks, and repels mosquitoes in dogs only. Advantage II for dogs and cats kill adult fleas, larvae, and eggs. It also controls lice

on dogs. The canine combination product with moxidectin (Advantage Multi for Dogs in the United States and Advocate in Europe) is used for the prevention of heartworm disease, adult fleas, adult and immature hookworms, adult roundworms, and adult whipworms. It has also been successfully used in the treatment of sarcoptic mange, cheyletiellosis, and mild cases of demodicosis (Plumb, 2015). Advantus flavored soft chews kill adult fleas within one hour. The feline combination product (Advantage Multi for Cats) is indicated for the prevention of heartworm disease, adult fleas, ear mites, adult and immature hookworms, and adult roundworms (Plumb, 2015).

Dosage Forms
- **Advantage II for Dogs**
- **Advantage II for Cats**
- **K9 Advantix II**
- **Advantage Multi for Dogs**
- **Advantage Multi for Cats**
- **Advantus soft chews for Dogs**
- **Seresto Collar for Dogs and Cats**

Adverse Side Effects. For imidacloprid alone, do not use in puppies younger than 7 weeks or in kittens younger than 8 weeks. Do not use the combination product (K9 Advantix) on cats. Caution should be used in households with both dogs and cats, especially when cats are in close contact with or will groom dogs in the household.

When used as directed, adverse effects are unlikely. Most problems are seen after oral dosing of topical products (Plumb, 2015).

(S)-Methoprene Combinations

Clinical Uses. Methoprene is added to premise sprays and topical products to eliminate insects (usually fleas) because it prevents the maturation of eggs and larvae.

Dosage Forms
- **Adams Flea and Tick Spot On for Dogs and Cats**
- **Adams Plus Flea and Tick Spot On for Dogs**
- **Adams Plus Flea and Tick Spray for Dogs and Cats**
- **Adams Flea and Tick Spray for Dogs and Cats**
- **Frontline Plus for Cats and Kittens**
- **Frontline Gold for Cats and Kittens**
- **Frontline Plus for Dogs and Puppies**
- **Frontline Gold for Dogs and Puppies**
- **Vet-Kem Ovitrol-Xtend Spot On for Cats**
- **Vet-Kem Ovitrol-Xtend Spot On for Dogs**

Adverse Side Effects. Methoprene can also be found in products that contain permethrin or phenothrin, which can be toxic to kittens.

Permethrin

Clinical Uses. This product acts as an adult insecticide and miticide. Permethrins have action against fleas, lice, ticks, *Cheyletiella*, *Sarcoptes scabiei* (Plumb, 2015).

Dosage Forms
- **Adams Flea and Tick Spot On**
- **K9 Advantix II**
- **Effitix Plus for Dogs**
- **Vectra 3D**

Adverse Side Effects. This agent can be toxic to cats. Only use those products indicated for use in cats.

Selamectin

Clinical Uses. Selamectin is used on dogs 6 weeks of age or older and provides protection against fleas and heartworms, and treats and controls ear mites. Additionally, in dogs, it is indicated for sarcoptic mange, and controls tick infestations due to American dog ticks (Plumb, 2015). Revolution Plus for cats is used on cats 8 weeks of age or older and weighing greater than 2.8 lb.

Dosage Forms
- **Revolution for Dogs and Cats**
- **Revolution Plus for Cats**

Adverse Side Effects. Do not use Revolution on sick, weak, or underweight dogs and cats. Use with caution in cats with a history of neurologic abnormalities.

Topical Pyrethrins and Pyrethrin Combinations

Clinical Uses. These acts as adult insecticides and miticides. They have action against fleas, lice, ticks, and *Cheyletiella* (Plumb, 2015).

Dosage Forms
- **Adams Plus Flea and Tick Shampoo With IGR**
- **Adams Plus Pyrethrin Dip**
- **Ecto-Soothe 3X Shampoo**
- **Pyrethrins Dip and Spray**
- **Vet-Kem Flea and Tick Shampoo**

Adverse Side Effects. Do not allow cats to groom themselves after products such as dips or sprays have been applied.

Topical Pyriproxyfen and Pyriproxyfen Combinations

Clinical Uses. This is a second-generation IGR that is added to premise sprays and topical products to act against fleas.

Dosage Forms
- **Advantage II for Dogs**
- **Advantage II for Cats**
- **K9 Advantix II**
- **Effipro Plus Topical Solution for Cats**
- **Effitix Plus Topical Solution for Dogs**
- **Frontline Gold for Cats and Kittens**
- **Frontline Gold for Dogs and Puppies**

Adverse Side Effects. When used alone, pyriproxyfen has low toxicity in mammals. Skin irritation or allergic reactions could occur.

Spinetoram

Clinical Uses. This is labeled for the prevention and treatment of flea infestations in cats and kittens 8 weeks of age or older.

Dosage Form
- **Cheristin**

Adverse Side Effects. None are reported by the manufacturer.

Fluralaner

Clinical Uses. Fluralaner kills adult fleas in dogs and cats. In dogs and puppies (6 months of age and older, weighing 4.4 lb or more) it is indicated for the treatment and prevention of flea (*Ctenocephalides felis*) and tick (*Ixodes scapularis* [black-legged tick], *Dermacentor variabilis* [American dog tick], and *Rhipicephalus sanguineus* [brown dog tick]) for 12 weeks. It is also indicated for the treatment and control of *Amblyomma americanum* (lone star tick) infestations for 8 weeks (Merck, 2016).

In cats and kittens (6 months of age and older, weighing 2.6 lb or more) it is indicated for the treatment and prevention of flea (*C. felis*) and tick (*I. scapularis* [black-legged tick]) infestations for up to 12 weeks. It is also indicated for the treatment and control of *D. variabilis* (American dog tick) infestations for 8 weeks (Merck, 2016). Bravecto Plus topical solution for cats contains fluralaner and moxidectin as the active ingredients. It provides 2-month protection against fleas (kills adult fleas, prevents and treats flea infestation) and ticks (kills Ixodes scapularis and Dermacentor variabilis), prevention of heartworm disease, and treatment of roundworms (Toxocara cati) and hookworms (Ancylostoma tubaeforme) (Merck, 2019).

Dosage Forms
- **Bravecto Chews for Dogs**
- **Bravecto Topical Solution for Dogs and Cats**
- **Bravecto Plus topical solution for cats** (Fluralaner and moxidectin)

Adverse Side Effects. The most common side effect is vomiting.

BOX 11.1 Case Scenario

Heidi, a 1-year-old spayed female German Shorthair Pointer was presented for scratching and itching.

The owner explained that Heidi has been scratching and itching for the past 2 days.

Additional history: Up to date on vaccinations. No other pets at home. Currently on Heartgard.

Physical examination findings: Heidi was full of energy, wagging her tail, alert, and responsive. Temperature, pulse and respirations were normal. Mucous membranes were pink and moist, CRT (capillary refill time): <2 seconds. Heart and lung sounds: within normal limits.

A small area (size of a dime) of alopecia was observed at the base of the tail, otherwise she appeared to be in good health. Examination of the skin revealed live fleas (four found) and moderate amount of flea dirt, using a flea comb. A fecal sample was also obtained for analysis. Fecal sample: no internal parasites observed.

Diagnosis: Fleas

The veterinary technician discharged Heidi and went over the instructions with the owner. She gave the owner Adams d-Limonene Flea & Tick Pet Shampoo to bathe Heidi and Nexgard chewables as a once-a-month oral flea and tick preventative. She further explained that the goal of flea control is to eliminate the fleas on Heidi, eliminate the existing fleas in her home, and prevent further re-infestation. The owner asked when she can bathe her and give her the Nexgard? She replied that she should give Heidi a bath when she gets home to rid her of the fleas that are currently on her, she should then give her the Nexgard with or without food each month as a flea and tick preventative. The owner asked how long it would take to kill the fleas? She replied within 24 hours. The owner asked if she should treat the environment as well? She stated that Nexgard can control flea infestations as it will kill the existing adult flea infestation, but it may take 2–3 months due to the existing life stages of fleas in the environment. She further explained that treatment of the environment is essential in preventing infestation as fleas spend most of their life cycle off the host. Cleaning the environment by vacuuming and treating with sprays or foggers should be done routinely.

Veterinary technicians play an important role educating clients and must have a thorough understanding of the flea life-cycle, clinical signs associated with flea infestation, and the different flea control products available.

Afoxolaner

Clinical Uses. Afoxolaner is given orally to treat and control flea and tick infestations in dogs. It is used in puppies 8 weeks of age or older and weighing greater than 4 lb (Plumb, 2015). It should not be used in cats.

Dosage Forms
- **Nexgard chewables for Dogs**

Adverse Side Effects. Possible side effects include nausea, vomiting, diarrhea, and lethargy. It should be used with caution in dogs with known seizure disorders.

Lufenuron

Clinical Uses. Lufenuron prevents flea eggs from hatching. Sentinel Spectrum also contains other ingredients which protect against heartworms, while treating and controlling adult stages of tapeworms, hookworms, roundworms, and whipworms (Virbac, 2018).

Dosage Forms
- **Sentinel Flavor Tabs for Dogs**
- **Sentinel Spectrum Chews for Dogs**

Adverse Side Effects. Side effects include vomiting, lethargy, pruritus, urticaria, diarrhea, anorexia, ataxia, and convulsions.

Nitenpyram

Clinical Uses. It is a flea adulticide in dogs and cats over 4 weeks of age, and weighing more than 2 lb; it kills fleas within 30 minutes.

Dosage Forms
- **Capstar**

Adverse Side Effects. Side effects in dogs and cats include lethargy, vomiting, itching, decreased appetite, diarrhea, hyperactivity, incoordination, seizures, and other effects.

Spinosad

Clinical Uses. Spinosad is given once a month, orally, to kill fleas. It is used on dogs and cats 14 weeks of age or older (cats must weigh >4.1 lb) (Plumb, 2015). Trifexis contains other ingredients which protect against heartworm and the treatment of hookworms, roundworms, and whipworms.

Dosage Forms. All of the following are veterinary-label products.

- **Comfortis chewable tablets for dogs and cats** (kills fleas only)
- **Trifexis chewable for dogs**

Adverse Side Effects. Vomiting is the most common side effect. It should not be used on pregnant or nursing animals.

REVIEW QUESTIONS

1. The skin consists of _____ layers and is part of the _____ system.
2. _____ is essential for healthy skin.
3. Name seven functions of the skin.
4. Shampoos are more effective if left on the skin about _____ to _____ minutes before rinsing.
5. Keratolytics and keratoplastics are known as _____ agents.
6. Name the four stages of wound healing.
7. What does an astringent do to the skin?
8. Patients are commonly presented for skin problems when in reality they may have a _____ illness.
9. Why are behavioral-type drugs used in treating skin illness?
10. All patients presented for dermatologic problems have an underlying systemic illness.
    a. True
    b. False
11. Increased skin irritation may result in hyperpigmentation of the skin.
    a. True
    b. False
12. Humans have multiple hairs per follicle, but animals have one hair per follicle.
    a. True
    b. False
13. The maturation phase marks the beginning of wound healing.
    a. True
    b. False
14. What is produced by fibroblasts so that the wound can begin to bind tissues?
15. Define and give an example of primary intention healing.
16. Define and give an example of secondary intention healing.
17. Skin scrapings are commonly used to identify what type of mites?
18. What tests are utilized as diagnostic procedures for dermatophytes?
19. Which product is an antiseptic commonly used as a surgical scrub?
20. What products contain fipronil or fipronil/(S)-methoprene as an active ingredient?
21. What products can be used to treat seborrhea oleosa?
22. Federal law prohibits the use of _____ products in any food-producing animal.
23. Nitenpyram is the active ingredient found in which product?
    a. Bravecto Chews
    b. Capstar
    c. Comfortis
    d. Nexgard
24. Revolution contains the active ingredient selamectin which is used to treat what type of external and internal parasites?
25. Seresto collars are used to kill and repel fleas and ticks on dogs for how many months and explain water resistance of the collar.

REFERENCES

Merck Animal Health. (2016). *Package insert for Bravecto*. United States.
Merck Animal Health. (2019). *Package insert for Bravecto*. United States.
Plumb, D. C. (2015). *Veterinary drug handbook* (8th ed.). Ames, IA: Wiley.
Virbac. (2018). *Package insert for Sentinel*. United States.

12

Antiinfective Drugs

OBJECTIVES

After studying this chapter, you should be able to

1. Discuss the mechanisms of action of antiinfective drugs and understand the concept of antimicrobial resistance.
2. Describe the use of aminocyclitols/aminoglycosides.
3. Describe the use of carbapenems, cephalosporins, and macrolides.
4. Describe the use of penicillins, tetracyclines, and lincosamides.
5. Discuss quinolines/fluoroquinolones, sulfonamides, and antibacterials.
6. Explain the clinical uses of antifungal agents.
7. Discuss antiviral drugs.
8. Explain how disinfectants and antiseptics are used.

OUTLINE

KEY TERMS

Aerobes
Anaerobes
Antibacterial
Antibiotic
Antimicrobial drugs
Antimicrobial residues
Antimicrobial resistance
Antiseptics
Bacteria
Bactericidal
Bacteriostatic
Beta-lactamase
Detergent
Disinfect

Disinfectant
Efficacy
Fungicidal
Fungistatic
In vitro
In vivo
Iodophor
Microorganism
Nephrotoxic
Ototoxic
Sporicidal
Tachypnea
Teratogenic
Thrombophlebitis

INTRODUCTION

Microorganisms are ubiquitous in the environment. Some microorganisms have pathogenic potential, but others do not. Animals usually make initial contact with an infectious agent somewhere on the body's surface (e.g., mucous membranes, skin, respiratory tract, or digestive tract). In the fight against infection, several hundred antimicrobial drugs have been developed since the early 1900s. These drugs have been used to fight disease in both humans and animals. **Antimicrobial drugs** are natural or synthetic products that prevent growth or kill microorganisms without harming the animal.

Not all antimicrobials have the same degree of effectiveness against **microorganisms**. A determination can be made to distinguish different types of bacteria with the use of a Gram stain. The Gram stain is a laboratory procedure in which dyes are used to stain **bacteria** (Fig. 12.1). Gram-positive bacteria stain dark blue to purple. Gram-negative bacteria stain pink to red. However, some bacteria cannot be identified through the Gram-stain technique. For differentiating acid-fast bacilli, carbol fuchsin stain can be used and then decolorized with ethyl alcohol and hydrochloric acid. Other bacteria must be identified by special techniques such as dark-field examination or Gimenez stain. Giemsa and Wright stains may be used to identify parasites and intracellular microorganisms. Bacteria with similar staining properties tend to respond to the same antimicrobial therapy. So, narrow-spectrum antibiotics are effective against a specific group of bacteria; either gram-positive or gram-negative. Broad-spectrum antibiotics are effective against both gram-positive and gram-negative bacteria; they act against a wide range of bacteria. Still other bacteria are classified by their ability to survive with or without oxygen. **Aerobes** are bacteria that must have

oxygen to live and replicate. Other bacteria are able to live and multiply without oxygen; these are known as **anaerobes**. Anaerobes may be hardy and difficult to eradicate.

MECHANISM OF ACTION

Through analysis of the effects that a drug's action has on bacteria (i.e., spectrum of activity), antimicrobial drugs can be divided into two categories: **bactericidal** (kills microorganisms) and **bacteriostatic** (inhibits replication). However, some strains of mutant bacteria have greater resistance to some antimicrobials. Resistant strains of bacteria can make antimicrobial therapy difficult. **Antimicrobial resistance** develops when microorganisms, such as bacteria and fungi no longer respond to a drug that previously were effective. Therefore, some infections become harder to control if bacteria become resistant to the antibiotic. So, when a drug is given at the recommended dosing and does not reach a concentration at the infection site that can effectively stop the growth or kill the bacteria, antimicrobial resistance occurs. In order to prevent mutant strains from developing, antimicrobial drugs must not be used indiscriminately. Some important factors that increase antimicrobial resistance include overuse, inappropriate use (giving antibiotics before they are needed), subtherapeutic dosing, and not following the full course of treatment. Veterinary technicians play an important role, when speaking to clients, to help assure that the drugs dispensed are used appropriately and they follow the full course of treatment.

Once a sample is collected from the infection site, a culture and sensitivity test is performed. Several tests are available for testing the susceptibility of an organism to a specific antimicrobial drug. Most commonly, the disk susceptibility test (Kirby-Bauer) is used in small laboratories, as well as in veterinary hospitals (Fig. 12.2). With this test, an agar plate with a standard amount of cultured organism is used. Using a dispenser, paper disks impregnated with various antimicrobial drugs are placed within the agar plate. Incubation is carried out, along with measurement of the zones of inhibition. These zones show which antimicrobial agents are susceptible or resistant to each particular antimicrobial and how effectively they may perform **in vitro**. The broth dilution susceptibility test is also used in many laboratories (Fig. 12.3). An organism is inoculated into a series of tubes or wells in a microculture plate. These tubes or wells contain different concentrations of antimicrobials. The lowest concentration of an antimicrobial drug that inhibits the growth of an organism is the minimum inhibitory concentration

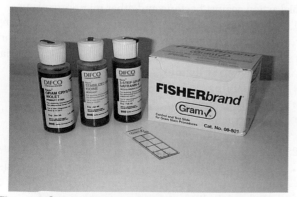

Fig. 12.1 Gram staining kit. (From Sirois, M. [2015]. *Laboratory procedures for veterinary technicians* [6th ed.]. Missouri: Elsevier.)

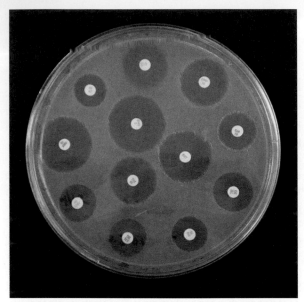

Fig. 12.2 Culture and sensitivity test plate showing the zone of inhibition. (From Bassert, J. M. [2018]. *Clinical textbook for veterinary technicians* [9th ed.]. St. Louis: Missouri.)

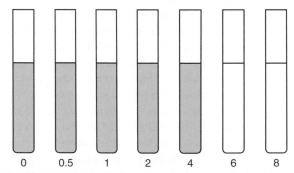

0	0.5	1	2	4	6	8

Fig. 12.3 The broth dilution susceptibility test. Note that the organism grew in broth containing 0, 0.5, 1, 2, and 4 mg/mL of antibiotic. The organism was inhibited in the tube that contained 6 mg/mL. The minimum inhibitory concentration is 6 mg/mL.

(MIC). The MIC represents the degree of susceptibility of an organism to a specific concentration of a particular antimicrobial drug. Levels below the MIC are ineffective, and levels above the therapeutic range are toxic. The antimicrobials that are effective in vitro may not always be the best choice for use **in vivo**. A clinician chooses which agent to use by considering the diagnosis and assessing each agent's pharmacodynamics and pharmacokinetics. This process allows a clinician to choose the most efficient and efficacious drug to treat a specific condition.

The use of veterinary drugs in food-producing animals has a potential to produce residues in milk, eggs, and meat and may become a health hazard to the consumer. Exposure to antimicrobials in food can potentially cause allergic reactions and antimicrobial resistance in humans. The reason for drug residues is failure to follow withdrawal times and improper usage. Animal drug withdrawal time is the amount of time required for the drug to be cleared from the animal's system before being slaughtered for human consumption or food products (milk and eggs) can be sold.

> **TECHNICIAN NOTES**
>
> **Special Considerations When Antimicrobial Drugs Are Used**
> - Do not use antimicrobial drugs for mild infection.
> - Antimicrobials should be used only for individuals at risk of severe infection.
> - Do not dismiss the principles of asepsis just because there are many antibiotics from which to choose.
> - The use of antimicrobials should be based on a definitive diagnosis.
> - Do not use a broad-spectrum antibiotic if the infecting organism is sensitive to a specific antibiotic.
> - Antimicrobial drugs should be administered in full therapeutic doses.
> - If an antimicrobial can be used topically or locally, do so. This reserves the use of systemic drugs for serious disease.
> - Be careful regarding antibiotic withdrawal times in animals to be slaughtered for human consumption and antibiotic withdrawal times in dairy cows.
> - Penicillin G benzathine is long-acting (48 hours) and is not approved for use in dairy animals.

Antimicrobials are classified according to their mechanism of action. There are five mechanisms of antimicrobial action against bacteria and other microorganisms.

1. **Inhibition of cell wall synthesis.** Drugs that interfere with bacterial cell wall formation can kill or inhibit bacterial organisms only when the bacteria are growing or dividing.
   - **Penicillins**
   - **Cephalosporins**
   - **Bacitracin**
   - **Vancomycin**
2. **Damage to the cell membrane.** Damaging the bacterial cell membrane alters its barrier and allows antimicrobial drugs to enter and leave the cell.
   - **Polymixin B**
3. **Inhibition of protein synthesis.** Antimicrobial drugs target bacterial protein synthesis by binding to

the ribosomes and disrupting the bacteria's metabolism leading to inhibition of growth or death.

- **Aminoglycosides**
- **Tetracyclines**
- **Macrolides**
- **Lincosamides**
- **Chloramphenicol**

4. **Inhibition of metabolic processes (inhibition of folic acid synthesis).** Antimicrobial drugs interfere with cellular processes (block or bind to bacterial enzymes) essential for the bacteria's survival.

- **Sulfonamides**

5. **Inhibition of nucleic acid synthesis.** Antimicrobial drugs bind to components involved with DNA and RNA synthesis and interfere with division and survival.

- **Fluoroquinolones**
- **Metronidazole**
- **Rifampin**

Ⓡ Aminocyclitols/Aminoglycosides

Pharmacodynamics/Pharmacokinetics. Aminocyclitols belong to a class of drugs that are sugar-derived and that demonstrate important biologic value. Aminocyclitols are components that make up aminoglycoside-type antibiotics. Aminoglycoside antibiotics act on susceptible bacteria presumably by irreversibly binding to the 30S ribosomal subunit, thus inhibiting protein synthesis. Antimicrobial activity of aminoglycosides is enhanced in an alkaline environment. Aminoglycoside antibiotics are inactive against fungi, viruses, and most anaerobic bacteria (Plumb, 2015). Aminoglycosides are only effective against aerobic bacteria.

Aminoglycosides are not absorbed well after oral or intrauterine administration. They can be absorbed from topical administration when used in irrigations during surgical procedures. After intramuscular (IM) administration to dogs and cats, levels peak from 30 minutes to 1 hour later. After absorption, aminoglycosides are distributed primarily in the extracellular fluid. They do not readily cross the blood–brain barrier nor do they penetrate ocular tissue. Aminoglycosides tend to accumulate in the inner ear and kidneys, which explains their toxicity to those organs. Elimination of aminoglycosides after parenteral administration occurs almost entirely by glomerular filtration (Plumb, 2015). See Table 12.1.

> **📋 TECHNICIAN NOTES**
>
> Aminoglycosides tend to take up residence in the ears and kidneys, making them **ototoxic** and nephrotoxic. Elimination mostly occurs by glomerular filtration.

Amikacin

Clinical Uses. Parenteral use is only Food and Drug Administration (FDA) approved in dogs and is used to treat serious gram-negative infections. Amikacin is FDA approved for intrauterine infusion in mares and for intraarticular injection in foals to treat septic arthritis.

Dosage Forms. All of the following are veterinary-label products.

- **Amikacin Sulfate Injection**
- **Amiglyde-V**
- **Amikacin Sulfate Intrauterine Solution**

Adverse Side Effects. This drug is ototoxic and nephrotoxic. Cats are very susceptible to the vestibular effects of amikacin. In the United States, amikacin is not FDA approved for use in cattle or other food animals.

Storage of the Drug. Amikacin can be stored at room temperature and is stable for up to 2 years. Solutions over time may become pale yellow, but this does not decrease the drug's efficacy.

Apramycin

Clinical Uses. Some countries use this drug to treat bacterial enteritis, colibacillosis, and salmonellosis in pigs, calves, and poultry (Plumb, 2015).

Dosage Forms

- **Apralan**

Adverse Side Effects. Do not use this drug in cats. Do not use in patients with myasthenia gravis.

Storage of the Drug. Apramycin powder should be stored in a cool dry place, in a tightly closed container. It should be protected from moisture. It should be stored at less than 25°C (or 77°F).

Gentamicin

Clinical Uses. This drug is used for treatment of infections caused by gram-negative, aerobic bacteria.

Dosage Forms. All of the following are veterinary-label products.

- **Gentocin Durafilm**
- **Gentocin solution, otic solution, topical spray**
- **Gentocin ophthalmic solution, ophthalmic ointment**
- **Otomax**
- **Mometamax otic solution**
- **Gentamax 100**
- **Gentaglyde solution**
- **Garasol Injection, solution**
- **Garacin Piglet Injection**
- **Gentamicin Sulfate injection, ophthalmic solution**
- **Gentamicin sulfate topical spray, solution**

TABLE 12.1 **Aminoglycoside Preparations, Indications, and Antagonistic Drugs.**

Drug	Indications	Antagonist	Comments
All aminoglycosides	Infections caused by susceptible pathogens, pneumonias, urinary tract infections, endometritis, and septicemias that are resistant to other antibiotics	Dimenhydrinate and ethacrynic acid affect hearing loss	Monitor patient for hearing loss
Tobramycin, gentamicin, neomycin		Neuromuscular blocking agents	Administer calcium and anticholinergic agents as prescribed
Gentamicin		Amphotericin B and cephalosporins produce nephrotoxicity	Monitor renal function test results frequently when combining these agents
Neomycin		Digitalis glycosides, penicillin V	Doses may need to be adjusted when combining these agents
Gentamicin, tobramycin		Carbenicillin, azlocillin, mezlocillin, piperacillin	Never mix these two types of antibiotics; if a patient is receiving combined therapy, administer the doses at least 1 hour apart

- **Gen-Gard Soluble Powder**
- **Garacin**
- Various other

Adverse Side Effects. Gentamicin should be used with extreme caution in patients with chronic renal failure (CRF). Do not use in patients that are debilitated, who have a fever, sepsis, or dehydration. Use this drug with caution in working dog breeds such as seeing-eye dogs, herding dogs, or dogs for the hearing impaired because it can cause ototoxicity. Do not use in animals with neuromuscular disorders or in patients with botulism. IM injections in horses may cause muscle irritation, so intravenous (IV) injections are preferred. Do not use gentamicin in rabbits.

Storage of the Drug. Gentamicin sulfate for injection and the oral solution should be stored at room temperature (15°C–30°C [59°F–86°F]). Do not store the drug in rusty containers, nor offer medicated-drinking water in rusty containers because the drug will be destroyed.

Neomycin

Clinical Uses. Neomycin is more **nephrotoxic** than the other aminoglycosides. It is also less effective against gram-negative organisms. Its use topically is mainly for the skin, eyes, and ears; orally, it is used to treat enteric infections, reduce microbe numbers in the colon before surgery, and reduce ammonia-producing bacteria in the treatment of hepatic encephalopathy.

Dosage Forms. All of the following are veterinary-label products.

- **Neomycin Sulfate Oral liquid, solution**
- **Neomycin sulfate**
- **Panalog cream, ointment**
- **Animax ointment, cream**
- **Tresaderm**
- **Tritop ointment**
- **Neomycin sulfate 325**
- **Neo-Sol 50**
- Various others

Adverse Side Effects. Rarely, neomycin has caused ototoxicity, nephrotoxicity, severe diarrhea, and malabsorption of the intestines.

Storage of the Drug. Neomycin should be stored at room temperature, in tightly sealed, light-resistant containers. Neomycin (in the dry state) is stable for at least 2 years at room temperature.

Spectinomycin

Clinical Uses. This is sometimes used in dogs, cats, and horses. Spectinomycin only has FDA approval for cattle, chickens, turkeys, and swine. This drug is active against a variety of aerobic gram-negative and gram-positive organisms, as well as mycoplasma.

Dosage Forms. All of the following are veterinary-label products.

- **Spectam Injectable**
- **Spectam Scour Halt**

- **Spectinomycin tablet, injectable, and oral liquid**
- **Spectramast sterile suspension**
- **SpectoGard Scour-Check**
- **SpectoGard water soluble powder**
- Various others

Adverse Side Effects. When spectinomycin is used correctly, adverse effects are uncommon. It probably has less ototoxicity and nephrotoxic activity than other aminoglycosides. Cattle that are injected subcutaneously (SC) have developed swelling at the site of injection.

Storage of the Drug. Store at room temperature. Avoid freezing.

Tobramycin

Clinical Uses. Tobramycin is used to treat systemic infections caused by gram-negative bacteria, pneumonia, soft tissue infections and has been used in nebulizing solutions for respiratory tract infections (Papich, 2016). It is also used for the prevention of cystine urolithiasis in patients that show no improvement after the use of dietary therapy combined with urinary alkalinization.

- **Tobramycin Sulfate Injection**
- **Tobramycin Sulfate Powder for Injection**
- **Tobramycin Solution for Inhalation** (TOBI)

Adverse Side Effects. According to Plumb (2015), increased liver enzymes, lethargy, dermatologic effects, aggressiveness, sulfur odor to the urine, or myopathy may be noted with this drug.

Storage of the Drug. Store tablets at room temperature in tightly sealed containers.

TECHNICIAN NOTES

- Because aminoglycosides enhance the effects of neuromuscular blocking drugs, it is best to refrain from using these drugs at the same time. Aminoglycoside blood levels should be determined before neuromuscular blocking drugs are used so that muscular collapse is prevented.
- Aminoglycosides are contraindicated in animals with renal insufficiency.
- Aminoglycosides are not approved for use in food-producing animals.
- Do not mix vials or syringes with other antibiotics.
- Aminoglycosides may cause problems such as ototoxicity or nephrotoxicity in animals, especially if the patient is receiving furosemide therapy when they are administered.

℞ Carbapenems

Pharmacodynamics/Pharmacokinetics. Carbapenems are a class of beta-lactam antibiotics with a wide range of antibacterial activity. Carbapenems inhibit bacterial cell wall synthesis, and they are usually bactericidal.

There are currently no pharmacokinetic data available for dogs and cats. In humans, these drugs are excreted in the urine or feces.

Ertapenem

Clinical Uses. Ertapenem may be useful in treating gram-negative bacterial infections and works well in the place of aminoglycosides when they should not be used. It is indicated primarily for resistant infections caused by bacteria resistant to other drugs (Papich, 2016).

Dosage Form. There are no veterinary-label products available.

- **Invanz** (human label)

Adverse Side Effects. The adverse effects in dogs and cats are unknown.

Storage of Drug. Ertapenem should be stored at room temperature.

Imipenem–Cilastatin

Clinical Uses. This drug combination is useful in equine or small animal medicine to treat serious infections when less expensive antibiotics perform poorly.

Dosage Forms. Only human-label products are available.

- **Primaxin**

Adverse Side Effects. Gastrointestinal (GI) problems such as vomiting, anorexia, and diarrhea may be seen along with central nervous system (CNS) toxicity, pruritus, and anaphylaxis. It may cause seizures if the IV dose is given too rapidly.

Storage of Drug. Store at room temperature. After reconstitution, the solution is stable for 4 hours at room temperature or 10 hours if refrigerated. Do not freeze solutions.

Meropenem

Clinical Uses. Meropenem is useful in treating resistant gram-negative bacterial infections, especially when aminoglycosides may pose a risk. It is also active against gram-positive bacteria, except methicillin-resistant strains of *Staphylococcus* (Papich, 2016).

Dosage Form. Only human-label products are available.

- **Merrem IV**

Adverse Effects. When given SC, meropenem may cause animals to have hair loss at injection sites.

℞ Cephalosporins

Pharmacodynamics/Pharmacokinetics. Cephalosporins are a group of broad-spectrum, semisynthetic antibiotics derived from *Cephalosporium acremonium,* a species of soil-inhabiting fungi, which share the nucleus 7-aminocephalosporanic acid. Cephalosporins that were named before 1975 are spelled with *ph,* and those named after 1975 are spelled with *f.* Cephalosporins are bactericidal beta-lactam antimicrobials that inhibit bacterial cell wall synthesis. First-generation cephalosporins are active mainly against gram-positive bacteria. They are indicated for the treatment of urinary tract infections, skin and soft tissue infections, pyoderma (other dermal infections), and pneumonia (Papich, 2016). Second-generation cephalosporins have a broader spectrum of activity, and third-generation cephalosporins are mainly used against gram-negative organisms. Fourth-generation cephalosporins have an extended spectrum and have increased resistance to hydrolysis and B-lactamases (Plumb, 2015). See Table 12.2.

TABLE 12.2	**Cephalosporin Preparations, Indications, and Antagonistic Drugs.**			
Drug	**Indications**	**Antagonist**	**Comments**
Cefadroxil	Infections caused by sensitive organisms in, for example, the respiratory tract, skin, urinary tract, soft tissue, bones, and joints	All cephalosporins: gentamicin	Ingestion of food does not impair absorption
Cephalexin	Infections of the skin, soft tissue, urinary tract infections, and pneumonia		Ingestion of food may delay absorption
Cefazolin	Infections of the skin, soft tissue, respiratory tract, and urinary tract		Highly protein-bound; very rarely nephrotoxic
Cephapirin	Mastitis		Intramammary infusion for mastitis
Cefoxitin (acephamycin)	Treatment of susceptible infections		Local reaction may occur at injection site
Ceftiofur HCl	Treatment of respiratory disease in cattle and swine; broad spectrum against gram-positive and gram-negative bacteria including beta-lactamase–producing strains		May be used in lactating dairy animals
Ceftiofur sodium	Treatment of respiratory disease in cattle, sheep, horses, and swine; urinary tract infections in dogs; and for control of early mortality associated with *Escherichia coli* organisms in day-old chicks and day-old turkey poults; broad spectrum against gram-positive and gram-negative bacteria including beta-lactamase–producing strains		May be used in lactating dairy animals
Cefotaxime	Infections of gram-negative bacteria and some *Streptococcus*		
Cefpodoxime	Infections of the skin and soft tissue		
Cefovecin	Infections of the skin, soft tissue, and urinary tract		May see changes in laboratory results
Cefepime	Broad spectrum of activity with gram-positive cocci, gram-negative bacilli and *Pseudomonas*		Some activity against some extended spectrum beta-lactamase–producing strains
Cefotetan	Infections of gram-negative bacteria and anaerobes		Resistance to cephalosporinase enzyme

Orally Active

- **Cephalexin** (Rilexine chewable tablets)
- **Cefadroxil** (Cefa-Tabs, Cefa-Drops)
- **Cefpodoxime** (Simplicef)
- **Cefepime** (Maxipime)

Parenterally Active

Cephalosporins that are active by parenteral administration are placed into four groups.

Group I First-Generation. This group is effective against gram-positive bacteria and less effective against gram-negative bacteria; the drugs show poor activity against *Pseudomonas*. They are more effective against *Staphylococcus* and *Streptococcus* than penicillin.

- **Cephalexin**
- **Cefadroxil**
- **Cephapirin**
- **Cefazolin**

Group II Second-Generation. This group is more effective against gram-negative bacteria than the first-generation drugs and slightly less effective against gram-positive bacteria.

- **Cefotetan**
- **Cefoxitin**

Group III Third-Generation. This group has high activity against gram-negative bacteria and *Pseudomonas*.

- **Cefovecin**
- **Cefpodoxime**
- **Ceftiofur**
- **Ceftriaxone**

Group IV Fourth-Generation. Cefepime has activity against gram-positive cocci, gram-negative bacilli including *Pseudomonas* and certain Enterobacteriaceae (Werth, 2019).

- **Cefepime**

Cephalexin

Clinical Uses. Cephalexin (Rilexine) is FDA approved for veterinary use in the United States. It has been used to treat dogs, cats, horses, rabbits, ferrets, and birds that are infected with *Staphylococcus*.

Dosage Forms
- **Rilexine chewable tabs** (veterinary label)
- **Keflex** (human label)
- Other generic brands

Adverse Side Effects. There is a low occurrence of problems associated with cephalexin. Cephalexin has

been known to cause salivation, tachypnea, and excitability in dogs and emesis and fever in cats.

Cefadroxil

Clinical Uses. Cefadroxil is useful in treating infections of the skin, soft tissue, genitourinary tract, and pneumonia in dogs and cats. Cefa-Tabs and Cefa-Drops are FDA approved for use in dogs and cats.

Dosage Forms
- **Cefa-Drops**
- **Cefa-Tabs**

Adverse Side Effects. These are usually not serious and occur rarely. They include hypersensitivity, GI effects, the potential for nephrotoxicity, and tachypnea, rarely.

Storage of the Drug. Cefadroxil should be stored at room temperature. After reconstitution, the suspension should be refrigerated and discarded after 14 days.

Cephapirin

Clinical Uses. An intramammary cephapirin sodium product is FDA approved in the United States for the treatment of mastitis.

Dosage Forms
- **Cefa-Lak**
- **ToMORROW** (cephapirin benzathine)
- **Cefa-Dri**
- **ToDay** (cephapirin sodium)

Adverse Side Effects. These rarely occur. Allergic reactions, rashes, fever, and lymphadenopathy may be seen.

Storage of the Drug. Cephapirin intramammary syringes should be stored at controlled room temperature.

Cefazolin

Clinical Uses. In the United States, there are no FDA approved cefazolin products for veterinary use. It is used for treatment of soft tissue, skin, and genitourinary tract infections (Papich, 2016).

Dosage Forms. Only human-label products are available.
- **Cefazolin Sodium Powder for injection**
- **Cefazolin Sodium for IV infusion**

Adverse Side Effects. These are usually not serious and do not often happen. Some signs that may be seen include hypersensitivity, fever, eosinophilia, and lymphadenopathy. Pain at the injection site may occur when given IM, and it may have the potential for nephrotoxicity.

Storage of the Drug. Cefazolin sodium powder and solutions for injection should be protected from light. The powder should be stored at room temperature. After reconstitution, the solution is stable for 24 hours when kept at room temperature or 96 hours if refrigerated. After reconstitution, if freezing is desired, the preparation is stable for at least 12 weeks.

Cefotetan Disodium

Clinical Uses. Cefotetan is a good choice for treating serious infections in which enteric gram-negative bacteria or anaerobes are suspected (Papich, 2016).

Dosage Form. Only human-label products are available.

• **Cefotetan Disodium Powder for Solution**

Adverse Side Effects. This drug appears to be well tolerated. The following may be seen: hypersensitivity, pain at the injection site, and gut flora alteration. Cefotetan may cause nephrotoxicity.

Storage of the Drug. The sterile powder for injection should be stored below 22°C (71.6°F). Darkening of the powder over time does not harm its efficacy. After reconstituting with sterile water, the solution is stable for 24 hours if stored at room temperature or 96 hours if refrigerated.

Cefoxitin

Clinical Uses. Cefoxitin can be used clinically when injectable cephalosporins are indicated; gram-negative bacteria or anaerobes including abdominal infections and soft tissue wounds (Papich, 2016).

Dosage Form. Only human-label products are available.

• **Cefoxitin** (Mefoxin)

Adverse Side Effects. These are usually not serious and rarely occur. Hypersensitivity and pain at the injection site may be seen, it may alter gut flora, and it has potential for nephrotoxicity.

Storage of Drug. Cefoxitin should be stored at temperatures less than 30°C (86°F).

Cefovecin

Clinical Uses. Cefovecin is FDA approved to treat skin infections in dogs and in cats to treat wounds and abscesses.

Dosage Form

• **Convenia**

Adverse Side Effects. This drug is well-tolerated in dogs and cats. In dogs, it may cause some changes in laboratory results such as increases in gamma glutamyl transpeptidase (GGT) and alanine aminotransferase (ALT). In cats, changes in laboratory results include mild increases in

ALT, increases in blood urea nitrogen (BUN), and moderately increased creatinine levels. In dogs, clinical signs including depression, lethargy, and vomiting may be seen.

Storage of the Drug. Store the powder and reconstituted product in the original container and keep refrigerated at 2.22°C to 7.78°C (36°F to 46°F). Use the entire contents within 56 days after reconstitution. Protect from light. Solution that darkens over time does not adversely affect the drug's potency.

Cefpodoxime Proxetil

Clinical Uses. This drug is FDA approved and used in the treatment of skin and soft tissue infections.

Dosage Forms

• **Simplicef**

• **Cefpodoxime Proxetil tablets**

Adverse Side Effects. Cefpodoxime proxetil may cause diarrhea, vomiting, and allergic reactions.

Storage of the Drug. Store at 20°C to 25°C (68°F to 77°F).

Ceftiofur Crystalline Free Acid

Clinical Uses. This drug is FDA approved and is used in swine for the treatment of respiratory disease. It is used in cattle for the treatment of bovine respiratory disease (BRD), shipping fever, and pneumonia. In dairy cattle, it is used for the treatment of subclinical mastitis.

Dosage Forms

• **Excede**

• **Excede for Swine**

Adverse Side Effects. Hypersensitivity reactions may occur.

Storage of the Drug. The ready-to-use injectable product should be stored at 20°C to 25°C (68°F to 77°F).

Ceftiofur Sodium

Clinical Uses. Ceftiofur sodium is FDA approved and is used in cattle for the treatment of respiratory disease and acute interdigital necrobacillosis. It is used in swine for the treatment of bacterial pneumonia. In sheep and goats, it is used for the treatment of pneumonia. In horses, it is used for the treatment of respiratory infections. It is used in dogs for the treatment of urinary tract infections and is used in chicks and poults for the control of early mortality. Withdrawal time in cattle is 4 days before slaughter. No milk discard time is needed. In sheep and goats, no withdrawal time for slaughter or withholding milk is needed. Do not use in horses intended for human consumption.

Dosage Form

• **Naxcel**

- **Ceftiofur Sodium Sterile powder**

Adverse Side Effects. These are usually rare. Pain may follow injection. Administration to horses under stress may be associated with acute diarrhea that could be fatal. Hypersensitivity reactions may occur.

Storage of the Drug. Unreconstituted powder should be stored at room temperature. Protect from light. Color change will not affect efficacy. After reconstitution, the solution is stable for up to 7 days when refrigerated.

> ### TECHNICIAN NOTES
>
> - Naxcel is approved for use in lactating dairy animals.
> - Remember to read package inserts regarding milk withholding time, withholding time in animals to be slaughtered, and milk withholding time after mastitis treatment.

Ceftriaxone

Clinical Uses. Ceftriaxone is used to treat serious infections. It has activity against *Borrelia burgdorferi,* which makes it an excellent choice for treating Lyme disease.

Dosage Form. Only human-label products are available.

- **Rocephin**

Adverse Side Effects. These include hematologic effects, "sludge" in bile, hypersensitivity reactions, increased liver enzyme, BUN, and creatinine levels, and urine casts. Pain on IM injection may occur.

Storage of the Drug. The powder for reconstitution should be stored at or below 25°C (77°F).

Cefepime

Clinical Uses. Cefepime is useful in treating serious infections in dogs or foals when aminoglycosides are contraindicated. Limited use in veterinary medicine.

Dosage Form. Only human-label products are available.

- **Maxipime**

Adverse Side Effects. Clinical signs that may be seen include loose stools in dogs. Intramuscular injections may be painful.

Storage of the Drug. The powder for injection should be stored between 2°C and 25°C (35.6°F and 77°F).

Macrolides

Pharmacodynamics/Pharmacokinetics. Many of the macrolides inhibit protein synthesis by penetrating the cell wall and binding to the 50S ribosomes subunits in susceptible bacteria. Many of them are considered bacteriostatic antibiotics and are used to treat gram-positive bacteria associated with respiratory disease. They have a broad spectrum of activity. The majority of these drugs are excreted from the body in the bile.

Azithromycin

Clinical Uses. This is a good broad-spectrum agent. Azithromycin is used to treat gram-positive bacteria and is effective against *Mycoplasma.* It has been used in cats to treat upper respiratory tract infections.

Dosage Form. Only human-label products are available.

- **Zithromax**

Adverse Side Effects. Azithromycin can cause vomiting in dogs when given at high doses. It has fewer GI effects than erythromycin.

Storage of the drug. Store tablets at temperatures less than 30°C (86°F).

Clarithromycin

Clinical Uses. Clarithromycin is used to treat *Helicobacter* spp. infections in cats and ferrets. It is useful in treating *Rhodococcus equi* infections in foals (Plumb, 2015).

Dosage Forms. Only human-label products are available.

- **Biaxin**
- **Prevpak;** a combination of lansoprazole, amoxicillin, and clarithromycin

Adverse Side Effects. Redness of the ears may occur when the drug is used in cats. GI disturbances may occur.

Storage of the Drug. Store the tablets at 15°C (59°F to 86°F).

Erythromycin

Clinical Uses

Erythromycin is FDA approved to treat infections in swine, sheep, and cattle. It may be used to treat esophageal reflux in dogs and cats.

Dosage Forms. The following are human-label products unless otherwise specified.

- **Gallimycin-100, 36 Sterile, 36 Dry**
- **Erythro 100, 200, 36 Dry**
- **Erythro 100 injection**
- **Erythromast 36**

Adverse Side Effects. These occur rarely. When injected IM, pain at the injection site may occur. Oral dosing may cause GI problems. In swine, rectal prolapse and rectal edema have been reported. The use of erythromycin in adult equines remains controversial; horses may develop severe, sometimes fatal diarrhea (Plumb, 2015).

Storage of the Drug. Store in tightly sealed containers at room temperature.

Tilmicosin

Clinical Uses. Tilmicosin is FDA approved for the treatment of bovine and ovine respiratory diseases caused by *Mannheima (pasteurella) haemolytica*. It is also used in cattle, sheep, and rabbits. This drug must be injected SC.

Dosage Form
- Micotil

Adverse Side Effects. These include injection site swelling and inflammation, lameness, collapse, anaphylaxis, decreased food and water consumption, and death (Elanco, 2010). Other adverse effects may include increased heart rate and decreased contractility (Papich, 2016). Tilmicosin is potentially lethal to humans, swine, and horses. In case of human injection, contact a physician immediately.

📋 TECHNICIAN NOTES

- Always use proper drug handling procedures to avoid accidental self-injection. Injection of this drug in humans has been associated with fatalities.
- Do not use an automatically powered syringe.
- Injection of this antibiotic has been shown to be fatal in swine, and may be fatal in horses and goats.
- Do not use in female dairy cattle 20 months of age or older. Use in lactating dairy cattle may cause milk residues.
- The withdrawal time of this drug is 42 days.
- Approved for use in cattle and sheep only (Elanco, 2010).
- Do not give IV to camelids.

Tulathromycin

Clinical Uses. Tulathromycin is FDA approved and is used in nonlactating dairy cattle to treat upper respiratory infections, bovine foot rot, and infectious bovine keratoconjunctivitis.

Dosage Form
- Draxxin
- Draxxin 25 Injection

Adverse Side Effects. These are minimal in cattle and swine. Allergic reactions are possible. SC or IM injections may cause local tissue reactions.

Storage of the Drug. Store below 25°C (77°F). The agent is stable up to 36 months.

Tylosin

Clinical Uses. The injectable form of the drug is FDA approved in dogs and cats. It is not used very often in those species. It is sometimes used to treat chronic colitis in small animals. Tylosin is commonly used to promote growth in cattle, swine, and chickens. It is used for treating BRD, diarrhea in pigs, and other diseases in poultry.

Dosage Form. Only veterinary-label products are available.
- Tylan
- Tylan 50 injection, 200 injection
- Tylosin injection
- Various others (combinations)

Adverse Side Effects. These include pain at injection site and possible GI upset.

Storage of the Drug. Store in well-closed containers at room temperature.

℞ Penicillins

History of Penicillin

Sir Alexander Fleming was born on August 6, 1881 in Scotland. He served as a captain during World War I. After seeing many of his comrades dying of bacteria-infected wounds, he desperately wanted to find a cure that could save lives. The main problem was finding an antibacterial substance that would not be toxic to animal tissue. In 1928, he was studying influenza virus in his somewhat disorganized laboratory. He saw a mold that had developed in a petri dish after being discarded in the sink before being disinfected. He noticed that the culture plate was one that contained *Staphylococcus* and that this mold had created a zone of inhibition around itself. He named the substance (mold) penicillin. Dr. Fleming died on March 11, 1955 (nobelprize.org, 1964).

Pharmacodynamics/Pharmacokinetics for Penicillins. Penicillin is the most commonly used antibiotic; it is bactericidal against susceptible bacteria. It is effective against most gram-positive bacteria and less effective against gram-negative bacteria. It acts by inhibiting mucopeptide synthesis in the cell wall, which results in a defective barrier and an osmotically unstable spheroplast (Plumb, 2015), making it more prone to lysis. Some penicillins are not absorbed well when administered orally but are rapidly absorbed after IM injections. After being absorbed by the body, penicillin is present throughout the body except for the cerebrospinal fluid, joints, and milk. Penicillin G is inactivated by stomach acid and therefore should not be given orally. Penicillin preparations, indications, and antagonistic drugs are found in Table 12.3.

TABLE 12.3 Penicillin Preparations, Indications, and Antagonistic Drugs.

Drug	Indications	Antagonist	Comments
Narrow-Spectrum Penicillins			
Penicillin G sodium	Infections caused by penicillin-sensitive organisms: bacterial pneumonia, upper respiratory tract infections, equine strangles, blackleg, infected wounds, urinary tract infections (at high doses)	Tetracyclines, chloramphenicol, and paromomycin	May add to sodium load
Penicillin G potassium	Same as for penicillin G sodium	Same as for penicillin G sodium	May produce hyperkalemia (IV); delayed absorption in horses (IM); unreliable absorption
Penicillin G procaine	Same as for penicillin G sodium	Same as for penicillin G sodium	Never give IV; contraindicated in some exotics and horses that race; preslaughter withdrawal and milk withholding periods
Penicillin G benzathine	Same as for penicillin G sodium	Same as for penicillin G sodium	Never give IV; preslaughter withdrawal required, and may persist in dairy cattle milk for 2 weeks
Narrow-Spectrum, Acid-Resistant Penicillins			
Penicillin V	Mild infections already controlled by parenteral therapy	Same as for penicillin G sodium	Should not be administered with food; less active against gram-negative bacteria than penicillin G
Beta-Lactamase–Resistant Penicillins			
Methicillin	Pyodermatitis, otitis externa, and other conditions caused by *Staphylococcus aureus*	Same as for penicillin G sodium	Not stable in solution; many incompatibilities in vitro
Cloxacillin	Same as for methicillin	Same as for penicillin G sodium	Frequently used in dry-cow intramammary preparations
Dicloxacillin and floxacillin	Same as for methicillin	Same as for penicillin G sodium	Absorbed from GI tract better than cloxacillin
Oxacillin	Same as for methicillin	Sulfonamides	Not absorbed as well as cloxacillin
Broad-Spectrum Penicillins			
Ampicillin and hetacillin	Infection of organs and tissues caused by ampicillin-sensitive bacteria	Chloramphenicol, erythromycin, tetracyclines, cephaloridine	Incompatible with many drugs and solutions; food impairs absorption; milk withholding and preslaughter withdrawal times
Amoxicillin	Same as for ampicillin	Same as for ampicillin	Absorbed from GI tract better than ampicillin
Carbenicillin sodium	Same as for ampicillin, but especially *Pseudomonas* infections	Same as for ampicillin	Freshly mixed solutions should be used
Broad-Spectrum Penicillins			
Carbenicillin indanyl sodium	Same as for carbenicillin sodium	Same as for ampicillin	Absorbed rapidly from the GI tract

Continued

TABLE 12.3   Penicillin Preparations, Indications, and Antagonistic Drugs.—cont'd

Drug	Indications	Antagonist	Comments
Potentiated Penicillins			
Amoxicillin-potassium clavulanate (4:1)	Wide range of infections when used in combination	Same as for ampicillin	Capsules/tablets that are not kept in air-tightly sealed containers lose activity; do not give to patients allergic to penicillins or cephalosporins
Inhibitor of Tubular Secretion of Penicillins			
Probenecid	Prolongs blood levels of penicillins that have very short plasma half-lives or that are extremely costly	Same as for ampicillin	

IV, Intravenous; *IM,* intramuscular; *GI,* gastrointestinal.

Penicillins are also called beta-lactam antibiotics. Penicillin and cephalosporin antibiotics have a beta-lactam ring in their molecular structure and are called beta-lactam antibiotics. Many bacteria synthesize beta-lactamases (bacterial enzymes) that degrade beta-lactam antibiotics (penicillin) before they reach the bacteria's cell wall. So, when penicillin encounters beta-lactamase, the beta-lactamase will break the beta-lactam ring causing penicillin to become inactive and have no effect on the bacteria. Beta-lactamase-resistant penicillin drugs include methicillin, cloxacillin, dicloxacillin, and oxacillin.

Penicillin drugs that are inactivated by beta-lactamase can be protected from the bacterial enzyme if they are combined with another drug producing a stronger, more potentiated, penicillin that is resistant to the beta-lactamase enzyme (Bill, 2017). Clavulanic acid (a beta-lactamase inhibitor) is combined with amoxicillin to produce a potentiated drug called Clavamox. Clavulanic acid acts by irreversibly binding to the beta-lactamase enzyme, protecting amoxicillin so that it can attach to the cell wall and kill the bacteria.

Amoxicillin

Clinical Uses. Amoxicillin is used to treat a wide range of infections in various species. Amoxicillin is a reasonable choice for treating abscesses in cats even before culture and susceptibility results are available.

Dosage Forms. All of the following are veterinary-label products.

- **Amoxi-Tabs**
- **Amoxi-Drop Oral suspension**
- **Amoxi injectable**
- **Amoxi-Bol**
- **Amoxi-Sol**
- **Amoxi-Mast**
- **Biomox**
- **Robamox**

Adverse Side Effects. These rarely occur. Allergic reactions may occur. Amoxicillin may cause GI upset when administered orally. High doses or prolonged doses have been associated with neurotoxicity. Liver enzymes may rise.

Storage of the Drug. Store at room temperature. After reconstitution, the oral suspension should be refrigerated (preferably). Discard unused portions after 14 days. Product should be shaken well before administering.

Amoxicillin/Clavulanate

Pharmacodynamics/Pharmacokinetics. Clavulanic acid acts by irreversibly bonding to beta-lactamases and penicillinases produced by bacterial agents. Clavulanate potassium is readily absorbed after oral dosing. It can cross the placenta but is not considered teratogenic. When amoxicillin is combined with clavulanic acid it is called a potentiated aminopenicillin.

Clinical Uses. This combination drug is used in the treatment of urinary tract, skin, and soft tissue infections in dogs and cats. It can also be used for treatment of canine periodontal disease, bacterial cystitis in female dogs, and hepatobiliary infections in dogs or cats (sometimes with a fluoroquinolone as an adjunct).

Dosage Forms
- **Clavamox Chewables**
- **Clavamox Drops**

Adverse Side Effects. Allergic reactions and GI upset may occur.

Storage of the Drug. Store at temperatures less than 23.9°C (75°F). After reconstitution, suspensions are stable for 10 days if refrigerated. Unused portions should be discarded after 10 days.

Ampicillin

Clinical Uses. Ampicillin is active against gram-negative bacteria. It is used to treat skin infections, wounds, abscesses, and urinary tract infections.

Dosage Forms
- **Polyflex**
- **Amp-Equine**
- **Princillin**

Adverse Side Effects. Hypersensitivity and GI upset may occur.

Storage of the Drug. Ampicillin can be stored at room temperature before reconstitution. After reconstitution, the drug is stable for 3 months if refrigerated.

Ampicillin/Sulbactam

Pharmacodynamics/Pharmacokinetics. Combining sulbactam with ampicillin extends its spectrum of activity to those bacteria that would otherwise cause ampicillin to be ineffective. This medication is best administered parenterally.

Clinical Uses. It is effective parenterally against beta-lactamase–producing bacterial strains of otherwise resistant bacteria.

Dosage Form
- **Unasyn** (human label)

Adverse Side Effects. Intramuscular injections are painful. IV injection may cause thrombophlebitis. Allergic reactions are possible.

Storage of the Drug. Unreconstituted powder should be stored at temperatures at or below 30°C (86°F).

Cloxacillin

Clinical Uses. Cloxacillin is used for intramammary infusions in dry and lactating dairy cattle. It is important to adhere to milk withdrawal times when using this drug.

Dosage Forms
- **Orbenin-DC**
- **Dry-Clox intramammary infusion**
- **Boviclox**
- **Dariclox**

Adverse Side Effects. Allergic reactions may occur.

Storage of the Drug. Store at temperatures less than 25°C (77°F).

Dicloxacillin

Clinical Uses. Dicloxacillin is administered per os (PO; by mouth) for the treatment of bone, skin, and other soft tissue infections in small animals.

Dosage Form
- **Dicloxacillin Capsules**

Adverse Side Effects. Allergic reactions may occur. This drug may cause GI upset when given orally.

Storage of the Drug. Store at temperatures less than 20°C (68°F).

Oxacillin

Clinical Uses. Oxacillin is used in the treatment of bone, skin, and other soft tissue infections in small animals.

Dosage Forms
- **Oxacillin Sodium Powder for Oral Solution**

Adverse Side Effects. These include allergic reactions and GI upset. Neurotoxicity can occur with prolonged use.

Storage of the Drug. Store at room temperature.

Penicillin G

Clinical Uses. Penicillin is the drug of choice for a variety of bacteria. It has a narrow-spectrum of activity and is used to treat *Staphylococcus*, *Streptococcus*, some gram-positive aerobes, and obligate anaerobes. Penicillin G should not be given orally as it is inactivated by stomach acid; it is used as an injectable.

Dosage Forms
- **Penicillin-G Procaine**
  - Dry-Mast
  - Albadry Plus suspension
  - Go-Dry, Masti-Clear
  - Crysticillin
  - Various others
- **Penicillin G Benzathine**
  - Flo-cillin
  - Combi-Pen 48
  - Dura-biotic

TECHNICIAN NOTES

- Veterinary personnel who are allergic to penicillin should be careful when handling this drug.
- Some species, such as snakes, birds, turtles, guinea pigs, and chinchillas, are sensitive to procaine penicillin G.
- Subcutaneous administration of penicillin G or benzathine penicillin should be avoided because of potential tissue injury and residue potential in food animals.
- Penicillin should not be used in horses intended for food.
- Carefully read labels concerning milk withholding times and the treatment of animals to be slaughtered for food.
- Penicillin G benzathine is long-acting (48 hours) and is not approved for use in dairy cattle.

Adverse Side Effects. Do not use in individuals that are sensitive to penicillins.

Storage of the Drug. Store at room temperature. After powder for injection is reconstituted, the solution should be kept refrigerated. Penicillin G and benzathine penicillin G should be stored at 8.89°C (48°F) or lower but not frozen.

Penicillin V

The aforementioned information regarding penicillin G closely resembles the efficacy of penicillin V. The main difference is that penicillin V is more readily absorbed when given PO than is penicillin G. It has a narrow-spectrum of activity and is used to treat infections caused by *Streptococcus*. It is not commonly used in veterinary medicine.

Dosage Form. Only human-label products are available.
- **Penicillin V potassium tablets and oral solution**

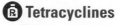

Tetracyclines

Pharmacodynamics/Pharmacokinetics. Tetracyclines usually act as time-dependent antibiotics and inhibit protein synthesis by reversibly binding to 30S ribosomal subunits of susceptible organisms, thereby preventing binding to those ribosomes of aminoacyl transfer-RNA (Plumb, 2015). Tetracyclines are generally considered to be bacteriostatic antibiotics. Tetracyclines have activity against most mycoplasma, spirochetes (including the Lyme disease organism), chlamydia, and rickettsia. With regard to gram-positive bacteria, the tetracyclines have activity against some strains of *Staphylococci* and *Streptococci*, but the resistance of these organisms is on the rise. Oxytetracycline and tetracycline have almost identical spectrums of activity and patterns of cross-resistance. Tetracyclines have antiinflammatory and immunomodulating effects. They can suppress antibody production and chemotaxis of neutrophils and inhibit lipases, collagenases, prostaglandin synthesis, and activation of complement component three. Tetracyclines are readily absorbed after being administered orally. Intramuscular administration carries a lower ability to be absorbed. Tetracyclines can cross the placenta, enter fetal circulation, and can be distributed into milk. Tetracyclines are eliminated from the body by glomerular filtration. The elimination half-life of tetracycline is about 5 to 6 hours in dogs and cats. See Table 12.4.

TABLE 12.4	Tetracycline Preparations, Indications, and Antagonistic Drugs.		
Drug	**Indications**	**Antagonist**	**Comments**
Oxytetracycline	Infections of organs or tissues caused by tetracycline-sensitive strains; anaplasmosis; often ineffective for endocarditis, empyema, meningitis, septic arthritis, and osteomyelitis	Antacids, milk, diuretics, methoxyflurane, penicillins, ferrous sulfate	Long withdrawal times in cattle; shock reaction may occur when given intravenously in horses; diarrhea also common in horses
Chlortetracycline	Same as for oxytetracycline	Antacids, milk, diuretics, methoxyflurane, penicillins	
Tetracycline	Same as for oxytetracycline	Same as for oxytetracycline	
Doxycycline, minocycline	Same as for oxytetracycline, but much better tissue penetration; doxycycline is especially useful for canine ehrlichiosis	Minocycline—same as for chlortetracycline; doxycycline—same as for oxytetracycline, barbiturates, and carbamazepine	These drugs are potent broad-spectrum tetracyclines

TECHNICIAN NOTES

Tetracyclines given to young animals may cause yellow to brown discoloration of bones and teeth.

Chlortetracycline

Clinical Uses. Chlortetracycline is used mostly in water or feed treatments or topically for ophthalmic use (Plumb, 2015).

Dosage Forms. The following are all veterinary-label products.

- **Aureomycin**
- **Aureomix**
- **Pennchlor**
- **ChlorMax, Coban**
- **Deracin**

Adverse Side Effects. When given in high doses, this drug may cause an increased BUN level and hepatotoxicity; it should be used with caution in patients with renal disease. High doses in ruminants can cause ruminal microflora depression. In small animals, high doses may cause nausea, vomiting, anorexia, and diarrhea. Cats do not tolerate oral tetracycline well. Long-term use in dogs may cause urolith formation. Horses stressed by surgery, anesthesia, or trauma may develop severe diarrhea. Long-term tetracycline therapy can result in overgrowth (superinfections) of nonsusceptible bacteria or fungi.

Storage of the Drug. Keep tetracyclines in tightly sealed containers protected from light.

Doxycycline

Clinical Uses. Doxycycline is commonly used in small animals to treat *Borrelia*, *Leptospira*, rickettsiae, chlamydia, *Mycoplasma*, *Bartonella*, and *Bordetella*. Doxirobe is used in dogs as an oral application for the prevention/treatment of periodontal disease.

Dosage Forms
- **Doxirobe Gel**
- **Vibramycin** (human label)

Adverse Side Effects. After oral administration, the most common effects seen in dogs and cats are vomiting, diarrhea, and anorexia. Giving the drug with food seems to help some of these problems. Oral doxycycline has been blamed for causing esophageal strictures in cats. Therefore, after giving an oral dose to cats, it should be followed by at least 6 mL water.

Storage of the Drug. Keep stored in tightly sealed, light-resistant containers at temperatures less than 30°C (86°F).

Minocycline Hydrogen Chloride

Clinical Uses. Minocycline is useful for the treatment of brucellosis, especially when used in conjunction with aminoglycosides.

Dosage Forms
- **Minocin**

Adverse Side Effects. After oral administration in dogs and cats, nausea and vomiting are the most commonly reported side effects.

Storage of the Drug. Keep oral preparations in tightly sealed containers at room temperature. Do not freeze the oral suspension. The injectable form should be stored at room temperature and protected from light.

Oxytetracycline

Clinical Uses. Oxytetracycline is commonly used in cattle. It may be helpful in the treatment of BRD, pink eye, and wound infections.

Dosage Forms
- **Terramycin**
- **Liquamycin LA**
- **Bio-Mycin**
- **Biocyl**
- **Oxyject**
- **Oxytet injectable**
- Various others

Adverse Side Effects. Oxytetracycline may cause ruminal depression in ruminants. It can also cause GI distress, staining of teeth in young animals, and long-term use may cause uroliths (Plumb, 2015).

Storage of the Drug. Store in tightly sealed, light-resistant containers at room temperature.

Tetracycline

Clinical Uses. Tetracycline is still used as an antimicrobial, although other forms are more commonly used in today's veterinary practices. Tetracycline is used in combination with niacinamide to help control sterile inflammatory skin conditions in dogs (Plumb, 2015).

Dosage Forms

- **Delta Albaplex** (a combination product with tetracycline, novobiocin, and prednisolone)
- **Albaplex**
- **Panmycin tablets, capsules, Aquadrops liquid**
- **Panmycin Hydrochloride**
- **Tetracycline HCL**
- Various others

TECHNICIAN NOTES

- Never give tetracycline intravenously to a horse.
- Absorption of tetracyclines through the GI tract is dramatically decreased by the presence of food, milk products, and antacids.
- Carefully read labels about use in animals to be slaughtered.
- Tetracycline is not approved for use in lactating dairy animals or poultry that produce eggs for human consumption.

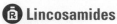 **Lincosamides**

Pharmacodynamics/Pharmacokinetics. Lincosamide antibiotics are broad-spectrum antibiotics that have activity against anaerobes, gram-positive aerobic cocci, and toxoplasma parasites, among others. Horses, rodents, ruminants, and lagomorphs are hypersensitive to lincosamides. Lincosamides are distributed to milk and can cause diarrhea in nursing animals. The pharmacokinetics of lincosamides have not been extensively studied in veterinary species (Plumb, 2015). The following information is from studies on the effect of the drugs on humans. Lincosamides are rapidly absorbed after oral dosage. Peak serum levels are reached about 2 to 4 hours after oral dosing. Intramuscular administration peaks about twice as long as that reached after oral dosing. Lincosamides are distributed into most tissues. The drugs can cross the placenta. Lincosamides are partially metabolized in the liver. Unchanged drug and metabolites are excreted in the urine, feces, and bile. The elimination half-life of lincomycin is about 3 to 4 hours in small animals (Plumb, 2015).

BOX 12.1   Case Scenario Bordetella bronchiseptica

Kiana, a 14-week-old intact female Husky puppy, was presented by the owner with a chief complaint of coughing.

History: The owner purchased the puppy 6 days ago from a pet store, noticed some nasal discharge when they first got her for which she is being treated with Clavamox. For the past 3 days she has been coughing (hacking but nonproductive), she appears more lethargic and only ate a small amount of food today. No vomiting or diarrhea. She has had two sets of distemper puppy vaccines. She is currently on fenbendazole for worms. No other animals in the household.

Physical examination findings: Kiana was quiet, alert, and responsive. Temperature: 103.2°F, Pulse: 110 bpm, no pulse deficits, Respirations: 30 bpm with minimal effort, mucous membranes: pink and moist, CRT (capillary refill time): <2 seconds. Heart sounds: normal, Lung sounds: increased bronchovesicular lungs sounds but no crackles or wheezes heard. Tracheal irritation and cough elicited upon palpation of the trachea. Obtained SpO$_2$: 98% on room air.

Diagnostic tests: Thoracic radiographs to assess signs of pneumonia versus infection, Baermann fecal test to rule out lungworm, complete blood count (CBC) and chemistry.

Diagnostic results: CBC and chemistry revealed inflammatory leukogram, increased ALKP (common for growing puppies to have elevated ALKP), Thoracic radiographs revealed a mild diffuse bronchointerstitial pattern, Baermann fecal: negative.

Diagnosis: Bordetella bronchiseptica

The Clavamox was discontinued and the owner was dispensed doxycycline twice daily for 2 weeks and butorphanol to be given every 12 hours as needed to suppress the cough.

The veterinary technician went over the discharge instructions with the owner and discussed the two different medications that were dispensed. She also told the owner to restrict Kiana's exercise for 2 weeks and because the disease is highly contagious, she should not take her to public places, like pet stores or dog parks. The veterinary technician scheduled a follow-up appointment in 2 weeks at which time thoracic radiographs will be done again to reveal if there is resolution of the bronchointerstitial pattern. The owner asked if Kiana could have the rest of her vaccinations? The veterinary technician stated that once the follow-up radiographs are taken and assessed they will determine at that appointment whether or not the third distemper series vaccine, Bordetella intranasal vaccine, and rabies vaccine will be given.

TECHNICIAN NOTES

- Carefully read labels about use in animals for slaughter.
- Lincosamides should not be administered to rabbits, hamsters, guinea pigs, or horses.

Clindamycin

Clinical Uses. Clindamycin is FDA approved for use in dogs and cats. It is commonly used to treat wounds, abscesses, and osteomyelitis caused by *Staphylococcus aureus*. It may also be used to treat toxoplasmosis. This drug is commonly used to treat stomatitis.

Dosage Forms. The following are all veterinary-label products.
- **Antirobe Capsules, Aquadrops**
- **Clintabs**
- **Clinsol**
- **Clindamycin HCL oral drops, oral liquid, capsules**

Adverse Side Effects. Clindamycin may cause GI upset and esophageal strictures in cats when administered without food or a water bolus. Cats may have hypersalivation or lip smacking after oral administration. Intramuscular injections cause pain at the injection site.

Storage of the Drug. Store at room temperature.

Lincomycin

Clinical Uses. Lincomycin is FDA approved for use in dogs, cats, swine, and in combination with other agents for chickens. It is used to provide treatment against anaerobes, gram-positive aerobic cocci, and toxoplasma parasites.

Dosage Forms
- **Lincocin**
- **Lincocin Aquadrops**
- **Lincomix Injectable**

 TECHNICIAN NOTES

- Lincomycin is not for use in avians used for egg laying, breeders, or turkeys.

Adverse Side Effects. Lincomycin may cause GI upset and pain at the injection site when given as an IM injection. Rapid IV administration can cause hypotension and cardiopulmonary arrest.

Storage of the Drug. Store at room temperature.

Pirlimycin

Clinical Uses. Pirlimycin is used for intramammary infusion for dairy cattle.

Dosage Form
- **Pirsue sterile solution**

 TECHNICIAN NOTES

Milk withdrawal time (when used at labeled doses) is 36 hours after the last treatment. Meat withdrawal time (when used at labeled doses) is 9 days.

Adverse Side Effects. No adverse effects have been reported at this time.

Storage of the Drug. Store syringes at or below 25°C (77°F).

Quinolones/ Fluoroquinolones

Pharmacodynamics/Pharmacokinetics. Quinolones are bactericidal agents. The mechanism of action is believed to be inhibition of bacterial DNA-gyrase (a type-II topoisomerase), which prevents DNA supercoiling and DNA synthesis (Plumb, 2015). These agents have activity against many gram-negative bacilli and cocci. They have variable activity against most *Streptococci*, so they are not usually recommended for these infections. Bacterial resistance is a concern. These drugs are well absorbed after oral dosing. Quinolones are distributed throughout the body. Highest concentrations are found in the bile, kidney, liver, lungs, and reproductive system. Quinolones are eliminated from the body by both renal and nonrenal routes.

Ciprofloxacin

Clinical Uses. Ciprofloxacin may be used when a larger oral dosage of IV product is desired (as an alternative to enrofloxacin.) This drug differs from enrofloxacin in its pharmacokinetics. In dogs, enrofloxacin's bioavailability is almost twice that of ciprofloxacin after oral administration. Ciprofloxacin is one of the metabolites of enrofloxacin. It is used to treat lower respiratory tract infections, skin infections, and urinary tract infections in dogs and cats.

Dosage Forms
- **Cipro**

Adverse Side Effects. Ciprofloxacin may cause hypersensitivity. Its use is contraindicated in growing animals because it may cause cartilage abnormalities. Use with caution in patients with renal or hepatic insufficiency and in patients that are dehydrated. It is preferable to administer the drug PO on an empty stomach.

Storage of the Drug Store in tightly sealed containers at temperatures less than 30°C (86°F), unless otherwise noted by the manufacturer.

TECHNICIAN NOTES

- Ciprofloxacin should not be given with dairy products or antacids as these products can decrease absorption of the drug.
- Fluoroquinolone should be used with caution when given at high doses to cats as it can cause retinal detachment.

Danofloxacin

Clinical Uses. Danofloxacin is labeled for use in cattle (not dairy or veal) to treat BRD. It can be used in cattle by administering two injections SC 48 hours apart. The FDA prohibits extralabel use in food animals.

Dosage Form
- **Advocin sterile injectable solution**

Adverse Side Effects. Hypersensitivity may occur. Lameness in calves has been reported. SC injections in cattle may cause local irritation to tissue.

Storage of the Drug. Store at or below 30°C (86°F).

Difloxacin

Clinical Uses. Difloxacin is approved for use in dogs for treatment of bacterial infections susceptible to the drug. It is not labeled for use in cats or other species.

Dosage Form
- **Dicural tablets**

Adverse Side Effects. This drug may cause hypersensitivity. Use caution in young growing animals because it may cause cartilage abnormalities. It may also cause seizure disorders, hepatic or renal insufficiency, dehydration, and GI distress.

Storage of the Drug. Store between 15°C and 30°C (59°F and 86°F).

Enrofloxacin

Clinical Uses. Enrofloxacin is used effectively against a variety of pathogens, although it is not effective against anaerobes. It is somewhat contraindicated in growing animals because it may cause cartilage abnormalities. It is approved for use in cattle (not calves). Extralabel use is prohibited.

Dosage Form
- **Baytril tabs, soft chewable tablets**
- **Baytril 100 injectable solution**
- **Baytril otic**
- **Enroflox injectable**

Adverse Side Effects. These include GI distress, CNS stimulation, crystalluria, and hypersensitivity. Intravenous administration can be risky in small animals.

Storage of the Drug. Store in tightly sealed containers less than 30°C (86°F).

Marbofloxacin

Clinical Uses. Marbofloxacin is effective against a variety of pathogens. It has no efficacy against anaerobes.

Dosage Form
- **Zeniquin**

Adverse Side Effects. Marbofloxacin may cause hypersensitivity and GI distress. It is not for use in young growing animals because of the potential for cartilage abnormalities.

Storage of the Drug. Store at or below 30°C (86°F).

Orbifloxacin

Clinical Uses. This drug is used in dogs and cats for bacterial infections susceptible to orbifloxacin. It can help in the treatment of susceptible gram-negative infections in horses.

Dosage Forms
- **Orbax**
- **Orbax tablets**

Adverse Side Effects. Orbifloxacin may cause GI upset.

Storage of the Drug. Store between 2.22°C and 30°C (36°F and 86°F).

Pradofloxacin

Clinical Uses. Pradofloxacin is a bactericidal antibiotic; activity against gram-negative, gram-positive, and anaerobic bacteria. It is approved for the treatment of skin infections in cats caused by strains of Pasteurella multocidia, Streptococcus canis, Staphylococcus aureus, S. felis, and S. pseudintermedius (Plumb, 2015).

Dosage Forms
- **Veraflox oral suspension for cats**

Adverse Side Effects. Pradofloxacin appears to be well tolerated at recommended dosages with occasional diarrhea. It is not approved for use in dogs.

Storage of the Drug. Store at room temperature.

TECHNICIAN NOTES

- The safety of fluoroquinolones in breeding or pregnant dogs and cats has not been determined.
- Fluoroquinolones cannot be used in cattle intended for dairy production or in veal calves.
- Fluoroquinolones cannot be used in laying hens that produce eggs for human consumption.
- Carefully read labels regarding withdrawal periods for animals intended for slaughter.

℞ Sulfonamides

Pharmacodynamics/Pharmacokinetics. Sulfonamides are bacteriostatic agents when used alone. It is thought that they prevent bacterial replication by competing with para-aminobenzoic acid (PABA) in the biosynthesis of tetrahydrofolic acid in the pathway to form folic acid. Only microorganisms that make their own folic acid are affected by sulfa drugs. Sulfonamides are readily absorbed from the GI tract of nonruminant animals. Peak levels occur 1 to 2 hours after administration. Levels tend to be highest in the liver, kidney, and lungs and lower in muscle and bone. Sulfonamides are excreted from the body by the kidneys with some action by the liver (Plumb, 2015).

Sulfachlorpyridazine

Clinical Uses. Sulfachlorpyridazine is used in the treatment of diarrhea in calves caused by *Escherichia coli* in those patients younger than 1 month. It is used to treat colibacillosis in swine.

Dosage Forms
- **Vetisulid tablets, Oral Suspension, injectable**

Adverse Side Effects. Sulfachlorpyridazine may precipitate in the urine. It may cause keratoconjunctivitis sicca in dogs, bone marrow depression, hypersensitivity reactions, focal retinitis, fever, vomiting, and nonseptic polyarthritis. It may be potentially teratogenic. IV injection given rapidly may cause muscle weakness, blindness, ataxia, and collapse. SC or IM injection may cause tissue irritation.

Storage of the Drug. Store at room temperature. Protect from light. Avoid freezing.

Sulfadiazine/Trimethoprim and Sulfamethoxazole/Trimethoprim

Clinical Uses. These combinations are used in dogs and horses to treat infections caused by susceptible organisms. They are effective for treating prostate infections and for infections caused by many strains of methicillin-resistant staphylococci.

Dosage Forms. All of the following are veterinary-label products.
- **Di-Trim tablets**
- **Di-Trim 24%, 48% injection**
- **Tribrissen 400 Oral Paste**
- **Tribrissen 48% Injection**
- **Tucoprim Powder**
- **Uniprim Powder**

Adverse Side Effects. Keratoconjunctivitis sicca, hypersensitivity, acute neutrophilic hepatitis with icterus, vomiting, anorexia, diarrhea, fever, hemolytic anemia, urticaria, polyarthritis, facial swelling, polydipsia, crystalluria, hematuria, polyuria, cholestasis, hypothyroidism, anemias, agranulocytosis, idiosyncratic hepatic necrosis in dogs, and potentially teratogenicity, are all possible.

Storage of the Drug. Store at room temperatures in tightly sealed containers.

TECHNICIAN NOTES

- It may be necessary to monitor tear production in animals that are on long-term treatment with sulfonamides.

Sulfadimethoxine

Clinical Uses. This drug is for use in dogs and cats for respiratory, genitourinary, enteric, and soft tissue infections. It is used in the treatment of coccidiosis in dogs, but the use of this drug is not FDA approved for this indication. Sulfadimethoxine is used in horses to treat *Streptococcus equi*. It is used in cattle to treat shipping fever complex, calf diphtheria, bacterial pneumonia, and foot rot. In poultry, sulfadimethoxine is added to drinking water to treat coccidiosis, fowl cholera, and infectious coryza.

Dosage Forms
- **Albon Injection 40%**
- **Albon Tablets, Concentrated solution, oral suspension**
- **Albon SR** (sustained release)
- **SulfaMed**
- Various others

Adverse Side Effects. Sulfadimethoxine may precipitate in the urine, may contribute to the risk of crystalluria, hematuria, and renal tubule obstruction. It causes the same adverse effects as seen with other sulfonamides.

Storage of the Drug. Store at room temperature in tightly sealed containers.

Sulfadimethoxine/Ormetoprim

Clinical Uses. This combination is FDA approved for the treatment of skin and soft tissue infections in dogs caused by *S. aureus* and *E. coli*. Rofenaid is used for enhanced broad-spectrum antibacterial activity and aids in the prevention of coccidiosis in chickens and turkeys.

Dosage Forms
- Primor
- Rofenaid 40
- Romet 30

Adverse Side Effects. These are the same as seen with other sulfonamides.

Storage of the Drug. Store in tightly sealed containers at room temperature.

℞ Antibacterials

Aztreonam

Clinical Uses. Aztreonam is used in small animals to fight serious infections caused by a wide variety of bacteria. It has been used for the treatment of infections caused by gram-negative microorganisms.

Dosage Forms
- Azactam
- Cayston

Adverse Side Effects. In humans, known side effects include colitis, pain or swelling after IM injection, and phlebitis after IV administration.

Storage of the Drug. Store powder for reconstitution at room temperature.

Chloramphenicol

Clinical Uses. Chloramphenicol is an amphenicol and is used to treat a variety of infections in small animals and horses, especially those caused by anaerobic bacteria. It is a broad-spectrum bacteriostatic antibiotic that is effective against gram-positive, gram-negative, and anaerobic bacteria including meningitis, chronic bronchitis, pyoderma, rickettsia, mycoplasma, and chlamydia.

Dosage Forms
- Chloramphenicol Capsules

- **Chloromycetin tablets, ophthalmic ointment**
- **Viceton tablets**
- **Mychel-Vet capsules, tablets, injection**

TECHNICIAN NOTES

- Chloramphenicol is very stable and residual amounts of the drug can be left in meat, milk, or eggs. Therefore, the FDA has prohibited the use of chloramphenicol in food animals because of human public health implications.
- Chloramphenicol is not recommended for dogs maintained for breeding purposes.
- Chloramphenicol should not be administered simultaneously with penicillin, streptomycin, or the cephalosporins.

Adverse Side Effects. Chloramphenicol may cause aplastic anemia in humans.

Storage of the Drug. Store in tightly sealed containers at room temperature.

Dapsone

Clinical Uses. Dapsone is useful in the treatment of mycobacterial diseases in dogs and possibly cats. It may be useful in the adjunct treatment of brown recluse spider (*Loxosceles reclusa recluse*) bites.

Dosage Form
- **Dapsone Oral Tablets** (human label)

Adverse Side Effects. Dapsone may cause hepatotoxicity, dose-dependent methemoglobinemia, hemolytic anemia, thrombocytopenia, neutropenias, GI disturbance, neuropathies, cutaneous drug eruptions, and photosensitivity. It may possibly be a carcinogen.

Storage of the Drug. Store at room temperature.

Florfenicol

Clinical Uses. Florfenicol is an amphenicol and is FDA approved for use in cattle in the treatment of BRD. It is also effective against rickettsia, mycoplasma, and chlamydia.

Dosage Forms
- **NuFlor**
- **NuFlor Gold**
- **NuFlor Concentrate Solution**
- **Aquaflor**
- **Resflor Gold**

TECHNICIAN NOTES

- Florfenicol is not approved for use in female dairy cattle 20 months or older and should not be used in veal calves, calves younger than 1 month old, or calves receiving an all-milk diet.
- Florfenicol is for IM injection only. Injections should be administered into the neck, and no more than 10 mL should be given per site.

Adverse Side Effects. Florfenicol may cause anorexia, decreased water consumption, and diarrhea. Reactions may be severe if injected at sites other than the neck. Anaphylaxis and collapse have been reported in cattle.

Storage of the Drug. Store between 2.22°C and 30°C (36°F and 86°F).

Fosfomycin

Clinical Uses. Fosfomycin is useful in the treatment of multidrug-resistant urinary tract infections in dogs.

Dosage Form
- **Monurol** (human label)

Adverse Side Effects. Very little information about adverse effects in animals is known. In humans, it may cause diarrhea. In cats, renal tubular damage may occur.

Storage of the Drug. Store at room temperature.

Isoniazid

Clinical Uses. Isoniazid is sometimes used for chemoprophylaxis in small animals that live in households with a human that has tuberculosis.

Dosage Forms
- **Nydrazid** (human label)
- **Rifater** (human label)
- **Rifamate** (human label)

Adverse Side Effects. Hepatotoxicity, CNS stimulation, peripheral neuropathy and thrombocytopenia, ataxia, seizures, salivation, diarrhea, vomiting, and arrhythmias have been reported.

Storage of the Drug. Store at temperatures below 40°C (104°F).

Metronidazole

Clinical Uses. Metronidazole is a nitroimidazole and is used in the treatment of *Giardia* in both dogs and cats. In horses, the drug has been used for the treatment of anaerobic infections.

Dosage Forms
- **Flagyl**
- **Metronidazole**

 TECHNICIAN NOTES

Metronidazole is prohibited for use in food animals by the FDA.

Adverse Side Effects. Metronidazole may cause neurologic disorders, lethargy, weakness, neutropenias, hepatotoxicity, hematuria, anorexia, nausea, vomiting, and diarrhea. In horses, there have been reported cases of *Clostridium difficile* and *Clostridium perfringens* diarrhea and death after the use of metronidazole.

Storage of the Drug. Store at room temperature.

Nitrofurantoin

Clinical Uses. Nitrofurantoin is used to treat urinary tract infections.

Dosage Forms
- **Macrodantin** (human label)
- **Macrobid** (human label)
- **Furadantin** (human label)

 TECHNICIAN NOTES

- Except for approved topical use, nitrofurantoin has been prohibited in food-producing animals.
- Nitrofurantoin should not be used in veal calves.

Adverse Side Effects. Nitrofurantoin may cause GI disturbance and hepatopathy.

Storage of the Drug. Store at room temperature and protect from the light.

Novobiocin

Clinical Uses. When used in combination with penicillin G, these two drugs are used in dry dairy cattle as a mastitis tube.

Dosage Forms
- **Albamix feed medication**
- **Albadry Plus suspension**
- **Albaplex capsules, tablets**
- **Delta Albaplex 3X tablets**
- **Drygard suspension**
- **Biodry suspension**

Adverse Side Effects. When used systemically, novobiocin may cause fever, GI disturbances, and blood dyscrasias.

Storage of the Drug. Store in tightly sealed containers at room temperature.

Rifampin

Clinical Uses. The principle use of rifampin in veterinary medicine is for treatment of *R. equi* infections in young horses. In small animals, it may be used in conjunction with antifungal agents in the treatment of histoplasmosis.

Dosage Forms
- **Rimactane** (human label)
- **Rifadin** (human label)

Adverse Side Effects. Rifampin may cause red-or-ange colored urine, tears, sweat, and saliva. There are no harmful consequences from this effect (Plumb, 2015).

Storage of the Drug. Store in tightly sealed containers at room temperature.

Tiamulin

Clinical Uses. Tiamulin is used in swine to treat pneumonia and swine dysentery.

Dosage Forms
- **Denagard 10, Dengard 5**
- **Denagard Liquid Concentrate**
- **TiaGard**
- **Deracin**

Adverse Side Effects. These are considered unlikely.

Storage of the Drug. Protect from moisture and store in a dry place.

Vancomycin

Clinical Uses. Vancomycin is used to treat methicillin-resistant *Staphylococcus* spp. (MRSA).

Dosage Form
- **Vancocin**

Adverse Side Effects. Nephrotoxicity and ototoxicity are the most serious potential adverse effects.

Storage of the Drug. Store in tightly sealed containers at room temperature.

See Table 12.5 for a summary of commonly used antimicrobial agents.

Antifungal Agents

Pharmacodynamics/Pharmacokinetics. Ketoconazole is fungistatic against susceptible fungi. It is believed that some antifungal agents increase cellular membrane permeability and cause secondary metabolic effects and growth inhibition. Some antifungals are readily absorbed after oral administration, whereas other antifungal agents must be given IV.

Amphotericin B

Clinical Uses. Amphotericin B is a systemic antifungal used for serious mycotic infections. It must be administered IV.

Dosage Forms
- **Fungizone** (human label)

TECHNICIAN NOTES

- Amphotericin B is administered intravenously through dilution in 5% dextrose.
- Renal function should be monitored closely during treatment.

Adverse Side Effects. Amphotericin B is nephrotoxic. Renal function monitoring must be done.

Storage of the Drug. Vials of amphotericin B powder for injection should be stored in the refrigerator and protected from light and moisture.

Fluconazole

Clinical Uses. Fluconazole is useful in the treatment of systemic mycoses such as cryptococcal meningitis, blastomycosis, and histoplasmosis.

Dosage Forms
- **Diflucan** (human label)
- **Viaflex Plus** (human label)

Adverse Side Effects. There is only limited experience with this drug in domestic animals. So far, it seems safe for use in dogs and cats. Some side effects include inappetence, vomiting, and diarrhea.

Storage of the Drug. Store at temperatures less than 30°C (86°F) in tightly sealed containers.

Flucytosine

Clinical Uses. This drug is active against strains of *Cryptococcus* and *Candida*.

Dosage Form
- **Ancobon** (human label)

Adverse Side Effects. Flucytosine may cause GI disturbances, dose-dependent bone marrow depression, cutaneous eruption, oral ulceration, and increased levels of hepatic enzymes.

Storage of the Drug. Store preferably at room temperature.

TABLE 12.5 Summary of Classes of Antibacterial Agents Commonly Used in Veterinary Patients.[a]

Class	Examples	Primary Spectrum of Activity	Side Effects and Notes Regarding Use
Penicillins MOA: interfere with development of bacterial cell wall (bactericidal)	Penicillins: narrow spectrum • Penicillin G • Penicillin V	• Gram-positive aerobes • Obligate anaerobes	• Diarrhea • Hypersensitivity reactions
	Penicillins: aminopenicillins • Ampicillin • Amoxicillin		
	Penicillins: potentiated aminopenicillins • Amoxicillin + Clavulanate	• Also effective against beta-lactamase–producing *Staphylococcus* • Gram-negative aerobes	
	Beta-lactamase resistant: • Cloxacillin • Dicloxacillin • Oxacillin	Spectrum of activity is slightly less than that of penicillins and aminopenicillins	
Cephalosporins MOA: interfere with development of bacterial cell wall (bactericidal)	Cephalosporins: first generation • Cefazolin • Cephalexin • Cefadroxil • Cephapirin	• Gram-positive aerobes • Penicillinase-producing *Staphylococcus*	• Diarrhea • Vomiting, anorexia • Hypersensitivity reactions
	Cephalosporins: second generation • Cefotetan • Cefoxitin	• More gram-negative efficacy than first-generation, but slightly less gram-positive efficacy	
	Cephalosporins: third generation • Cefpodoxime • Ceftiofur • Ceftriaxone • Cefovecin	• Even more gram-negative efficacy, with significantly less gram-positive efficacy	
Aminoglycosides MOA: inhibit bacterial ribosomal protein production (bactericidal)	Gentamicin Amikacin Neomycin	• Gram-negative aerobes	• Kidney toxicity • Otic toxicity • Avoid use in dehydrated patients • Poor gastrointestinal (GI) absorption, mainly administered parenterally
Sulfonamides MOA: inhibit bacterial production of folic acid (unpotentiated sulfonamides: bacteriostatic; potentiated sulfonamides: bactericidal)	Sulfonamides • Sulfadiazine • Sulfamethoxazole • Sulfadimethoxine Potentiated sulfonamides • Sulfadiazine + trimethoprim • Sulfamethoxazole + trimethoprim • Sulfadimethoxine + ormetoprim	• Gram-positive aerobes • Gram-negative aerobes • Some protozoa	• Diarrhea • Bone marrow suppression • Hypersensitivity reactions in dogs involving joints, bone marrow, skin, liver, and dry eye • Teratogenic

Continued

Class	Examples	Primary Spectrum of Activity	Side Effects and Notes Regarding Use
Fluoroquinolones MOA: disrupts bacterial DNA supercoiling and storage (bactericidal)	Enrofloxacin Orbifloxacin Marbofloxacin Ciprofloxacin Difloxacin Pradofloxacin	• Gram-negative aerobes • *Brucella* • *Chlamydia* • *Mycobacterium* • Mycoplasma • Rickettsia	• Diarrhea • Young animals—cartilage damage • Cats—blindness • Seizures (in patients with history of seizures) • Should not be used during pregnancy • Ciprofloxacin contraindicated in horses
Amphenicols MOA: bind to ribosomes and inhibit bacterial protein synthesis (bacteriostatic at standard doses)	Chloramphenicol Florfenicol	• Gram-positive aerobes • Gram-negative aerobes • Obligate anaerobes • *Rickettsia* • *Chlamydia* • *Mycoplasma*	• Diarrhea • Bone marrow suppression • Gloves to be worn when handling tablets to avoid accidental absorption • Chloramphenicol use illegal in food-producing animals • Florfenicol approved for use in cattle
Macrolides MOA: inhibit bacterial protein synthesis (bacteriostatic)	Erythromycin Clarithromycin Tilmicosin Azithromycin Tylosin	• Gram-positive aerobes • Obligate anaerobes • Penicillinase-producing *Staphylococcus* • *Mycoplasma*	• Diarrhea • Erythromycin and tylosin may cause fatal diarrhea in horses
Lincosamides MOA: inhibit bacterial protein synthesis (bacteriostatic at lower concentrations, bactericidal at higher concentrations)	Clindamycin Lincomycin Pirlimycin	• Gram-positive aerobes • Obligate anaerobes • *Mycoplasma*	• Diarrhea • Contraindicated in horses
Tetracyclines MOA: bind to bacterial ribosomes and inhibit protein synthesis (bacteriostatic)	Tetracycline Oxytetracycline Doxycycline Minocycline	• Gram-positive aerobes • *Chlamydia* • *Rickettsia* • *Borrelia* • *Mycoplasma*	• Diarrhea • Esophageal strictures in cats • Decreased oral absorption when given with calcium- and iron-containing products, antacids, and sucralfate • Bind to enamel of developing teeth in neonates, causing yellow discoloration • Doxycycline (intravenous) contraindicated in horses
Nitroimidazoles MOA: disrupt bacterial synthesis of DNA and nucleic acids (bactericidal/protozoacidal)	Metronidazole Ronidazole	• Obligate anaerobes • Protozoa	• Neurotoxicity (dose related) • Use illegal in food-producing animals

aIncluding spectrum of activity, mechanism of action (MOA), and clinically important side effects.
Modified 2019 from Bassert, J. M. (2018). *McCurnin's clinical textbook for veterinary technicians* (9th ed.) St. Louis: Missouri.

Griseofulvin

Clinical Uses. Griseofulvin is used in dogs and cats to treat dermatophytic fungal infections of the skin, hair, and claws. It is used to treat ringworm in horses. Griseofulvin is a fungistatic drug that is FDA approved for systemic administration to treat superficial fungal diseases including *Trichophyton* and *Microsporum* species.

Dosage Forms
- **Fulvicin U/F tablets, powder, Bolus**
- **Griseofulvin powder**

 TECHNICIAN NOTES

- Griseofulvin should not be administered to pregnant or breeding animals.
- Absorption of griseofulvin is enhanced by administration with a fatty meal.

Adverse Side Effects. Griseofulvin may cause anorexia, vomiting, diarrhea, anemia, neutropenia, leukopenia, thrombocytopenia, depression, ataxia, hepatoxicity, dermatitis/photosensitivity, and toxic epidermal necrolysis. Cats are more susceptible to adverse side effects.
Storage of the Drug. Store at less than 40°C (104°F).

Itraconazole

Clinical Uses. Itraconazole may be used to treat systemic mycoses. It is probably more effective than ketoconazole but is much more expensive than ketoconazole. Itraconazole is considered by many to be the drug of choice for treating blastomycosis.

Dosage Forms
- **Itrafungol**
Adverse Side Effects. Anorexia in dogs and hepatic toxicity may occur.
Storage of the Drug. Store between 15°C and 25°C (59°F and 77°F).

Ketoconazole

Clinical Uses. Ketoconazole is used to treat fungal infections in dogs, cats, and other small species. Use of ketoconazole in cats is controversial, and some say it should never be used in that species. It can also be used for the medical treatment of hyperadrenocorticism in dogs.

Dosage Forms
- **Ketoconazole tablets** (human label)
Adverse Side Effects. Ketoconazole may cause GI disturbances and hepatic toxicity. Ketoconazole may cause infertility in male dogs.

Storage of the Drug. Store in tightly sealed containers at room temperature.

Nystatin

Clinical Uses. Nystatin is a topical antifungal ointment or cream used to treat *Candida* infections.
Dosage Forms
- **Panalog ointment, cream**
- **Animax ointment, cream**
- **Derma-Vet ointment, cream**
Adverse Side Effects. Nystatin may cause hypersensitivity.
Storage of the Drug. Store at room temperature in tightly sealed, light-resistant containers.

Voriconazole

Clinical Uses. Voriconazole is used to treat a variety of fungal infections in veterinary patients. There is some interest in treating birds for aspergillosis with this drug.
Dosage Forms
- **Vfend** (human label)
Adverse Side Effects. Accurate information in veterinary medicine is limited. Liver enlargement may occur. Cats tend to have many more side effects.
Storage of the Drug. Store below 30°C (86°F).

℞ Antiviral Agents

Antiviral agents are used to treat viruses. The current drugs on the market are used in the treatment of herpes simplex types 1 and 2, cytomegalovirus, Epstein-Barr, and varicella-zoster viruses. Elimination half-lives in dogs, cats, and horses for acyclovir are about 3 hours.

Acyclovir

Clinical Uses. Acyclovir is useful in treating herpes infections in a variety of avian species and in cats with corneal or conjunctival herpes infections. It should be used with caution in veterinary patients because information about using this drug is not well established in animal patients. Acyclovir is being investigated as a treatment for equine herpes virus type-1 myeloencephalopathy in horses, but its clinical efficacy has not been proven at this time (Plumb, 2015).
Dosage Forms
- **Zovirax;** generics also (human label)
Adverse Side Effects. Acyclovir may cause GI disturbances when given orally.
Storage of the Drug. Store in tightly sealed, light-resistant containers at room temperature.

Famciclovir

Clinical Uses. Famciclovir may be useful in the treatment of feline herpes infections

Dosage Form
• **Famvir** (human label)

Adverse Side Effects. These are not well documented. Famciclovir appears to be well tolerated when used for up to 3 weeks.

Storage of the Drug. Store at room temperature.

Interferon Alfa

Pharmacokinetics/Therapeutics. Interferon has antiviral, antiproliferative, and immunomodulating effects. This is thought to occur by its effects on the synthesis of RNA, DNA, and cellular proteins. Interferon alfa is used in cats to treat feline viruses and a variety of dermatologic conditions. The mechanisms for its antineoplastic activities are not well understood but are probably also related to these effects (Plumb, 2015). This drug must be diluted in saline and may be available through compounding pharmacies.

Dosage Forms
• **Intron A** (human label)
• **Alferon N** (human label)

Adverse Side Effects. In cats, no adverse effects are common.

Storage of the Drug. Refrigeration is necessary.

Lysine

Clinical Uses. Lysine may be effective in suppressing feline herpesvirus (FHV-1) infections in cats. Lysine is an amino acid that is thought to compete with arginine for incorporation into many herpes viruses (Plumb, 2015).

Dosage Forms
• **Viralys Gel**
• **Viralys Powder**
• **L-Lysine Powder-Pure**

Adverse Side Effects. These are unlikely when mixed with food.

Storage of the Drug. Store at room temperature.

Oseltamivir

Clinical Uses. Oseltamivir has been suggested as a treatment for canine parvovirus infections. Some studies have been performed to ascertain the effectiveness of this drug in equines infected with equine influenza.

Dosage Form. In 2006, the FDA banned the extralabel use of oseltamivir and other influenza antivirals in chickens, turkeys, and ducks (Plumb, 2015).
• **Tamiflu** (human label)

Adverse Side Effects. No information in animals is available.

Storage of the Drug. Store at or below 25°C (77°F).

Zidovudine

Clinical Uses. Zidovudine may be useful in treating feline immunodeficiency virus (FIV) or feline leukemia virus (FeLV).

Dosage Form. Only human-label products are available.
• **Retrovir**

Adverse Side Effects. In cats, reductions in red blood cells, packed cell volume, and hemoglobin are the most commonly reported adverse effects. Diarrhea and weakness have also been reported.

Storage of the Drug. Store at room temperature.

® Disinfectants/Antiseptics

There are many different types of disinfectants that are used in veterinary medicine: chlorines, phenols, quaternary ammonium compounds, and many others. Disinfectants are antimicrobial agents that are used on inanimate (nonliving) objects to destroy microorganisms such as bacteria, viruses, and fungi. Antiseptics are antimicrobial agents that are used on living tissue to inactivate or destroy microorganisms such as alcohols and biguanide compounds. Sometimes the same compound may act as an antiseptic and a disinfectant, depending on the drug concentration, conditions of exposure, number of organisms, etc. To achieve maximal efficiency, it is essential to use the proper concentration of the drug for the purpose intended (Wickstrom, 2015).

Biguanide Compounds

Chlorhexidine is the most common disinfectant in this group. In high dilutions, it is bactericidal, fungicidal, and active against enveloped viruses (e.g., feline infectious peritonitis virus and FeLV). Other viruses, spores, and mycobacteria are relatively resistant.

Clinical Uses. These include disinfecting surgical instruments, anesthetic equipment, and kennels. It is also available as a surgical scrub and a teat dip.

Dosage Forms
• **Chlorhexidine solution, scrub**
• **Nolvadent oral solution**
• **Nolvasan solution**
• **Nolvasan surgical scrub**
• **Virosan solution**

Adverse Side Effects. Adverse side effects are uncommon.

Chlorines and Iodines

Chlorines and iodines are halogens that inactivate pathogens by oxidizing free sulfhydryl groups on bacterial enzymes. Chlorines are bactericidal, exhibit high levels of activity against viruses, and are fungicidal and tuberculocidal unless highly diluted. Iodines and iodophors are bactericidal, exhibit high levels of activity against viruses, are fungicidal and tuberculocidal, and are effective against bacterial spores.

Clinical Uses. Chlorines are recommended for floors, plumbing fixtures, spot disinfection, and fabrics not harmed by bleaching. Iodine tincture is used for skin preparations and thermometers. Iodophors are used to disinfect thermometers, utensils, rubber goods, and dishes and for presurgical skin preparation.

Dosage Forms
- **Sodium hypochlorite**
- **Clorox bleach**
- **Iodine tincture (7%)**
- **Betadine surgical scrub**
- **Povidone solution**

Adverse Side Effects. The strong vapor of chlorines may irritate the eyes and mucous membranes. Skin irritation may result from failure to rinse a chlorine-disinfected surface. Chlorine bleaches colored fabrics and is corrosive to most metals. Tinctures of iodine contain alcohol and are drying to the skin. They stain and may corrode metal. Iodophors may corrode metal. Iodine solutions stain and may corrode metal, and high concentrations (3.5%) may irritate living tissue.

 TECHNICIAN NOTES

- These compounds are inactivated by organic material.
- Always check labels for dilution requirements (more is *not* better).
- Iodophors are less staining and irritating than other iodine compounds.

Ethylene Oxide

Ethylene oxide works via substitution of cell alkyl groups for labile hydrogen atoms. It sterilizes against bacteria, fungi, and viruses. This gas, which should be handled carefully when used by veterinary personnel, may irritate the lungs and cause chemical burns if skin contact occurs. The gas is flammable and is considered to be a human carcinogen. When inanimate objects are sterilized, this gas must be used with proper ventilation and according to proper Occupational Safety and Health Administration (OSHA) standards.

Clinical Uses. Ethylene oxide is used to sterilize inanimate objects such as blankets, pillows, mattresses, instruments with lenses, rubber goods, thermolabile plastics, books, and papers.

Adverse Side Effects. Adverse side effects are uncommon if ethylene oxide is used according to proper OSHA standards and with good ventilation.

 TECHNICIAN NOTES

- Special equipment is required when ethylene oxide is used as a sterilization gas.
- After rubber boots are sterilized with this gas, it is best to let them "air" for several hours before donning them, to prevent chemical burns to the skin of the feet.
- Proper ventilation (refer to OSHA standards) must be employed when this gas is used.

Phenolics: Saponated Cresol and Semisynthetic Phenols

The mode of action of phenolics is protein coagulation. They destroy selective permeability of cell membranes; leakage of cell constituents results. They are effective against bacteria, fungi, and some viruses, but they are not sporicidal and are only weakly effective against nonenveloped viruses (e.g., parvovirus). Cresol must be used in soft water and is slow-acting. Organic matter, soap, or hard water (except cresol) does not inactivate phenolics. They have high detergency and a residual effect if allowed to dry on surfaces.

Clinical Uses. These include use as a general disinfectant for laundry, floors, walls, and equipment.

Dosage Forms
- **Amphyl**
- **Lysol Disinfectant Spray**

Adverse Side Effects. Adverse side effects are uncommon, but repeated and prolonged skin exposure may result in accumulation in tissue and eventual toxic effects such as neurotoxicity or teratogenicity.

 TECHNICIAN NOTES

Some phenolics have objectionable odors.

Quaternary Ammonium Compounds: Cationic Detergents

Cationic detergents concentrate at the cell membrane and are thought to act by dissolving lipids in cell walls

TABLE 12.6   Disinfectant Preparations and Their Activity.

Disinfectant Group	Proprietary Products	Recommendations	Bactericidal	Virucide	Fungicidal	Sporicidal at Room Temperature
Quaternary ammonium compounds	Roccal-D Plus	Dairy equipment, floors, walls, rubber goods	M	M	M	N
Phenolics	Panteck Cleanser	Laundry rinse, floors, walls, equipment	M	M	H	N
	Lysol I.C. Disinfectant Spray					
Halogens	*Chlorines:* Clorox, Purex	Floors, spot disinfection	M	H	H	S
	Iodophors: Betadine, Povidone solution	Presurgical skin preparation, thermometers, dairy operation	H	H	M	S
Glutaraldehyde	Cidex	Instruments	H	H	H	M
Chlorhexidine	Nolvasan, Virosan	Instruments, surgical scrub, dairy operation	M	M	M	N
Alcohols	Isopropyl alcohol 70%	Instruments, thermometers, skin preparation	H	N	S	N

H, High activity; *M,* moderate activity; *N,* no activity; *S,* slight activity.

and membranes. They are more active against gram-positive than against gram-negative organisms. They are bacteriostatic at high dilutions, but spores, viruses, mycobacteria, and *Pseudomonas aeruginosa* are relatively resistant. Organic debris, hard water, and anionic soaps and detergents inactivate quaternary ammonium compounds.

Clinical Uses. These include cleaning of inanimate objects such as floors, walls, and rubber goods.

Dosage Forms

• **Roccal-D Plus**

Adverse Side Effects. Adverse side effects are uncommon.

 TECHNICIAN NOTES

Read labels carefully because some quaternary ammonium compounds do not effectively disinfect against some common viruses (e.g., parvovirus).

See Table 12.6 for a summary of disinfectant preparations and their activity.

Other Disinfectants/Antiseptics

Soaps. Soaps, or anionic detergents, have only slight bactericidal activity but are effective in the mechanical removal of organisms. They are not sporicidal or tuberculocidal and have limited virucidal activity. They often contain germicides, such as triclosan, that decrease the number of resident flora after washing. Their mode of action is the same as that of cationic detergents.

Organic Mercury Compounds. These compounds such as merbromin (Mercurochrome) and thimerosal (Merthiolate) may be used as antiseptics. They have only slight bactericidal activity.

Alkalis. Alkalis such as lye and quicklime may be used for disinfecting stables and premises.

Hydrogen Peroxide. Hydrogen peroxide is an oxidizing agent that is available as a 3% aqueous solution and may be used for cleaning and disinfecting wounds and as a mouthwash for septic stomatitis.

Glutaraldehyde. Glutaraldehyde is a dialdehyde that is bactericidal, virucidal, fungicidal, and sporicidal. It is not inactivated by organic debris. Its uses include disinfecting surgical instruments, anesthetic equipment, floors, walls, and nonfood contact surfaces.

REVIEW QUESTIONS

1. Different types of bacteria can be distinguished with the use of a _____ stain.
2. Gram-positive bacteria will stain what color?
3. Gram-negative bacteria will stain what color?
4. _____ is approved for use in lactating dairy animals.
5. _____ can cause staining of teeth in young animals.
6. _____ should never be given intravenously to horses.
7. Some aminoglycosides may be _____ toxic and/or _____ toxic.
8. Griseofulvin is used to treat _____.
9. A drug's _____ of activity is the range of bacteria affected by its action.
10. Aerobes are bacteria that require oxygen to live.
    a. True
    b. False
11. A fungicidal agent inhibits the growth of fungi.
    a. True
    b. False
12. A bacteriostatic agent inhibits the growth of bacteria.
    a. True
    b. False
13. Penicillin-G benzathine is a long-acting antibiotic that is approved for use in dairy animals.
    a. True
    b. False
14. Doxycycline is classified as a(n)_____.
    a. penicillin
    b. cephalosporin
    c. aminoglycoside
    d. tetracycline
15. Enrofloxacin is a _____.
    a. penicillin
    b. cephalosporin
    c. fluoroquinolone
    d. tetracycline
16. Describe the difference between a disinfectant and an antiseptic.
17. What is the term for an agent that kills bacteria?
18. What class of antibiotic drug should only be given to adult (mature) animals as administration in young animals can result in alterations in cartilage growth?
    a. Aminoglycosides
    b. Fluoroquinolones
    c. Lincosamides
    d. Penicillins
19. Which one of the following drugs would be contraindicated in an animal with otitis interna and renal disease?
    a. Aminoglycosides
    b. Macrolides
    c. Fluoroquinolones
    d. All of the above
20. Which one of the following is a good antibiotic choice for treating stomatitis?
    a. Metronidazole
    b. Doxycycline
    c. Clindamycin
    d. Erythromycin
21. Some bacteria produce an enzyme called _____ that degrades penicillin.
22. A bacteria can mutate or develop resistance to drugs due to:
    a. overuse of an antibiotic
    b. low doses of antibiotics
    c. not following the full course of antibiotics
    d. all of the above
23. Monitoring tear production may be indicated when a patient is on long-term treatment of which antibiotic?
    a. Penicillin
    b. Sulfonamides
    c. Tetracycline
    d. Lincomycin
24. A Border collie pup weighing 15 lb is presented to the veterinarian. The dog is infected with *Isospora canis*. The veterinarian orders sulfadimethoxine for treatment. The dosage is 55 mg/kg PO initially on the first day of therapy, then 27.5 mg/kg PO for 9 days. On hand in the pharmacy are 250-mg tablets. How many tablets should be dispensed for this patient?
    a. 10.5 tablets
    b. 20.5 tablets
    c. 15.5 tablets
    d. 30.5 tablets

25. A Holstein cow diagnosed with bovine respiratory syncytial virus (BRSV) needs to be treated. The veterinarian orders tilmicosin at a dosage of 10 mg/kg SC. On hand in the pharmacy is a parenteral product with a concentration of 300 mg/mL. If the cow weighs 900 lb, how many milliliters should be obtained for treatment?

a. 12.6 mL
b. 15.6 mL
c. 13.6 mL
d. 14.6 mL

REFERENCES

Bill, R. L. (2017). *Clinical pharmacology and therapeutics for veterinary technicians* (4th ed.). St. Louis, MO: Elsevier.

Elanco. (2010). *Package insert for Micotil*. Indianapolis, Indiana: Elanco.

Nobelprizeorg. Sir Alexander Fleming – Biographical. NobelPrize.org. Nobel Media AB 2020. Sat. 23 May 2020. https://www.nobelprize.org/prizes/medicine/1945/fleming/biographical/. From Nobel Lectures, Physiology or Medicine 1942-1962, Elsevier Publishing Company, Amsterdam, 1964.

Papich, M. (2016). *Saunders handbook of veterinary drugs* (4th ed.). St. Louis: MO.

Plumb, D. C. (2015). *Veterinary drug handbook* (8th ed.). Ames, IA: Wiley-Blackwell.

Werth BJ. Cephalosporins. (2018). In "The Merck veterinary manual" (online edition) http:merckveterinarymanual.com/. Accessed August 2019.

Wickstrom ML. Overview of Antiseptics and Disinfectants. (2015). In "The Merck veterinary manual" (online edition) http:merckveterinarymanual.com/. Accessed April 2020.

13

Antiparasitic Drugs

OBJECTIVES

After studying this chapter, you should be able to

1. List and discuss the five types of symbiotic relationships of parasites.
2. Define *parasitiasis* and describe the differences between ectoparasites and endoparasites.
3. Identify the different classes of parasiticides and any contraindications for each particular class.
4. Discuss protozoa and describe antiprotozoal drugs.
5. Discuss heartworm disease, including the clinical signs, heartworm disease treatment, the risks involved, the role of *Wolbachia*, and the American

Heartworm Society 2018 recommended heartworm management protocol in dogs.
6. Name common heartworm preventative products and identify the products that treat and control other parasites.
7. Discuss ectoparasites and various application systems used to control them in animals.
8. Name the ingredients found in common insecticides.
9. Discuss the use of organophosphates.

OUTLINE

KEY TERMS

Anthelmintic

Bots

Caval syndrome

Ectoparasite

Endoparasite

Helminths

Microfilaria

Nematodes

Organophosphate

Parasitiasis

Parasitosis

Symbiosis

Vermicide

Vermifuge

Wolbachia

INTRODUCTION

Controlling parasites in companion animals is a high priority for veterinary medicine. Some people get squeamish when talking about worms, but once the subject is broached, most clients listen intently to what is being said. Veterinary technicians play an important role in educating clients about the life cycle of parasites and the current products used to eradicate them, and in explaining how important the health of the public is to veterinary medicine in terms of the removal of those parasites with zoonotic potential. This interaction gets the point across and shows how important it is to keep pets free of parasites.

TECHNICIAN NOTES

- Veterinary technicians can educate both adults and children by allowing them to view parasite eggs under the microscope during their pet's physical examination.
- Allowing a child to view parasite eggs under the microscope may be all it takes to spark the interest of a future veterinary technician.

A formalin-preserved heart infected with *Dirofilaria immitis* adults provides a great visual aid when the subject of heartworm prevention is discussed. Serum bottles with *Toxocara canis* or *Dipylidium caninum* adults also make good visual aids when client education is provided.

Parasites live on this earth in many diverse forms and relationships. Parasites lead a symbiotic life (symbiosis). Five types of symbiotic relationships have been identified: (1) predator-prey, (2) phoresis, (3) mutualism, (4) commensalism, and (5) parasitism (Hendrix, 2017). An example of a predator-prey relationship is that of a hawk that finds, captures, and eats a mouse that is running in a field. The word form *phore*, from which phoresis is derived, means *to carry*. An example of phoresis is the bacterium *Moraxella bovis*, the etiologic agent of infectious bovine keratoconjunctivitis, or pinkeye, being mechanically carried from the eyes of one cow to those of another on the sticky footpads of the face fly, *Musca autumnalis* (Hendrix, 2017). Mutualism occurs when both members of a symbiotic relationship gain from each other. An example of mutualism is the ciliated protozoa that live in the rumen of a cow. The cow benefits by having bulk and fiber digested more readily, and the ciliates benefit because the rumen provides a warm, liquid environment in which to live. Commensalism is a type of symbiotic relationship in which one symbiont benefits, but the other symbiont is not harmed. An example of commensalism is mistletoe growing in the top of a tree. Lastly, parasitism occurs when one species lives at the expense of another. An example of parasitism is *Trichuris vulpis* that live in the cecum of the canine.

Sometimes, an animal may harbor a parasite on or within its body that is potentially pathogenic, but the animal does not exhibit any outward signs (i.e., clinical disease) of parasitism. This is known as parasitiasis. If, however, the animal harbors a parasite on or within its body, and injury occurs to the animal because of the parasite, this is known as parasitosis. Parasites living on the outside of an animal's body are known as ectoparasites (e.g., fleas and ticks), and parasites living on the inside of an animal's body are known as endoparasites (e.g., canine heartworms). An animal with ectoparasites is said to be infested, and an animal with endoparasites is said to be infected. Sometimes, a parasite may wander from its normal location in the host's body to another location where it does not normally live. These parasites are said to be aberrant (erratic). Although most veterinary personnel use the lay term given to parasites when speaking with a client, it is also important for veterinary technicians to know the genus and species name of the most common parasites. The Linnaean classification scheme is fundamental in keeping parasites organized (i.e., kingdom, phylum, class, order, family, genus, and species).

Each parasite has its own individual life cycle, which may consist of several stages. Every parasite has at least a definitive host and, depending on the species, may have one or more intermediate hosts. The host that contains the adult (sexually mature) stage of the parasite is known as the definitive host, and the host that contains the immature (not sexually mature) stage of the parasite is known as the intermediate host. Knowing the life cycle of parasites helps veterinarians determine which drugs to use and how many doses will be needed to eradicate the parasite from the host animal's body.

 TECHNICIAN NOTES

Veterinary technicians need to understand and be able to explain to the client the reason for specific dosing intervals, application methods, and the importance of breaking the life-cycle to control the parasites by cleaning the environment.

Some parasites have zoonotic potential. This means they may be transmissible from animals to humans. Veterinary technicians should be familiar with which parasites have this ability so they can properly educate clients. Examples of parasites with zoonotic potential include *Toxoplasma gondii*, *Trichinella spiralis*, *Ancylostoma caninum*, and *T. canis* (Hendrix, 2017).

The Companion Animal Parasite Council (www.capcvet.org) recommends fecal centrifugation techniques to accurately diagnose endoparasitism. Additionally, the amount of feces collected for evaluation is important and should consist of at least 1 g. The specific gravity of flotation solution is equally important, in that ideally it should be 1.18 to 1.20.

 TECHNICIAN NOTES

Educating clients about how to collect a freshly voided fecal sample from a pet will result in more accurate fecal evaluations. (Tell them to bring a sample in a resealable plastic bag to each of their pets' appointments.)

Ectoparasites represent an ongoing problem faced by companion animal and livestock owners. Numerous products are manufactured for the removal of fleas and ticks from an animal's body. Because so many products are available, veterinary technicians play an important role in educating clients about the effectiveness of each product. Client education is important in the area of ectoparasites because misuse of over-the-counter insecticides can be fatal. Clients should be taught to ask veterinary personnel about the correct use of shampoos, dips, sprays, powders, and topical parasiticides (e.g., fipronil and imidacloprid) before a purchase is made.

Parasitology is a fascinating subject. However, for most clients, it is not fascinating at all because they just want their pet to be free of worms and bugs. It is up to veterinary personnel to have knowledge about available products and to remember that—as technology evolves—lifelong learning must be pursued so that professionals can remain current with how each drug or parasiticide works. Veterinary personnel have a double responsibility because it is up to them to protect both pets and their owners from those parasites with zoonotic potential and to educate clients accordingly. Veterinary medicine truly has a twofold purpose: the medical treatment of animals *and* protection of the public from health risks associated with zoonotic diseases and parasites. In some ways, veterinary medicine is more important than human medicine when it is considered from this standpoint because it represents the first defense in the protection of human health. Reading package inserts helps veterinary personnel to understand how a particular drug works. Tables 13.1 to 13.4 list products and their uses for various species.

ENDOPARASITES

Endoparasites found in the gastrointestinal (GI) tracts of animals benefit not only from the foodstuffs the animal ingests but also from body fluids (e.g., blood). Horses with increased numbers of endoparasites in the GI tract may develop colic. Puppies and kittens with increased numbers of intestinal parasites may develop fatal anemia if not treated early. Adult heartworms can cause disruption of the normal movement of blood within the heart chambers, resulting in clinical signs similar to congestive heart failure. Without treatment, a dog with active heartworm infection will die.

In the following section, some of the most common anthelmintics used in veterinary practice today are

TABLE 13.1 **Parasiticides Used for Treatment and Control of Internal Parasites in Dogs and Cats.**

Drug	Toxocara, Toxascaris	Ancylostoma, Uncinaria	Strongyloides	Trichuris	Dirofilaria Adults	Dirofilaria Microfilariae	Taenia	Dipylidium	Giardia[a]	Coccidia
Albendazole	+	+	−	+	−	−	+	−	+	−
Amprolium	−	−	−	−	−	−	−	−	−	+
Butamisole hydrochloride	−	+	−	+	−	−	−	−	−	−
Eprinomectin	+	+	−	−	−	+	−	−	−	−
Epsiprantel	−	−	−	−	−	−	+	+	−	−
Febantel	+	+	−	+	−	−	+	−	−	−
Febantel/praziquantel	+	+	−	+	−	−	+	+	−	−
Fenbendazole	+	+	−	+	−	−	+	−	−	−
Ivermectin	+	+	−	+	−	+	−	−	−	−
Melarsomine dihydrochloride	−	−	−	−	+	−	−	−	−	−
Metronidazole	−	−	−	−	−	−	−	−	+	−
Milbemycin oxime	+	+	−	+	−	+	−	−	−	−
Moxidectin	+	+	−	+	−	+	−	−	−	−
Piperazine salts	+	−	−	−	−	−	−	−	−	−
Praziquantel	−	−	−	−	−	−	+	+	−	−
Praziquantel/pyrantel pamoate	+	+	−	−	−	−	+	+	−	−
Praziquantel/pyrantel pamoate/febantel	+	+	−	+	−	−	+	+	−	−
Pyrantel pamoate	+	+	−	−	−	−	−	−	−	−
Selamectin	+	+	−	−	−	+	−	−	−	−
Sulfadiazine/trimethoprim	−	−	−	−	−	−	−	−	−	+
Sulfadimethoxine	−	−	−	−	−	−	−	−	−	+
Thiabendazole	−	−	+	−	−	−	−	−	−	−

[a]Paromomycin, an antibiotic, is being used to manage *Cryptosporidium* infections and resistant *Giardia* infections in dogs and cats.

+, Indicated for use; −, not indicated for use.

Modified from McCurnin, D. M., & Bassert, J. M. (2002). *Clinical textbook for veterinary technicians* (5th ed.). Philadelphia: WB Saunders.

TABLE 13.2 Parasiticides Used to Treat Internal Parasites in Horses.

Drug	Gasterophilus	Ascarids	Strongylus Vulgaris	Strongylus Edentatus	Small Strongyles	Pinworms	Strongyloides
Cambendazole	−	+	+	+	+	+	+
Dichlorvos	+	+	+	+	+	+	−
Febantel	−	+	+	+	+	+	+
Fenbendazole	−	+	+	+	+	+	+
Ivermectin	+	+	+	+	+	+	+
Moxidectin	+	+	+	+	+	+	−
Oxibendazole	−	+	+	+	+	+	+
Oxfendazole	−	+	+	+	+	+	+
Phenothiazine	−	−	+	+	+	−	−
Piperazine salts	−	+	−	−	+	+	−
Pyrantel salts	−	+	+	−	+	−	−
Thiabendazole	−	−	+	+	+	+	+
Thiabendazole/ piperazine	−	+	+	+	+	+	+
Thiabendazole/ trichlorfon	+	+	+	+	+	+	+
Trichlorfon	+	+	−	−	−	+	−
Trichlorfon/pheno-thiazine/piperazine	+	+	+	−	+	+	−

+, Indicated for use; −, not indicated for use.
From McCurnin, D. M., & Bassert, J. M. (2002). *Clinical textbook for veterinary technicians* (5th ed.). Philadelphia: WB Saunders.

discussed. Anthelmintics are drugs used to eliminate helminths (internal parasite worms) from the animal. Anthelmintics fall into two categories, vermicides and vermifuges. A **vermicide** kills the parasite (worm) and a **vermifuge** paralyzes the parasite (worm) and gets expelled from the GI tract into the feces. As a veterinary technician, you may come into contact with products not mentioned in this section. The charts in this section list various products, their trade names, and their effectiveness. Since anthelmintics are so numerous, many veterinarians keep only a few products to meet their needs and to limit inventory. Some products are available under many different names. Experience will provide familiarity with various available brands.

℞ Antinematodal

Antinematodal drugs are anthelmintics used to treat nematodes (roundworms) such as *Toxocara* spp. and *Toxascaris* spp. The term "ascarids" is also used to describe nematodes.

Benzimidazoles

Benzimidazoles interfere with the worm's (nematodes) energy level on a cellular basis. They bind to beta tubulin and prevent its entry into microtubules that are needed for energy metabolism. Without energy, the worm dies.

Clinical Uses. Benzimidazoles are used in the following species:
- *Horses.* Effective against strongyles, pinworms, and ascarids.
- *Cattle.* Ascarids, several species of strongyles and other stomach worms; albendazole is also effective against adult liver flukes and tapeworms; fenbendazole is also effective against lungworms.
- *Sheep and goats.* Ascarids, several species of strongyles and other stomach worms; fenbendazole is also effective against lungworms.
- *Dogs.* Hookworms, roundworms, and whipworms; some are effective against *Taenia pisiformis* but not *D. caninum.*
- *Swine. Strongyloides* and lungworms.
- Many of the benzimidazoles are used as anthelmintics for exotics such as snakes and birds.

Dosage Forms. This class includes the following products:
- **Thiabendazole** (Equizole, TBZ, Omnizole, Equivet)

TABLE 13.3	Parasiticides Used to Treat Internal Parasites in Cattle, Sheep, and Goats.					
	PARASITE					
Drug	Haemonchus	Ostertagia	Trichostrongylus	Cooperia	Nematodirus	Strongyloides
Albendazole	+	+	+	+	+	−
Clorsulon	−	−	−	−	−	−
Decoquinate	−	−	−	−	−	−
Eprinomectin	+	+	+	+	+	+
Fenbendazole	+	+	+	+	+	+
Ivermectin	+	+	+	+	+	+
Lasalacid	−	−	−	−	−	−
Levamisole	+	+	+	+	+	+
Moxidectin	+	+	+	+	+	−
Monensin	−	−	−	−	−	−
Phenothiazine	+	+	+	−	−	−
Sulfonamides	−	−	−	−	−	−
Thiabendazole	+	+	+	+	+	+

+, Indicated for use; −, not indicated for use.
Modified from McCurnin, D. M., & Bassert, J. M. (2002). *Clinical textbook for veterinary technicians* (5th ed.).
Philadelphia: WB Saunders.

TABLE 13.4	Parasiticides Used for Control of External Parasites on Cattle, Sheep, and Goats.											
	PARASITE											
Drug	Cattle Grub	Horn Fly	Face Fly	Other Flies	Maggots	Chewing Lice	Sucking Lice	Psoroptic Mite	Other Mites	Ear Ticks	Other Ticks	Sheep Ked
Carbaril	−	+	+	+	−	+	+	−	−	+	+	−
Coumaphos	+	+	+	+	+	+	+	+	−	+	+	+
Chlorpyrifos	−	+	−	−	−	+	+	−	−	−	−	−
Dichlorvos	−	+	+	+	−	−	−	−	−	−	+	−
Eprinomectin	+	+	−	−	−	+	+	+	+	−	−	−
Famphur	+	−	−	−	−	+	+	−	−	+	+	−
Doramectin	−	−	−	−	−	+	+	−	−	−	−	−
Fenthion	+	−	−	−	−	+	+	−	−	+	+	−
Fenvalerate	−	+	+	−	−	−	−	−	−	+	−	−
Ivermectin	+	−	−	−	−	−	+	+	+	+	+	−
Methoxychlor	−	+	+	+	−	+	+	−	−	+	+	−
Moxidectin	+	+	−	−	−	+	+	+	+	−	−	−
Permethrin	−	+	+	−	−	−	−	−	−	−	+	−
Phosmet	+	+	−	−	−	+	+	+	+	+	+	−
Pyrethrins	−	+	+	+	−	−	−	−	−	−	−	−
Rotenone	−	−	−	−	−	+	+	−	−	−	−	+
Trichlorfon	+	+	−	−	+	+	+	−	−	+	+	−

+, Indicated for use; −, not indicated for use.
From McCurnin, D. M., & Bassert, J. M. (2002). *Clinical textbook for veterinary technicians* (5th ed.). Philadelphia: WB Saunders.

TABLE 13.3 Parasiticides Used to Treat Internal Parasites in Cattle, Sheep, and Goats—cont'd

| | | | PARASITE | | | | |
Bunostomum	Trichuris	Oesophagostomum	Chabertia	Dictyocaulus	Moniezia	Fasciola	Coccidia
+	−	+	+	+	+	+	−
−	−	−	−	−	−	+	−
−	−	−	−	−	−	−	+
+	+	+	−	+	−	−	−
+	+	+	+	+	−	−	−
+	−	+	+	+	−	−	−
−	−	−	−	−	−	−	+
+	+	+	+	+	−	−	−
+	−	+	−	+	−	−	−
−	−	−	−	−	−	−	+
−	−	+	−	−	−	−	−
−	−	−	−	−	−	−	+
+	−	+	+	−	−	−	−

- **Oxibendazole** (Anthelcide EQ)
- **Fenbendazole** (Panacur, Safeguard)
- **Febantel** (Drontal Plus, Rintal)
- **Cambendazole** (Camvet)
- **Oxfendazole** (Benzelmin, Synanthic)
- **Albendazole** (Valbazen)

Adverse Side Effects. These are uncommon but include vomiting and diarrhea. Albendazole may have potential teratogenic effects (bone marrow suppression) and should not be used during the first 30–45 days of pregnancy (Plumb, 2015).

TECHNICIAN NOTES
- Read labels carefully regarding use in lactating dairy animals and animals to be slaughtered.
- None of these products is approved for use in cats.

Tetrahydropyrimidines

Clinical Uses. Tetrahydropyrimidines are used in the following species:
- *Horses.* Ascarids, strongyles, pinworms
- *Cattle, sheep, and goats.* Strongyles
- *Dogs and cats.* Hookworms, roundworms
- *Swine.* Roundworms, strongyles

Dosage Forms. This class includes the following products:
- **Pyrantel pamoate** (Nemex, Strongid, Anthelban)
- **Pyrantel tartrate** (Banminth 48)
- **Morantel tartrate** (Nematel, Rumatel)

Adverse Side Effects. These are uncommon but may include increased respiration, profuse sweating, and incoordination.

TECHNICIAN NOTES
Read labels carefully regarding use in lactating dairy animals and animals to be slaughtered.

Imidazothiazoles

Clinical Uses. Imidazothiazoles are used in the following species:
- *Horses.* Ascarids, strongyles
- *Cattle, sheep, and goats.* Strongyles, lungworms
- *Dogs and cats.* Febantel—hookworms, roundworms, whipworms; levamisole has been used in dogs as a microfilaricide
- *Swine.* Strongyles, *Strongyloides*, lungworms, nodule worms
- These products also may be used effectively in some exotic species.

BOX 13.1   Case Scenario

Mitsy, a 10-week-old intact female DSH (domestic short haired) kitten, was presented for the chief complaint of worms in the stool.

History: The owner was given the kitten by her neighbor 2 days ago. Mitsy was given her first set of vaccines 2 weeks ago. The owner noted when cleaning out the litter box, yesterday, she saw something that looked like spaghetti. Mitsy is the only cat in the household and she does not go outside. She has a good appetite and has been drinking water but her belly looks like it is getting a little bigger. No vomiting or diarrhea.

Physical examination findings: Mitsy was very playful. TPR was normal, heart and lung sound were normal, mucous membranes were pink and moist, and her CRT (capillary refill time) was <2 seconds. Her skin and hair coat looked good with no fleas or flea dirt seen. No ocular or nasal discharge noted.

    A fecal sample was obtained and a fecal flotation was performed. The fecal test revealed *Toxocara cati* (roundworm).

Diagnosis: *Toxocara cati*

    The owner asked the veterinary technician what that meant. She explained that roundworms are intestinal parasites that are very common in cats. Mitsy most likely ingested the larvae that passed through the infected mother's milk, and became infected soon after birth.

    The roundworms migrate to the intestines, soaking up nutrients from the cat's diet. The larvae of *Toxocara cati* roundworms can infect people, as well as cats. This happens when eggs are ingested. So, it is important that the stool be removed from the litter box daily and always wash your hands after handling the litter box material. Proper prevention of a roundworm infection is important to prevent human health problems.

    Pyrantel pamoate was given orally to Mitsy and the veterinary technician continued to explain that the worms will pass into the stool. The medication will only paralyze or anesthetize the adult worms and will not kill the immature forms of the worm or the migrating larvae, therefore, at least two or three treatments are needed; they are typically repeated at 2- to 3-week intervals. So, Mitsy will be dewormed again with each follow-up visit when given her booster vaccinations.

Dosage Forms. This class includes the following products:
- Febantel (Rintal)
- Levamisole

    Adverse Side Effects. These include transient foaming at the mouth.

 TECHNICIAN NOTES

Read labels carefully regarding use in lactating dairy animals and animals to be slaughtered.

Avermectins

Avermectins are derived from the bacterium *Streptomyces avermitilis*. Avermectins kill by interfering with nervous system and muscle function, thus breaking down neurotransmission. The drug binds and activates glutamate-gated chloride channels that are present in neurons and myocytes, which results in neuromuscular paralysis and death. In mammals, glutamate-gated chloride channels are absent. Therefore, invertebrates are susceptible to these drugs. Avermectins do not cross the blood-brain barrier unless given at high doses.

    Ivermectin. Ivermectin has a wide spectrum of activity and has been used extra-label for internal and external parasites in exotics and wildlife.

    Clinical Uses
- *Horses.* Large and small strongyles, pinworms, ascarids, hairworms, large-mouth stomach worms, neck threadworms, bots, lungworms, intestinal threadworms, and summer sores secondary to *Habronema* or *Draschia* spp.
- *Cattle.* Gastrointestinal roundworms, lungworms, cattle grubs, sucking lice, and mites.
- *Swine.* Gastrointestinal roundworms, lungworms, lice, and mange mites.
- *Dogs.* Effective preventive for *D. immitis*; Heartgard Plus contains pyrantel pamoate and is effective against hookworms and roundworms.
- *Cats.* Effective preventive for *D. immitis* and for the removal of hookworms.
- *Birds and snakes.* Effective against some endoparasites and ectoparasites.

    Dosage Forms
- Heartgard
- Heartgard Plus
- Heartgard for Cats

- **Eqvalan**
- **Iverheart Max**
- **Ivomec**
- **Zimecterin** (horses)

Adverse Side Effects. Adverse side effects may occur in collies with MDR1 (Multidrug Resistance-1) genetic defect and poorly functioning P-gp; potential for severe toxicity.

Selamectin. See section on preventatives in this chapter.

Milbemycin oxime. See section on preventatives in this chapter.

Moxidectin
Clinical Uses
- *Horses.* Large and small strongyles, encysted cyathostomes, ascarids, pinworms, hairworms, large-mouth stomach worms, and bots.
- *Cattle.* Gastrointestinal roundworms, lungworms, cattle grubs, mites, lice, and horn flies.
- *Dogs.* Effective preventive for *D. immitis.*

Dosage Forms
- **Quest 2% Equine Oral Gel**
- **Cydectin Pour-On** (cattle)
- **ProHeart 6** (subcutaneous injection for dogs)
- **ProHeart 12** (subcutaneous injection for dogs)
- **Advantage Multi** (dogs and cats)

Doramectin
Clinical Uses
- *Cattle.* Gastrointestinal roundworms, lungworms, eyeworms, grubs, biting and sucking lice, horn flies, and mange mites.
- *Swine.* Gastrointestinal roundworms, lungworms, kidney worms, sucking lice, and mange mites.

Dosage Forms
- **Dectomax Injectable Solution**
- **Dectomax Pour-On**

Eprinomectin
Clinical Uses
- Indicated for various GI roundworms, cattle grubs, lice, mange mites, and lungworms
- No meat or milk withdrawal times for this agent
- May also be useful in the treatment of ear mites in rabbits (*Psoroptes cuniculi*)
- Restricted use in lactating cows

Dosage Form
- **Eprinomectin**—Eprinex (topically applied avermectin antiparasiticide for cattle)

- **LongRange for cattle** (subcutaneous injection for beef cattle)

Adverse Side Effects. These are uncommon. Toxic signs include mydriasis, ataxia, tremors, and depression.

TECHNICIAN NOTES
- Although not approved, Ivomec is sometimes used for the treatment of ear mites in cats and scabies in dogs.
- Crumbling or breaking of the tablets or use of a chewable version is not recommended because of the small amount of medication in heartworm preventives.
- Read labels carefully regarding use in lactating dairy animals and animals for slaughter. Moxidectin is approved for use in dairy cattle of all ages and at all stages of lactation, except for veal calves.

Other Agents
Piperazine
Clinical Uses
- *Dogs and cats.* Roundworms
- Used effectively in exotics such as birds and snakes
- Commonly combined in large-animal dewormers to broaden its spectrum and enhance its efficacy

Dosage Forms
- **Pipa-Tabs**

TECHNICIAN NOTES
- Piperazine does not kill the hookworms, tapeworms, and whipworms but paralyzes them and expelled in the feces.

Adverse Side Effects. Adverse side effects include diarrhea, vomiting, and ataxia.

Praziquantel/Pyrantel Pamoate/Febantel
Clinical Uses
- *Dogs.* Effective for the removal of tapeworms, hookworms, roundworms, and whipworms.

Dosage Form
- **Drontal Plus**

Adverse Side Effects. These are uncommon.

TECHNICIAN NOTES
- Do not use in dogs weighing less than 2 lb or in puppies younger than 3 weeks.
- Do not use in pregnant animals.

Emodepside

See section on topical solutions in this chapter.

 ## Anticestodal

Anticestodal drugs are used to treat cestodes (tapeworms). Removal of tapeworms in dogs and cats is necessary due to the potential for zoonotic diseases.

Bunamidine

Clinical Uses

- *Dogs. T. pisiformis, D. caninum, Echinococcus granulosus,* and *Echinococcus multilocularis*
- *Cats. D. caninum, Taenia taeniaeformis*
  Dosage Form
- Scolaban
  Adverse Side Effects. These are uncommon but include vomiting, anorexia, diarrhea, and lethargy.

> **TECHNICIAN NOTES**
>
> - No adverse reactions have been reported in pregnant or breeding animals.
> - This product is not for use in puppies younger than 4 weeks or kittens younger than 6 weeks.

Praziquantel

Clinical Uses. Praziquantel is used to treat tapeworms in dogs and cats. It is also effective against *Taenia* and *Echinococcus.*

- *Dogs and cats. D. caninum*
  Dosage Form
- **Droncit** (Injection and oral forms)
- Various others (combination of other antiparasitics)
  Adverse Side Effects. Diarrhea and vomiting may occur.

> **TECHNICIAN NOTES**
>
> - It is important to inform owners that fleas are directly involved with the tapeworm's life cycle and therefore preventing flea infestations is vital.

Epsiprantel

Clinical Uses

- *Dogs. T. pisiformis* and *D. caninum*
- *Cats. T. taeniaeformis* and *D. caninum*
  Dosage Form
- **Cestex** (oral form)
  Adverse Side Effects. These are uncommon.

> **TECHNICIAN NOTES**
>
> - Safety in pregnant or breeding animals has not been established
> - This product is not for use in puppies or kittens younger than 7 weeks.

 ## Antitrematodal

Antinematodal drugs are used to treat trematodes (flukes), such as *Paragonimus, Fasciola,* and *Dicrocoelium.*

Clorsulon

Clinical Uses. Clorsulon is a narrow-spectrum antiparasitic used in livestock against liver flukes.

- *Cattle.* Liver flukes
- Effective against immature and adult flukes
  Dosage Form
- **Curatrem**
  Adverse Side Effects. These are uncommon.

> **TECHNICIAN NOTES**
>
> - This product is not approved for use in female dairy cattle of breeding age.
> - Read label regarding use in animals to be slaughtered.

Albendazole

Clinical Uses. Albendazole is an oral suspension dewormer for cattle and sheep. It is used for the control of liver flukes, tapeworms, stomach worms, intestinal worms, and lung worms. It should not be administered during the first 45 days of pregnancy in cattle. Do not use in female dairy cattle of breeding age or lactating goats (Plumb, 2015).

- *Cattle.* Liver flukes
- Effective against adult flukes and many intestinal worms
  Dosage Form
- **Valbazen**

Praziquantel

Clinical Uses. Praziquantel is used against a variety of trematodes and cestodes.

- *Dogs and cats.* Lung flukes
  Dosage Form
- **Droncit** (tablet, injection)
- Various other (combined with other antiparasitics)
  Adverse Side Effects. Diarrhea and vomiting may occur.

Topical Solutions
Emodepside/Praziquantel
Clinical Uses
- A topical solution for the treatment and control of hookworms, roundworms, and tapeworms in cats 8 weeks of age or older
- Emodepside is a cyclic depsipeptide
- Praziquantel is an isoquinoline cestocide
- To be applied every 30 days for preventive purposes
  #### Dosage Form
- Profender

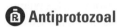
- Pregnant women should wear gloves when applying Profender to their cats.

Antiprotozoal
Protozoa are single-celled organisms found at various body sites that have the ability to replicate rapidly. Coccidia and *Giardia* are the protozoa that are most commonly associated with diarrhea in many species of animals. Protozoa are most commonly transmitted via contaminated feed and/or water. Prevention of these parasites includes providing uncontaminated food and water and clean housing and avoiding overcrowding. *Babesia* is a hematozoan (i.e., a protozoan) that is transmitted by ticks and affects many species of animals. An injectable treatment for babesiosis is available for dogs.

Drugs for Treating Coccidia and Other Protozoa
Dosage Forms
- **Monensin** (Coban 60); turkeys and chickens
- **Monensin** (Rumensin), various others
- **Lasalocid** (Bovatec)
- **Amprolium** (Corid); calves
- **Clopidol** (Coyden 25); chickens
- **Diclazuril** (Clincox); horses
- **Maduramicin ammonium** (Cygro); chickens
- **Narasin/nicarbazine** (Maxiban 72); chickens, various others
- **Ponazuril** (Marquis); horses
- **Robenidine hydrochloride** (Robenz); chickens
- **Sulfadimethoxine** (Albon); chickens, turkeys, dogs, and cats
- **Sulfadimethoxine/ormetroprim** (Primor)
- **Sulfadiazine/trimethoprim** (Tribrissen)
- **Sulfamethoxazole/trimethoprim** (Septra, Bactrim)

- **Sulfadiazine/pyrimethamine**—used to treat *T. gondii*
  Adverse Side Effects. These are uncommon.

 TECHNICIAN NOTES
- Read labels carefully regarding use in food-producing animals and animals to be slaughtered.
- Veterinary technicians need to be aware that sulfa drugs can cause KCS (Keratoconjunctivitis sicca) and need to inform owners when sulfa drugs are dispensed.

Drugs for Treating *Giardia*
Dosage Forms
- **Metronidazole** (Flagyl); dogs and cats
- **Albendazole** (Valbazen); dogs and cats
- **Fenbendazole** (Panacur, Safe-Gard in dogs, cattle and horses)

Adverse Side Effects. These are uncommon, but vomiting and diarrhea may occur in some animals treated with metronidazole.

TECHNICIAN NOTES
- Metronidazole is not recommended for use in pregnant animals.
- Oral metronidazole is bad tasting and may be difficult to administer to cats. It can be compounded in different flavors.
- Metronidazole is prohibited from being used in any animal used for human consumption.

Drugs for Treating *Babesia*
Imizol is available for the treatment of clinical signs of babesiosis and/or evidence of *Babesia* organisms in the blood. This product is indicated for use in dogs, and treatment consists of two injections given over a 2-week interval.

Atovaquone is effective in treating dogs with *Babesia gibsoni* infections. When used in combination with azithromycin, it can be used to treat cytauxzoonosis in cats.

Diminazene aceturate is used in several species to treat for trypanosomiasis, babesiosis, or cytauxzoonosis. This drug is available in several countries but not the United States.

Imidocarb dipropinate can be used to treat *Babesia* and related parasites. It has also been used to treat cytauxzoonosis in cats, although results on its efficacy are not yet available (Plumb, 2015).
Dosage Forms
- **Imidocarb dipropinate** (Imizol)

Adverse Side Effects. These may include injection pain and mild cholinergic signs such as salivation, nasal drip, and vomiting. Other less common side effects include panting, restlessness, diarrhea, and mild injection site inflammation.

TECHNICIAN NOTES

Severe cholinergic signs may be reversed with atropine sulfate.

HEARTWORM DISEASE

Heartworm disease is commonly found throughout the United States. It is a mosquito-borne infectious disease that primarily affects dogs and wild Canidae, although cats and ferrets also may become infected. *D. immitis* is the filarial nematode that causes heartworm disease. *Acanthocheilonema reconditum* (formerly known as *Dipetalonema reconditum*) (Hendrix, 2017) is a subcutaneous filarial nematode that does not require treatment because it is nonpathogenic.

The dog and some wild canids are the definitive host for heartworm and serve as the main reservoir of infection. The mosquito is the vector for transmission of *D. immitis* and becomes infected when taking a blood meal from a host with microfilaria. The cat is not a natural host for *D. immitis*, therefore when bitten by a mosquito the infective larvae usually do not survive. However, if a large number of infective larvae are injected by the mosquito then some may develop into adults. Over the past several years, the number of cats in which heartworm disease has been diagnosed has increased.

Clinical signs of heartworm disease in the dog include coughing, dyspnea, exercise intolerance, syncope, ascites, and abnormal lung and heart sounds. The clinical signs in the cat are vague or can consist of coughing, increased respiratory effort, dyspnea, anorexia, vomiting, weight loss, collapse, and sudden death. The inflammatory process in the lungs of a cat affects the airways, producing coughing and asthma-like or allergic bronchitis signs which can be mistaken for feline asthma (AHS, 2020a, 2020b).

In dogs, as the number of adult worms increase, they can be present in the right ventricle. Dogs with a large number of worms can develop caval syndrome where the worms move into the right ventricle to the right atrium and the vena cava, interfering with blood flow and valvular function. If surgical extraction of the worms is not performed promptly in dogs diagnosed with Caval syndrome, death can occur within 2 days. (AHS, 2020a, 2020b).

In the cat, heartworm infections usually consist of one or two adult worms (<6 adult worms) that survive 2 to 3 years or longer, which is much shorter than that in dogs which can be up to 7 years. Live adult worms can migrate to the pulmonary arteries producing an inflammatory process. This inflammatory process in the lungs is often misdiagnosed as asthma or allergic bronchitis but is actually part of a syndrome called heartworm-associated respiratory disease (HARD) (AHS, 2020b).

D. immitis has its own parasite, the bacteria Wolbachia, which contribute to heartworm disease. *Wolbachia* are gram-negative intracellular bacteria living in the body of both the immature and adult worms; they play an important role in the worm's survival and pathogenesis of the disease. Therefore, part of the treatment regimen for heartworm disease includes doxycycline, an antibiotic, that kills *Wolbachia*. The American Heartworm Society (AHS) recommends doxycycline to be given for 1 month prior to treatment for adult heartworms. This will reduce the number of immature heartworms, and may also reduce the number of adult heartworms.

Cats are usually not treated for adult heartworm due to a possible thromboembolism from dead worms in the pulmonary arteries. Instead, treatment focuses on supportive care and allowing for a self-cure. Prednisone can be administered to infected cats with lung disease and whenever antibody and/or antigen positive cats display clinical signs (AHS, 2020b).

American Heartworm Society 2020 Recommended Heartworm Management Protocol in Dogs

Day 0—In a dog diagnosed and verified as heartworm positive:
- Apply an EPA-registered canine topical product labeled to repel and kill mosquitoes.

If the dog is symptomatic:
- Stabilize the patient.
- Begin Prednisone on a tapering dose for 4 weeks.
- Exercise restriction during the entire treatment and recovery period.

Day 1—Administer a dose of a monthly heartworm preventative.
- Pretreat with antihistamines and glucocorticoids if not already on prednisone, to decrease the risk of anaphylaxis if large numbers of microfilaria are present.

Days 1–28—Administer doxycycline for 4 weeks to decrease pathology associated with dead worms and to disrupt heartworm transmission.

Day 30—Administer a dose of a monthly heartworm preventative.
- Apply a topical product to repel and kill mosquitoes.

Day 31–60—A 30 day waiting period following doxycycline before administering melarsomine to allow time for the *Wolbachia* surface proteins to dissipate before killing the adult worms.

Day 61—Administer a dose of a monthly heartworm preventative.

- Administer the first dose of melarsomine injection intramuscular.
- Begin prednisone on a low dose for 4 weeks.
- Decrease activity level to cage restriction and leash walk in yard.

Day 90—Administer a dose of a monthly heartworm preventative.

- Administer the second dose of melarsomine injection intramuscular.
- Begin prednisone on a tapering dose for 4 weeks.

Day 91—Administer the third dose of melarsomine injection intramuscular.

- Continue exercise restriction for 6 to 8 weeks after last dose of melarsomine injection.

Day 120—Test for microfilaria.

- If positive treat with a microfilaricide and retest in 4 weeks.
- Continue a year-round heartworm preventative program.

Day 365—Antigen test 9 months after last melarsomine injection.

- Screen for microfilaria.
- If still antigen positive, retreat with doxycycline followed by two doses of melarsomine 24 hours apart. (AHS, 2020a, 2020b)

Prevention is the key word for controlling heartworm disease. Dogs not undergoing an approved heartworm disease prevention program should be tested for the presence of adult heartworms before preventive treatment is begun. Clients should be educated about the importance of treating an existing infection if one exists, preventing infection or reinfection, and ensuring periodic testing that may be necessary. (Many veterinarians will not prescribe heartworm prevention without an annual heartworm antigen test.) Products for the prevention of *D. immitis* infection in cats are available. No adulticide products have been approved for use in cats. Table 13.5 provides a comparison of several heartworm preventives that are on the market at this time.

Adulticides
Melarsomine Dihydrochloride

Melarsomine is the only approved adulticide for use in dogs. It is an arsenic compound administered by deep intramuscular injection in the lumbar region. The administration schedule is based on classification of the severity of heartworm disease.

Dosage Form
- **Immiticide**

Adverse Side Effects. Some dogs experience reactions such as pain, swelling, and tenderness at the injection site. Firm nodules may form at the injection site. Coughing, gagging, depression, lethargy, anorexia, fever, lung congestion, and vomiting are common reactions.

TECHNICIAN NOTES

- The manufacturer recommends use of a 23-gauge, 1-inch needle for dogs up to 22 lb and a 22-gauge, 1½-inch needle for dogs larger than 22 lb.
- Safety in breeding, lactating, or pregnant bitches has not been determined.
- Melarsomine is contraindicated in dogs with severe heartworm disease (Class 4, according to manufacturer disease classification).
- Clients must be informed of the potential for morbidity and mortality associated with heartworm treatment.
- Exercise in dogs should be restricted after treatment has been provided.

Microfilaricides

Microfilaricides should be given approximately 4 weeks after administration of the last adulticide if they still test positive for microfilaria. They are used to kill circulating microfilaria. Although not approved as microfilaricides, ivermectin and milbemycin oxime have been used, as well as levamisole.

Preventives
Fluralaner Plus Moxidectin
Clinical Uses

- *Cats.* Must be 6 months of age or older weighing at least 2.6 lb.
- To be applied topically once every 2 months.
- Used for the treatment of fleas and ticks, prevention of heartworm, and treatment of roundworm and hookworm infections.

Dosage Form
- **Bravecto Plus topical solution for cats**

Adverse Side Effects. These include vomiting, hair loss, itching, diarrhea, lethargy, dry skin, elevated ALT, and hypersalivation (Merck, 2020).

Imidacloprid Plus Moxidectin
Clinical Uses

- *Dogs.* Must be 7 weeks or older and weighing at least 3 lb.
- *Cats.* Must be 9 weeks or older and weighing at least 2 lb.
- To be applied topically on a monthly basis.

TABLE 13.5 Common Heartworm Prevention Products.

Product	Method of Administration	Age Restrictions	Effect on Other Parasites
Bravecto Plus for Cats	Topical application every 2 months	Kittens: 6 months of age	Fleas, Ticks, Roundworms, Hookworms
Heartgard Plus for Dogs and Cats	Chewable tablet given monthly	Puppies: 6 weeks of age Kittens: 6 weeks of age	Dogs: roundworms, hookworms Cats: hookworms
Heartgard chewables for Dogs and Cats	Chewable tablet given monthly	Puppies: 6 weeks of age Kittens: 6 weeks of age	Dogs: roundworms, hookworms Cats: hookworms
Interceptor Plus	Chewable tablets given monthly	Puppies: 6 weeks of age	Dog: roundworms, hookworms, whipworms, tapeworms
Interceptor for Dogs and Cats	Tablet given monthly	Puppies: 4 weeks of age Kittens: 6 weeks of age	Dogs: roundworms, hookworms, whipworms Cats: roundworms, hookworms
Iverhart Max for Dogs	Chewable tablet given monthly	Puppies: 8 weeks of age	Roundworms, hookworms, tapeworms
Iverhart Plus for Dogs	Chewable tablet given monthly	Puppies: 6 weeks of age	Roundworms, hookworms, tapeworms
Revolution Plus for Cats	Topical application monthly	Kittens: 8 weeks of age	Fleas, kills 3 types of ticks, ear mites, roundworms, hookworms
Revolution for Dogs and Cats	Topical application monthly	Puppies: 6 weeks of age Kittens: 8 weeks of age	Dogs: sarcoptic mange mites, ear mites, fleas, American dog ticks (Dermacentor) Cats: fleas, ear mites, roundworm, hookworms
Sentinel for Dogs	Tablet given monthly	Puppies: 4 weeks of age	Hookworms, roundworms, whipworms
Sentinel Spectrum for Dogs	Chewable tablet given monthly	Puppies: 6 weeks of age	Fleas, roundworms, hookworms, whipworms, tapeworms
Simparica Trio	Chewable tablet given monthly	Puppies: 8 weeks of age	Fleas, Ticks, Roundworms, Hookworms
ProHeart 6	Injectable that lasts 6 months	Dogs: 6 months of age	Hookworms
ProHeart 12	Injectable that lasts 12 months	Dogs: 12 months of age	Hookworms
Trifexis for Dogs	Chewable tablet given monthly	Puppies: 8 weeks of age	Fleas, roundworms, hookworms, whipworms
Coraxis for Dogs	Topical application monthly	Puppies: 7 weeks of age	Roundworms, hookworms, whipworms
Advantage Multi for Dogs and Cats	Topical application monthly	Puppies: 7 weeks of age Kittens: 9 weeks of age	Dogs: fleas, roundworms, hookworms, whipworms, Sarcoptic mange Cats: fleas, ear mites, roundworms, hookworms
Centragard for Cats	Topical application monthly	Kittens: 7 weeks of age	Roundworms, hookworms, tapeworms

Dosage Form
- **Advantage Multi for Dogs and Cats**

Ivermectin

Clinical Uses
- *Dogs.* Monthly preventive; the Plus formula contains pyrantel pamoate and is effective against hookworms and roundworms.

- *Cats.* Monthly preventive for *D. immitis* and for the removal of hookworms.
- Eliminates the tissue stage of heartworm larvae.
  ### Dosage Forms
- **Heartgard chewables for dogs and cats**
- **Heartgard Plus chewables for dogs**
- **Iverheart Plus**
- **Iverheart Max**

Adverse Side Effects. These are uncommon. Toxic signs include mydriasis, depression, and ataxia.

Milbemycin Oxime
Clinical Uses
- *Dogs.* Monthly, orally administered, preventive; also controls hookworms, roundworms, and whipworms.
- Eliminates the tissue stage of heartworm larvae.
- Sentinel product contains lufenuron for flea control.
Dosage Forms
- **Interceptor**
- **Interceptor Plus**
- **Sentinel**
- **Sentinel Spectrum**
- **Trifexis**
Adverse Side Effects. These are uncommon.

Moxidectin
Clinical Uses
- *Dogs.* Preventive used for *D. immitis.*
- Eliminates the tissue stage of heartworm larvae.
- Moxidectin is currently an approved microfilaricide.
Dosage Form
- **Proheart 6** (injectable given subcutaneously)
- **Proheart 12** (injection given subcutaneously)
- Advantage Multi
Adverse Side Effects. Adverse side effects may include lethargy, vomiting, ataxia, anorexia, diarrhea, nervousness, weakness, polydipsia, and itching.

Selamectin
Clinical Uses
- *Dogs and cats.* Used as a monthly preventive.
- Available as a solution for topical administration.
- Indications include prevention of heartworm disease caused by ***D. immitis***, prevention and control of flea infestations, treatment and control of ear mites *(Otodectes cynotis)* infestation, treatment and control of sarcoptic *(Sarcoptes scabiei)* mange in dogs, and hookworm and roundworm treatment in cats.
Dosage Form
- **Revolution**
Adverse Side Effects. These are uncommon but include transient, localized alopecia at the application site of some treated cats.

ECTOPARASITES

Most ectoparasites are ubiquitous in the environment; therefore, control is often difficult. Environmental factors such as housing (indoor or outdoor) and geographic location may affect the incidence of many ectoparasites such as fleas and ticks. When trying to control ectoparasites, the veterinary technician must be familiar with the products used to eradicate these parasites and must be able to educate clients about how to properly combat their pet's infestation. Not only do ectoparasites cause misery to their host, but many dermatologic problems also arise from their infestation. Additionally, increased infestation of fleas may affect humans because fleas are not host specific. Table 13.6 provides a comparison of various topical products on the market at this time.

℞ Application Systems
Prediluted Sprays
Consumers like the convenience of sprays, and sprays are available for animal and environmental use. These formulations are available only for the use specified on the label and should be used accordingly. Sprays are available as water-based and alcohol-based formulations. Water-based sprays do not penetrate oily coats or fabrics as well and do not dry as quickly as alcohol-based sprays. However, alcohol-based sprays may be irritating and drying to the skin. Alcohol-based sprays do usually kill ectoparasites quickly. Environmental sprays are usually residual. Most pet sprays require application daily or every 2 to 3 days for adequate parasite control.

Adverse Side Effects. These vary among products. Carefully read warning labels.

TECHNICIAN NOTES
- Spray the pet from head to tail, including the legs and abdomen. Avoid only the eyes, mouth, and nose. For best results, spray against the natural lay of the hair.
- Educate clients about environmental control and how to treat the pet.
- Read labels before applying to young, sick, or pregnant animals. Some products are not safe for certain species (e.g., cats).
- Water-based flea sprays are best used on young animals because alcohol-based sprays tend to evaporate quickly and may cause loss of body heat. It is best to apply water-based sprays only to the dorsal area and then to spread the spray by combing through the haircoat. In this way, the young animal does not lose body heat.

TABLE 13.6 Comparison of Products Indicated for Flea and Tick Control.

	Active Ingredient(s)	Age Approved for Use	Approved for Pregnant or Lactating Animals	Time Need to Kill Fleas After First Application	Effectiveness on Ticks	Other Parasites Affected	How Often Applied
ACTIVYL	Indoxacarb	Puppies: 8 weeks Kittens: 8 weeks	No	24–72 hours	No	None	Monthly
ADVANTAGE II	Imidacloprid, Pyriproxifen	Puppies: 7 weeks Kittens: 8 weeks	Consult with veterinarian	12 hours	No	Lice	Monthly
K-9 ADVAN-TIX II	Imidacloprid, Permethrin, Pyriproxifen	Puppies: 7 weeks	No	12 hours	Yes	Repels flies and mosquitos, kills lice	Monthly
ADVANTUS	Imidacloprid	Puppies: 10 weeks	Not tested	1 hour	No	None	Daily
ADVANTAGE MULTI	Imidacloprid, Moxidectin	Puppies: 7 weeks Kittens: 9 weeks	No	12 hours	No	**Dogs:** Roundworms, hook-worms, whipworms, heart-worm, sarcoptic mange **Cats:** Roundworms, hookworms, ear mites, heartworm	Monthly
BREVECTO CHEW	Fluralaner	Puppies: 6 months	Yes	12 hours	Yes, kills ticks for 12 weeks, but kills Lone Star ticks for 8 weeks	Sarcoptic mange, mites, demodectic mange	Every 12 weeks
BRAVECTO PLUS FOR CATS	Fluralaner, Mox-idectin	Kittens: 6 months	No	12 hours	Yes, Black-legged tick and American Dog tick for 2 months	Roundworms and hook-worms	Every 2 months
BRAVECTO TOPICAL	Fluralaner	Puppies: 6 months Kittens: 6 months	No	8 hours	**Dogs:** Yes, kills ticks for 12 weeks, but kills Lone Star ticks for 8 weeks **Cats:** Yes, kills Black-legged tick for 12 weeks and American Dog tick for 8 weeks		Dog: Every 12 weeks
CAPSTAR	Nitenpyram	Puppies: 4 weeks Cats: 4 weeks	Yes	Begins killing within 30 minutes	No	None	As needed
CHERISTIN	Spinetoram	Kittens: 8 weeks	Consult with veterinarian	Begins killing within 30 minutes	No	None	Monthly
CREDELIO	Lotilaner	Puppies: 8 weeks	No	4 hours	Yes	None	Monthly
EFFIPRO PLUS	Fipronil	Puppies: 8 weeks Kittens: 8 weeks	Yes	12 hours	Yes	Mosquitos and chewing lice	Monthly
EFFITIX TOPICAL	Fipronil, Perme-thrin	Puppies: 8 weeks Do Not use on cats	Consult with veterinarian	6 hours	Yes	Kills and repels mosquitos, Repels biting flies, kills lice	Monthly

Product	Active Ingredients	Minimum Age	Safe for Cats / Consult	Flea Kill Time	Repels/Kills	Protects Against	Frequency
EFFITIX PLUS	Fipronil	Puppies: 8 weeks Do Not use on cats	Consult with veterinarian	6 hours	Yes	Kills and repels mosquitos, repels biting flies, kills lice	Monthly
FRONTLINE PLUS	Fipronil, Methoprene	Puppies: 8 weeks Kittens: 8 weeks	Yes	12 hours	Yes	Kills chewing lice, aids in the control of sarcoptic mange	Monthly
FRONTLINE GOLD	Fipronil, Methoprene, Pyriproxyfen	Puppies: 8 weeks Kittens: 8 weeks	Yes	Begins killing within 30 minutes	Yes	Kills chewing lice	Monthly
IVERHART MAX	Ivermectin, Pyrantel pamoate, Praziquantel	Puppies: 8 weeks	No	—	No	Roundworms, hookworms, tapeworms, heartworm	
NEXGARD	Afoxolaner	Puppies: 8 weeks	No	8 hours	Yes	No	Monthly
REVOLUTION	Selamectin	Puppies: 6 weeks Kittens: 8 weeks	Yes	Within 38 hours	Yes	Dogs: heartworm, ear mites, sarcoptic mange Cats: heartworm, roundworms, hookworms, ear mites	Monthly
SENTINEL	Lufenuron, Milbemycin	Puppies: 4 weeks	Yes	Prevents flea eggs from hatching and maturing but does not kill adult fleas	No	Heartworm, roundworms, hookworms, whipworms	Monthly
SENTINEL SPECTRUM	Lufenuron, Milbemycin, Praziquantel	Puppies: 6 weeks	No	Prevents flea eggs from hatching and maturing but does not kill adult fleas	No	Roundworms, hookworms, tapeworms, whipworms, heartworm	Monthly
SERESTO	Imidacloprid, Flumethrin	Puppies: 7 weeks Kittens: 10 weeks	No	Within 24 hours	Yes	Lice, controls sarcoptic mange	Every 8 months
SIMPARICA	Sarolaner	Puppies: 6 months	No	Within 3 hours	Yes	None	Monthly
SIMPARICA TRIO	Sarolaner, moxidectin, and pyrantel	Puppies: 8 weeks	No	4 hours	Yes	Roundworms and hookworm	Monthly
TRIFEXIS	Spinosad, Milbemycin	Puppies: 8 weeks	Consult with veterinarian	Within 30 minutes	No	Heartworm, roundworms, hookworms, whipworms	Monthly
VECTRA 3D	Dinotefuran, Permethrin, Pyriproxifen	Puppies: 8 weeks	Consult with veterinarian	6 hours	Yes	Repels and kills mosquitos, mites, biting flies, lice	Monthly
VECTRA for CATS	Dinotefuran, Pyriproxifen	Kittens: 8 weeks	No	6 hours	Yes	Repels and kills mosquitos, mites, biting flies, lice	Monthly

Emulsifiable Concentrates

Dips. Concentrates have to be diluted with water. Dips usually are used after a shampoo and generally are considered residual.

Adverse Side Effects. These vary among products. Read labels carefully for animal and user safety and precautions.

> **TECHNICIAN NOTES**
>
> - Removal of excess water or drying of the coat before dipping is recommended to prevent further dilution of the product.
> - For best results, do not rinse after applying the dip.
> - Organophosphate dips should *never* be applied to cats.

Yard and Kennel Sprays. These are designed for environmental use and should not be used on animals. These products are residual.

Adverse Side Effects. These vary among products. Directions for application should be followed carefully for the safety of the user and of animals.

Shampoos. These products may contain insecticides or medications, or they may be effective only for cleaning the coat. Some shampoos are available as concentrates and require dilution before use. Shampoos are not considered to be residual. Shampoos should be rinsed well; water hardness/softness affects how quickly some shampoos rinse away.

Adverse Side Effects. These vary among products. Shampoos that contain carbamates or organophosphates should not be used with other products of the same origin.

> **TECHNICIAN NOTES**
>
> - Read labels carefully. Shampoos may seem harmless, but they can be harmful if used improperly.
> - It is recommended that most shampoos be left on the haircoat for 5 to 10 minutes before rinsing.
> - If shampoo is not rinsed well, a hot spot may develop on the pet's skin.

Dusts. The popularity of these products has decreased with the availability of effective sprays. In addition, dusts do not provide a quick kill.

Adverse Side Effects. These include irritation to mucous membranes and drying of the skin and haircoat.

Foggers. Foggers work best in large, open rooms. Remind clients that foggers do not go around corners, under couches, or into closets. Combining foggers with a premises spray enhances results. Labels should always be read carefully.

Monthly Flea and Tick Products

Fipronil. Fipronil is a topical solution that provides flea and tick control, according to the manufacturer, the product collects in the oils of the skin and hair follicles. It controls less severe flea infestations for up to 3 months and ticks for 1 month. Fipronil kills newly emerged adult fleas and all stages of ticks.

Dosage Forms
- **Frontline Plus**
- **Frontline Gold**
- **EFFIPRO**
- **EFFIPRO Plus**
- **EFFITIX Plus**
- **EFFITIX Topical**

Adverse Side Effects. Adverse side effects include hypersensitivity (rare) and possible irritation at the site of administration (Plumb, 2015).

> **TECHNICIAN NOTES**
>
> - The product remains effective after bathing, water immersion, or exposure to sunlight.
> - Do not use on kittens younger than 12 weeks or on puppies younger than 10 weeks.
> - This product may be harmful to debilitated, aged, pregnant, or nursing animals.
> - Do not use more often than once every 30 days.
> - It is recommended that gloves be worn when applying this product.

Imidacloprid. Imidacloprid is a topical solution that provides flea control and, according to the manufacturer, is not absorbed into the bloodstream or other internal organs. It controls less severe flea infestations for up to 4 weeks and kills newly emerged adult fleas.

Dosage Form
- **Advantage II**
- **Advantage Multi**
- **Advantus**
- **K-9 Advantix II**

Adverse Side Effects. Adverse side effects are uncommon.

TECHNICIAN NOTES

- This product remains effective after bathing, water immersion, or exposure to sunlight.
- Do not use on kittens younger than 8 weeks or on puppies younger than 7 weeks.
- This product should not be used in pregnant animals.
- This product may be used weekly for severe infestations.
- It is not necessary to wear gloves when applying this product.

TECHNICIAN NOTES

- Do not use in puppies or kittens younger than 6 weeks. Sentinel is approved for use in puppies 4 weeks old.
- Oral products are considered to be safe for use in pregnant, breeding, or lactating animals.
- The safety of the injectable product in reproducing animals has not been established.

Imidacloprid and Permethrin. This combination is a once-a-month topical product for dogs that is used to treat ticks and fleas and to repel mosquitoes. It can be used on puppies 7 weeks or older. K9 Advantix is effective after swimming.

Dosage Form
- **K9 Advantix II**

Lotilaner. Lotilaner is a monthly chewable tablet for the treatment and prevention of fleas and ticks. It is used in dogs and puppies 8 weeks of age or older weighing 4.4 pounds or greater (Elanco, 2019).

Dosage Form
- **Credelio** chewable tablets

Adverse Side Effects. These include weight loss, elevated blood urea nitrogen, increased urination, and diarrhea (Elanco, 2019).

Lufenuron. Lufenuron is a monthly flea control administered orally; it is absorbed into fatty tissue and slowly released into the bloodstream. Sentinel also contains milbemycin for the prevention of heartworms and the control of some intestinal parasites in dogs. Lufenuron controls fleas by preventing the development of chitin, the substance that makes up the flea's exoskeleton. This product does not kill adult fleas. Fleas must take a blood meal to ingest the product.

Dosage Forms
- **Program 6 month injectable for cats**
- **Sentinel**
- **Sentinel Spectrum**

Adverse Side Effects. Adverse side effects are uncommon. Cats may develop a small lump at the injection site.

Indoxacarb. Indoxacarb is a monthly, topical spot-on treatment for fleas in dogs and cats.

Dosage Form
- **Activyl**

Fluralaner. Fluralaner is a chewable tablet or topical solution, given once every 12 weeks, for the treatment of fleas and ticks. Bravecto Plus for cats contains fluralaner and moxidectin for the treatment of fleas and ticks, prevention of heartworm, and treatment and control of roundworms and hookworms. It is a topical solution applied once every 2 months (Merck, 2020).

Dosage Form
- **Bravecto chew for dogs**
- **Bravecto Topical solution for dogs**
- **Bravecto Topical solution for cats**
- **Bravecto Plus Topical solution for cats**

Afoxolaner. Afoxolaner is a monthly chewable tablet for the treatment of fleas and ticks on dogs.

Dosage Form
- **NexGard**

Adverse Side Effects. Use with caution in animals with a history of seizures. Adverse side effects are vomiting.

Permethrin. Permethrin is a topical solution that provides flea and tick control; according to the manufacturer, migration of permethrin occurs on the skin surface. It controls fleas, deer ticks, and brown dog ticks for up to 4 weeks and American dog ticks for 2 to 3 weeks. Dogs should be tested for heartworm disease before initial treatment is provided. Permethrin is not only an insecticide; it is also a repellent.

Dosage Form
- **K-9 Advantix II**
- **Activyl Plus**
- **OTC Horse sprays**
- **Pour-ons and Spot-ons for livestock and horses**
- **Impregnated into cattle ear tags**

Adverse Side Effects. Adverse side effects include skin sensitivity and lethargy.

Sarolaner. Sarolaner (Simparica) is a chewable tablet, given monthly, for the treatment and prevention of fleas and ticks. It can be used in dogs 6 months of age or older weighing 2.8 pounds or greater. In addition, Simparica Trio contains a combination of sarolaner, moxidectin, and pyrantel. It is a monthly chewable tablet for the treatment of fleas and ticks, prevention of heartworm disease, and the treatment and control of roundworm and hookworm infestations in dogs and puppies 8 weeks of age or older weighing 2.8 pounds or greater (Zoetis, 2019).

Dosage Form
- **Simparica** for dogs only
- **Simparica Trio** for dogs only

Adverse Side Effects. Adverse effects include vomiting, tremors, lethargy, seizures, anorexia, ataxia, pruritis, hypersalivation, and hyperactivity (Zoetis, 2019).

Selamectin. Selamectin is a topical solution applied monthly that prevents or controls flea infestation in dogs and cats. It kills adult fleas and prevents flea eggs from hatching. In addition, selamectin is also indicated for prevention of heartworm disease in dogs and cats, treatment and control of ear mite infestations in dogs and cats, and treatment of hookworm and roundworm infections in cats.

Dosage Form
- **Revolution**

Adverse Side Effects. These are uncommon but include transient, localized alopecia at the application sites of some treated cats.

Spinosad. This is a monthly tablet for prevention of flea infestations. It can be used on dogs 14 weeks or older.

Dosage Form
- **Comfortis chewable tablets for dogs**

Spinetoram. This is a monthly topical application for flea and tick control in cats.

Dosage Form
- **Cheristin for cats**

Insecticides
Pyrethrins

These are extracted from pyrethrum or chrysanthemum flowers. They are generally considered safe for most mammals. Pyrethrins have a quick-kill effect and low residual activity (stabilized or microencapsulated pyrethrins have increased residual effects). They are commonly found in pet sprays, dips, shampoos, dusts, foggers, premises sprays, and yard and kennel sprays and are often used in conjunction with other insecticides. Pyrethrins are always used with synergists to maximize their effects.

Synthetic Pyrethroids

Kirk (1986) identifies pyrethroids as "synthesized chemicals modeled on the chrysanthemate molecule of natural pyrethrins, with various substitutions and modifications." Pyrethroids are commonly used in pet sprays, dips, foggers, premises sprays, and yard and kennel sprays. Most have a quick-kill effect, and some have limited residual effects. Their safety is comparable with that of natural pyrethrins. Synergists are not always needed with pyrethroids.

Dosage Forms. The following are common pyrethroids:
- **Tetramethrin**
- **Deltamethrin**
- **Permethrin**

Carbamates

Carbamates act as cholinesterase inhibitors and should not be used with other cholinesterase inhibitors, phenothiazine derivatives, and succinylcholine. They are found in dusts, sprays, shampoos, and flea and tick collars.

Dosage Forms. The following are common carbamates:
- **Carbaryl**
- **Propoxur** (mainly small-animal products)

Adverse Side Effects. These include excessive salivation, vomiting, diarrhea, muscle tremors, and miosis.

> **TECHNICIAN NOTES**
>
> - Read labels carefully.
> - Atropine and 2-PAM (pralidoxime) are antidotal.

Organophosphates

Organophosphates consist of a group of insecticides that inactivate acetylcholinesterase. Without this enzyme, parasites (especially ectoparasites) are unable to move because these chemicals stop nerve transmission. Many of these pesticides tend to break down when exposed to light, air, soil, and other environmental factors. However, some traces have been known to be residual in drinking water and food. Although they may degrade rather quickly, these substances have a high level of toxicity and may cause problems in people and animals exposed to large doses. SLUDDE is a good mnemonic to use for remembering the effects of toxic doses of these drugs: *Salivation, Lacrimation, Urination, Defecation, Dyspnea,* and *Emesis.* Atropine may be used as an antidote.

Organophosphates act as cholinesterase inhibitors and should not be used with other organophosphates, carbamates, phenothiazine derivatives, or succinylcholine. They are found in dips, pet sprays, dusts, yard and kennel sprays, premises sprays, and systemics.

Dosage Forms. The following are common organophosphates:
- **Chlorpyrifos** (tickicide, insecticide)
- **Dichlorvos** (insecticide, larvicide)
- **Diazinon** (lousicide, larvicide, insecticide)
- **Fenthion** (insecticide, larvicide)
- **Phosmet** (insecticide, lousicide)

Adverse Side Effects. These include excessive salivation, vomiting, diarrhea, muscle tremors, and miosis.

> **TECHNICIAN NOTES**
>
> - These products should not be used in dogs prone to seizures.
> - Read labels carefully for user and animal safety.
> - Atropine and 2-PAM (pralidoxime) are antidotal.

Formamidines

Amitraz is the most commonly used formamidine in veterinary medicine. Of note, amitraz is not an organophosphate.

Dosage Forms. The following products contain amitraz:
- **Mitaban** (treatment for canine demodicosis)
- **Preventic Tick Collar for Dogs**
- **Taktic** (large-animal insecticide)

Adverse Side Effects. These include transient sedation, lowered rectal temperature, increased blood glucose level, and seizures.

> **TECHNICIAN NOTES**
>
> Read labels carefully.

Nitenpyram

These are oral tablets for canines and feline 4 weeks or older. Nitenpyram belongs to the chemical class neonicotinoids. It is used to kills adult fleas and starts working within 30 minutes of administration. It is safe for dogs or cats that are pregnant and/or nursing.

Dosage Form
- **Capstar**

Synergists

Synergists are compounds that are added to pyrethrins and some pyrethroids to increase the efficacy of their insecticidal effects.

Dosage Forms. The following are common synergists:
- **Piperonyl butoxide**
- **N-Octyl bicycloheptene dicarboximide** (MGK 264)

Adverse Side Effects. Piperonyl butoxide has shown evidence of toxicity in cats due to licking their treated fur and a low incidence of chronic neurologic side effects (e.g., tremors, incoordination, and lethargy); sprays have levels equal to or greater than 1.5% (Kirk, 1986).

Repellents

Repellants are commonly used in human, equine, and companion animal products. Most repel gnats, mosquitoes, and flies; when combined with pyrethrins and pyrethroids, they repel new fleas and ticks longer than the active ingredient alone. In horses and cattle, they are used to prevent flies from laying eggs on the skin, decreasing bot infestations.

Dosage Forms. The following are common repellents:

- **2,3,4,5-bis (2-butylene) tetrahydro-2-furaldehyde** (MGK 11)
- **Di-*n*-propyl isocinchomeronate** (MGK 326)
- **Butoxypolypropylene glycol**—used in equine fly repellents

Insect Growth Regulators and Insect Growth Hormones

Maturation and pupation of flea larvae normally require a low level of natural insect growth regulators (IGRs). Products that contain IGRs mimic natural IGRs. They cause a high level of IGRs and interrupt the natural development of flea eggs or flea larvae without killing the flea. IGRs are found in pet sprays, flea collars, and premises sprays.

Dosage Forms. The following are common IGRs:
- **Methoprene incorporated into Frontline products**
- **Pyriproxyfen (Nylar) incorporated into Advantage II and Advantix II**

Other Insecticides

Rotenone. Rotenone is very toxic to fish and swine. It is commonly used in combination with other insecticides.

Dosage Forms
- **Rotenone Shampoo**
- **Ear Mite Lotion**

Ivermectin. Ivermectin is a systemic injectable for the control of ectoparasites and some helminths. Studies show efficacy against *S. scabiei* and *O. cynotis*; however, it is not approved for these uses in dogs or cats.

Dosage Forms
- **Ivomec 1% Injection for Cattle**
- **Ivomec 1% Sterile Solution for Swine**

ᴅ-Limonene. This is an extract of citrus peel and is found in flea sprays, shampoos, and dips. It provides a quick kill but is not residual.

Dosage Forms
- **Adams ᴅ-Limonene Flea and Tick Shampoo**
- **Neem Supreme**

Benzyl Benzoate. Benzyl benzoate is effective against many ectoparasites and may be combined with other agents.

Petroleum Distillate. Petroleum distillate is usually added to pyrethrin and pyrethroid products as the solvent.

REVIEW QUESTIONS

1. Name five types of symbiotic relationships.
2. What is parasitiasis?
3. What is parasitosis?
4. What are ectoparasites?
5. What are endoparasites?
6. An animal with endoparasites is said to be _____, and an animal with ectoparasites is said to be _____.
7. What is an anthelmintic?
8. _____ dips should never be used on cats.
9. IGR is an acronym for _____.
10. Praziquantel is a drug that is used to rid the body of _____.
11. Explain the difference between an anthelmintic that is a vermicide and a vermifuge.
12. What is the name of the antidote used for organophosphate poisoning?
13. Drontal plus contains what three ingredients to remove roundworms, hookworms, tapeworms, and whipworms?
14. Ivermectin, moxidectin, and doramectin are in the _____ class.
    a. avermectin
    b. ivermectin
    c. tetrahydropyrimidine
    d. microfilaricide
15. All the following are monthly heartworm preventives, except _____.
    a. milbemycin oxime
    b. selamectin
    c. Heartgard Plus
    d. diethylcarbamazine
16. _____ is a topical solution that controls ascarids, hookworms, and tapeworms in felines.
    a. Selamectin (Revolution)
    b. Emodepside/praziquantel (Profender)
    c. Fipronil (Frontline)
    d. Lufenuron (Program)
17. An arsenic compound administered by deep intramuscular injection in the lumbar region is _____.
    a. caparsolate
    b. clorsulon
    c. melarsomine dihydrochloride
    d. Ivomec

18. Albendazole is the active ingredient found in
   _____.
   a. Droncit
   b. ProMeris
   c. Synanthic
   d. Valbazen
19. An organophosphate is a substance that can interfere with the function of the nervous system by
   inhibiting the enzyme cholinesterase.
   a. True
   b. False
20. Advantage has greater efficacy against _____, and
   Frontline has greater efficacy against _____.
   a. ticks; fleas
   b. fleas; ticks
21. _____ are parasitic worms, including intestinal
   roundworms, filarial worms, lungworms, kidney
   worms, heartworms, and others.
   a. Cestodes
   b. Trematodes
   c. Acanthocephalans
   d. Nematodes
22. When a dog has heartworm disease, what is meant
   by the term Wolbachia?
23. A 1700-lb Angus bull needs to be dewormed with
   albendazole liquid. On hand in the pharmacy is
   albendazole (113.6 mg/mL). The dose is 10 mg/kg
   PO. How many milliliters should be obtained to
   treat this bull?

   a. 48 mL
   b. 68 mL
   c. 58 mL
   d. 38 mL
24. A heifer-calf that weighs 120 lb is found to have
   Eimeria zurnii. The veterinarian orders amprolium
   for treatment of the calf. On hand in the pharmacy
   is Corid liquid (9.6%). The dosage is 10 mg/kg PO
   for 5 days. After the treatment, the veterinarian
   wants to use the drug for prophylaxis. The dosage
   for this is 5 mg/kg for 21 days. How many milliliters
   of the drug should be dispensed to provide prophy-
   lactic treatment for this calf?
   a. 58.8 mL
   b. 60 mL
   c. 49.65 mL
   d. 50 mL
25. A dog is found to have *Dipylidium caninum*. The
   dog weighs 22.4 lb. The dosage is 68 mg for a dog
   this size. On hand in the pharmacy is the right drug
   to use, and it has a concentration of 34 mg per tablet. What drug should be used for this patient? How
   many tablets should be dispensed for one dose?
   a. Doxycycline; two tablets
   b. Praziquantel; two tablets
   c. Diethylcarbamazine; two tablets
   d. Furosemide; two tablets

REFERENCES

American Heartworm Society (AHS). (2020a). *Current canine guidelines for the prevention, diagnosis, and management of heartworm infections in dogs.* American Heartworm Society. https://d3ft8sckhnqim2.cloudfront.net/images/pdf/2020_AHS_Canine_Guidelines.pdf?1580934824. Accessed May 2020.

American Heartworm Society (AHS). (2020b). *Current feline guidelines for the prevention, diagnosis, and management of heartworm infections in cats.* American Heartworm Society. https://d3ft8sckhnqim2.cloudfront.net/images/pdf/2020_Feline_Guidelines_Summary.pdf?1580934824. Accessed May 2020.

Elanco. (2019). *Package insert for Credelio*, Greenfield, Indiana.

Hendrix, C. M. (Ed.). (2017). *Diagnostic veterinary parasitology* (5th ed.) St. Louis: Mosby.

Kirk, R. W. (1986). *Current veterinary IX: Small animal practice.* Philadelphia: WB Saunders.

Merck. (2020). *Package insert for Bravecto Plus for cats*, Madison, New Jersey.

Plumb, D. C. (2015). *Veterinary drug handbook* (8th ed.). Ames, IA: Wiley-Blackwell.

Zoetis. (2019). *Package insert for Simparica*, Kalamazoo, Michigan.

14

Drugs Used to Relieve Pain and Inflammation

OBJECTIVES

After studying this chapter, you should be able to

1. Define terms related to the pharmacology of drugs used to relieve pain and inflammation, understand the difference between physiologic and pathologic pain, and explain the concepts of preemptive and multimodal pain therapy.
2. Describe the anatomy and physiology associated with pain production and relief, list and discuss the four steps involved in the production of pain sensation, and list physical signs associated with the expression of pain in animals.
3. Discuss nonpharmacologic modalities for pain management in animals.
4. Describe the use of NSAIDs in animal pain management, including listing and discussing the indications, side effects, and uses of specific NSAID options.

5. Discuss the use of opioid analgesics to control pain in animals.
6. List and discuss the use of other drugs used as pain control agents.
7. Describe the mechanism of action of antihistamines and differentiate between the action of H_1 and H_2 histamine receptors.
8. List indications for muscle relaxants.
9. List the two major categories of corticosteroids and describe the effects of each, describe how the hypothalamic–pituitary–adrenal axis controls the release of corticosteroids in the body, and list indications and side effects of corticosteroids.
10. Describe the mechanism of action and list some indications of local, regional, and topical anesthetic agents.

OUTLINE

KEY TERMS

Addison's disease
Analgesia
Ceiling effect
Cushing's disease
Histamine
Iatrogenic
Modulation
Multimodal analgesia
Nerve block
Neuropathic pain
Nociceptors

Pathologic pain
Perception
Physiologic pain
Preemptive analgesia
Prostaglandin
Regional anesthesia
Somatic pain
Transdermal application
Transduction
Transmission
Visceral pain

INTRODUCTION

Pain has been defined by the International Association for the Study of Pain as "an unpleasant sensory and emotional experience associated with actual or potential tissue damage." It may occur alone or in combination with inflammation. Pain sensation arises in the terminal ends of sensory nerve fibers called *nociceptors,* which are located in every tissue of the body. Nociceptors (pain receptors) may be activated through mechanical, thermal, and chemical stimulation to create a nerve impulse. Chemical stimulation may be derived from an exogenous source or from endogenous chemicals such as eicosanoids (prostaglandins), bradykinin, serotonin, and others released in response to tissue damage. These substances may create a "sensitizing soup," which may create a lower threshold for nociceptors, amplifying the pain response (Muir, 2015).

Physiologic pain can be beneficial in that it can allow the animal to avoid damaging stimuli. Pathologic pain results from tissue or nerve damage and may be further classified according to its origin, severity, or duration. Visceral pain arises from hollow abdominal organs, peritoneum, heart, liver, and lungs while somatic pain arises from the musculoskeletal system. Somatic pain may be further described as superficial (arising from the skin) or deep (arising from periosteum, tendon, or joint tissues). Neuropathic pain can arise due to injury to the peripheral or central nervous system (CNS) and is described in humans as "burning" or "shooting" (Gaynor, 2015). Pain can have varying degrees of severity (none, mild, moderate, or severe) and is classified as acute or chronic. Acute pain is of sudden onset (injury) and varies in severity from mild to severe and is usually associated with tissue damage. Chronic pain persists beyond the normal healing time or associated with progressive disease where healing has not occurred.

Severe or chronic pain may have an emotional content that activates sympathetic stimulation. It can be harmful because it can lead to stress and related problems such as gastrointestinal (GI) lesions, immunosuppression, delayed healing, hypertension, fatigue, abnormal behavior, and potential dysrhythmias. The ethical treatment of animals includes the "five freedoms": freedom from pain, hunger and malnutrition, discomfort, disease and injury, and freedom to express normal behavior.

Assessment of pain in animals can be very difficult because of the dependence on nonverbal communication in veterinary medicine. Furthermore, animals differ from people in their pain response. It is important for

THE OHIO STATE UNIVERSITY VETERINARY TEACHING HOSPITAL

PAIN MANAGEMENT PLAN

PATIENT ID CARD

"Pain assessment is considered part of every patient evaluation, regardless of presenting complaint."

Date: _____   Department: _____

| Pulse rate: | Temperature: | °C / °F | |
| Respiratory rate: | Weight: | lbs / kg | Attitude: |

Is pain present upon admission? Y ☐ N ☐   Pain on palpation only? Y ☐ N ☐   Cause of pain:

Signs of pain (Check all that apply):

Behavior:	Normal ☐	Depressed ☐	Excited ☐	Agitated ☐	Guarding ☐	Aggressive ☐
Vocalization:	None ☐	Occasional ☐	Continuous ☐	Other ☐		
Posture:	Normal ☐	Frozen ☐	Rigid ☐	Hunched ☐	Recumbent ☐	Reluctant to move ☐
Gait:	Sound ☐	Lame weight bearing ☐		Lame non-weight bearing ☐	Non-ambulatory ☐	

Other signs of pain: Previous Analgesic History:

Descriptors (Circle):

Restless	Not grooming
Agitated	Obtund
Trembling	Inappetant
Nervous	Biting or Licking area

Classification of pain (Check):

Acute ☐
Acute recurrent ☐
Chronic (>weeks) ☐
Chronic progressive ☐

Superficial ☐
Deep ☐
Visceral ☐

Inflammatory ☐
Neuropathic ☐
Both (Infl/Neuro) ☐
Cancer ☐

Primary hyperalgesia ☐
Secondary hyperalgesia ☐
Central analgesia ☐

Anatomical location of pain (Circle):

Ventral   Dorsal

Left

Right

Comments:

Diagnosis:

Fig. 14.1 Form for determining pain level in veterinary patients. (From Gaynor, J. [2008]. *Handbook of veterinary pain management.* St. Louis: Elsevier.)

wild animals to control the expression of pain to avoid predation or abandonment. Response to pain varies among individuals and may include increased heart rate, increased respiratory rate, mydriasis, salivation, vocalization, changes in facial expression, aggressive behavior, guarding of the painful site, restlessness, unresponsiveness, failure to groom, abnormal gait, and abnormal stance. A patient that is pain-free will be quiet and calm (Paddleford, 1999). Consult the *Handbook of Veterinary Pain Management* for pictures and descriptions of pain behaviors in animals. Pain scales and evaluation instruments (Figs. 14.1 through 14.3) have been developed to make pain evaluation more objective. Veterinary technicians play an important role in pain management and must be familiar with the clinical signs (behavioral and physiologic) associated with pain, provide analgesia for animal patients, and provide client education. Understanding the physiology of pain, analgesic medications available, and nonpharmacologic interventions is crucial in the quality of patient care. Table 14.1 illustrates clinical signs associated with pain in dogs and cats.

Drugs used to control pain (analgesics) include nonsteroidal antiinflammatory drugs (NSAIDs), opioids, α-2 agonists, ketamine, and others. The body is able to produce its own opiate-like analgesic agents called *endorphins* and *enkephalins*. Efforts to synthesize these substances for commercial production have been unsuccessful.

At one time people believed that masking pain with analgesics could interfere with the diagnosis or treatment course of a disease. It is now known that animals in pain should be treated for humane reasons and so that the harmful side effects that accompany pain can be reduced. The treatment regimen may vary according to assessment of the severity and the origin of the pain. For best results, pain management intervention should be **preemptive** (before tissue damage) and include **multimodal analgesia** when possible.

Inflammation is a basic process that occurs in the body in response to tissue injury caused by physical, chemical, or biologic trauma. The objectives of this process are (1) to counteract the injury by removing or walling off the cause of the injury and (2) to repair or replace the damaged tissue. Clinical manifestations (cardinal signs) of

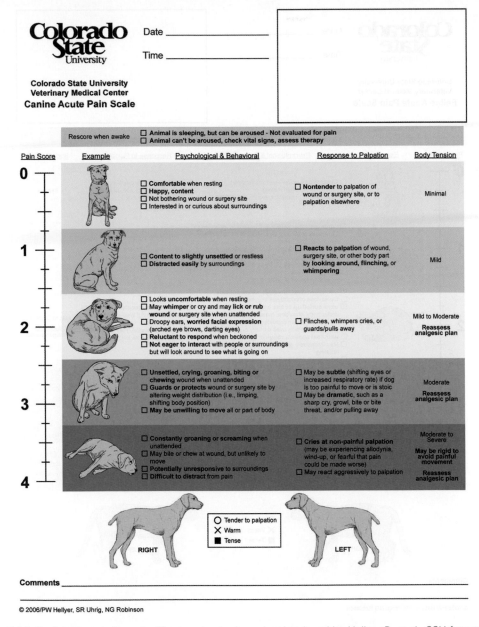

Fig. 14.2 Canine acute pain scale. (Acute animal pain scales developed by Hellyer P, et al. *CSU for assessment of pain in dogs and cats*. www.IVAPM.org. Accessed October 21, 2015.)

inflammation include redness, heat, swelling, pain, and loss of function. Although the process is designed to be protective, it can continue to become a source of further injury or damage (e.g., allergy, shock, or "proud flesh").

Damage to cells from any source results in the release of several chemical mediators that may initiate or prolong the inflammatory response. These chemicals include **prostaglandins**, leukotrienes, **histamine**, cytokines, and other mediators. These substances cause helpful responses such as dilation and increased permeability of blood vessels that result in increased blood flow to the injured tissue. Enhanced blood flow brings

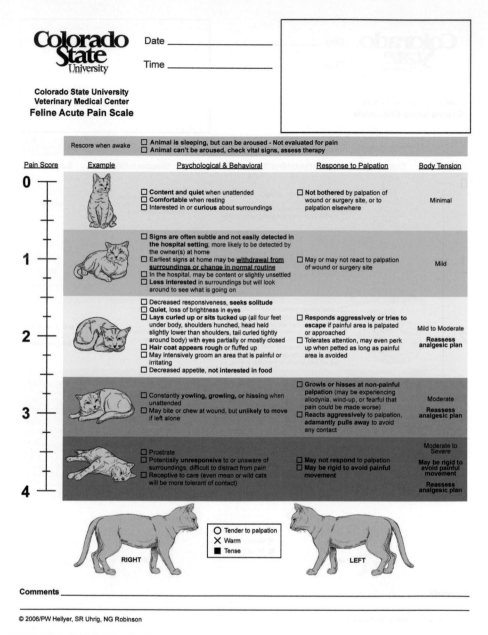

Fig. 14.3 Feline acute pain scale. (Acute animal pain scales developed by Hellyer P, et al. *CSU for assessment of pain in dogs and cats.* www.IVAPM.org. Accessed October 21, 2015.)

plasma to dilute the offending agent, fibrin to immobilize it, and phagocytic cells to remove it. Redness, heat, swelling, and, to some extent, the pain of inflammation result from increased amounts of blood in the damaged tissue. The chemical mediators serve other beneficial functions such as attracting phagocytic cells to the area of concern (chemotaxis) and several potentially harmful

functions such as initiation of bronchoconstriction (histamine), anaphylactic shock, pain (histamine), cell death, platelet aggregation, and intestinal spasm. The inflammatory process can be acute (anaphylaxis) or chronic (flea allergy and arthritis).

Drugs that are used to minimize the inflammatory process include NSAIDs, glucocorticosteroids, and several

TABLE 14.1 Behavioral and Physiologic Signs Associated With Pain in the Dog and Cat.

Hunched back	Aggression when touched	Unwillingness to move	Bradycardia
Tail between legs	Decreased grooming	Difficulty lying down	Tachycardia
Head in down position	Vocalization (Whimpering/ Moaning/Hissing)	Avoiding stairs	Panting
	Hiding	Circling/Pacing	Tachypnea
	Decrease use of litter box	Lameness	Dilated pupils
	Scratching	Non–weight bearing of limb	
	Chewing at painful area	Stilted gait/Stiffness	
	Decreased appetite		
	Decreased social interactions		
	Depressed		
	Changes in urination/ defecation		

miscellaneous agents such as dimethyl sulfoxide (DMSO). Another process mediated by a chemical (or chemicals) released from damaged cells is fever. Fever is an increase in body temperature to above normal; it is an important clinical indicator of disease. The purpose of fever may include destruction of invading microorganisms by heat inactivation and facilitation of biochemical reactions in the body (most chemical reactions are accelerated by increased heat).

Heat is generated by the metabolic activity of muscles and glands and is dissipated through radiation or conduction loss from the skin, sweat evaporation, and evaporation during panting. A "thermostat" in the hypothalamus regulates these mechanisms, which control body temperature.

A substance that can initiate a fever is called a *pyrogen*. An exogenous pyrogen is a foreign substance (e.g., bacteria, viruses) that when introduced into the body causes the release of an endogenous pyrogen (a chemical mediator such as prostaglandin) from white blood cells; this endogenous pyrogen causes resetting of the hypothalamic thermostat. The hypothalamus then activates processes to generate or conserve body heat: shivering to generate more heat, constriction of blood vessels in the skin to prevent radiation and conduction loss, and decreased sweating or panting to reduce evaporation loss. Damaged cells in some instances may release endogenous pyrogens in the absence of exogenous pyrogens. Drugs used to control fever are primarily NSAIDs.

ANATOMY AND PHYSIOLOGY

The production of pain sensation arises through a four-step process: transduction, transmission, modulation, and perception (Fig. 14.4). The first step called *transduction* occurs in nociceptors (pain receptors), which are terminal sensory nerve endings found in almost every tissue of the body. The nociceptor creates action potentials (electric impulses) in peripheral sensory nerves when activated by noxious stimuli. The second step is the transmission of the impulses to the CNS by two fiber systems: type C unmyelinated fibers are responsible for dull, poorly localized pain (in humans), and type A delta fibers are responsible for sharp, localized pain (Ganong, 2003). Type A and type C fibers carry impulses to the dorsal horn of the spinal cord (Fig. 14.5). This information then, in the third step, undergoes modulation (suppression or amplification) and is transmitted up the cord via the spinothalamic tract through the thalamus to the cerebral cortex, where processing occurs and recognition results in pain perception. If any part of this neuronal chain or the cortical interpretive area is nonfunctional, pain sensation does not occur. Multimodal therapy takes advantage of this concept to intervene at different sites within the pathways. Because an active cortex is required, the perception of pain can occur only in a conscious animal. It should be remembered that reflexive activity (e.g., withdrawal reflex) without pain recognition can occur as a result of nociceptor stimulation (see Chapter 4).

The perception of pain can be enhanced by phenomena called *hyperalgesia* and *central sensitization* (Boothe, 2012). Hyperalgesia occurs when the area of tissue injury becomes more sensitive and the threshold for subsequent stimuli decreases. This sensitivity can spread to surrounding uninjured tissue (secondary hyperalgesia). When the neurons of the spinothalamic tract of the spinal cord are stimulated repeatedly, they apparently become sensitized and discharge at a much lower threshold. This activity is called *central sensitization*, or *"wind-up,"* and is the rationale for the idea that pain control is enhanced if an analgesic is given before pain is generated.

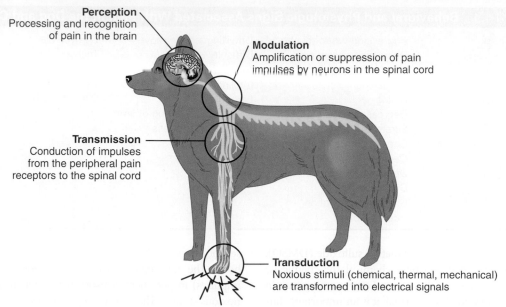

Fig. 14.4 Pain sensation results from four basic steps. (From Thomas, J. [2017]. *Anesthesia and analgesia for veterinary technicians* [5th ed.]. St. Louis: Elsevier.)

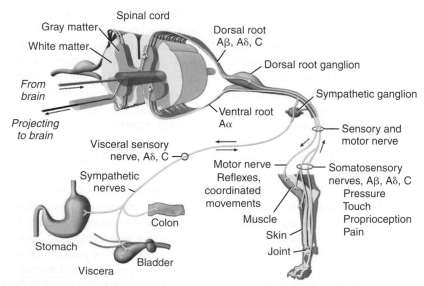

Fig. 14.5 Pain pathways and relevant receptors. (From Gaynor, J. [2015]. *Handbook of veterinary pain management* [3rd ed.]. St. Louis: Elsevier.)

When spinal cord lesions occur, superficial pain is inhibited before deep pain or lesion severity worsens. The absence of deep pain is often a poor prognostic sign.

As mentioned previously, pharmacologic intervention for pain control may target a single, or multiple, points of intervention in the pain process. Transduction can be inhibited by local anesthetics, opioids, NSAIDs, and other substances. Transmission of nerve impulses can be inhibited by local anesthetics and alpha-2 agonists. Modulation of pain impulses can occur in the spinal cord through the effects of

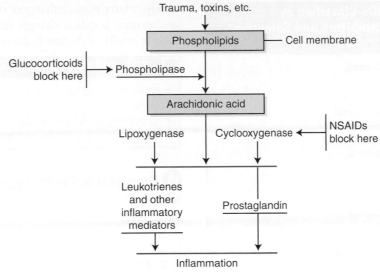

Trauma, toxins, etc.

Phospholipids — Cell membrane

Glucocorticoids block here → Phospholipase

Arachidonic acid

Lipoxygenase   Cyclooxygenase ← NSAIDs block here

Leukotrienes and other inflammatory mediators   Prostaglandin

Inflammation

Fig. 14.6 Actions of nonsteroidal antiinflammatory drugs *(NSAIDs)* and glucocorticoids that interrupt the inflammatory response.

local anesthetics, opioids, alpha-2 agonists, tricyclic antidepressants, NSAIDs, anticonvulsants, and other drugs. Pain perception in the cortex can be inhibited by the use of anesthetics, opioids, benzodiazepines, and alpha-2 agonists.

℞ Nonpharmacologic Modalities for Pain Management

A comprehensive pain management plan should involve pharmacologic and nonpharmacologic interventions. The 2015 American Animal Hospital Association (AAHA)/ American Association of Feline Practitioners (AAFP) pain management guidelines are evidence based and support veterinary professionals in incorporating pain management into practice, improving patient care (AAHA, 2015). Some nonpharmacologic interventions include acupuncture, laser therapy, pulse electromagnetic field therapy (PMFT), physical therapy, environmental modifications, and thermal modifications. Further information on nonpharmacologic modalities can be found on the AAHA website; aaha.org under guidelines.

℞ Nonsteroidal Antiinflammatory Drugs

NSAIDs are very useful analgesic drugs that have been shown to work synergistically with opioids when used together. NSAIDs are thought to work by inhibiting an enzyme called cyclooxygenase (COX), which synthesizes prostaglandin. Two forms (COX-1 and COX-2) of COX exist. COX-1 maintains physiologic functions

such as modulation of renal blood flow, platelet function, and gastric mucosal integrity. Therefore, the disadvantage of administering NSAID is COX-1 inhibition resulting in reduced renal blood flow, bleeding, and GI ulceration. COX-2 is considered the induced (by tissue injury) form that promotes the formation of prostaglandin from cell membrane arachidonic acid (Fig. 14.6). So, COX-2 is associated with tissue trauma and inflammation. COX-2 is also involved in thermoregulation (Edwards, 2019). Generally, inhibition of COX-2 is responsible for effectiveness of NSAIDs and reduces inflammation and fever whereas inhibition of COX-1 is associated with side effects. NSAIDs that selectively inhibit COX-2 are thought to produce fewer GI side effects. Recent research has suggested that this scheme may be an oversimplification and that COX-2 may be induced constitutively in some tissues (Budsberg, 2015). COX-1 versus COX-2 selectivity may depend on the drug, the dose, and the species (Claude, 2013). Ideally, NSAIDs that spare COX-1 and selectively inhibit COX-2 would reduce inflammation and eliminate the negative effects. Box 14.1 lists NSAIDs classified as nonspecific COX inhibitors and selective COX-2 inhibitors.

Glucocorticoids exert their effects by blocking phospholipase, an enzyme necessary for the production of both prostaglandins and leukotrienes (intervention is provided earlier in the sequence of the formation of inflammatory mediators). Because the inflammatory

BOX 14.1 NSAIDs Classified as Nonspecific COX Inhibitors and Selective COX-2 Inhibitors

Nonspecific COX inhibitors:
Aspirin
Phenylbutazone
Flunixin meglumine (Banamine)
Ibuprofen

Selective COX-2 inhibitors:
Carprofen (Rimadyl)
Etodolac
Deracoxib (Deramaxx)
Firocoxib (Previcox, Equioxx)
Meloxicam (Metacam)
Robenacoxib (Onsior)

reaction is blocked earlier by glucocorticoids, they are more effective antiinflammatory agents than are NSAIDs (Langston & Mercer, 1988). NSAIDs are often preferred, however, because they have fewer side effects and they promote analgesia and fever reduction. At this time, it is not known why glucocorticoids do not induce the analgesic and antipyretic effects of NSAIDs. It is also unknown why some NSAIDs provide relief of only mild pain (aspirin) and others provide relief of moderate to severe pain (flunixin). Some clinicians speculate that NSAIDs may act to varying degrees centrally to modulate spinal transmission of pain impulses (Paddleford, 1999).

The most common side effects of the NSAIDs are GI ulceration and bleeding, which probably result from interference with the normal mucous coating of the stomach. Other side effects may include hepatotoxicity, nephrotoxicity, inhibition of cartilage metabolism, bone marrow suppression, and bleeding tendencies (from reduced platelet aggregation).

Cats tend to be less tolerant of NSAIDs than other species due to their slower liver metabolism. Therefore, NSAIDs will be in their active form for a longer period of time.

All pets should undergo a thorough physical examination and history, as well as appropriate laboratory tests, before NSAIDs are initiated. Clients should be advised to stop the use of these drugs and to contact their veterinarian if they observe side effects in their pets that are receiving NSAIDs. Pets receiving long-term treatment with NSAIDs should have periodic evaluations of liver and kidney function performed. Clients should be advised to watch their pets for anorexia, vomiting, changes in bowel movements, bloody or tarry stools, lethargy or other changes in behavior, seizures, jaundice, changes in urination (frequency, color, or smell), or changes in the condition of the skin.

TECHNICIAN NOTES
- NSAIDs should be used with caution in geriatric animals.
- Combining NSAIDs or combining NSAIDs with corticosteroids should be done with great caution or avoided.

Nonspecific Cyclooxygenase Inhibitor NSAIDs
Salicylates

Aspirin, a salicylate, is also known as acetylsalicylic acid. Its actions include the following:
- Relief of pain (analgesia)
- Reduction in fever (antipyrexia)
- Inhibition of inflammation (antiinflammatory effect)
- Reduction in platelet aggregation (blood-thinning effect)

These effects are thought to occur as a result of the ability of aspirin to inhibit an enzyme (COX) that is responsible for the synthesis of prostaglandin. Prostaglandin is a chemical mediator of the processes that lead to pain, fever, inflammation, and platelet aggregation. Its inhibition results in diminishing of each process.

Clinical Uses. Clinical uses of aspirin exist for most animal species and may include the following:
- Relief of mild to moderate pain caused by musculoskeletal conditions such as arthritis and hip dysplasia
- Postadulticide treatment for heartworm disease
- Analgesia/antipyrexia
- Treatment of cats with hypertrophic cardiomyopathy
- Treatment of endotoxic shock

Dosage Forms. These include plain uncoated tablets, buffered uncoated tablets, enteric-coated forms, and boluses (large-animal applications). Many generic or brand names are available in many different strengths, including the following:
- **Aspirin bolus; horses and cattle**
- **Aspirin tablets; dogs**
- **Aspirin granules; horses**

Adverse Side Effects. Adverse side effects of aspirin include gastric irritation, which can lead to ulceration and bleeding. Cats are highly susceptible to aspirin overdosage because of their inability to metabolize it rapidly; they should receive this drug only under the supervision of a veterinarian.

TECHNICIAN NOTES

- Enteric-coated aspirin, such as Bayer, may be used to prevent gastric irritation.
- "Baby" aspirin contains 81 mg.
- Aspirin has no withdrawal time in food animals.

Pyrazolone Derivatives

Phenylbutazone. Phenylbutazone, a pyrazolone derivative, is an NSAID that is approved for use in horses and dogs and commonly used in veterinary medicine. The injectable form of phenylbutazone must be given intravenously; if accidentally given outside the vein it can cause tissue necrosis and severe inflammation. Its actions include the following:

- Analgesia for mild to moderate pain
- Antiinflammatory action
- Antipyrexia

Clinical Uses. These include relief of inflammatory conditions of the musculoskeletal system of horses and dogs. Phenylbutazone is used extensively in horses for the treatment of lameness and for the relief of pain associated with colic. It sometimes is used in dogs and cattle for its antiinflammatory, analgesic, and antipyretic effects.

Dosage Forms. Dosage forms of phenylbutazone include parenteral injection, tablets, boluses, an oral paste, an oral gel, and powder.

- **Phenylbutazone tablets, boluses, paste, injection**
- **Butazolidin bolus, tablets, granules, injectable**
- **Phenylzone Paste**
- **EquiBute tablets, injectable**
- **Phen-Buta Vet tablets, injectable**
- **Phenylbute Paste**
- Various others

Adverse Side Effects. These include GI bleeding, anorexia, and bone marrow suppression.

TECHNICIAN NOTES

- Phenylbutazone injection should be administered by the intravenous route only. Subcutaneous and intramuscular injection may lead to sloughing of tissue.
- Prolonged use or an overdose can lead to bone marrow suppression.
- Prolonged use also may lead to ulcer formation.
- Animals that are receiving long-term treatment with phenylbutazone should be monitored carefully because of possible bone marrow suppression and potential ulcer formation.

Flunixin Meglumine

Flunixin is an NSAID that is labeled for use in horses and cattle. It has extralabel uses in other species. Its actions are related to its ability to inhibit COX and include the following:

- Analgesia
- Antipyrexia
- Antiinflammatory effects

Clinical Uses. Clinical uses of flunixin in horses include alleviation of pain associated with musculoskeletal disorders and colic. (Flunixin apparently has great ability to inhibit visceral pain.) It also has analgesic effects. In cattle, it is used for the control of pyrexia associated with bovine respiratory disease, endotoxemia, and acute bovine mastitis (Merck, 2017). Other uses in horses and other species (extralabel) include treatment of the following:

- Disk disease
- Endotoxic shock (it blocks the effects of endotoxins associated with colic in horses)
- Calf diarrhea
- Parvovirus disease
- Reducing fever
- Ophthalmic conditions (anterior uveitis)
- Postsurgical pain

Dosage Forms. Dosage forms of flunixin include injectable, oral paste, and oral granule formulations.

- **Banamine Injection**
- **Banamine-S**
- **Banamine Oral Paste**
- **Banamine Oral Granules**
- **Flunazine Injection**
- Various others

Adverse Side Effects. These are limited in horses but may include swelling at the injection site and sweating. In dogs, vomiting, diarrhea, nephrotoxicity, and gastric ulceration may occur with long-term use.

TECHNICIAN NOTES

- Flunixin is labeled for intravenous and intramuscular use in horses.
- Some equine clinicians believe that flunixin relieves abdominal pain so well in horses that it may cause a sense of false security about the condition of an animal with colic.
- Small-animal patients receiving flunixin should be well-hydrated and should be given intravenous fluids and ulcer prophylaxis (Paddleford, 1999).

Diclofenac Sodium

Clinical Uses. Diclofenac sodium is a topically applied NSAID cream or ointment labeled for use in horses for the control of pain and inflammation associated with lameness. It is also available, through a compounding pharmacy, in an ophthalmic formulation (solution or ointment) to treat certain types of uveitis in animals.

Dosage Forms
- **Surpass**

Adverse Side Effects. There is a low incidence of adverse side effects.

TECHNICIAN NOTES

- Gloves must be worn when applying this product to avoid absorption.

Propionic Acid Derivatives

Ketoprofen. Ketoprofen is a propionic acid derivative with analgesic, antipyretic, and antiinflammatory activities. It is Federal Drug Administration (FDA) approved for use in horses in the United States but has been used a great deal in dogs and cats in Europe and Canada. Its use in dogs and cats in the United States is extralabel.

Clinical Uses. In horses, ketoprofen is used for treatment of pain and inflammation associated with musculoskeletal disorders. It has been used for postoperative and chronic pain in dogs and cats extralabel.

Dosage Forms
- **Ketofen** (horses), injection

Adverse Side Effects. Side effects may include GI bleeding or ulceration, renal dysfunction, and generalized bleeding.

Ibuprofen. Ibuprofen is reported to have the potential for serious side effects in dogs and cats and is not recommended for use in these species.

Selective Cyclooxygenase-2 Inhibitor NSAIDs

Propionic Acid Derivatives

Carprofen. Carprofen is a propionic acid derivative NSAID that has been approved for oral and injectable use in dogs. It has a half-life of 8 hours and is a selective COX-2 inhibitory drug. It is used to manage pain and inflammation and has antipyretic activity.

Clinical Uses. Uses include the relief of pain associated with degenerative joint disease and postoperative pain resulting from soft tissue or orthopedic repair.

Dosage Forms
- **Rimadyl** tablets, caplets, injection, and chewable tablets
- **Carprieve** injection, caplets, chewable tablets
- **Novox** caplets
- **Carprofen** injection, caplets, flavored tablets, and chewable tablets

Adverse Side Effects. Side effects such as vomiting, diarrhea, and GI ulceration. Renal and hepatic side effects are rare. Laboratory monitoring for hepatic damage, especially in geriatric animals, should be performed.

Etodolac

Etodolac is a NSAID that has analgesic, antiinflammatory, and antipyretic activity.

Clinical Use. This drug is used for the management of pain and inflammation associated with osteoarthritis in dogs (Plumb, 2015).

Dosage Form
- **Generic tablets**

Adverse Side Effects. Side effects include anorexia, vomiting, diarrhea, and lethargy. Keratoconjunctivitis sicca (KCS) has also been reported as a side effect.

Deracoxib

Deracoxib is an analgesic and a nonsteroidal antiinflammatory agent of the coxib (COX-1–sparing) class.

Clinical Use. Deracoxib is labeled for the control of pain and inflammation associated with osteoarthritis, postoperative orthopedic surgery, and postoperative dental surgery in dogs. This drug should not be used in cats.

Dosage Form
- **Deramaxx tablets**

Adverse Side Effects. Side effects, as with other NSAIDs, include GI effects. By feeding the animal around the same time of drug administration can reduce vomiting. Other effects may include GI, renal, and hepatic toxicity.

Firocoxib

Firocoxib is an NSAID that belongs to the coxib (COX-1–sparing) class.

Clinical Uses. It is approved for the treatment of pain and inflammation associated with osteoarthritis and orthopedic surgery in dogs and horses.

Dosage Forms
- **Previcox Chewable Tablets** with once-daily dosing for dogs
- **Equioxx oral paste, chewable, and injection for horses**

BOX 14.2 Case Scenario

A 9-month-old male German Shepherd is presented to the veterinary hospital for limping and lameness on his right front leg.

History: The owner stated that he started limping about 2 days ago. The lameness seems to worsen when being walked and sometimes appears to shift to the other front leg.

Additional History: Up to date on vaccines. Not currently on any medications except heartworm preventative and flea and tick products. No history of trauma. Owner is feeding a high-quality diet. He is eating and drinking normally.

Initial assessment: BAR (Bright, Alert, Responsive), full of energy and very curious. Vital signs are within normal limits. He has a normal respiratory effort although panting, mucous membranes: pink and moist, CRT (capillary refill time): <1 second, and hydration status was normal.

Physical examination findings: Moderate pain elicited on deep palpation of the diaphysis of the long bone on the right front limb. No muscle atrophy noted.

Diagnostic workup: Radiographs of the right front limb, CBC and chemistry panel, and 4DX serology test.

Diagnostic results: The serology test was negative for Heartworm, Lyme, Ehrlichia and Anaplasma. The CBC and chemistry panel were within normal limits, although a slight eosinophilia was noted on the CBC. Radiographs revealed areas of increased medullary opacity (hazy/cloudy densities in the marrow cavity) of the long bone on the right front leg.

Diagnosis: Panosteitis

Treatment: The veterinarian prescribed Previcox (firocoxib) to be given once daily to provide adequate pain relief. A follow-up appointment is scheduled for 2 weeks for a progress evaluation and to determine if there are any concurrent orthopedic problems. The veterinary technician described some of the clinical signs associated with discomfort and pain that she should monitor for at home. She also informed the owner to limit his activity over the next couple of weeks and to notify the hospital if any limping or lameness is observed, especially on other limbs. The veterinary technician further explained how it can develop in other long bones after clinical signs subside in the original affected limb and he may have recurrent episodes until he reaches the age of 2 years. The prognosis is very good as it usually resolves on its own.

At the next appointment the owner stated that he was doing much better and no limping or lameness was observed for the past few days. No pain elicited on palpation of the long bones on all limbs. The owner was told to contact the hospital if he should have another episode of limping or lameness.

This scenario illustrates the important role a veterinary technician plays in pain management and being able to discuss clinical signs associated with pain with the owner.

Adverse Side Effects. Side effects include abdominal pain, nausea, black tarry or bloody stool, and change in behavior. Side effects in horses include diarrhea and excitation.

Meloxicam

Meloxicam is a COX-2 receptor NSAID; called a preferential COX-2 inhibitor. It inhibits COX-2 much more strongly than COX-1. It has antiinflammatory, analgesic, and antipyretic properties.

Clinical Uses. Meloxicam is used to control pain associated with surgical procedures, arthritis, and other causes. Metacam is approved for use as a single (one-time) subcutaneous injection in cats for surgical pain.

Dosage Forms
- **Metacam Oral Suspension**
- **Metacam Injection**
- **Meloxidyl oral suspension**
- **OroCAM, transmucosal oral spray for dogs**

Adverse Side Effects. These are similar to other NSAIDs.

Robenacoxib

Robenacoxib is a coxib (COX-1–sparing) NSAID, highly selective COX-2 inhibitor. It is used for the relief of pain and inflammation associated with osteoarthritis, orthopedic, and soft-tissue surgery in dogs and cats. This drug is approved for use for up to 3 days in cats.

Clinical Uses. Robenacoxib is used for the treatment of pain and inflammation associated with chronic osteoarthritis in dogs and cats and acute pain associated with musculoskeletal conditions in cats.

Dosage Form
- **Onsior,** tablets and injection

Adverse Side Effects. Side effects may include vomiting or diarrhea. The package insert should be consulted for potential interactions with some other drugs.

Other NSAIDs

Dimethyl Sulfoxide

Dimethyl sulfoxide is a clear liquid that was originally developed as a commercial solvent. It is noted for its antiinflammatory action, although not an antiprostaglandin drug, and its ability to act as a carrier of other agents through the skin. Its antiinflammatory actions may be related to its ability to trap products associated with the inflammatory response. DMSO causes vasodilation when applied topically.

Clinical Uses. Clinical uses of DMSO are varied; however, the only labeled use for DMSO is for topical application to reduce acute swelling resulting from trauma or as an antiinflammatory in otic preparations. DMSO has reportedly been used as the following:
- An adjunct to intestinal surgery (intravenously)
- A treatment for cerebral edema or spinal cord injury (intravenously)
- A treatment for perivascular injection of chemotherapeutic agents or other irritating substances (topical)
- A carrier of drugs across the skin

Dosage Forms. Dosage forms of DMSO include a solution (90%) and a gel (90%).
- **Domosol Gel and Solution (90%)**
- **Synotic Otic solution (DMSO and a steroid)**
- **Synasac solution**

Adverse Side Effects. Adverse side effects of DMSO are probably minimal with limited use or exposure but may include the following: garlic taste, which occurs very shortly after the agent is applied to the skin; skin irritation accompanied by a burning sensation; and induction of birth defects (teratogenic) in some species. When administered intravenously to horses it may cause hemolysis and hemoglobinuria (Plumb, 2015).

TECHNICIAN NOTES

- Rubber gloves should be worn while applying DMSO.
- Bandaging over an application of DMSO may cause skin irritation.
- Dimethyl sulfoxide should be used carefully when cholinesterase inhibitors have also been used.

Acetaminophen

Acetaminophen is an analgesic with limited antipyretic and antiinflammatory activities.

Clinical Uses. Clinical uses of acetaminophen are limited in veterinary medicine, and acetaminophen use should be discouraged because of the risk of potential toxicity and the availability of acceptable substitutes. Use in cats is contraindicated because of their deficiency of glucuronyl transferase, which makes them susceptible to methemoglobinemia and hepatic necrosis (Edwards, 2019).

Dosage Forms. Dosage forms of acetaminophen include tablets, caplets, and liquid formulations.
- **Tylenol**

TECHNICIAN NOTES

- Acetaminophen should never be given to cats.
- Over-the-counter products should be checked carefully for the presence of acetaminophen before they are used in cats.
- The drug used to treat acetaminophen toxicity is N-acetylcysteine (Mucomyst).

Adverse Side Effects. Adverse side effects of acetaminophen use in cats include the formation of methemoglobinemia, cyanosis, anemia, and liver damage. Cats have a limited ability to biotransform acetaminophen and may succumb to a single dose.

Buscopan Compositum

Buscopan Compositum is a product that contains butylscopolammonium bromide and metamizole sodium (dipyrone).

Clinical Uses. This product is FDA approved for the management of abdominal pain associated with equine colic.

Dosage Form
- **Buscopan**

Adverse Side Effects. The major adverse side effect is a transient elevated heart rate.

Grapiprant

Grapiprant is a non-steroidal, non-cyclooxygenase inhibiting antiinflammatory drug. It is a selective antagonist of specific prostaglandin receptors (EP4), reducing pain and inflammation. By interfering with only the EP4 receptor, it suppresses pain while reducing the effects on the gastrointestinal tract, kidney, and blood clotting mechanisms (Brooks, 2019).

Clinical Uses. It is a NSAID that controls pain and inflammation associated with osteoarthritis in dogs 9-months of age or older weighing 8 pounds or greater.

Dosage Form
- **Galliprant**

Adverse Side Effects. Some adverse side effects are vomiting, diarrhea, decreased appetite, decreased activity level, soft stools with or without blood.

Polysulfated Glycosaminoglycan

This is a semisynthetic mixture of glycosaminoglycans derived from bovine cartilage. This drug reduces degenerative changes induced by noninfectious or traumatic joint disease and promotes activity in the synovial membrane. It is FDA approved for intramuscular injection and is labeled for use in horses and dogs.

Dosage Form
- **Adequan**
- **Adequan Canine**

Adverse Side Effects. Mild side effects include pain at injection site, diarrhea, depression, lethargy, and abnormal bleeding.

Hyaluronate Sodium

Hyaluronate sodium is a high viscosity mucopolysaccharide used for the treatment of synovitis associated with osteoarthritis in horses. It increases the thickness of the joint fluid and acts as a lubricant.

Dosage Forms. Read the package insert for routes of administration.
- **Legend injectable solution, Multi Dose**
- **Equron**
- **Hyalovet**
- **Hyvisc**

Ⓡ Opioid Analgesics

Opioids and opioid receptors are discussed in a general fashion in Chapter 4. This section addresses only use of opioids to control pain.

Opioids relieve pain by binding with specific receptor sites in the brain, spinal cord, and peripheral tissue. By altering neurotransmitter release, they alter nerve impulse formation and transmission at many levels within the CNS. The ultimate effect is that the opioids block or inhibit pain impulses to higher CNS centers responsible for the perception of pain. Opioids are commonly used in injured or debilitated animals and are the most effective class of drug for managing acute pain and even chronic pain.

Opioid Agonists

Opioid agonists remain one of the most effective drug classes for relieving moderate to severe pain (Wagner, 2015). Opioid agonists are drugs that bind with all opioid receptor sites and produce opioid effects including analgesia and sedation. Adverse side effects of opioid agonists include bradycardia, respiratory depression, excitement, panting, vomiting, and constipation. Opioid agonists include etorphine, fentanyl, hydromorphone, meperidine, methadone, morphine, and oxymorphone. Even though some of these drugs are considered more potent than morphine, morphine is still considered to be one of the most effective of the opioids. All agonists are Class II controlled substances. Naloxone is an opioid antagonist (reversal agent) that is used in cases of severe adverse effects or overdose.

Clinical Uses. Opioid agonists are used to control moderate to severe pain in animals.

Dosage Forms
- **Morphine sulfate**
- **Oxymorphone**
- **Hydromorphone**
- **Meperidine (Demerol)**
- **Fentanyl, transdermal and injectable**

Adverse Side Effects. Side effects can include respiratory depression, sedation, bradycardia, excitement, and addiction. Systemic hypertension and histamine release are additional adverse effects seen with morphine. Cats are more sensitive to the excitatory effects of opioid agonists than are other species; therefore lower doses are used.

Transdermal Fentanyl Use. Transdermal application of fentanyl has been successfully used in humans for control of chronic pain. Fentanyl transdermal patches are FDA approved for use in dogs and are used for the control of postoperative and chronic pain in dogs and cats.

Caution should be exercised when transdermal patches are used; the main concerns are to ensure that the animal does not eat or lick the patch (causing possible overdosage) and that accidental exposure to humans (especially children) does not occur. When the patch is applied, gloves should be worn; the skin over the dorsum of the neck should be clipped, cleansed, and allowed to dry well; good skin contact with the patch should be achieved; and a snug bandage should be applied to hold the patch in place. The patch should never be cut or exposed to heat (e.g., heating blankets) because this interferes with the rate of release of fentanyl. The patch should be carefully disposed of after use. Adverse side effects are respiratory depression, bradycardia, rash at the site of application, urinary retention, and constipation (Plumb, 2015).

Opioid Agonists–Antagonists

The opioid agonist–antagonist drugs bind with opioid kappa receptors but antagonize opioid mu receptors. Opioid agonists–antagonists include butorphanol (Class IV), pentazocine (Class IV), and nalbuphine. These drugs are considered effective for mild to moderate pain and have few side effects.

Clinical Uses. The primary use is for the relief of mild to moderate pain. Butorphanol has a short duration of action of approximately 60–90 minutes. Butorphanol is also approved for use as an antitussive, to help alleviate chronic nonproductive coughing, in dogs and cats.

Dosage Forms
- **Butorphanol** (Torbugesic) injection
- **Butorphanol** (Torbutrol) tablets and injection
- **Pentazocine** (Talwin-V)

Adverse Side Effects. Side effects include sedation, ataxia, and salivation (pentazocine).

Opioid Partial Agonists

The opioid partial agonists bind with the mu receptors but only partially activate them. Buprenorphine is the primary drug in this category and has a longer duration of action than morphine. There is a ceiling effect to this drug, meaning, higher doses do not provide any additional pain relief but may increase the side effects. Buprenorphine is readily absorbed across mucous membranes and can be effectively administered to cats by the sublingual/buccal route.

Clinical Uses. Uses include relief of mild to moderate pain in cats, dogs, horses, and small mammals.

Dosage Form
- **Buprenex;** human label
- **Simbadol**

Adverse Side Effects. Side effects include sedation and respiratory depression.

Opioid Antagonist

Nalaxone is an antagonist (reversal agent) that works by blocking opioids at the receptors.

Clinical Uses. It rapidly reverses sedation and adverse side effects. The onset of action occurs within 1–2 minutes after intravenous injection.

Dosage Form
- **Nalaxone** (Narcan)

 TECHNICIAN NOTES

- Nalaxone is an opioid antagonist used to reverse opioid overdoses and adverse side effects.

℞ Other Drugs Used as Pain Control Agents
α-2 Adrenergic Agents

α-2 agonists are a group of sedative, analgesic drugs that exert their effects by interacting with α-2 adrenergic receptors in the CNS. Unlike primary analgesics like opioids and NSAIDs, α-2 agonists are considered adjuvant analgesics (Lamont, 2015). α-2 agonists, unlike most primary analgesics, can have important cardiovascular side effects.

Clinical Uses. These agents provide sedation, analgesia, muscle relaxation, and reduce anxiety. They may be used as a sedative–analgesic for short, noninvasive procedures, as a component of an injectable anesthetic protocol, as a preanesthetic sedative–analgesic agent, as a postoperative sedative–analgesic agent (bolus or constant rate infusion [CRI]), as a CRI during inhalation anesthesia, as an epidural or intrathecal agent, and others.

Dosage Forms.
- **Xylazine** (Xylazine Injection, Rompun, AnaSed)
- **Dexmedetomidine** (Dexdomitor)
- **Medetomidine** (Domitor)—not currently available in the United States but still available in Canada
- **Romifidine** (Sedivet)
- **Detomidine** (Dormosedan)

Adverse Side Effects. Side effects include bradycardia, transient hypertension, hypotension, muscle tremors, atrioventricular block, vomiting, and hypothermia.

 TECHNICIAN NOTES

- Atipamezole (Antisedan) is an α-2 antagonist drug commonly used to reverse dexmedetomidine.
- Yohimbine is an antagonist drug used to reverse the effects of xylazine.

Ketamine

Ketamine is classified as a dissociative anesthetic/ *N*-methyl-D-aspartate (NMDA) receptor antagonist. NMDA receptors are involved in relaying pain information to the brain. NMDA receptor antagonism may help to prevent the "windup" phenomenon, allow use of lower doses of opioids, and prevent severe acute pain and chronic pain.

Clinical Uses. Microdoses of ketamine are used (primarily as a CRI) as a part of multimodal analgesic protocols.

Dosage Form
- **Ketamine hydrochloride injection**
- **Ketaset injection**
- **Vetalar injection**

Adverse Side Effects. At microdoses, there are few side effects, although tachycardia is possible.

Tramadol

Tramadol is a mu-receptor, opiate-like agonist (Plumb, 2015) that also inhibits the reuptake of norepinephrine and serotonin, causing it to act like an α-2 agonist (Gaynor, 2015). Tramadol is a Schedule IV controlled drug.

Clinical Uses. Tramadol may be useful as an alternative analgesic agent or as an adjunct for postoperative or chronic pain in dogs and horses.

Adverse Side Effects. Side effects may include anxiety, tremors (seizures), vomiting, diarrhea, or sedation.

Miscellaneous Pain Control Agents

- *Lidocaine.* Lidocaine is a local anesthetic that provides systemic analgesia when given intravenously. Lidocaine is also used as an intravenous antiarrhythmic and in combination with opioids, α-2 agents, and/or ketamine (e.g., morphine, lidocaine, ketamine [MLK], hydromorphone, lidocaine, ketamine [HLK], fentanyl, lidocaine, ketamine [FLK], and others) for analgesia or as an adjunct to inhalation anesthesia.
- *Amantadine.* Amantadine may be helpful with controlling "windup," neuropathic pain, and opioid tolerance.
- *Gabapentin.* Gabapentin is helpful in controlling pain related to neuropathic pain, osteoarthritis, and cancer.
- *Tricyclic antidepressants.* Agents like amitriptyline block the reuptake of serotonin and norepinephrine (possible α-2 effect) and may enhance opioid analgesia.

- *Benzodiazepines.* Diazepam has been used as an adjunctive analgesic in birds.

℞ Antihistamines

Antihistamines are drugs that are used to inhibit the effects or spreading of the inflammatory process. These drugs do not inhibit the formation of prostaglandins or other inflammatory mediators. They work by preventing histamine from combining with tissue receptors or by displacing histamine from receptor sites.

Antihistamines may be useful in controlling allergic responses because histamine is a major chemical mediator of the allergic response.

Histamine is a chemical that is released from mast cells when they are adequately stimulated by immunoglobulin E (IgE) antibodies to allergens (Fig. 14.7). Histamine then combines with tissue receptors and causes dilation of small blood vessels, increased permeability of capillaries, smooth muscle spasm, and increased secretion of glands. Two types of antihistamine receptors have been identified: H_1 and H_2.

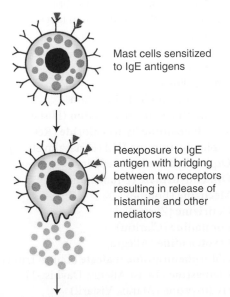

Mast cells sensitized to IgE antigens

Reexposure to IgE antigen with bridging between two receptors resulting in release of histamine and other mediators

Activation of H_1 receptors with dilation of blood vessels, increased capillary permeability, pain, and other inflammatory responses

Fig. 14.7 The release of histamine from mast cells when stimulated by immunoglobulin E *(IgE)* antibodies.

Antihistamines competitively block the binding of histamine to H_1 receptors, which may block progression of the allergic response. Some antihistamines also block H_1 receptors that may contribute to motion sickness or nausea. Some antihistamines have a high affinity for H_1 receptors in the brain and cause a sedative effect.

Stimulation of H_2 receptors causes increased flow of hydrochloric acid by the gastric mucosa. H_2 blockers reduce the secretion of hydrochloric acid and may be used to treat GI irritation and ulceration.

Clinical Uses. Antihistamines are used to treat the following:

- Pruritus
- Urticaria and angioedema associated with acute allergic reactions
- Laminitis in horses and cattle
- Downer cow syndrome
- Motion sickness
- Reverse sneeze syndrome
- Anaphylactic shock
- Upper respiratory tract conditions

Dosage Forms. These include injectables, oral preparations, and topical agents. Many brand names are available under veterinary and human labels. A partial list of the formulations follows.

H_1 Blockers

Dosage Forms
- **Pyrilamine maleate injection**
- **Pyrilamine maleate injection** (Histavet-P)
- **Tripelennamine hydrochloride** (ReCovr Injection)
- **Diphenhydramine HCl** (Histacalm Shampoo, Spray)
- **Diphenhydramine** (Benadryl)
- **Dimenhydrinate** (Dramamine)
- **Meclizine** (Bonine)
- **Cetirizine** (Zyrtec)
- **Loratadine** (Claritin)
- **Fexofenadine** (Allegra)
- **Chlorpheniramine maleate** (Chlor-Trimeton)
- **Clemastine** (Tavist Allergy, Dayhist-1)
- Hydroxyzine (Atarax, Vistaril)
- **Trimeprazine** (Temaril-P)

H_2 Blockers

Dosage Forms
- **Cimetidine** (Tagamet)
- **Famotidine** (Pepsid)

- **Ranitidine** (Zantac)
- **Nizatidine** (Axid)

Adverse Side Effects. Adverse side effects of the antihistamines include drowsiness, weakness, dry mucous membranes, urinary retention, and CNS stimulation on overdose.

 TECHNICIAN NOTES

Antihistamines are not as effective in controlling pruritus in animals as they are in humans.

Ⓡ Muscle Relaxants

Skeletal muscle relaxants may be used as an aid in the treatment of acute inflammatory and traumatic conditions of muscle and the spasms that may result from these situations. They are thought to work by decreasing muscle hyperactivity without interfering with normal muscle tone. This action may be brought about by selective action on the internuncial neurons of the spinal cord.

Methocarbamol

Robaxin-V is labeled for use in dogs, cats, and horses.

Clinical Uses. This product is used to treat patients with the following:
- Intervertebral disk syndrome
- Strains and sprains
- Myositis and bursitis
- Muscle spasms
- Tying up in horses

Dosage Forms
- **Robaxin-V tablets and Robaxin-V injectable**

Other Muscle Relaxants

Dantrolene

Dosage Form
- **Dantrium**

Adverse Side Effects. These include excessive salivation, emesis, muscle weakness, and ataxia when overdosed. The package insert states that adverse side effects are seldom encountered.

Ⓡ Corticosteroids

Corticosteroid drugs are used in veterinary medicine to treat inflammatory, pruritic, and immune-mediated diseases. These drugs are also used to treat shock, laminitis, anorexia, adrenal insufficiency, and various other conditions. The technician should remember that corticosteroid therapy involves treatment of the signs of disease; it is seldom, if ever, curative.

TABLE 14.2 Duration of Action of Corticosteroids.

Short Acting (<12 h)	Intermediate Acting (12–36 h)	Long Acting (>48 h)
Hydrocortisone	Prednisone	Betamethasone
Cortisone	Prednisolone	Dexamethasone
	Methylprednisolone	Flumethasone
	Triamcinolone	Paramethasone

Natural corticosteroids are hormones that are produced by the adrenal cortex, whereas corticosteroids used clinically are synthetic reproductions (analogues) of naturally occurring hormones. Corticosteroids are classified according to their activity as mineralocorticoids or glucocorticoids and according to their duration of action as short, intermediate, or long-acting (Table 14.2). Mineralocorticoids such as aldosterone regulate electrolyte and water balance in the body. Glucocorticoids such as cortisone exert antiinflammatory and immunosuppressive effects and influence the metabolism of carbohydrate, fat, and protein. No corticosteroid has complete glucocorticoid or mineralocorticoid activity, but each has a predominant activity that determines its classification. Because mineralocorticoids are seldom used clinically, this discussion focuses on glucocorticoids.

Control of the release of naturally occurring corticosteroids (i.e., cortisol, corticosterone, and deoxycortisol) is complex and occurs through the hypothalamic–pituitary–adrenal axis (Fig. 14.8). Control is exerted through this axis by two basic mechanisms. The first is a feedback mechanism that is related to the level of cortisol in the bloodstream. When the level of cortisol in the blood is lowered, the hypothalamus sends a chemical messenger called *corticotropin-releasing factor (CRF)* to the anterior pituitary gland. This causes the pituitary to release a substance called *adrenocorticotropic hormone (ACTH)* into the bloodstream. The blood then carries ACTH to the adrenal cortex, where it stimulates this structure to release cortisol to raise the amount in the blood to appropriate levels. On the other hand, a high level of blood cortisol inhibits release of CRF by the hypothalamus, and the blood level is thus prevented from reaching excessive levels. It should be noted that the hypothalamus cannot distinguish between naturally occurring cortisol and synthetic analogues administered by veterinarians.

The second mechanism for control of release of cortisol by the adrenal gland involves the stress response. External and internal stressors such as crowding, weaning, transporting, disease, surgery, trauma, pain, fear, anxiety, and many others can stimulate the hypothalamus—through impulses from higher brain centers—to release CRF. The control mechanism then proceeds in the fashion illustrated in Fig. 14.8.

One of the major indications for the clinical use of corticosteroids is for their antiinflammatory effects. These effects are brought about by their ability to block the enzyme phospholipase, which promotes the reaction that results in the formation of prostaglandin—a primary mediator of the immune response. Corticosteroids also protect cells from inflammatory trauma by various mechanisms that include but are not limited to the following:

- Stabilizing cell membranes to help prevent their breakdown
- Stabilizing lysosomal membranes so they do not release their harmful enzymes
- Disrupting histamine synthesis
- Inhibiting interleukin synthesis
- Reducing exudative processes

Corticosteroids are also used clinically for their immunosuppressive effects. They are used to suppress the immune system in allergic conditions such as flea allergy dermatitis, atopy, autoimmune hemolytic anemia, rheumatoid arthritis, and uveitis. The immunosuppressive effect comes from the ability of corticosteroids to do the following:

- Inhibit antibody formation
- Decrease the concentrations of lymphocytes and eosinophils
- Suppress the migration of neutrophils
- Inhibit phagocytosis

Although immunosuppressive qualities are very useful clinically, they can also mask the signs of serious infection that are simultaneously present.

Corticosteroids are useful in the treatment of lymphoid tumors because they cause a direct lymphotoxic effect (Barton, 2012).

All steroid compounds are synthesized from a basic parent compound that has been described as resembling three rooms and a bath (Fig. 14.9). Steroids are formed in three regions of the adrenal gland. Those regions and their respective products include the following:

- Zona glomerulosa—mineralocorticoids
- Zona fasciculata—glucocorticoids
- Zona reticularis—sex hormones (androgen and estrogen)

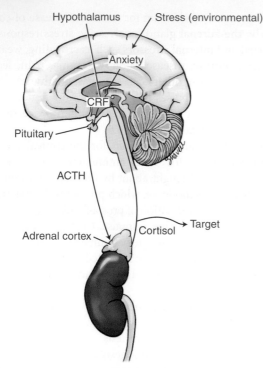

Fig. 14.8 Release of corticosteroids is under the control of the hypothalamic–pituitary–adrenal axis. *ACTH,* Adrenocorticotropic hormone; *CRF,* corticotropin-releasing factor.

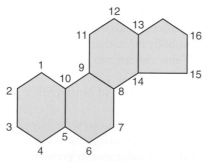

Fig. 14.9 The configuration of the parent molecule of all steroid molecules, including corticosteroids.

An increased number of double bonds in the parent compound, the addition of certain side chains, or the addition of fluorine atoms to the parent molecule usually increases the antiinflammatory effects of corticosteroids.

Clinical Uses. Corticosteroids are used in treatment of the following conditions:

- Allergic reactions/conditions
- Inflammatory conditions of the musculoskeletal system
- Shock/toxemia
- Laminitis
- Inflammatory ocular conditions such as conjunctivitis and uveitis
- Addison's disease
- Autoimmune disease such as autoimmune hemolytic anemia, lupus, and rheumatoid arthritis
- Lymphocytic neoplasms

Dosage Forms. Corticosteroids are available in injectable, oral, and topical forms and in preparations that contain antibiotic, antifungal, and corticosteroid products. These products may be applied to the skin or mucous membranes, injected into lesions, given orally, or administered parenterally. When emergency conditions call for administration of corticosteroids, the intravenous route is normally used with a water-soluble product in a water-soluble vehicle. Water-soluble products can be injected via the intramuscular or subcutaneous route when life-threatening conditions do not exist. Long-acting depot (repositol) products are prepared in a poorly soluble vehicle to prolong their effects. The justification for these long-acting products has been questioned by some clinicians.

A list of some of the many available corticosteroid products follows here.

Injectables

- **Dexamethasone**—Azium Dexameth-A-Vet; Dexium; Dexamethasone sterile solution
- **Dexamethasone Sodium Phosphate**—Dex-A-Vet; Dexium-SP
- **Desoxycorticosterone**—Percorten-V
- **Betamethasone** —BetaVet; Betasone
- **Flumethasone** —Flucort solution
- **Isoflupredone** —Predef 2 × aqueous suspension
- **Methylprednisolone**—Depo-Medrol
- **Prednisolone sodium phosphate**—Prednis-A-Vet
- **Prednisolone sodium succinate**—Solu Delta Cortef
- **Triamcinolone**—Vetalog parenteral

Oral

- **Dexamethasone**—Azium powder, tablets, boluses, oral solution; Naquasone bolus; Dexium tablets; Pet Derm III tablets
- **Desoxycorticosterone Pivalate**—Zycortal suspension
- **Flumethasone**—Flucort tablets; Anaprime suspension
- **Methylprednisolone**—Cortaba tablets; Medrol tablets

- **Prednisolone**—Temaril-P tablets, capsules; Delta Albaplex tablets, 3 × tablets
- **Prednisolone generic tablets**
- **Triamcinolone**—Vetalog oral powder

Topical

- **Animax ointment, cream**
- **Corticalm lotion**
- **Gentocin Topical Spray, Otic solution**
- **Panalog cream**
- **Neo-Predef ointment**
- **Otomax**
- **Relief HC spray**
- **Synalar Otic Solution**
- Various others

Adverse Side Effects. Adverse side effects of corticosteroids are numerous and include the following:
- Polyuria and polydipsia
- Thinning of the skin and muscle wasting (atrophy) that result from the ability of corticosteroids to convert protein into glucose (seen with long-term administration)
- Depressed (delayed) healing
- Polyphagia and resultant weight gain
- Iatrogenic (caused by the veterinarian) hyperadrenocorticism, iatrogenic Cushing's disease
- Hypoadrenocorticism (iatrogenic) resulting from suppression of the hypothalamic–pituitary–adrenal axis by long-term administration of exogenous corticosteroids followed by sudden cessation of treatment (Addison's disease)
- Gastric ulcers with or without bleeding
- Osteoporosis (long-term)
- Abnormal behavior

Clinicians must give careful consideration to the use of corticosteroids because their administration is fraught with many potential side effects. Much information has been written about the appropriate use of corticosteroids in veterinary medicine, and a selection of the principles of use follows:
- Alternate-day dosing may help prevent iatrogenic hypoadrenocorticism.
- Administration should never be stopped abruptly but should be tapered off gradually.
- Very large doses may be used in emergency situations.
- Corticosteroids generally are not used for the treatment of corneal ulcers.

- When corticosteroids are injected into joint spaces, extreme care should be given to aseptic technique.

 TECHNICIAN NOTES

- It is important to discuss with clients not to abruptly stop corticosteroid treatment as it can cause iatrogenic Addison's disease.

Ⓡ Local, Regional, and Topical Anesthetic Agents

Many clinical situations call for the use of local or topical anesthesia to prevent or relieve pain. These agents are discussed here in this chapter on pain relief rather than in the traditional context of anesthesia.

In some situations, general anesthesia is not available or is too dangerous for a client. In others, repair of a small laceration may not justify the use of general anesthesia. In equine medicine, lameness may be diagnosed by administering a **nerve block** to an area and then observing abatement of the lameness. In bovine medicine, it may be useful to administer a regional nerve block to prevent straining while replacing a prolapsed uterus. In cats, it may be useful to apply a local anesthetic to the larynx to facilitate placement of an endotracheal tube.

Local anesthetics work by preventing the generation and conduction of nerve impulses in peripheral nerves. These anesthetics are administered by the following routes:
- Topically to the skin or mucous membranes of the ear, eye, larynx, or other appropriate area
- By infiltration in a localized area, such as the margin of a wound, to anesthetize nerve endings (Fig. 14.10)
- By injection into joint spaces (intra-articular)
- For intravenous regional nerve block; may be used for foot surgery in cattle by applying a tourniquet to the proximal area of a limb and then infusing a local anesthetic into the limb
- Around nerve bodies
  - Epidural anesthesia—injection of a local anesthetic into the epidural space (see Fig. 14.10) of the spinal canal to provide anesthesia to the area around the anus and perineum for obstetric manipulations and to stop straining for the replacement of a prolapsed uterus
  - Nerve block—local anesthetic deposited around a specific nerve (Fig. 14.11) to facilitate minor procedures (e.g., lameness diagnosis, dental procedures, declawing (Fig. 14.12), dehorning, lid or lip suturing)

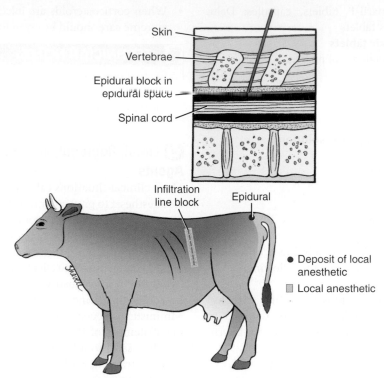

Fig. 14.10 The use of local anesthetics can provide local and regional anesthesia.

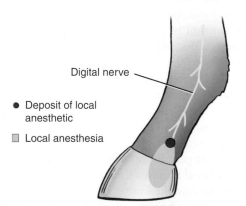

Fig. 14.11 Local anesthesia for diagnosis of lameness in horses.

- Paravertebral block—placement of a local anesthetic around a spinal nerve near where it leaves the intervertebral space; this procedure blocks a larger area and may be used for procedures such as cesarean section and rumenotomy

The onset and duration of action of the agents vary. Lidocaine has a rapid onset of action (5 to 10 minutes) and a somewhat short duration (1 to 2 hours).

Lidocaine may cause a stinging sensation when injected. The onset of bupivacaine effect takes 20 minutes, but it lasts 3 to 5 hours. The effects of local anesthetics can be prolonged by adding epinephrine, which causes vasoconstriction, thereby prolonging absorption time by reducing blood supply in the area. Some clinicians prefer to use xylazine or a narcotic agent for administering epidural anesthesia.

Clinical Uses. Local anesthetics are used for the following purposes:

- Infiltration of local areas
- Epidural anesthesia
- Topical application in the eye, ear, and larynx, among others
- Nerve block
- Antiarrhythmic effects

Dosage Forms. Local anesthetic agents are available in injectable and topical forms. A partial list of these agents follows here.

Injectable

- **Lidocaine** (LidoJect)
- **Bupivacaine** (Marcaine, Nocita)

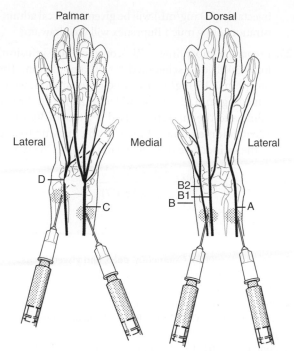

Fig. 14.12 Local anesthesia for a declaw procedure. Branches of the ulnar (*A, D*), radial (*B, B1, B2*), and median (*C*) nerves are infiltrated with local anesthetic before a declaw procedure of the front limbs in a cat. (From Muir, W. W., & Hubbell, J. A. [2013]. *Handbook of veterinary anesthesia* [5th ed.]. St. Louis: Elsevier.)

- **Procaine HCl**
- **Lidocaine hydrochloride injection**
- **Mepivacaine** (Carbocaine-V)

Topical

- **Proparacaine** (Ophthaine)—used for ophthalmic procedures

Adverse Side Effects. Local anesthetics can have adverse side effects if the total maximum dose for the species being treated is exceeded. Side effects may include restlessness, excitement, hypotension, and seizures.

📋 TECHNICIAN NOTES

- Lidocaine with epinephrine should never be used if an antiarrhythmic is indicated.
- Exceeding the total recommended dose of local analgesics may cause toxicity.

REVIEW QUESTIONS

1. Pain sensation arises in free nerve endings called _____.
2. List some signs associated with pain in animals.
3. NSAIDs that preferentially inhibit _____ are thought to produce fewer GI side effects.
4. What is the most common side effect of the NSAIDs?
5. Why are cats so susceptible to aspirin overdose?
6. Phenylbutazone should be administered parenterally by the subcutaneous route only.
   a. True
   b. False
7. What Class II opioid is administered via transdermal patch?
8. Corticosteroid therapy involves treatment of the signs of disease and often cures the disease as well.
   a. True
   b. False
9. What function do mineralocorticoids serve in the body?
10. List some principles that should be followed concerning corticosteroid therapy.
11. What does the term *iatrogenic* mean?
12. Describe the side effects of short-term and long-term corticosteroid use.
13. What is the mechanism of action of local anesthetic agents?
14. What are some indications for the use of local anesthetics?
15. The body is able to produce its own opiate-like analgesic agents called _____.
    a. histamine
    b. endorphins
    c. prostaglandins
    d. cytokines
16. Flunixin meglumine is a(an) _____.
    a. propionic acid derivative
    b. antihistamine
    c. muscle relaxant
    d. NSAID
17. DMSO causes _____ when applied topically.
    a. vasoconstriction
    b. vasodilation
18. List the four steps involved in the production of pain sensation.
19. Define *windup* as it applies to pain production.

20. Pain resulting from tissue injury is called _____pain.

21. List a class of drug that would alter pain recognition and perception.

22. Pain control that utilizes a combination of drugs acting at different sites in the pain production pathways is called _____therapy.

23. An 80-lb dog will be treated with carprofen for osteoarthritis at 4.4 mg/kg once a day. Rimadyl chewable tablets (100 mg) will be used. How many tablets will you give with each dose?

24. An 8-lb cat will be treated for postsurgical pain with buprenorphine at a dosage of 0.02 mg/kg. Buprenex injectable (0.3 mg/mL) will be given by buccal administration. How much Buprenex will you draw up?

25. Prepare a morphine CRI (constant rate infusion) for a 30-lb dog scheduled for an amputation. The morphine (15 mg/mL) will be given at a dosage of 2 mcg/kg/min. It will be added to a 500 mL bag of saline and the mixture infused at a rate of 30 mL/h. What volume of morphine will you draw up to add to the saline? Use the CRI formula from Chapter 3:

$$M = \frac{\{D \times W \times V\}}{\{R \times 16.67\}}$$

REFERENCES

American Animal Hospital Association (AAHA). (2015). *AAHA/AAFP pain management guidelines for dogs and cats.* aaha.org/aaha-guidelines/pain-management-config/pain-management-Intro/. Accessed August 2019.

Barton, C. L. (2012). Chemotherapy. In D. M. Boothe (Ed.), *Small animal clinical pharmacology and therapeutics.* Philadelphia: WB Saunders.

Boothe, D. M. (2012). Control of pain in small animals. In D. M. Boothe (Ed.), *Small animal clinical pharmacology and therapeutics.* Philadelphia: WB Saunders.

Brooks, W. (2019). Grapiprant. Veterinary Information Network. Available at: veterinarypartner.vin.com. Accessed April 2020.

Budsberg, S. C. (2015). Nonsteroidal antiinflammatory drugs. In J. S. Gaynor, & W. W. Muir (Eds.), *Handbook of veterinary pain management* (2nd ed.). St Louis: Elsevier.

Claude, A. (2013). Acute pain management. In *The small animal practice: Pharmaceutical options, in Proceedings. Tennessee Veterinary Medical Association.* Murfreesboro, TN.

Edwards S. Nonsteroidal anti-inflammatory drugs. In *The Merck Veterinary Manual* (online edition). http:merckveterinarymanual.com/. Accessed September 2019.

Ganong, W. F. (2003). Cutaneous, deep, and visceral sensation. In W. F. Ganong (Ed.), *Review of medical physiology* (21st ed.). New York: McGraw-Hill.

Gaynor, J. S. (2015). Definitions of terms describing pain. In J. S. Gaynor, & W. W. Muir (Eds.), *Handbook of veterinary pain management* (2nd ed.). St. Louis: Elsevier.

Lamont, L. A. (2015). α-2 agonists. In J. S. Gaynor, & W. W. Muir (Eds.), *Handbook of veterinary pain management* (2nd ed.). St Louis: Elsevier.

Langston, V. C., & Mercer, H. D. (1988). Non-steroidal anti-inflammatory drugs. In *Proceedings. 17th Semin Vet Tech. West Vet Conf: Las Vegas.*

Merck Animal Health. (2017). *Drug insert for Banamine*, Madison, New Jersey.

Muir, W. W. (2015). Physiology and pathophysiology of pain. In J. S. Gaynor, & W. W. Muir (Eds.), *Handbook of veterinary pain management* (2nd ed.). St. Louis: Elsevier.

Paddleford, R. R. (1999). *Analgesia and pain management. Manual of small animal anesthesia.* Philadelphia: WB Saunders.

Plumb, D. C. (2015). *Veterinary drug handbook* (7th ed.). Ames, IA: Wiley-Blackwell.

Wagner, A. E. (2015). Opioids. In J. S. Gaynor, & W. W. Muir (Eds.), *Handbook of veterinary pain management* (2nd ed.). St. Louis: Elsevier.

15

Therapeutic Nutritional, Fluid, and Electrolyte Replacements

OBJECTIVES

After studying this chapter, you should be able to

1. Define terms related to fluid, electrolyte, and selected therapeutic nutritional preparations.
2. Describe the distribution of water and electrolytes in the body.
3. Describe the composition of body and therapeutic fluids.
4. Define *osmotic pressure* and *tonicity* as they apply to fluids.
5. Discuss the basic principles of fluid therapy and the indications for fluid therapy.
6. Understand the indicators of dehydration and estimating the degree of dehydration in animals.
7. Determine the amount of fluid to administer to a patient based on their clinical indications.
8. Discuss the different routes of fluid administration and indications for their use.
9. Accurately calculate the rate of intravenous fluid administration using standard and micro administration sets.
10. Describe parameters and methods used to monitor a patient on fluid therapy and discuss when to discontinue fluid therapy.
11. Prepare fluid administration equipment.
12. List and describe the types of solutions used in fluid therapy.
13. Discuss the use of fluid additives.
14. List and describe selected oral electrolyte preparations.
15. Discuss parenteral nutrition and describe selected parenteral vitamin–mineral products.

OUTLINE

KEY TERMS

Buffer
Colloid
Dissociation
Electrolyte
Empirical
Hyperkalemia
Hypernatremia
Hypertonic solutions
Hypokalemia
Hyponatremia

Hypotonic solutions
Hypovolemia
Isotonic solutions
Metabolic acidosis
Metabolic alkalosis
Oncotic pressure
Osmotic pressure
Solute
Transcellular fluid
Turgor

INTRODUCTION

Veterinary technicians have an important role in fluid, electrolyte, and therapeutic nutritional therapy for patients. They administer parenteral or oral fluid or nutritional products and monitor patients' responses under the direction of a veterinarian. Fluid therapy is tailored to each patient and must be constantly reevaluated according to the variations in patient status. Technicians must have a thorough knowledge of the products and their use because the use of these products can be critically important to the outcome of a case.

ANATOMY, PHYSIOLOGY, AND CHEMISTRY

Distribution of Body Water and Electrolytes

Measurements of total body water (TBW) have shown that water represents 50% to 70% of the total body weight in adult animals; 60% is often used as the average figure.

As much as 80% of a neonatal animal's body weight may be water, which is a factor that makes fluid loss in young animals potentially very serious. An increase in body fat decreases the amount of TBW and makes it important to estimate fluid needs on the basis of lean body mass to avoid overhydration.

TBW is distributed in several compartments within the body (Fig. 15.1). Sixty percent of TBW is found within cells and is called *intracellular fluid (ICF)*. ICF makes up 40% of total body weight (approximately two-thirds of TBW). The fluid found outside the cells is called *extracellular fluid (ECF)* and accounts for 20% of total body weight.

ECF (discounting the relatively small **transcellular fluid** component) distributes itself between the interstitial fluid (15% of body weight) and the intravascular fluid or plasma (5% of body weight). The intravascular fluid volume is estimated at 90 mL/kg for dogs and 45 mL/kg for cats.

Body fluid compartments should be thought of as volumes of fluid and electrolytes in dynamic equilibrium,

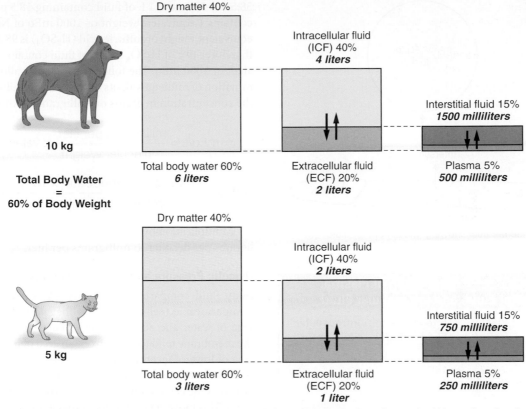

Dry matter 40%

Intracellular fluid
(ICF) 40%
4 liters

Interstitial fluid 15%
1500 milliliters

10 kg

**Total Body Water
=
60% of Body Weight**

Total body water 60%
6 liters

Extracellular fluid
(ECF) 20%
2 liters

Plasma 5%
500 milliliters

Dry matter 40%

Intracellular fluid
(ICF) 40%
2 liters

Interstitial fluid 15%
750 milliliters

5 kg

Total body water 60%
3 liters

Extracellular fluid
(ECF) 20%
1 liter

Plasma 5%
250 milliliters

Fig. 15.1 Body fluid compartments. (From DiBartola, S. P. [2008]. *Fluid, electrolyte and acid-base disorders in small animal practice* [3rd ed.]. St Louis: Saunders.)

with fluids and electrolytes moving back and forth across semipermeable cell membranes. Changes in the quantity of fluid or electrolytes in one compartment usually result in changes in these quantities in other compartments. Fluids administered intravenously to an animal first enter the intravascular space of the ECF, move into the interstitial space, and then enter the ICF (Fig. 15.2). In most cases, loss of fluid occurs first from the ECF and then from other compartments.

Composition of Body and Therapeutic Fluids

Body water contains an array of solutes that vary in quantity from compartment to compartment. A solute is a substance that dissolves in a solvent; this solvent is usually water in biologic systems. The molecules of substances called electrolytes break down (dissociate) into charged particles called *ions*. Electrolytes are positively charged (cations) or negatively charged (anions). The number of cations always equals the number of anions in healthy animals (Table 15.1). In the ECF, the most abundant cation is sodium, and the most abundant anions are chloride and

bicarbonate. In the ICF, the major cations are potassium and magnesium, and the major anions are phosphates and proteins. Therapeutic fluids are described as balanced if they resemble ECF in composition and unbalanced if they do not. Lactated Ringer's solution (LRS) is an example of a balanced solution, and saline is an example of an unbalanced solution. Table 15.2 lists the composition of some of the solutions used in fluid therapy.

It is important for technicians to have a basic understanding of the way in which solute particles such as electrolytes are quantified in fluids. One of the oldest ways of measuring solute concentration is by describing the weight of the solute per 100 mL of solution (g%). A 0.9% sodium chloride (NaCl) solution (saline) would contain 0.9 g/100 mL or 900 mg/100 mL. Other clinically significant ways of describing the quantity of solute particles include the use of concepts of (1) the milliequivalent, (2) osmolality, (3) osmolarity, and (4) tonicity.

The milliequivalent is the unit of measurement that is used to express the concentration of electrolytes, such as sodium, potassium, and calcium, in solutions. The

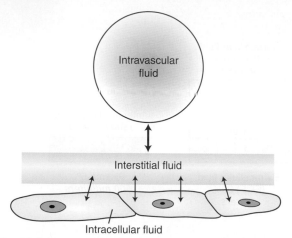

Fig. 15.2 Schematic showing movement of fluid between compartments.

TABLE 15.1	Composition of Plasma, Interstitial Fluid, and Intracellular Fluid.		
Ion	**Plasma (mEq/L)**	**Interstitial Fluid (mEq/L)**	**Intracellular Fluid (mEq/L)**
Cations			
Na^+	142	145.1	12.0
K^+	4.3	4.4	140
Ca^{2+}	2.5	2.4	4.0
Mg^{2+}	1.1	1.1	34
Total	**149.9**	**153.0**	**190**
Anions			
Cl^-	104	117.4	4
HCO_3^-	24	27.1	12
H_2PO_4	2	2.3	40
Protein	14	none	50
Other	5.9	6.2	84
Total	**149.9**	**153.0**	**190**

concentration of these substances is usually expressed as milliequivalents per liter (mEq/L) in fluids and milliequivalents per milliliter in supplements. The milliequivalent describes the tendency of a particle to combine with another particle and is defined as 1:1000 of an equivalent. An *equivalent weight* is defined as the weight in grams of an element that will combine with 1 g of hydrogen ion. For all practical purposes, the equivalent weight of a compound is equal to the gram molecular weight of the substance divided by the total positive valence of the material in question (Blankenship et al., 1976). For example, the equivalent weight of NaCl is

58.5/1 = 58.5, and 1 L of fluid containing 58.5 g of NaCl contains 1 equivalent weight or 1000 mEq of NaCl. The equivalent weight of sulfuric acid (H_2SO_4) is 98.1/2 = 49; therefore, 49 g of H_2SO_4 in 1 L of fluid contains 1 equivalent or 1000 mEq. The following formulas allow determination of milliequivalents of solute in a solution when the concentration in grams or milligrams is known:

$$mEq/L = \frac{\text{milligrams per liter}}{\text{molecular weight}} \times \text{valence}$$

or

$$mEq/L = \frac{\text{milligrams per deciliter} \times 10^*}{\text{molecular weight}} \times \text{valence}$$

*Multiplication by 10 in the numerator converts milligrams per deciliter to milligrams per liter.

Osmotic Pressure and Tonicity of Fluids

Body fluid compartments usually are separated by a semipermeable (cell) membrane that permits the passage of water and some solutes. Solutes that can cross the membrane tend to move from an area of higher to an area of lower concentration by the process called *diffusion* and continue toward equilibrium. Solutes that cannot cross the cell membrane tend to attract water toward them. This movement of water across a cell membrane is called *osmosis*, and the ability of particles to attract water is called **osmotic pressure**.

Osmolality is a determination of the osmotic pressure of a solution on the basis of the relative number of solute particles in 1 kg of the solution. The greater the number of particles, the greater the pressure generated. The unit of measurement of osmolality is the osmol (osm), and 1 osm of any substance is equal to 1 g molecular weight divided by the number of particles formed by the **dissociation** of that substance. A substance that dissociates into two particles in solutions creates twice as much osmotic pressure as one that does not dissociate. The milliosmole (mOsm) is used when fluids are described because the quantities being measured are very small in biologic systems. One kilogram of a solution containing 29.25 g (58.5/2 particles) of NaCl would generate 1 osm/kg, or 1000 mOsm/kg of osmotic pressure.

Osmolarity refers to the number of particles per liter of solvent rather than per kilogram of solvent, as with osmolality. Very little difference is observed, however, between osmolality and osmolarity of animal fluids, and the terms frequently are used interchangeably. A 1-L solution that

TABLE 15.2 Composition of Solutions Used in Fluid Therapy.

	Glucose[a] (g/L)	Na+ (mEq/L)	Cl- (mEq/L)	K+ (mEq/L)	Ca2+ (mEq/L)	Mg2+ (mEq/L)	Buffer[b] (mEq/L)	Osmolarity (mOsm/L)	kcal/L
Dextrose Electrolyte Solution Composition									
5% Dextrose in water (D5W)	50	0	0	0	0	0	0	252	170
10% Dextrose	100	0	0	0	0	0	0	505	340
2.5% Dextrose in 0.45% NaCl	25	77	77	0	0	0	0	280	85
5% Dextrose in 0.45% NaCl	50	77	77	0	0	0	0	406	170
5% Dextrose in 0.9% NaCl	50	154	154	0	0	0	0	560	170
0.45% NaCl	0	77	77	0	0	0	0	155	0
0.85% NaCl (normal saline)	0	145	145	0	0	0	0	290	0
0.9% NaCl	0	154	154	0	0	0	0	310	0
3% NaCl	0	513	513	0	0	0	0	1027	0
Lactated Ringer's solution	0	130	109	4	3	0	28(L)	273	9
2.5% Dextrose in lactated Ringer's solution	25	130	109	4	3	0	28(L)	398	94
5% Dextrose in lactated Ringer's solution	50	130	109	4	3	0	28(L)	524	179
2.5% Dextrose in half-strength lactated Ringer's solution	25	65.5	55	2	1.5	0	14(L)	263	89
Normosol-M in 5% dextrose[c]	50	40	40	13	0	3	16(A) 27(A)	364	175
Normosol-R[c]	0	140	98	5	0	3	23(G)	296	18

Continued

TABLE 15.2 Composition of Solutions Used in Fluid Therapy.—cont'd

	Glucose[a] (g/L)	Na+ (mEq/L)	Cl- (mEq/L)	K+ (mEq/L)	Ca2+ (mEq/L)	Mg2+ (mEq/L)	Buffer[b] (mEq/L)	Osmolarity (mOsm/L)	kcal/L
Plasma-Lyte R[d]	0	140	103	10	5	3	47(A) 8(L)	312	17
Plasma-Lyte 148 / A	0	140	98	5	0	3	27(A)	294	
Plasma-Lyte M	0	40	40	13	0	0	0	363	
Plasma-Lyte M in 5% dextrose[c]	50	40	40	16	5	3	12(A) 12(L)	376	178
Plasma	1	145	105	5	5	3	24(B)	300	—
Additives and Solutions									
20% Mannitol	200(M)	0	0	0	0	0	0	1099	—
7.5% NaHCO₃	0	893(B)	0	0	0	0	893(B)	1786	0
8.4% NaHCO₃	0	1000(B)	0	0	0	0	1000(B)	2000	0
10% CaCl₂	0	0	2720	0	1360	0	0	4080	0
14.9% KCl	0	0	2000	2000	0	0	0	4000	0
50% Dextrose	500	0	0	0	0	0	0	2780	1700

[a]All glucose, with one exception: M, mannitol.
[b]Buffers used: A, acetate; B, bicarbonate; G, gluconate; L, lactate.
[c]CEVA Laboratories.
[d]Baxter Healthcare.
Modified, 2019 From Chew, D. J., & DiBartola, S. P. (1986). Saunders manual of small animal nephrology and urology. Philadelphia: WB Saunders Co.

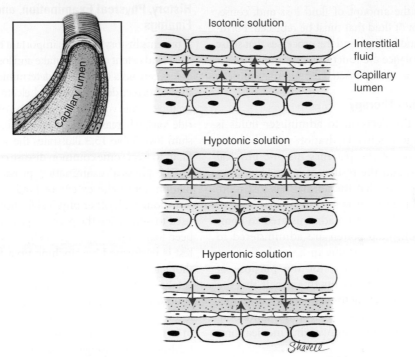

Fig. 15.3 Schematic showing the potential osmotic effects of intravenous fluids on water movement between the interstitial space and the capillary lumen (intravascular space).

contains a full gram molecular weight (58.5 g) of NaCl would generate 2 osm, or 2000 mOsm/L, of osmotic pressure.

Not all solutes contribute to osmotic activity (exert a "pull" on water molecules). Those particles that are capable of generating pressure are called *effective osmoles,* and those that are not are called *ineffective osmoles.* Sodium and glucose provide most of the effective osmoles in commercial fluid preparations. The total effective osmolarity/osmolality of a solution is called *tonicity.* The osmolality of dog and cat serum is approximately 300 mOsm/L. Commercial fluids with an osmolality of 300 mOsm/L are **isotonic** (e.g., Ringer's solution). Those with an osmolality greater than 300 mOsm/L are **hypertonic** (e.g., 10% dextrose), and those with an osmolality less than 300 mOsm/L are **hypotonic** (e.g., 0.45% saline).

An illustration of the importance of the osmolality of fluids is as follows: if a higher concentration of sodium exists than in the interstitial space, then water would be drawn from the intracellular space into the interstitial space. Once in the interstitial space, fluid would move between the intravascular space and the interstitial space to maintain balance between these two compartments.

Flow into and out of the intravascular space occurs at the capillary level, whose membranes are permeable to small particles like sodium and glucose but are generally impermeable to large molecules like colloids and plasma proteins. A large amount of solute within the intravascular space will create high osmotic/oncotic pressure and cause water to be retained within or drawn into the vasculature. Another factor influencing the movement of fluids between compartments is the fluid hydrostatic pressure within the compartment. When the hydrostatic pressure of the fluid exceeds the osmotic/oncotic pressure (pull) of the solute, fluid leaves the compartment. Fig. 15.3 illustrates the potential movement of water into and out of the vasculature based on the osmolality of the vascular fluid.

Osmotic destruction of red blood cells by the fluids is avoided because most therapeutic fluids are composed of solute concentrations similar to that found in body fluids.

PRINCIPLES OF FLUID THERAPY

Fluid therapy is a critical but somewhat inexact component of veterinary medical care. It is critical because it is often lifesaving, but it is inexact because its application revolves around estimating the amount of fluid loss and, consequently, the amount of fluid that must be replaced. Fortunately, if the heart and kidneys and the processes that sense and control fluid balance are functioning normally, many errors of estimation are compensated for automatically.

Indications for Fluid Therapy

A basic factor in the decision to administer fluids is the animal's hydration status. Hydration status is determined by evaluation of the patient's history, physical examination status, and the results of basic laboratory tests. If it is determined that the animal has lost more water than it has taken in, it is said to be in a state of *dehydration,* and fluids must be administered to compensate. In addition, fluids often are administered to maintain normal hydration status in animals that are losing excessive fluid quantities, for the purpose of replacing electrolytes and nutrients in animals that are not eating properly, correcting hypovolemia, correcting acid–base and electrolyte imbalances, and maintaining an open intravenous line for administering medications.

Fluid Balance

In healthy animals, the intake of fluid and electrolytes is adjusted to offset losses that occur. Sources of water intake include (1) water that is drunk, (2) water that is ingested in food, and (3) water that results from the metabolism of food (metabolic water). Normal routes of water loss include (1) urine, (2) fecal water, (3) sweat (horses), and (4) respiration. Respiratory loss potentially can be important in dogs because of panting, and sweating can be important in horses. Fluid losses are frequently characterized as sensible—those that can be measured easily (e.g., urine, vomiting, diarrhea), and insensible—those that cannot be measured easily (e.g., respiratory losses).

 TECHNICIAN NOTES

Insensible losses can be estimated at one-third of maintenance requirements.

Decreased fluid intake often accompanies anorexia, and increased fluid loss occurs in disease states that cause polyuria, vomiting, and diarrhea. Third-space shifts or sequestrations of body water occasionally may cause quantities to be taken from circulation as they are trapped in body cavities or lost through skin lesions (e.g., intestinal obstruction, body cavity effusions, or hemorrhages). Extensive burns, which are uncommon in veterinary medicine, also can cause extensive fluid loss.

History, Physical Examination, and Laboratory Findings

A patient's history provides important information about the route and extent of water intake and loss. Knowing the route of loss can aid a clinician in determining the type of fluid to use to correct dehydration and electrolyte imbalances. For example, acute vomiting leads to loss of potassium and chloride ions, whereas acute diarrhea causes primarily a potassium loss. Table 15.3 illustrates the selection of crystalloid fluids to treat some common disease conditions.

The physical examination provides important information about the extent of fluid loss. The skin **turgor** test, along with other physical findings (see Table 15.4), is used to determine the percentage of body weight that has been lost via fluid (percent dehydration). The skin turgor test is performed by pinching up a fold of skin over the thoracic or lumbar area and then determining how long it takes to return to a normal position. If the neck area is used in small animals, the extra skin may cause misleading results. The point of the shoulder should be used in horses because the skin of the neck area can again be misleading. The longer the skin takes to return to normal, the greater the degree of dehydration. Animals with little body fat may appear to be more dehydrated than they really are (slow return to normal skin position) because of low body fat levels, whereas obese animals may appear to be well-hydrated when they are not because increased fat increases skin elasticity. Dehydrated animals may exhibit dry mucous membranes, as well as increased skin tenting.

It is important to differentiate between dehydration and hypovolemia when assessing physical findings. *Hypovolemia* refers to what is occurring in the vascular system, whereas *dehydration* refers to changes in the intracellular and interstitial system. Correction of hypovolemia is often more urgent than treating mild to moderate dehydration because proper organ perfusion and function depend on adequate perfusion by the vascular system. Signs used to detect hypovolemia are based on perfusion and include pale mucous membrane color, increased capillary refill time, hypotension, tachycardia, weak peripheral pulses, cool peripheral extremities, and hypothermia.

Simple laboratory tests may be performed to aid in assessing hydration status because most of the evaluations mentioned earlier are subjective. These tests include packed cell volume (PCV), total plasma protein (TPP), and urine specific gravity determination. Dehydration generally results in an increase in PCV, TPP, and urine specific gravity. PCV always should be evaluated with TPP because anemia can make a dehydrated

TABLE 15.3 Fluid and Electrolyte Disorders and Fluids Used in Their Correction.

Condition	SERUM Na+	Cl−	K+	HCO₃	Volume	Fluid of Choice
Diarrhea	D	D	D	D	D	Plasma-Lyte A + KCL Lactated Ringer's + KCl, Normosol-R
Pyloric obstruction	D	D	D	I	D	0.9% NaCl
Dehydration	I	I	N	N/D	D	Plasma-Lyte A + KCL Lactated Ringer's, 0.9% NaCl, Normosol-R
Congestive heart failure	N/D	N/D	N	N	I	0.45% NaCl + 2.5% dextrose, 5% dextrose
End-stage liver disease	N/I	N/I	D	D	I	Plasma-Lyte A + KCL, 0.45% NaCl + 2.5% dextrose + KCl
Acute renal failure						Plasma-Lyte A, Normosol-R, lactated Ringer's, 0.9% NaCl
Oliguria	I	I	I	D	I	0.9% NaCl
Polyuria	D	D	N/D	D	D	Plasma-Lyte A, lactated Ringer's + KCl, Normosol-R
Chronic renal failure	N/D	N/D	N	D	N/D	Lactated Ringer's solution, Plasma-Lyte A, 0.9% NaCl
Adrenocortical insufficiency	D	D	I	N/D	D	0.9% NaCl
Diabetic ketoacidosis	D	D	N/D	D	D	0.9% NaCl (±KCl)

D, Decreased; *I,* increased; *N,* normal.
From Battaglia, A. M. (2016). *Small animal emergency and critical care for veterinary technicians* (3rd ed.). St Louis: Elsevier.

TABLE 15.4 Clinical Signs of Dehydration.

	Dry Oral Mucous Membranes	Increased Skin Tenting	Tachycardia	Decreased Pulse Pressure	Sunken Eyes	Alteration of Consciousness
5%	√	√				
7%	√	√	√			
10%	√	√	√	√		
12%	√	√	√	√	√	√

patient appear to be normally hydrated. Plasma lactate levels may be elevated in cases with poor tissue perfusion. Technicians should consult more advanced references for interpretation of laboratory findings related to hydration status and hypovolemia.

Determining the Amount of Fluid to Administer

Clinical indications for fluid therapy include resuscitation (shock), replacement (dehydration), and maintenance (maintaining normal fluid balance).

Shock Doses of Fluids

A patient's shock dose is a volume of fluid equivalent to an animal's total blood volume. Shock doses of isotonic crystalloid fluids cited in the 2013 American Animal Hospital Association and the American Association of Feline Practitioners (AAHA/AAFP) are:

- **Dogs: 80–90 mL/kg IV (dosed to effect)**
- **Cats: 50–55 mL/kg IV (dosed to effect)**

Fluid administration is normally given in increments (e.g., one-quarter of the calculated shock dose) over 15 minutes and reassess the patient for improvement. If needed, another bolus of shock doses may be given and the patient reassessed. If 50% of the calculated shock volume of isotonic crystalloids has not caused sufficient improvement in perfusion, then switching to or adding a colloid may be needed.

For example, if a 10-kg dog presents in shock, the shock dose of fluids in milliliters is calculated as follows:

$$\frac{80 \text{ mL}}{\text{kg}} \times 10 \text{ kg} = 800 \text{ mL}$$

The dog would need a fraction (¼ dose) of the total dose over a specified period of time (15 minutes).

$$800 \text{ mL} \times \frac{1}{4} = 200 \text{ mL}$$

Replacement Fluids

Three values that are calculated to determine the fluid replacement volume to administer are (1) the hydration deficit, (2) the maintenance requirement, and (3) the ongoing losses.

The hydration deficit, which is the amount of fluid that must be replaced to bring the animal back to a normal hydration status, is calculated by multiplying the estimated percent of dehydration (as a decimal) by the patient's body weight in kilograms. The percentage of dehydration is estimated from the history, physical examination, and laboratory findings. The following equation is used to determine the volume of fluid required to replace hydration deficits:

% dehydration (as a decimal) × body weight (kg)
= Volume to deliver in liters

For example, if a 10-kg beagle is determined to be 5% dehydrated, the hydration deficit is calculated as follows:

$$0.05 \times 10 = 0.5 \text{ L}$$
$$0.5 \text{ L} \times 1000 \text{ mL/L} = 500 \text{ mL}$$

Or the following equations can be used:

% dehydration (as a decimal) × body weight (kg)
× 1000 = Volume to deliver in mL

% dehydration (as a decimal) × body weight (lb)
× 500 = Volume to deliver in mL

The length of time for the volume to be replaced is determined by the veterinarian; replacement is usually over 12–24 hours.

Maintenance Fluids

The second value needed to calculate the volume of fluids to administer is the maintenance value. Maintenance fluid therapy is used to replenish normal fluid balance and is indicated for animals that have lost fluids via normal urination, evaporation, or metabolism. Maintenance fluid therapy is not indicated in animals with hypotension, ongoing losses, or volume depletion. Recommended maintenance fluid rates (mL/kg/h) for the dog and cat as cited in the 2013 AAHA/AAFP Fluid Therapy Guidelines are as follows:

- *Dogs:* **2–6 mL/kg/h**
- *Cats:* **2–3 mL/kg/h**

Other formulas that are used to determine the daily maintenance fluid requirement include 40–60 mL/kg/day or 30 mL/lb/day.

For example: What is the maintenance requirement for a 10-kg dog in milliliters per hour?

The formula for the maintenance requirements in milliliters per hour is calculated as follows:

Rate per hour (mL) = Animal's weight in kg
× volume (mL) per kg

$$\text{Minimum rate per hour} = 10 \text{ kg} \times \frac{2 \text{ mL}}{\text{kg}}$$

Minimum rate per hour = 20 mL

$$\text{Maximum rate per hour} = 10 \text{ kg} \times \frac{6 \text{ mL}}{\text{kg}}$$

Minimum rate per hour = 60 mL

The calculations above show both the minimum and maximum fluid rates in milliliters because the fluid rate is given as a range. When determining the amount of fluid to be given over 24 hours, the rate per hour (in this case, 20 mL will be used) is multiplied by 24 hours which equal 480 mL per day.

$$\frac{20 \text{ mL}}{\text{h}} \times \frac{24 \text{ h}}{\text{day}} = 480 \text{ mL/day}$$

The maintenance fluid requirements are added to the hydration deficit.

Ongoing Losses

The final calculation to be made is that for ongoing losses. Ongoing losses include vomiting, diarrhea, blood loss, and excessive panting. If it is estimated that the beagle is losing 100 mL of fluid per day through vomiting, then an additional 100 mL of fluid would have to be added to the total calculated volume.

The total volume that the beagle would need to be given in 24 hours is as follows:

Total fluid volume/day = Maintenance
+ Ongoing losses + Hydration deficit

480 mL for normal maintenance
+ 100 mL for ongoing losses
+ 500 mL to correct the hydration deficit
1080 mL/day

| Maintenance Fluid Requirements: FELINE | | |
Body weight (kg)	Feline total water (mL/day)	Feline (mL/h)
1.0	80	3
1.5	108	5
2.0	134	6
2.5	159	7
3.0	182	8
3.5	204	9
4.0	226	9
4.5	247	10
5.0	267	11
5.5	287	12
6	307	13
6.5	326	14
7	344	14
7.5	363	15
8	381	16
8.5	398	17
9	416	17
10	450	19

Cat: *Formula* = 80 × body weight (kg)$^{0.75}$ per 24 hours
Rule of thumb: 2–3 mL/kg/h

| Maintenance Fluid Requirements: CANINE | | |
Body weight (kg)	Canine total water (mL/day)	Canine (mL/h)
1.0	132	6
2.0	222	9
3.0	301	13
4.0	373	16
5.0	441	18
10	742	31
20	1248	52
30	1692	71
40	2100	87
50	2481	103

Dog: *Formula* = 132 × body weight (kg)$^{0.75}$ per 24 hours
Rule of thumb: 2–6 mL/kg/h

This tip sheet is part of the *2013 AAHA/AAFP Fluid Therapy Guidelines for Dogs and Cats* Implementation Toolkit, sponsored by a generous educational grant from Abbott Animal Health.

Fig. 15.4 2013 AAHA/AAFP Fluid Therapy Guidelines for Dogs and Cats. (From AAHA/AAFP *Fluid Therapy Guidelines for Dogs and Cats: Implementation Toolkit*. [aahanet.org; American Animal Hospital Association].)

The 1080 mL per day should provide the dog with adequate fluids to correct for normal maintenance, ongoing losses, and dehydration.

AAHA/AAFP fluid therapy guidelines for dogs and cats supplemental information sheet (Fig. 15.4) provides a rapid estimation of fluid volumes based on maintenance needs. The animal's weight is found, and the appropriate column is then consulted for the volume of fluid needed. This information sheet does not take ongoing losses into account but provides a quick determination of fluid volume needed.

BOX 15.1 Case Scenario

Penny, a 4-year-old, spayed female, Cocker Spaniel weighing 33 lb (15 kg), presented to the veterinary hospital for vomiting and anorexia for the past 2 days.

Physical examination findings: Penny was lethargic and depressed. Temperature: 100.5°F, Pulse: tachycardia, good pulse quality, Respirations: tachypnea, lung sounds clear, mucous membranes: pink and tacky, CRT (capillary refill time): slightly prolonged (2–3 seconds), skin turgor: delayed, Blood pressure: 100 mm Hg. She is estimated to be 8% dehydrated.

An intravenous catheter was placed in preparation for intravenous fluids.

In this case, the patient has evidence of poor perfusion and therefore a rate of 20 mL/kg will be given as a bolus, at a quarter of the dose, over 15 min.

Calculation: 20 mL/kg × 15 kg = 300 mL

300 mL × $\frac{1}{4}$ dose = 75 mL bolus over 15 min.

The patient was reassessed and the parameters improved but were not within normal limits. Therefore, another bolus of 75 mL was given over 15 min. After reassessing the patient again, the heart rate, blood pressure, and CRT improved.

The patient had vomited twice (approximately 100 mL total) during the first 4 h.

Since the patient is 8% dehydrated, the fluid deficit for dehydration will be determined by:

Volume to replace in liters = % dehydration (as a decimal) × body weight (kg)

Volume in liters = (0.08) × 15 kg = 1.2 L or 1200 mL/day.

To determine the maintenance fluid requirements:

Maintenance requirements (mL) = body weight (kg) × 50 mL/kg/day

Maintenance volume in mL = 15 kg × 50 mL/kg/day = 750 mL/day

To determine ongoing losses due to vomiting: Ongoing losses were approximately 100 mL lost through vomiting.

Total rate = Maintenance + ongoing losses + hydration deficit

Total rate = 1200 mL + 100 mL + 750 mL

Total rate = 2050 mL/day

To determine the rate per hour you divide by 24 h.

2050 mL/24 h = 85 mL/h

The patient's perfusion status was monitored frequently including heart rate, respiratory rate, pulse quality, mucous membrane color, capillary refill time, mentation status, temperature, and weight.

The PCV/TP and urine specific gravity measurements were performed to determine if the values returned to normal indicating improvement in overall hydration and normal fluid level returning to the intravascular space.

The next day, the patient started to drink and eat small amounts of food and the maintenance fluids were discontinued.

Routes of Fluid Administration

The route by which fluids are administered depends on several factors such as the nature of the condition being treated, its duration, and its severity. The routes that may be used include (1) intravenous, (2) subcutaneous, (3) intraperitoneal, (4) intraosseous, and (5) oral. Fluids given by routes one, two, three, or four are administered by the parenteral route and may be referred to as parenteral fluids.

The intravenous route is preferred when the loss has been great or the disorder is severe. The intravenous route allows quicker, more precise delivery of fluids than the other routes. This route does require placement of an intravenous catheter and closer monitoring because of potential complications such as obstruction or kinking of the catheter, septicemia, embolism, and phlebitis. Catheters should be flushed with saline or heparinized saline

every 4 to 6 hours if intravenous fluids are not being administered and should be removed and replaced every 72 to 96 hours so that complications are minimized.

The subcutaneous route is useful when a patient's needs are not severe. The amount of fluid that can be administered subcutaneously depends on the size of the animal and the amount of loose skin that it has. Between 50 and 200 mL generally can be infused at a subcutaneous site. Great care should be taken not to administer enough fluid to dissect the skin loose from its blood supply because this can cause sloughing of skin over the site. Hypertonic or irritating fluids should not be given by the subcutaneous route.

The oral route is a practical means of administering fluids as long as an animal has no severe disorders of the gastrointestinal system. This route allows normal physiologic processes to control the amount of fluid and the amount and type of electrolytes absorbed. This route is not satisfactory when large volumes of fluid must be given rapidly.

The intraperitoneal route allows for administration of large volumes of fluid, but absorption is slow. Peritonitis is a potential complication, and this route is not commonly used.

The intraosseous (femur, ilium, or humerus) route is sometimes used in very small animals or in those with poor access to veins. This route allows rapid delivery of fluids and blood but requires greater technical expertise for placing the delivery needle. Careful attention should

be paid to sterile technique when this route is used so that osteomyelitis does not occur.

Rate of Administration

Once the volume of fluid needed and the route of administration have been decided, the time frame must be established for delivering the fluids. Rapid losses of fluid usually call for rapid replacement. Flow rates may depend on the type of fluid being administered (crystalloid vs. colloid), the conditions being treated, and the equipment available.

For treatment of patients with shock, crystalloid fluids may be administered rapidly (80–90 mL/kg/h in dogs and 50–55 mL/kg/h in cats). The use of a pressure administration cuff may allow more rapid infusion in these cases (Fig. 15.5). Colloids and mixtures of crystalloids and colloids are generally administered at a slower rate than crystalloids alone. Advanced references should be consulted for specific rates. Fluid warming devices (Figs. 15.6A and B) may be used to warm fluid during administration, if indicated. Fluids ideally should be infused continuously during a 24-hour period. One method of determining fluid flow rate is to calculate the hydration deficit, add maintenance and ongoing losses, and set the drip rate to administer the total during a

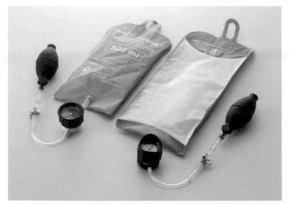

Fig. 15.5 Pressure administration cuff.

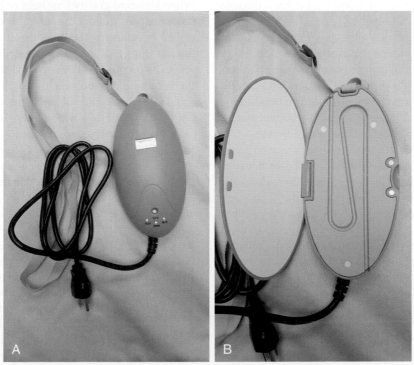

Fig. 15.6 (A) Intravenous fluid warmer. (B) Intravenous fluid warmer internal area showing intravenous line placement.

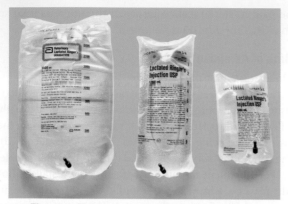

Fig. 15.7 Fluid containers. (Abbott IV Solutions.)

24-hour period. Some clinicians prefer to administer the hydration deficit during the first few hours and then to give the remainder over a longer period. Some divide the total calculated volume into three equal parts and administer each in an 8-hour period. In many practices, fluid administration can be monitored for a part of the day only. In this case, the total 24-hour fluid volume can be administered during the period that the patient can be monitored. (Common sense and medical judgment, however, must be exercised.) Portions of the total volume may be administered subcutaneously when appropriate.

Fluids are administered from plastic bags through intravenous administration sets (Figs. 15.7 and 15.8). Two sizes of administration sets that are commonly used in veterinary medicine are the standard or macrodrip set (15 drops/mL) and the minidrip or microdrip set (60 drops/ mL). Other sizes (10 drops/mL and 20 drops/mL) are also available. Microdrip sets are suited for use in administering fluids to cats and small dogs. The size of the administration set must be known to calculate the drip or flow rate.

To calculate the drip rate, first divide the total number of milliliters to be administered by the 24 hours to obtain a volume in milliliters per hour. Then, divide by 60 minutes to obtain milliliters per minute. Then, multiply the milliliters per minute by the drops per milliliter of the administration set that has been chosen to arrive at the number of drops (gtt) per minute (gtt/min). You may continue to drops per second by dividing by the drops per minute by 60 seconds to obtain drops per second. For example, if the beagle needs 1080 mL of fluid during a 24-hour period and a standard (15 gtt/mL) administration set is used, then the calculation is as follows:

$$\frac{\text{Volume of infusion}}{24 \text{ hours}} = \text{Volume in milliliters per hour}$$

$$\frac{1080 \text{ mL}}{24 \text{ h}} = \frac{45 \text{ mL}}{\text{h}}$$

$$\frac{45 \text{ mL}}{\text{h}} \times \frac{1 \text{ h}}{60 \text{ mins}} = 0.75 \text{ mL/min}$$

$$\frac{0.75 \text{ mL}}{\text{min}} \times \frac{15 \text{ drops}}{\text{mL}} = 11.25 \text{ drops/min}$$

$$\frac{11.25 \text{ drops}}{\text{min}} \times \frac{1 \text{ min}}{60 \text{ sec}} = 0.19 \text{ drops/sec}$$

0.19 drops per second is approximately 0.2 drops per second which is not measurable through the chamber; therefore the drip rate per second must be converted to the nearest whole drops. To convert the answer to drops per 5 seconds gives a drip number that would be closer to a whole number.

To figure out how many drops every 5 seconds, you would multiply 0.2 drops per second by 5 seconds to get the drip rate of 1 drop every 5 seconds.

$$\frac{0.2 \text{ drops}}{\text{second}} \times \frac{5}{5} = \frac{1 \text{ drop}}{5 \text{ seconds}}$$

Monitoring Fluid Administration

When standard gravity flow bags or bottles are used, the fluids are placed above the patient and drip rates are controlled by adjusting the roller clamp on the administration set (Figs.15.8 and 15.9). Labeled tape may be placed vertically on fluid bottles or bags to allow monitoring of the volume delivered (Fig. 15.10). Bottles or bags also should be labeled with all pertinent information, including the presence of any additives. It may be helpful to place a horizontal piece of tape across the fluid container to indicate when fluid delivery is to be stopped.

Infusion pumps (Figs. 15.11A and B) are commonly used in practice to ensure precise fluid administration. The flow rate is simply programmed into the machine to deliver the fluid volume over a set amount of time (Fig. 15.12A) or intravenous controllers (mL/min) can be used (see Fig. 15.12B). A volume control system or Buretrol device may be used for administering small volumes of fluid (Fig. 15.13). A clamp allows the volume control chamber to be filled with a predetermined amount of fluid from the bag or bottle. The line then is clamped off to prevent entry of additional fluid from the bag. The chamber can be refilled if desired. Also, the use of a syringe pump can be used for administering small volumes of fluid to provide more accuracy.

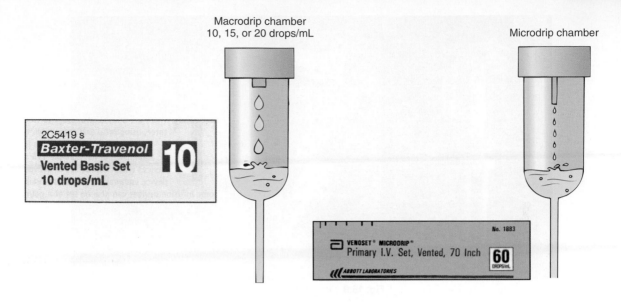

Macrodrip chamber
10, 15, or 20 drops/mL

Microdrip chamber

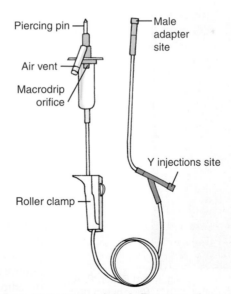

Fig. 15.8 Intravenous administration set. (From Mulholland, J. [2011]. *The nurse, the math, the meds.* St. Louis; Elsevier.)

Fluids administered too rapidly or in too great a volume can be life threatening. Careful monitoring of the physical status of the animal is essential. Lung sounds, respiratory rate and effort, pulse rate and quality, skin turgor, urine output, and the overall status of the animal should be monitored regularly, along with the PCV and the TPP. Additionally, urine specific gravity, blood pressure, and electrolytes should be monitored. When a large volume of fluids is administered rapidly, it is prudent to insert a

urinary catheter to monitor urine output and establish that the kidneys are functioning normally. Some clinicians also choose to insert a jugular catheter to monitor central venous pressure as a way of preventing fluid volume overload.

Signs of overhydration may include restlessness, serous nasal discharge, increased lung sounds (crackles), tachycardia, dyspnea, pitting subcutaneous edema, and an increased "Jello-like" feel in the subcutaneous

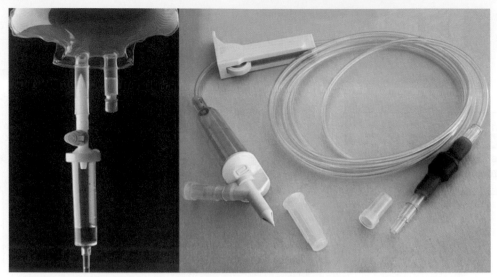

Fig. 15.9 Intravenous drip set.

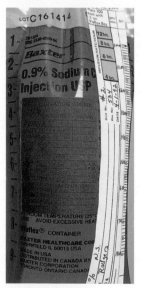

Fig. 15.10 Labeling (vertical) of fluid bag. (From Potter, P. A., Perry, A. G., Stockert, P. A., & Hall, A. [2011]. *Basic nursing* [6th ed., p. 511]. St. Louis: Mosby.)

tissue (Haskins, 2000). Fluid infusion should be slowed or stopped and the veterinarian contacted at the first appearance of these signs.

Discontinuation of Fluid Therapy

Fluid therapy is discontinued when clinical signs improve and laboratory test results return to normal. When repeated evaluations of body weight, urine output, PCV, TPP, urine specific gravity, and central venous pressure show progressive improvement, fluid therapy may be tapered or discontinued. As the animal recovers, fluid therapy may be cut back by decreasing the fluid volume given by 25% to 50% per day.

Preparing Fluid Administration Equipment

When preparing to administer intravenous fluids, follow a standard protocol. After gathering supplies and preparing the injection site, check to see that the fluid type is correct and that it is not out of date. Then, determine that the container is not cracked or chipped and that the solution is clear. Fluids should never contain precipitates or appear cloudy. After inspecting the container's cap to make sure that it is intact, remove the metal cap (bottle) or insertion port cover (bag), while taking care not to contaminate the port. Close the flow clamp on the administration set, and remove the cover from the administration set spike. Insert the administration set spike into the rubber stopper (bottle) or insertion port (bag). Hang the bottle or bag, and fill the fluid drip chamber half way (see Fig. 15.9), open the flow clamp and allow fluid to run through the line until all bubbles are cleared. Close the flow clamp and attach the adapter to the intravenous catheter using sterile technique. After the flow clamp is opened to determine that the catheter and the line are patent, the drip rate may be adjusted as required.

If at any time the flow rate slows or stops, check the following: (1) the catheter for correct placement

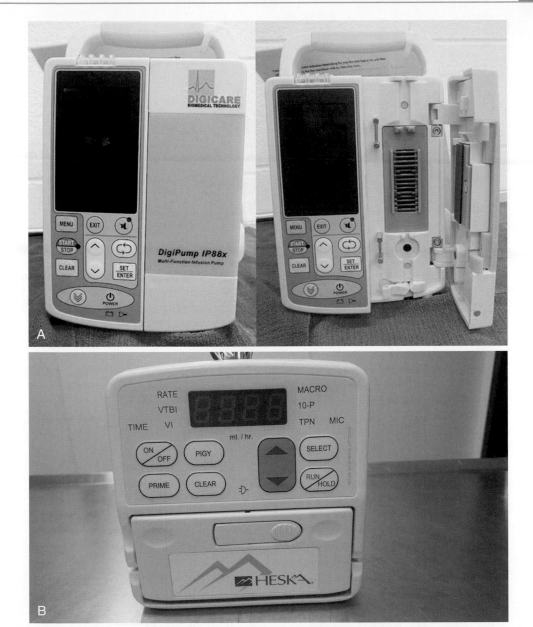

Fig. 15.11 (A) Fluid infusion pump. (From Sonsthagen, T. [2014]. *Veterinary instruments and equipment: A pocket guide* [3rd ed.]. St. Louis: Elsevier.) (B) Fluid infusion pump.

and patency, (2) the position of the patient to determine whether limb position or flexion has occluded the flow, (3) the flow clamp to see whether it is in the open position, (4) the tubing to determine whether it is kinked or crimped, and (5) the fluid level in the bottle.

Two fluid solutions may be administered simultaneously with the use of a piggyback setup of the containers (Fig. 15.14). The secondary bag is hung higher than the primary bag, and the secondary administration set line is connected to the Y port of the primary administration set.

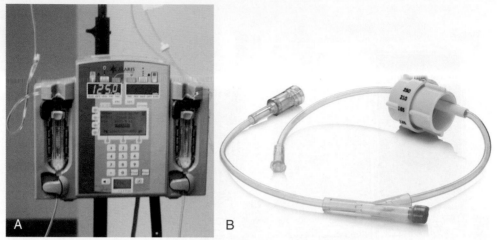

Fig. 15.12 (A) Intravenous infusion pump. (B) Intravenous infusion controller. (A, From Kee, J. L., & Marshall, S. M. [2009]. *Clinical calculations: With applications to general and specialty areas* [6th ed.]. St. Louis: Saunders. B, Courtesy Hospira, Inc., Lake Forest, IL. In Mulholland, J. [2011]. *The nurse, the math, the meds.* St. Louis: Elsevier.)

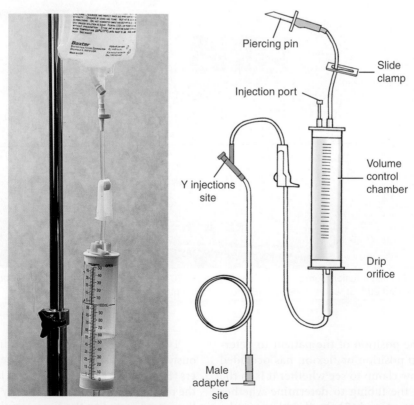

Fig. 15.13 Volume control administration set. (From Perry, A. G., & Potter, P. A. [2010]. *Clinical nursing skills and techniques* [7th ed.]. St. Louis: Mosby.)

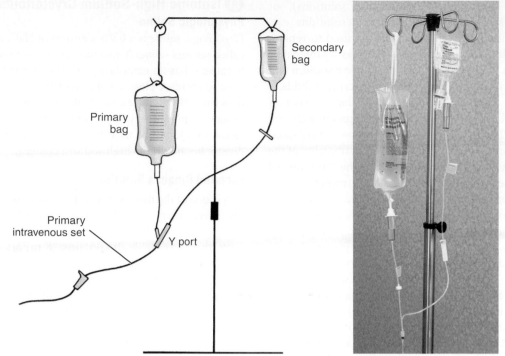

Fig. 15.14 Piggyback setup of fluids. (From Lilley, L. L, Collins, S. R., Harrington, S., & Snyder, J. S. [2014]. *Pharmacology and the nursing process* [7th ed.]. St. Louis: Mosby.)

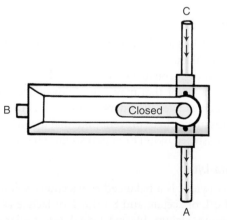

Fig. 15.15 Operation of a three-way valve. The handle points toward the closed port allowing fluid to flow in through port C and out through port A. The handle may be positioned toward each of the ports to change the direction of entry and exit.

Technicians should understand the use of a three-way valve. The three-way valve permits three-way connections to be made. Flow of fluid through the valve depends on the position at which the control handle is placed. The handle points toward the line that is closed. Fig. 15.15 illustrates the operation of a three-way valve.

TYPES OF SOLUTIONS USED IN FLUID THERAPY

Parenteral fluids can be broadly classified as crystalloids or colloids. Crystalloids may be further classified as isotonic high-sodium, hypotonic low-sodium, or hypertonic saline solutions. Colloids can be subdivided into synthetic starch-based colloids and natural colloids.

Ⓡ Crystalloid Solutions

Crystalloids are solutions that contain electrolyte and nonelectrolyte substances capable of passing through cell membranes, therefore entering all body fluid compartments. Administration of crystalloid solutions results in rapid equilibration (within 30 minutes to 1 hour) of fluid between the intravascular and interstitial spaces. Crystalloid solutions are used routinely in veterinary medicine because of their versatility and relatively low cost. Crystalloid solutions can be classified further as isotonic high-sodium (replacement solutions), hypotonic low-sodium (maintenance solutions), or hypertonic saline solutions. Replacement solutions (e.g., LRS) resemble ECF in content and are used to replace lost body fluids and electrolytes, whereas maintenance solutions (e.g., Plasma-Lyte M) contain less sodium and more potassium than are found in replacement fluids.

Clinical Uses. Isotonic crystalloids have a sodium content and osmolality close to ECF (approximately 300 mOsm/L). Therefore, an isotonic solution is a balanced electrolyte solution that is similar to the osmolality of the patient's plasma. A large percentage of the fluid infused will leave the intravascular space within 30 minutes. These fluids are versatile and may be used for treating dehydration, hypovolemic shock, vomiting, diarrhea, pancreatitis, metabolic acidosis (e.g., LRS), metabolic alkalosis (e.g., 0.9% NaCl), and other conditions. Examples of isotonic fluids include 0.9% NaCl, lactated ringers, Normosol-R, and Plasma-Lyte A. They should be used with caution or not used at all in patients in which sodium retention may be a problem (e.g., heart disease or renal disease).

Hypotonic solutions (crystalloids) have a sodium content and an osmolality less than ECF, so infused fluid tends to hydrate the extracellular space. This occurs because the extracellular space has a higher osmolality that pulls the fluid out of the vasculature into this space (see Fig. 15.3). Examples of hypotonic fluids include 0.45% NaCl, dextrose 5% in water (D_5W), and dextrose 2.5% with 0.45% saline. These fluids are used to treat hypernatremia or conditions in which sodium retention is a problem and are not suitable to treat hypovolemic shock since they quickly leave the intravascular space.

Hypertonic solutions (crystalloids) have an osmolality greater than that of ECF and cause fluid to move out of the intracellular/interstitial space and into the intravascular space. Examples of hypertonic fluids include 3% NaCl, 5% NaCl, and 7% NaCl. They are used to treat hypovolemic shock (by increasing intravascular volume) and may be beneficial in treating intracranial edema (by "pulling" excess fluid out of the brain into the vasculature). Hypertonic solutions should be avoided in animals that have hypernatremia, cardiac disease, or are dehydrated.

Dosage Forms. Dosage forms are numerous. Fluids are available in glass bottles, plastic bottles, and plastic bags that hold 250, 500, and 1000 mL. Containers that hold 3000 and 6000 mL are available for some solutions (see manufacturer product guides). The following section briefly describes the commonly used crystalloid solutions. See Table 15.2 for a listing of the composition and other characteristics of each.

Ⓡ Isotonic High-Sodium Crystalloids
Physiologic Saline

Physiologic saline is a 0.9% solution of NaCl and is also called *normal saline*. It also may be called *isotonic saline* because it has an osmolarity of 308 mOsm/L. Saline is used to increase plasma volume or to correct a sodium deficiency (hyponatremia). It also may be used to bathe tissues during surgery to prevent them from drying out. Saline should not be used in animals with known heart disease because of its high sodium content.

Lactated Ringer's Solution

LRS is one of the most versatile and commonly used fluids in veterinary medicine. It is a balanced electrolyte replacement solution that can be administered by any route that is available. It contains 28 mEq/L of lactate, which is converted by the liver to bicarbonate to act as a buffer against acidosis. Theoretically, LRS should not be administered with blood because the calcium contents could cause clotting to occur. LRS is not currently considered appropriate for use in critical patients (Crowe, 2007). It is not appropriate to use LRS in liver disease because the lactate may not be metabolized to bicarbonate. LRS should not be used when hypercalcemia or cancer is present.

Normosol-R

Normosol-R is a balanced, multiple-electrolyte solution with a dual buffering system (acetate and gluconate). Acetate and gluconate are metabolized outside the liver, which is a factor that may confer advantages in conditions such as liver disorders. Normosol is calcium free and thus may help to prevent potential incompatibilities with transfused blood or added sodium bicarbonate.

Plasma-Lyte

Plasma-Lyte R is a balanced replacement solution with 47 mEq/L of acetate and 8 mEq/L of lactate as buffers. It contains calcium. Plasma-Lyte A is a similar solution except that it contains no calcium or lactate. Plasma-Lyte M contains low sodium, low chloride, and higher potassium than the other Plasma-Lyte solutions and is used as a replacement or maintenance solution.

Ⓡ Hypotonic Low-Sodium Crystalloids
Dextrose 5% in Water

Dextrose 5% in water (D_5W) is a nonbalanced solution that contains only dextrose (50 g/L) and water.

Administering dextrose 5% is equivalent to administering pure water because the dextrose is metabolized to carbon dioxide and water. Dextrose 5% provides approximately 170 kcal/L (a quantity that cannot be relied on to meet the daily caloric needs of most small animals), although it may supplement other caloric sources. Dextrose 5% generally should not be given by the subcutaneous route because it may osmotically "draw" fluid from the vascular space. Dextrose in water should not be used as a maintenance solution because overdilution may cause an electrolyte imbalance. It is often mixed with a saline solution when hypotonic low-sodium solutions are indicated.

Dextrose 2.5% With 0.45% Saline

This solution contains 77 mEq/L each of sodium and chloride and 25 g/dL of dextrose (85 kcal/L). This solution may be used for patients who may be at risk if they take in too much sodium or for those with potential fluid retention.

Half-Strength Lactated Ringer's Solution With 2.5% Dextrose

This solution is a hypotonic low-sodium solution (66 mEq/L) containing small amounts of chloride (55 mEq/L) along with small amounts of potassium, calcium, dextrose, and lactate. It provides a slightly more balanced approach to the use of hypotonic low-sodium fluids.

Adverse Side Effects. Adverse side effects of fluid administration are primarily associated with overhydration. Signs of overhydration may include restlessness, shivering, serous nasal discharge, coughing, and pulmonary edema. High-sodium fluids should not be used in patients with heart disease, renal disease, inflammation, and/or edema.

Hypertonic Saline Solutions

Hypertonic saline solutions are available from commercial sources in 3%, 4%, 5%, 7%, 7.5%, and 23.4% preparations. These solutions are especially useful in treating hypovolemic shock with the use of small volumes of the solution. The 7.5% solution is considered the upper limit of concentration to avoid phlebitis.

Adverse Side Effects. These may include phlebitis, tissue irritation, re-hemorrhage in traumatic shock, electrolyte imbalances, and—when the administration rate is too fast—hypotension, bronchoconstriction, and bradycardia.

TECHNICIAN NOTES

- Fluids that contain preservatives such as benzyl alcohol should never be given to cats because of the likelihood of toxic reactions.
- Some clinicians warn against administering fluids with preservatives to puppies and adult dogs.

Colloid Solutions

Colloid solutions contain large molecular weight particles that are unable to cross cell membranes and therefore are confined to the vascular space. Unlike crystalloid solute, these colloid particles are effective osmoles that are able to hold fluid in the vascular space and draw fluid from the interstitial space into the vascular space (expand the plasma volume).

Colloids are classified as synthetic or natural colloids. Synthetic colloids include dextrans, hydroxyethyl starches (HESs), oxyglobin, and gelatins. Natural colloids contain proteins and include whole blood, plasma, and albumin.

Clinical Uses. Colloid solutions are used for expansion of the plasma volume in the treatment of patients with hypovolemia not due to dehydration, septic shock, or hypoalbuminemia. Colloids are useful in treating patients prone to edema because smaller fluid volumes are required for effective treatment.

Colloid administration can provide great patient benefit in select cases, but because of potential harmful side effects, they should be given judiciously.

Synthetic Colloids

Dextrans. Dextran is a large molecular weight branched polysaccharide solution with osmotic effects similar to albumin. Examples of dextrans include dextran 40 (10% solution) and dextran 70 (6% solution). Dextrans remain in the vascular space for 3 to 58 hours, respectively (Battaglia, 2016). These products should be used with caution in patients subject to vascular overload. Dextran is contraindicated in patients with coagulopathies.

Hydroxyethyl Starch. HES or hetastarch is a large molecular weight starch that is used in the treatment of hypovolemia and hypoproteinemia. It may also reduce intravascular inflammation and reduce vascular permeability and leakage. Hetastarch expands the plasma volume longer (12–36 hours). It is prepared as a 6% HES solution in 0.9% saline (Hespan), a 6% HES solution in lactated electrolyte (Hextend), a 6% HES solution in 0.9% saline (Voluven, VetStarch). These products also can cause volume overload, coagulopathies, and hypersensitivity reactions. The primary disadvantage of hetastarch is its expense.

Oxyglobin. Oxyglobin is a purified solution of bovine hemoglobin in altered LRS. It provides a substitute for hemoglobin and enhances oxygen carrying capacity for up to 40 hours. It is useful in anemic patients and those with reduced oxygen carrying capacity. Oxyglobin has been shown to act as an effective plasma volume expander as well as a carrier of oxygen. It has an extended shelf life and does not require crossmatching because intact red blood cells are not present. Oxyglobin may cause vasoconstriction and increased blood pressure, and care should be taken when choosing the volume and rate of administration. It is an expensive product that has faced limited availability problems.

Gelatins. Gelatins are derived from bovine collagens (modified beef collagen). They are indicated for short-term volume expansion and remain in the vasculature for 1 to 2 hours (Battaglia, 2016). Examples of gelatins include Haemacel and Gelofusine.

Natural Colloids

The natural colloids are high molecular weight solutions obtained from species-specific donor animals. Natural colloids act in a similar way to synthetic colloids by causing an increased intravascular volume and may contribute clotting factors in coagulopathies and provide blood cells in large volume loss. They include albumin (canine or human origin), fresh frozen plasma, frozen or stored plasma, and whole blood.

Albumin. Albumin provides over 75% of the oncotic pressure of plasma. Administration of albumin may be useful in critically ill patients needing intravascular volume expansion, especially if that animal is hypoalbuminemic, edematous, or suffering from vascular leakage of fluid. Human (Albuminar, Albutein, Flexbumin, Albuminate, and Plasbumin) and canine (Albumin, Canine) commercial albumin products are available. Caution should be used when administering the human albumin product because of "significant concerns with adverse effects" (Plumb, 2015). Few reports are available on the clinical use of the canine product.

Fresh Frozen Plasma. If the plasma is collected from centrifuged whole blood and frozen within 6 hours of collection, it is considered to be fresh frozen. Fresh frozen plasma contains albumin (and other plasma proteins) and clotting factors. It may be used to treat rodenticide coagulopathies, patients needing factor VII or von Willebrand factor, or disseminated intravascular coagulation. Fresh frozen plasma can be stored up to a year with preservation of the unstable clotting factors. After 1 year of storage fresh frozen plasma becomes stored plasma because of the loss of clotting factors. Freezing of plasma destroys the platelets.

Frozen or Stored Plasma. When frozen after 6 hours of collection plasma may not be suitable for treating factor VII or von Willebrand coagulopathy; however, it can be used to treat rodenticide coagulopathy (Rudloff, 2013) and patients with decreased protein levels.

Whole Blood. The primary use of whole blood is the treatment of patients with anemia. Fresh whole blood can also be used in patients with coagulation or platelet disorders because it contains all the coagulation factors and platelets. Transfusions are generally given in cases of anemia when the PCV drops below 20% or the hemoglobin level drops below 7 g/dL. Transfusions should be started slowly (e.g., 1 mL/kg) for the first 10 to 15 minutes, and the patient should be monitored closely for signs of transfusion reactions like panting, urticaria, or vomiting. If no signs of an acute transfusion reaction, the transfusion rate can then be increased to 2 mL/kg/h for the duration of the transfusion. The transfusion should be completed within 4 hours. Blood should be warmed to body temperature before administering through a line with a filter to remove small clots. The quantity of blood to transfuse can be calculated by using the following formula for a dog:

$$\text{Volume to transfuse (mL)} = 90 \text{ mL/kg}$$
$$\times \text{BW (kg)} \times \frac{\text{desired PCV} - \text{Patient PCV}}{\text{PCV of donor blood}^*}$$

[*]Measure or assume PCV equals 45% for whole blood
The blood volume of a dog is approximately 90 mL/kg.
The quantity of blood to transfuse can be calculated by using the following formula for a cat:

$$\text{Volume to transfuse (mL)} = 60 \text{ mL/kg}$$
$$\times \text{BW (kg)} \times \frac{\text{desired PCV} - \text{Patient PCV}}{\text{PCV of donor blood}^*}$$

[*]Measure or assume PCV equals 45% for whole blood

The blood volume for a cat is approximately 60 mL/kg.

For example, if a 20-kg dog has a PCV of 15% and the desired PCV is 25%, one would administer 396 mL; approximately 400 mL of blood.

$$\text{Volume to transfuse (mL)} = 90 \text{ mL/kg}$$
$$\times \text{ BW (kg)} \times \frac{\text{desired PCV} - \text{Patient PCV}}{\text{PCV of donor blood}^*}$$

* Measure or assume PCV equals 45% for whole blood

$$\text{Volume to transfuse (mL)} =$$
$$90 \text{ mL/kg} \times 20 \text{ kg} \times \frac{25\% - 15\%}{45\%}$$

$$\text{Volume to transfuse (mL)} = 1800 \text{ mL} \times 0.22$$

$$\text{Volume to transfuse (mL)} = 396 \text{ mL}$$

Adverse Side Effects. Adverse side effects of colloid administration include volume overload, coagulopathies, and hypersensitivity reactions. Allergic reactions may be seen in concentrated albumin or blood transfusions.

> **TECHNICIAN NOTES**
> * Colloids are not intended for maintenance or long-term use.
> * References should be checked when the appropriate flow rate for colloid solutions is determined.

> **TECHNICIAN NOTES**
> * The rate of administration of hypertonic saline solution is a very important consideration because exceeding this rate may cause serious side effects.
> * Hypertonic saline should be infused through a well-secured intravenous catheter to prevent extravasation of irritating fluids.

 Fluid Additives

In some instances, special substances may be added to intravenous fluid solutions to enhance the solutions' therapeutic effects. These substances may be added to correct acid–base abnormalities and electrolyte imbalances, to supplement calories, and to provide supplemental vitamins to replace those washed out by fluid therapy. The details of the additives must always be written on the fluid bag as well as in the medical record. It is recommended that fluid infusion pumps be utilized, when additives are added to fluids, to ensure administration rates are accurate.

Sodium Bicarbonate

Sodium bicarbonate is an alkalizing agent that may be added to correct metabolic acidosis and certain other conditions. Supplementation becomes necessary because lactate or acetate in fluid preparations often cannot correct severe metabolic acidosis. Normal serum bicarbonate is 24 mEq/L. Required amounts for supplementation may be calculated by measuring a patient's bicarbonate level and subtracting that value from 24 (normal). The difference is called the *bicarbonate deficit*. The bicarbonate deficit is multiplied by 0.3 and then by the animal's weight in kilograms to determine the number of milliequivalents of sodium bicarbonate to administer:

$$\text{Bicarbonate supplementation (mEq)}$$
$$= \text{Bicarbonate deficit} \times 0.3 \times \text{weight (kg)}$$

A 20-kg dog with a bicarbonate level of 14 mEq/L would require 60 mEq bicarbonate supplementation.

$$\text{Bicarbonate supplementation (mEq)}$$
$$= 24 - 14 = 10 \times 0.3 \times 20 = 60$$

When access to laboratory measurement of bicarbonate or carbon dioxide is not available, empirical estimations of supplementation levels are made on the basis of clinical judgment.

Bicarbonate concentration in commercial products is measured in milliequivalents per milliliter.

Clinical Uses. These include the treatment of metabolic acidosis and as an adjunctive therapy for the treatment of hypercalcemia or hyperkalemia. Sodium bicarbonate use is contraindicated in patients with metabolic or respiratory alkalosis and should be used with caution in patients with congestive heart failure, hypertension, oliguria, hypocalcemia, or hypokalemia.

Dosage Forms. Veterinary-approved forms include the following:
* **An 8.4% (1 mEq/mL) solution for injection** (veterinary label)
* **A choice of 4%, 4.2%, 5%, 7.5%, and 8.4% solutions for injection** (human label)

Adverse Side Effects. These may include metabolic alkalosis, hypokalemia, hypocalcemia, and hypernatremia.

TECHNICIAN NOTES

- Sodium bicarbonate is incompatible with several solutions and should be mixed only after consulting product inserts or appropriate references.
- Some references indicate that sodium bicarbonate should not be added to solutions that contain calcium because of the potential for precipitates to form.
- Replacement of the total number of milliequivalents should be made over several hours.

Potassium Chloride

Potassium chloride is a solution that is used to supplement potassium deficits (**hypokalemia**). Anorexia, diuresis, and diarrhea are some of the common causes of hypokalemia. Normal serum potassium levels are between 3.5 and 5.5 mEq/L. Signs of hypokalemia include weakness, lethargy, muscle weakness, and vomiting. Clinical signs of hypokalemia vary on the severity of the condition. Table 15.5 provides a guide for potassium supplementation that is based on the measured serum level of potassium. Intravenous potassium supplements must be diluted before administering and given slowly.

Clinical Uses. Potassium chloride is used for the treatment or prevention of potassium deficits.

Dosage Forms. Dosage forms for intravenous use include the following:

- **Potassium chloride for injection** (2 mEq/mL) (veterinary label)
- **Potassium chloride for injection** (2 mEq/mL) (human label)

Adverse Side Effects. These may include hyperkalemia, which is manifested by muscle weakness, and cardiac conduction disturbances, which can be life threatening. Potassium supplements may be contraindicated in hyperkalemia, renal failure, Addison's disease, or acute dehydration.

TECHNICIAN NOTES

- Potassium chloride solutions must be diluted before administration.
- The rate of infusion of potassium is critical and must not exceed a rate faster than 0.5 mEq/kg/h (DiBartola, 2011). Consult product inserts or other references for appropriate rates.

TABLE 15.5 **Potassium Supplementation Guide.[a]**

Serum K$^+$ (mEq/L)	mEq K$^+$ (To Add to 250 mL Fluid)	mEq K$^+$ (To Add to 1 L Fluid)	Maximum Infusion Rate of Intravenous Fluids (0.5 mEq/kg/h)
<2.0	20	80	6
2.1–2.5	15	60	8
2.6–3.0	10	40	12
3.1–3.5	7	28	18
>3.5, <5.0	5	20	25

[a]For dogs or cats with hypokalemia or for those with potassium depletion and normal serum potassium levels. This regimen is designed to be infused in maintenance volume of fluids.

Calcium Supplements

Calcium gluconate or calcium chloride is given as an intravenous infusion to correct hypocalcemia. Intravenous calcium must be administered slowly to avoid possible cardiac arrhythmias, cardiac arrest, or hypotension.

Clinical Uses. Calcium supplements are used for the treatment of hypocalcemia that may result from various conditions, which may include parathyroid gland disorders, milk fever, eclampsia, and excessive sweating in horses. Calcium in combination with phosphorus, magnesium, potassium, and dextrose is used to treat cattle with conditions such as grass tetany, milk fever, and downer cow syndrome.

Dosage Forms. A variety of veterinary-label and human-label products are available. The following is a partial list.

- **Calcium gluconate injection (generic and proprietary) 10%,** in ampules, syringes, vials, and bottles (veterinary label)
- **Calcium gluconate (various proprietary names) 23%,** in 100- and 500-mL bottles (veterinary label)
- **Calcium chloride injection (generic and proprietary) 10%,** in ampules, vials, and syringes (human label)
- **Numerous combination products** (Cal Dextro, Norcalciphos) that contain calcium, phosphorus, magnesium, potassium, and dextrose

Adverse Side Effects. Adverse side effects that result from hypercalcemia may include hypotension, cardiac arrhythmias, and cardiac arrest. These effects are usually a result of too rapid an infusion of calcium. Calcium gluconate may interact with other drugs such as cardiac glycosides and tetracycline antibiotics.

 TECHNICIAN NOTES

- Any product that contains calcium should be given by slow intravenous administration to prevent cardiac complications.
- Products that contain 23% calcium are labeled for large-animal use.

50% Dextrose

When caloric supplementation is indicated, 50% dextrose often is used as a stock solution to be added to other fluids to provide a desired percent solution of dextrose. It usually is not possible to meet the total caloric needs of a small animal patient through dextrose supplementation of intravenous fluids. Supplementation often is indicated, however, in patients that are hypoglycemic because of fever, sepsis, insulin overdose, insulinoma, liver disease, and other conditions. Varying amounts of dextrose may be added in an attempt to keep the blood glucose level near the normal range (80 to 100 mg/dL).

Intravenous administration of 50% dextrose is used in ruminants as a treatment for uncomplicated ketosis.

To prepare a 2.5% solution of dextrose, add 50 mL (25 g) of 50% dextrose to 1 L of fluids. Fifty milliliters of the original fluid solution should be removed before 50% dextrose is added to keep the dilution correct. To prepare a 5% solution, add 100 mL of 50% dextrose to 1 L of fluids. A formula that may be used to determine the quantity of a stock solution to be used in the preparation of percent solutions follows:

$$\frac{\text{Desired strength (concentration)}}{\text{Available strength (concentration)}}$$
$$= \frac{\text{How much you are going to use (Stock to use)}}{\text{How much you are going to make (Desired amount)}}$$

or

V_1 (Vol of stock) $\times C_1$ (Stock concentration)
$= V_2$ (Desired Vol) $\times C_2$ (Desired Concentration)

$$V_1 \times C_1 = V_2 \times C_2$$

For example, to make 250 mL of a 5% solution of dextrose using a stock supply of 50% dextrose, set up the formula in the following way:

$$\frac{5\%}{50\%} = \frac{X}{250}$$
Crossmultiplying $50X = 1250$
$$X = 25 \text{ mL}$$

or

V_1 (Vol of stock) $\times C_1$ (Stock concentration)
$= V_2$ (Desired Vol) $\times C_2$ (Desired Concentration)

$$V_1 \times 500 \text{ mg/mL} = 250 \text{ mL} \times 50 \text{ mg/mL}$$

$$V_1 = 12{,}500 \text{ mg/}500 \text{ mg/mL}$$

$$V_1 = 25 \text{ mL}$$

Therefore, to prepare 250 mL of 5% solution, draw up 25 mL of 50% dextrose and add 225 mL of a diluting fluid.

Clinical Uses. These include caloric supplementation in small animal patients and treatment of ketosis in ruminants.

Dosage Forms. Various manufacturers supply 50% dextrose. The most commonly used package is a 500-mL plastic bottle.

Adverse Side Effects. These are few if the product is used according to directions.

 TECHNICIAN NOTES

A 50% solution of dextrose contains 500 mg/mL.

Vitamin Supplements

Patients that have been given large amounts of fluid undergo diuresis, which may cause a corresponding loss of water-soluble vitamins (B complex and C), which makes fluid supplementation desirable. Animals with polyuria resulting from renal failure also lose water-soluble vitamins and benefit from supplementation of their parenteral fluids. Recommendations for supplementation vary from 0.5 to 2 mL per liter of fluids.

Clinical Uses. Vitamin supplements are used for restoration of normal levels of the water-soluble vitamins.

Dosage Forms. Several manufacturers produce vitamin B complex. Care should be taken to ensure that the form selected may be given intravenously. Many are labeled for intramuscular or subcutaneous use only.

Adverse Side Effects. These include hypersensitivity reactions to thiamine in the complex.

ORAL ELECTROLYTE PREPARATIONS

In severely dehydrated animals, fluids must be given by the intravenous route to be effective. In mild to moderate cases of dehydration, however, the oral route is a practical alternative to replenish water and electrolytes.

Oral electrolytes are packaged as powders that are mixed with water to form a solution that can be given free choice or by stomach tube. In some instances, oral pastes or fluids packaged for intravenous use may be given orally. The oral route of administration is especially useful for cases in which the veterinarian wishes to direct the pet or livestock owner in the home or farm treatment of the animal.

Diarrhea in young dairy calves, commonly called *calf scours,* is caused by bacteria, viruses, or nutritional factors and is a condition often treated with oral electrolyte solutions. The diarrhea is commonly a result of the type or amount of milk replacer that the calf is being fed. A calf is treated by eliminating the milk replacer from its diet and by giving it an oral electrolyte solution with glucose or glycine for 24 to 48 hours. Glucose and glycine provide a source of calories and may enhance absorption of the electrolytes. The solution may be administered via an esophageal feeder—a device that has a plastic bag (for mixing the electrolyte solution) attached to a rigid delivery tube (Fig. 15.16). The tube has a ball of sufficient diameter on the distal end to prevent introduction of the tube into the trachea.

Oral electrolyte solutions or pastes often are given to performance horses to replace electrolytes lost through sweating. Horses participating in endurance races, 3-day events, and other athletically demanding events benefit from electrolyte replenishment.

Administration of oral electrolyte solutions also may be helpful as a follow-up to intravenous fluid therapy for dogs recovering from viral enteritis or other diseases that cause prolonged vomiting or diarrhea. Hypokalemia in dogs and cats may be treated with oral potassium products.

Clinical Uses. These include electrolyte and water replenishment.

Dosage Forms. Dosage forms are numerous, and the following is only a partial listing:
- BlueLite – various species
- Calf Quencher

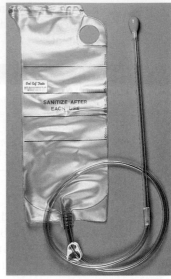

Fig. 15.16 Esophageal feeder. (From Sonsthagen, T. [2014]. *Veterinary instruments and equipment* [3rd ed.]. St Louis: Elsevier.)

- **Dexolyte**
- **Entrolyte (powder)**
- **Equi-Phar electro-amino paste**
- **Equi-Phar electrolyte solution with dextrose**
- **K9 Restart**
- **Pet-A-Lyte oral solution**
- **Re-Sorb (powder)**
- **Tumil-K (powder, gel, and tablets for dogs and cats)**
- **Vedalyte 8X**

Adverse Side Effects. These are rare if care is taken not to cause inadvertent administration into the respiratory system.

> **TECHNICIAN NOTES**
>
> Some of the oral electrolyte products for farm animals also contain antibiotics.

PARENTERAL NUTRITION

The term *parenteral* indicates the administration of nutrients by a route other than the gastrointestinal tract. Parenteral nutrition is described in human medicine as total or partial in reference to whether all nutrient requirements are supplied. Diseased and debilitated patients require a daily intake of adequate calories and protein to maintain good immune function, tissue synthesis, and normal metabolic activities. Those patients that are unable or have no desire to eat normally may need parenteral nutrition.

The term *total parenteral nutrition* does not apply to veterinary patients because there is no need to meet the needs for all essential fatty and amino acids, fat- and water-soluble vitamins, and macro and trace minerals, as there is in people (Remillard et al., 2000). In veterinary medicine, an attempt is made to meet the animal patient's resting energy requirement and most of the requirements for amino and fatty acids and to provide some of the required vitamins and minerals.

Parenteral nutrition solutions must be compounded for the individual patient. A mixture of all required nutrients, called a total nutrient admixture (TNA) or parenteral nutrition (PN), can be prepared for the veterinary patient in one fluid bag for convenience. The preparation of these solutions is beyond the scope of most veterinary clinics, but they may be available through human hospitals, veterinary schools, or specialty practices. For a list of products used in the formulation of parenteral nutrition and worksheets for calculations, consult Kirk's *Current Veterinary Therapy, XV.*

PARENTERAL VITAMIN/MINERAL PRODUCTS

Parenteral vitamin/mineral products are used to prevent or treat various conditions in veterinary medicine. They are used as therapeutic agents in large animal medicine more often than in small animal medicine. White muscle disease, "tying up," polyneuritis, pinkeye, reproductive problems, bracken fern poisoning, and polioencephalomalacia are only a few of the conditions prevented or treated with vitamin products in large animal practice. In small animal practice, routine vitamin and mineral supplementation is not considered necessary if the animal receives a balanced diet. Many small animal clinicians regard overuse of vitamin/mineral products as a bigger problem than vitamin/mineral deficiencies. Warfarin poisoning (vitamin K) and certain dermatologic conditions (zinc) are exceptions.

Oral multivitamin/mineral products are numerous and are not listed here.

Water-Soluble Vitamins
Vitamin B Complex
B-complex vitamins consist of a group of water-soluble vitamins that include thiamine, riboflavin, niacinamide (niacin), d-panthenol (pantothenic acid), pyridoxine, cyanocobalamin (B_{12}), biotin, choline, and folic acid. B vitamins serve as coenzymes for many metabolic reactions in the body. B complex often is added to intravenous fluids (discussed earlier) and may be given parenterally in an attempt to enhance the biochemical response of stressed or debilitated animals.

Clinical Uses. These vitamins are administered to replace or supplement a deficiency of B-complex vitamins.

Dosage Forms
- **B-Complex Plus**
- **Vitamin B Complex**
- **Vitamin B Complex Fortified**
- **Vitamin B Complex Injectable**

Adverse Side Effects. These can include allergic reactions and pain at the injection site.

📋 **TECHNICIAN NOTES**

- Check the label before giving B complex intravenously.
- Observe the animal for allergic reactions.
- B-complex injections may cause pain at the injection site.

Thiamine Hydrochloride (Vitamin B_1)

Thiamine is a water-soluble B-complex vitamin that acts as a coenzyme for biochemical reactions involved in carbohydrate metabolism. Deficiency of thiamine may occur as a consequence of decreased intake or synthesis or from increased destruction, which may result from bracken fern poisoning, thiamine-destroying factors in the rumen, or thiaminase in raw fish. Polioencephalomalacia of ruminants also has been associated with thiamine deficiency.

Clinical Uses. Thiamine is administered for the treatment of thiamine deficiency in all domestic species and as an aid in the treatment of lead poisoning in cattle.

Dosage Forms
- **Thiamine Hydrochloride Injection** (generic)
- **Vitamin B_1 Injection**
- **Vitamin B_1 Powder**

Adverse Side Effects. These may include hypersensitivity reactions and muscle soreness at intramuscular injection sites.

Cyanocobalamin (Vitamin B_{12})

Vitamin B_{12} is a B-complex vitamin that contains cobalt and is thought to act as a coenzyme in protein synthesis. Pernicious anemia is a condition that occurs in humans as the result of a failure to absorb B_{12} adequately. A deficiency in any case results in anemia because red blood cells fail to mature properly in the absence of B_{12}. B_{12} deficiencies are rare in veterinary medicine.

Clinical Uses. Vitamin B_{12} is administered for the management of B_{12} deficiencies.

Dosage Forms
- **Vita-Jec Vitamin B_{12}**
- **Vitamin B_{12} injection**

Adverse Side Effects. These may include allergic reactions to administration.

Ⓡ Fat-Soluble Vitamins

Vitamin A

Vitamin A is an organic alcohol that is converted from plant substances called *carotenoids* (e.g., beta carotene) in the intestine and liver and is stored primarily in the liver. It is needed for proper growth and maintenance of surface epithelium, for proper bone growth, and for maintenance of visual pigments in the retina. A deficiency of vitamin A may be associated with many clinical signs, including poor growth and reproductive performance, susceptibility to infectious disease, and poor vision in dim light. Many of the commercial vitamin A products are combined with vitamin D or E.

Clinical Uses. Vitamin A is administered for the prevention or treatment of vitamin A deficiencies.

Dosage Forms
- **Vitamin A-D Injectable**
- **Vitamin A-D Injection**
- **Vita-Jec Injection**
- **Vitamin A-D**

Adverse Side Effects. These are uncommon if label directions are followed.

Vitamin D

Vitamin D exists in two forms: D_2 and D_3. Vitamin D_2 is formed when a plant substance (ergosterol) is exposed to sunlight; D_3 is formed when a provitamin precalciferol in the skin is converted by sunlight. A deficiency of vitamin D is characterized by the development of rickets in young animals or osteomalacia in adults. Vitamin D often is combined commercially with vitamin A or E.

Clinical Uses. Vitamin D is administered for the treatment or prevention of vitamin D deficiencies.

Dosage Forms. Refer to the dosage forms for vitamin A.

Adverse Side Effects. These are uncommon if label directions are followed.

Vitamin E

Vitamin E (alpha-tocopherol) is involved (with selenium) in the metabolism of sulfur and acts as an antioxidant. Vitamin E is used in the prevention or treatment of selenium/vitamin E deficiency syndromes, such as white muscle disease (ewes, lambs, and calves), mulberry heart disease (sows and pigs), and myositis (horses).

Clinical Uses. Vitamin E is administered for the prevention and treatment of vitamin E deficiencies.

Dosage Forms
- **Bo-Se;** selenium, vitamin E injection (approved for use in calves, swine, and sheep)
- **E-SE;** selenium, vitamin E injection (approved for use in horses)
- **Mu-Se;** selenium, vitamin E injection (approved for use in nonlactating dairy cattle and beef cattle)
- **L-Se;** selenium, vitamin E injection (approved for use in lambs and baby pigs)
- **Seletoc;** selenium, vitamin E injection (approved for use in dogs)

Adverse Side Effects. These include allergic reactions and soreness at injection sites.

Vitamin K

Vitamin K is a fat-soluble vitamin required for the formation of prothrombin; for this reason, it is very important to the clotting process. Vitamin K is discussed in Chapter 20.

REVIEW QUESTIONS

1. Define hyperkalemia.
2. Intravascular fluid (plasma) makes up approximately _____ of body weight.
   a. 2%
   b. 5%
   c. 15%
   d. 40%
3. Explain the concept of a balanced solution for fluid therapy.
4. What are three units of measurement used for quantifying electrolytes in fluids?
5. Give examples of sensible and insensible fluid losses.
6. Underestimation of the degree of dehydration is sometimes a problem in _____ animals.

7. The three volumes that are calculated to arrive at the total fluid therapy volume are _____ _____.

8. Calculate the total volume of fluid needed (in 24 hours) for a 44-lb dog that is 6% dehydrated and is losing 100 mL of fluid daily through vomiting. The maintenance fluid rate is 2 mL/kg/h.

9. What drip rate, in drops/min, should be used to deliver (over a 24-hour period) the fluid for the dog in question 8 (using a standard administration set)?

10. Describe how you would set up the first bag of fluids for the dog in question 8.

11. Tell how you would prepare 500 mL of 5% dextrose from a 50% stock solution.

12. What is the purpose of the lactate in lactated Ringer's solution?

13. Give an example of a balanced solution and an example of an unbalanced solution.

14. _____ is a determination of the osmotic pressure of a solution based on the relative number of solute particles in 1 kg of the solution.

15. What is the longest time an IV catheter should remain in place before it is replaced?

16. What precaution should be observed when fluids are administered subcutaneously?

17. Any product that contains the electrolyte _____ _____ should be given by slow IV administration to prevent cardiac complications.

18. _____ is decreased body pH caused by excess hydrogen ions in the extracellular fluid.
    a. Metabolic acidosis
    b. Metabolic alkalosis
    c. Hypernatremia
    d. Hyponatremia

19. _____ are solutions containing electrolyte and nonelectrolyte substances that are capable of passing through cell membranes and therefore capable of entering all body fluid compartments.
    a. Colloids
    b. Hypertonics
    c. Calcium supplements
    d. Crystalloids

20. Vitamin A is an organic alcohol that is converted from plant substances called *carotenoids* in the intestine and liver and is stored primarily in the _____. It is needed for maintenance of visual pigments in the retina.
    a. liver
    b. pancreas
    c. stomach
    d. intestines

21. An adult dog weighing 44 lb needs maintenance fluids given. A standard drip set will be used for infusion of fluids. What is the volume of fluids needed for one day? What is the drip rate in drops/minute?
    _____

22. What maintenance volume of fluid is needed for one day for an 11-lb cat that is 5% dehydrated? What flow rate in mL/h would you use? _____
    _____

23. An 88-lb dog is seen with vomiting and diarrhea and is estimated to be 7% dehydration. The estimated fluid loss as vomitus and diarrhea is 200 mL/day. What is the total fluid volume needed for a 24-hour period? Using a standard drip set, what is the drip rate in drops/second? _____
    _____

24. What is the total fluid volume needed for one day (24 hours) for a 9-lb puppy that is 5% dehydrated and losing 50 mL per day as diarrhea? A microdrip set will be used, what is the flow rate in mL/h that you would use? _____
    _____

25. What is the fluid volume needed for 24 hours for a 120-lb dog that is seen with 10% dehydration and no ongoing fluid loss? What fluid volume will you use in milliliters to deliver one fourth of the total fluid volume over a 24-hour period? Using a standard drip set, what is the flow rate in drops/minute?
    _____

REFERENCES

American Animal Hospital Association and the American Association of Feline Practitioners (AAHA/AAFP). (2013). *Fluid therapy guidelines for dogs and cats: Implementation Toolkit*. aahanet.org. (Accessed September, 2019).

Battaglia, A. M., & Steele, A. M. (2016). *Small animal emergency and critical care for veterinary technicians* (3rd ed.). St. Louis: Elsevier.

Blankenship, J., & Campbell, J. B. (1976). Solutions. In J. Blankenship, & J. B. Campbell (Eds.), *Laboratory mathematics: Medical and biological applications*. St. Louis: Mosby.

Crowe, D. T. (2007). Emergency medicine. In *Proceedings Tennessee Veterinary Medical Association Annual Conference*. Brentwood, TN.

DiBartola, S. P. (2011). *Fluid therapy in small animal practice* (4th ed.). St. Louis: Elsevier.

Haskins, S. C. (2000). Fluid overload: How to identify and manage. In *Proceedings International Veterinary Emergency and Critical Care Symposium*. Orlando, FL.

Plumb, D. C. (2015). *Veterinary drug handbook* (8th ed.). Ames, IA: Wiley-Blackwell.

Remillard, R. L., Armstrong, P. J., & Davenport, D. J. (2000). Assisted feeding in hospitalized patients: Enteral and parenteral nutrition. In M. S. Hand, C. D. Thatcher, R. L. Remillard, et al. (Eds.), *Small animal clinical nutrition*. Marceline, MO: Walsworth Publishing Co.

Rudloff, E. (Fluid therapy series: Colloids in-depth. http://abbottanimalhealthce.com/. (Accessed February 24, 2013).

16

Blood-Modifying, Antineoplastic, and Immunosuppressant Drugs

OBJECTIVES

After studying this chapter, you should be able to

1. Explain the role of erythropoietin in red blood cell formation, describe the significance of iron in the hemoglobin molecule, and list the potential indications for and limitations of hematinics.
2. Describe the clotting mechanism in general terms, as well as list four anticoagulants and discuss their methods of action.
3. List examples of topical hemostatics.
4. Discuss parenteral hemostatic agents and name the antagonist for heparin overdose.
5. List the indications for the use of vitamin K_1 and discuss the possible adverse side effects of its use.
6. Define fibrinolysis and name a fibrinolytic agent.
7. Describe the phases of the cell cycle.
8. List six categories of antineoplastic drugs and give an example of each. Also, discuss safety precautions involved in the use of antineoplastic drugs.
9. Discuss alkylating agents, anthracyclines, antimetabolites, antitubulin agents, and miscellaneous antineoplastic drugs.
10. Define *biologic response modifier* (BRM) and list two examples of BRMs.
11. List indications for the use of immunosuppressive drugs and provide five examples.

OUTLINE

KEY TERMS

Alkylating agents
Cell cycle–nonspecific
Cell cycle–specific
Cytotoxic
Disseminated intravascular coagulation (DIC)
Endothelial layer
Erythropoietin
Fibrinolysis

Hybridoma
Metastasis
Myeloma
Myelosuppression
Thrombocytopenia
Thromboembolism
Thrombus
Vesicant

INTRODUCTION

In the first section of this chapter, drugs or agents that influence blood formation or its processes (e.g., clotting and fibrinolysis) such as hematinics, anticoagulants, anticoagulant antagonists/hemostatics, and fibrinolytic agents are discussed. Veterinary technicians should have a complete working knowledge of the applications and potential misuse of anticoagulants because they are used routinely in veterinary practice.

The second section covers antineoplastic and immunosuppressant drugs. Antineoplastic drug categories include alkylating agents, antimetabolites, mitotic inhibitors (vinca alkaloids), antibiotics, hormones, and miscellaneous agents. Safe handling techniques for these potentially dangerous agents are listed. Select immunosuppressant drugs and their clinical applications are discussed at the conclusion of this section.

BLOOD-MODIFYING DRUGS/AGENTS

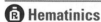 Hematinics

Red blood cells are formed in the bone marrow in response to stimulation by erythropoietin, a chemical released by the kidneys when hypoxia is present in this organ (Ganong, 2003) (Fig. 16.1). Their primary function is to carry oxygen to the tissues. This activity is greatly enhanced by the hemoglobin component of red blood cells. Only a small portion of oxygen is carried in solution in the plasma.

Hemoglobin is made up of a protein and an iron-containing pigment (Fig. 16.2). The iron in hemoglobin must be in the ferrous (Fe^{2+}) state to combine with oxygen in the most efficient way. If the iron in hemoglobin is in the ferric (Fe^{3+}) state, hemoglobin cannot combine with oxygen and is called *methemoglobin*. Adequate

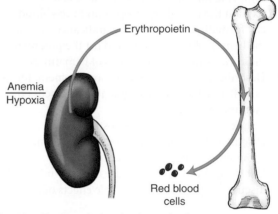

Fig. 16.1 Erythropoietin stimulates the bone marrow to produce red blood cells.

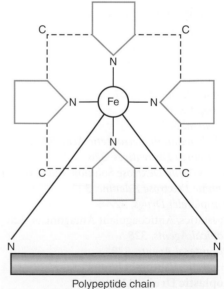

Fig. 16.2 The structure of hemoglobin.

amounts of iron, cobalt, copper, B vitamins, trace minerals, and protein are needed for normal hemoglobin and red blood cell formation.

Anemia can result from excessive loss of red blood cells, formation of inadequate numbers of red blood cells, or inadequate amounts of hemoglobin in the red blood cells. Iron-deficiency anemia, a relatively common form in humans, is rare in animals that consume balanced diets. One exception, however, is anemia in baby piglets, a condition that results from inadequate assimilation of iron from the placenta of the sow for future hemoglobin formation by the piglet. The piglet is born without adequate stores of iron for its rapid growth phase, and sow's milk is relatively low in this element. Iron-deficiency anemia is a problem of pigs raised in confined environments (concrete or slatted floors) because those raised outdoors usually obtain adequate iron from the soil.

Hematinics are substances that tend to promote an increase in the oxygen-carrying capacity of the blood. Hematinics are used to prevent or treat anemia, and the primary ingredient in most of these products is iron, a vital component of hemoglobin. Some also contain copper and B vitamins to enhance red blood cell formation. The response to hematinic administration is relatively slow, and this factor makes use of hematinics ancillary to whole blood transfusion in acute anemia.

Iron Compounds

Many injectable and oral iron preparations are available for veterinary use under generic and proprietary labels. The form of iron in these products may be iron dextran, ferrous sulfate, peptonized iron, gleptoferron, ferric hydroxide, and others, and the form apparently has little effect on use. Copper, B vitamins, liver fraction (an iron source), and palatability enhancers often are also added to the oral products. Injectable forms are labeled for intramuscular injection and contain only iron. They may cause discoloration of muscle tissue at the site of injection.

Clinical Uses. Iron compounds are used for prevention or treatment of anemia in piglets or as a nutritional supplement, depending on the form.

Dosage Forms
- **Iron dextran complex** (Armedexan, Anem-x, Ferrextran, Ferrodex, Pigdex-100, Imposil)
- **Ferrous Sulfate Oral Elixir**
- **Pet Tinic**

Adverse Side Effects. These are rare but may include muscle weakness, prostration, or muscle discoloration at the injection site.

TECHNICIAN NOTES

Pork quality assurance programs often recommend that iron injections be given in neck muscle rather than in the hind limb, ham muscle (a higher quality cut) because of potential meat staining and subsequent condemnation.

Erythropoietin

Erythropoietin, a protein produced by the kidneys, stimulates the division and differentiation of committed erythroid precursors (stem cells) in the bone marrow. A synthetic product, Epogen, has the same properties as erythropoietin and is available commercially. It is approved for human use and is produced by recombinant DNA technology. It is labeled for the treatment of anemia related to chronic renal failure or for that associated with azidothymidine treatment in patients with human immunodeficiency virus infection. No veterinary-approved product is available.

Clinical Uses. Erythropoietin is used in dogs and cats for the treatment of anemia associated with chronic renal failure or other causes.

Dosage Forms
- **Epogen**
- **Procrit**

Adverse Side Effects. In humans, adverse side effects may include hypertension, iron deficiency, polycythemia, and seizures. The use of human-coded proteins in dogs or cats could potentially cause allergic reactions.

Androgens

The treatment for anemia associated with chronic renal failure has traditionally been androgen therapy. Results obtained with the use of androgens for chronic anemia have been inconsistent.

Clinical Uses. Androgens are used for the treatment of chronic (nonregenerative) anemia.

Dosage Forms
- **Winstrol-V**
- **Equipoise**
- **Danazol**

Adverse Side Effects. These have included enlargement of the prostate, hepatic toxicity, and sodium and water retention.

Blood Substitutes

Researchers have looked for an oxygen-carrying substitute for red blood cells practically since it was learned that the hemoglobin in those cells was the transporting vehicle.

Oxyglobin (Hemoglobin-Based Oxygen Carrier Solution; HBOC) is a red blood cell substitute that consists of a polymerized bovine product with a hemoglobin concentration of 13 g/dL in a modified lactated Ringer's solution. This solution has obvious benefits over blood products that include availability, a long shelf life, universal compatibility, and freedom from disease-producing agents.

This hemoglobin solution picks up and distributes oxygen in a manner similar to red blood cells, but the oxygen-carrying function is shifted to cross-linked hemoglobin molecules in the plasma. Oxygen is carried by molecules in the plasma, thus diffusion of this gas across cell membranes occurs more efficiently than when it is carried by red blood cells because one fewer membrane must be crossed.

This product is stable for 3 years at room temperature or in the refrigerator. It is compatible with any other intravenous (IV) fluid, but other solutions should not be mixed in the same bag. A separate line should be used for these other solutions. No consideration is needed regarding blood typing or crossmatching when this product is used.

Oxyglobin also has osmotic properties similar to dextran 70 and hetastarch.

Clinical Uses. This product is labeled for the treatment of anemia in dogs regardless of the cause. It has been used in cats and foals but is not labeled for such use.

Dosage Form
- **Oxyglobin**

Adverse Side Effects. Potential side effects include pulmonary edema, discolored urine, discolored membranes, ventricular arrhythmias, fever, and coagulopathy. Oxyglobin can cause volume overload or vasoconstriction and should not be used in patients with cardiac or renal disease.

📋 TECHNICIAN NOTES

- The recommended administration rate should not be exceeded.
- Do not administer with other fluids or drugs through the same IV set.
- Do not combine with other fluids in the same bag.

℞ Anticoagulants

Blood coagulation is an obviously essential process that is designed to inhibit the loss of vital blood constituents from the circulatory system. Two separate systems or pathways may initiate the clotting mechanism—the intrinsic (intravascular) and extrinsic (extravascular) systems.

The intrinsic pathway is activated by injury to the endothelial layer of a blood vessel, which disrupts blood flow and causes a chain of chemical reactions leading to a thrombus, or clot. This process helps to repair damage to blood vessel walls that occurs from routine wear and from pathologic processes.

The extrinsic pathway is activated by injury to tissue and vessels, which release tissue thromboplastin. Thromboplastin stimulates the clotting mechanism. Vasoconstriction occurs in damaged blood vessels, causing a slowing of blood flow and facilitating clot formation. Platelet aggregation and adherence are also important steps in the clotting process.

The intrinsic and extrinsic pathways converge into a common pathway in the final steps of clot formation (Fig. 16.3). At least 13 clotting factors participate in this series of reactions (called a *cascade*) in which the product of the preceding reaction promotes the next reaction (Table 16.1). The final step in the process is the conversion of fibrinogen to fibrin by thrombin. If any of the clotting factors in the cascade (Fig. 16.4) are deficient or missing, clotting does not occur.

A balance must be maintained in the body between clot formation and clot breakdown. Destruction of clots—fibrinolysis—occurs through the action of an enzyme called *plasmin*. Plasmin digests fibrin threads and other clotting products to cause clot lysis and the release of fibrin degradation products into the circulation.

Anticoagulants inhibit clot formation by tying up or inactivating one of the clotting factors to interrupt the cascade reaction. They are used clinically to prevent coagulation of blood (or other body fluid) samples that are collected for testing, to preserve blood for transfusions, to inhibit clotting in IV catheters, and to prevent or treat thromboembolic disorders (e.g., thromboembolic cardiomyopathy in cats).

Heparin may be used paradoxically to treat the bleeding disorder disseminated intravascular coagulation (DIC), also known as consumptive coagulopathy (Fig. 16.5). DIC is not a primary disease but a secondary complication of an underlying disease. Some underlying conditions associated with DIC are immune-mediated disease, intravascular hemolysis, and shock.

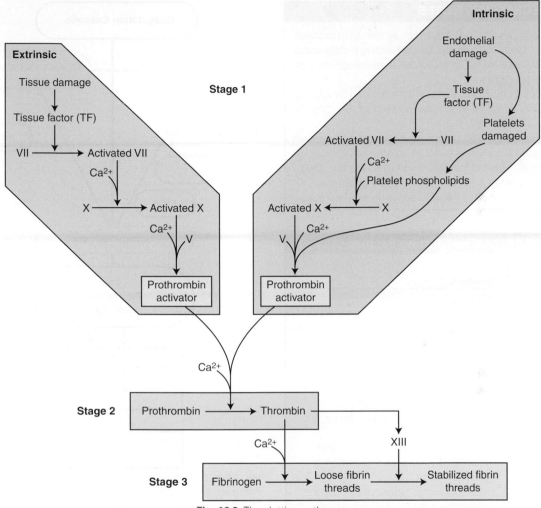

Fig. 16.3 The clotting pathways.

Heparin

Heparin is an anticoagulant that is found in many tissues of the body and is thought to be stored in mast cells. It is obtained from pig intestinal mucosa, and its strength is expressed in terms of heparin units. Heparin acts as an anticoagulant by preventing the conversion of prothrombin (factor II) to thrombin. Without thrombin, fibrinogen is not converted to fibrin and a clot does not form. Heparin does not break down clots but can prevent clots from increasing in size. It is administered therapeutically by intravenous or subcutaneous injection.

Clinical Uses. Heparin has various uses in veterinary medicine. It is used in vitro as an anticoagulant to preserve blood samples for testing by heparinizing (drawing heparin into the syringe and then forcing all visible quantities out) a syringe before the blood sample is drawn. It also is diluted in saline or sterile water for injection to form a flush solution for preventing clots in intravenous catheters. Heparin is sometimes used to preserve donated blood for transfusions when small quantities are needed (e.g., for cats or small dogs). It is used in vivo to aid in the treatment of DIC and **thromboembolism** and has been advocated for the treatment of laminitis in horses.

Dosage Forms. Forms approved for use in humans are used in veterinary medicine:
- **Heparin sodium injection**

Adverse Side Effects. These usually manifest as bleeding or **thrombocytopenia**.

📋 TECHNICIAN NOTES

- Heparin should not be used as an anticoagulant when blood is collected for performing a differential count because white blood cell morphology may be adversely affected.
- A heparin flush solution may be prepared by diluting heparin in saline at a concentration of 5 Units/mL (Crow et al., 1987).
- Approximately 750 Units of heparin should be drawn into a 60-mL syringe to act as an anticoagulant when blood is collected for transfusion (Norsworthy, 1992).
- Heparin blood collection tubes have a green top.
- Protamine sulfate is the antidote for heparin overdose.

TABLE 16.1   The Clotting Factors.

Coagulation Factor	Synonym
I	Fibrinogen
II	Prothrombin
III	Tissue factor (thromboplastin)
IV	Calcium ions
V	Proaccelerin, labile factor, or accelerator globulin
VI	Activated factor V
VII	Serum prothrombin conversion accelerator (SPCA), stable factor, or proconvertin
VIII	Antihemophilic factor (AHF), antihemophilic factor A, or antihemophilic globulin factor B
IX	Christmas factor, plasma thromboplastin component (PTC), or antihemophilic factor B
X	Stuart-Prower factor, thrombokinase
XI	Plasma thromboplastin antecedent (PTA) or antihemophilic factor C
XII	Hageman factor, glass factor, or contact factor
XIII	Fibrin-stabilizing factor (FSF) or fibrinase

Ethylenediaminetetraacetic Acid

Ethylenediaminetetraacetic acid (EDTA) is an anticoagulant that prevents clotting by chelation of calcium (factor IV). With calcium ions tied up by EDTA, clotting cannot occur. It is used in vitro to preserve blood samples and is the anticoagulant of choice when a differential count is needed (it preserves white cell morphology well). EDTA is prepared in lavender-topped collection tubes.

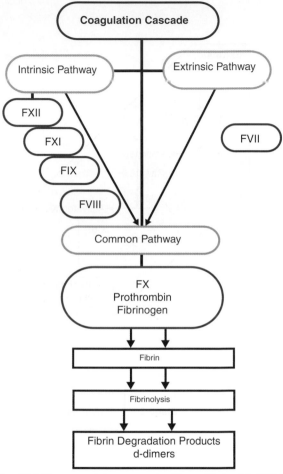

Fig. 16.4 The coagulation cascade. (From Sirois, M. [2011]. *Principles and practice of veterinary technology* [3rd ed.]. St. Louis: Elsevier.)

The calcium salt of EDTA (calcium disodium versenate) is also used in vivo as a chelating agent to treat lead poisoning and other heavy metal toxicity. This function does not involve the clotting mechanism.

Dosage Forms

- **Calcium disodium EDTA** is available through a veterinary compounding pharmacy.

Adverse Side Effects. Adverse side effects include vomiting, diarrhea, and renal toxicity.

Coumarin Derivatives

Coumarin derivatives such as dicumarol and warfarin are oral anticoagulants that bind vitamin K, therefore inhibiting the synthesis of prothrombin (factor II) and factors VII, IX, and X. These compounds are indicated for long-term treatment of thromboembolic conditions.

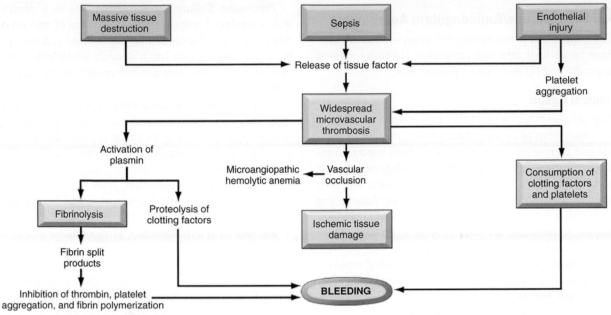

Fig. 16.5 Schematic diagram of the pathophysiology of disseminated intravascular coagulation. (From Zachary, JF. [2012]. *McGavin MD: Pathologic basis of veterinary disease* [5th ed.]. St. Louis: Elsevier.)

They are used clinically to a greater extent in human medicine than in veterinary medicine.

Dicumarol may be found in moldy sweet clover and has been associated with fatal hemorrhagic disease in cattle. Warfarin and related compounds are used in many rat poisoning products.

Clinical Uses. Coumarin derivatives are used for the long-term management of thromboembolic conditions.

Dosage Form
- **Coumadin**
- **Sofarin**

Adverse Side Effects. Adverse side effects are related to hemorrhages.

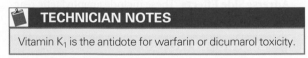

TECHNICIAN NOTES

Vitamin K₁ is the antidote for warfarin or dicumarol toxicity.

Acid Citrate Dextrose Solution and Citrate Phosphate Dextrose Adenine

Acid citrate dextrose (ACD) solution contains dextrose, sodium citrate, and citric acid and prevents clotting by chelating calcium. It is prepared in bottles or plastic bags for blood collection under both veterinary and human labels. Bottles are available for collecting 250 and 500 mL of blood. ACD solution preserves blood for 3 to 4 weeks.

Citrate phosphate dextrose adenine (CPDA-1) solution is available in plastic bags for collection of 450 mL of blood. CPDA-1 also prevents clotting by chelating calcium and preserves blood for as long as 6 weeks.

Eight milliliters of ACD or CPDA-1 can be drawn into a syringe to collect 50 mL of blood when small quantities are needed (Norsworthy, 1992).

Dosage Form
- **ACD solution**
- **CPDA-1 solution**

Antiplatelet Drugs

Antiplatelet drugs such as aspirin appear to impair clotting through inhibition of platelet stickiness and clumping. This activity is thought to be mediated through inhibition of the proaggregatory prostaglandin called *thromboxane* (Pugh, 1991).

Aspirin has been used both to prevent thromboembolism associated with heartworm treatment in dogs and to treat cardiomyopathy in cats.

TECHNICIAN NOTES

Aspirin must be used with caution in cats. Cats are deficient in glucuronyl transferase (the enzyme needed to metabolize aspirin) and have a prolonged excretion time (Khan, 2019).

℞ Hemostatics/Anticoagulant Antagonists

Substances that promote blood clotting—hemostatics—may be divided into two categories: (1) those applied topically and (2) those given parenterally.

Topical Agents

Topical agents act by providing a framework in which a clot may form or by coagulating blood protein to initiate clot formation. Framework substances used in topical hemostatics include gelatins and collagens, whereas styptics, hemostatic powders, and solutions are substances that initiate clotting through coagulation. The framework substances are absorbed after clot formation. Topical hemostatics are used to control capillary bleeding or bleeding from other small vessels.

Clinical Uses. These include the control of capillary bleeding at surgical sites or in superficial wounds.

Dosage Forms
- **Gelfoam absorbable gelatin sponge**
- **Benacel absorbable hemostatic dressing**
- **Vetspon absorbable hemostatic gelatin sponge**
- **Hemopad Absorbable Collagen Hemostat**
- **Surgicel Absorbable Hemostat**
- **Hemostat Powder** (ferrous sulfate powder)
- **Clotisol** (ferric sulfate)
- **Silver nitrate sticks**
- **Thrombogen topical thrombin solution**
- **Celox;** Celox granules represent a new generation of hemostatic agents. Celox is made of chitosan, a natural polysaccharide that is broken down by naturally occurring enzymes. Celox granules are reported to control bleeding in hypothermic conditions and in heparinized blood.
- **QuikClot Gauze Dressings;** QuikClot gauze dressings are kaolin-impregnated gauze dressings used to control traumatic bleeding in conjunction with compression.

Adverse Side Effects. These are usually minimal but may include delayed wound healing.

Parenteral Agents

Parenterally administered hemostatic agents act as anticoagulant antagonists because they do not directly activate clotting. These substances promote the synthesis of clotting factors that have been depleted through poisoning or disease, or they tie up (inactivate) anticoagulants that have been overdosed. These drugs are not used to control surgical or traumatic bleeding.

Protamine Sulfate. Protamine sulfate is a protein that is produced from the sperm or testes of salmon or related species (Plumb, 2015). Protamine has a strongly basic pH, and heparin has a strongly acidic pH. Protamine combines with heparin to form inactive complexes (salt).

Clinical Uses. Protamine sulfate is used for the treatment of heparin overdose and may be useful in treating bracken fern poisoning in cattle (Plumb, 2015). Slow intravenous administration is recommended.

Dosage Form
- **Protamine sulfate injection, USP**

Adverse Side Effects. Hypotension and bradycardia can occur if given too rapidly.

Vitamin K$_1$ (Phytonadione). Phytonadione is a synthetic substance that is identical to naturally occurring vitamin K$_1$. Vitamin K is necessary for the production (in the liver) of active prothrombin (factor II), proconvertin factor (factor VII), plasma thromboplastin component (factor IX), and Stuart factor (factor X). It is used clinically for treating cases in which vitamin K has been tied up or destroyed and in bleeding disorders associated with poor formation of vitamin K–dependent clotting factors. Immediate coagulant effect should not be expected after administration of vitamin K because several hours may pass before synthesis of new clotting factors occurs.

Clinical Uses. In veterinary medicine, vitamin K$_1$ is used for the treatment of rodenticide toxicity, for bleeding disorders related to faulty synthesis of vitamin K–dependent clotting factors, and for unknown anticoagulant toxicity.

Dosage Forms
- **Mephyton**
- May be obtained from a veterinary compounding pharmacy.

Adverse Side Effects. These include anaphylactic reactions (intravenous use) and bleeding at the injection site.

 TECHNICIAN NOTES

Many consider intravenous administration of phytonadione to be contraindicated because of the possibility of anaphylactic reactions.

Aminocaproic Acid. Aminocaproic acid inhibits fibrinolysis through its effects on plasminogen activator and possibly via antiplasmin activity. It may be used to inhibit bleeding in certain conditions like thrombocytopenia. It is contraindicated in patients with active intravascular clotting.

Dosage Form
- **Amicar**
- May be obtained from a veterinary compounding pharmacy.

Adverse Side Effects. Adverse side effects are uncommon, but may include vomiting, diarrhea, and decreased appetite.

Ⓡ Fibrinolytic. (Thrombolytic) Drugs

Thrombolytic drugs are used to break down or dissolve thrombi. Occlusion of an artery by a thromboembolus can cause necrosis of tissue distal to the blockage if the obstruction is not removed quickly. In humans, damage to heart muscle that occurs when a coronary artery is occluded in a heart attack is a classic example of this process. Pulmonary thromboemboli sometimes occur in dogs after heartworm treatment and may accompany cardiomyopathy in cats.

Thrombolytic agents may help to remove or reduce the size of the occluding thromboembolus and minimize tissue damage. This action is brought about by stimulating conversion of plasminogen to the enzyme plasmin, which lyses the clots. The sooner the therapy is initiated after thromboembolism has occurred, the better the chances of success. Thrombolytic activity of one of the products (alteplase) is activated by the presence of fibrin so that recent clots are targeted.

The expense of these drugs often precludes their use in veterinary medicine.

Clinical Uses. Clinical uses include treatment of pulmonary embolism, treatment of arterial thrombosis and emboli, treatment of coronary thrombosis, and IV catheter clearance.

Dosage Forms
- **Streptokinase** (Streptase)
- **Urokinase** (Abbokinase)

Adverse Side Effects. These are related to bleeding episodes, especially if anticoagulants have also been used.

ANTINEOPLASTIC DRUGS

Antineoplastic drugs are administered to animals in an attempt to cure or lessen the effect of neoplasms. Neoplasia is the abnormal growth of tissue into a mass that is not responsive to normal cellular control mechanisms.

The term *tumor* by definition indicates any tissue mass or swelling that may or may not be neoplastic. *Tumor* is often used broadly in common discussion to indicate a neoplasm. A neoplasm may be benign or malignant. In general, benign tumors (neoplasms) do not cause high mortality because they grow locally and do not invade adjacent tissue. These tumors may cause morbidity, however, by compressing or occluding organs. The term *cancer* is used to indicate a malignant neoplasm that is capable of causing destruction of the tissue of origin and is also capable of metastasis to other tissue (Fig. 16.6). Malignant tumors are very damaging to tissue and often lead to the death of the patient if treatment is not provided. A third type of neoplasm is an in situ tumor, which is a small tumor in epithelial tissue that appears to contain cancer cells but does not cross the basement membrane and invade adjacent tissue. Treatment of neoplasia involves several methods, including the use of drugs (chemotherapy), surgery, radiation, and immune modulation. Regardless of the method used, the goals of treatment are to keep the neoplasia under control, increase survival time, and improve the quality of life of the patient.

If one is to understand the use of chemotherapy drugs, a basic understanding of cancer formation is in order. Cancer has been called a "complex mutagenic disease" (Withrow & Vail, 2007) in which genetic mutations give a cell or cells the ability to replicate in an unlimited way (initiation), form a mass of cells (promotion), and invade adjacent tissue (progression). Oncologists speculate that five to six genetic mutations are the minimum number that must occur to give a cell the six fundamental characteristics of cancer. These six characteristics are (1) self-sufficiency in the production of cell growth signals, (2) insensitivity to antigrowth signals, (3) the ability to evade programmed cell death (apoptosis), (4) unlimited potential to replicate, (5) sustained ability to promote angiogenesis (blood vessel formation for the cancer mass), and (6) the capacity to invade tissue and metastasize.

Several mechanisms are thought to be involved in the production of the six hallmarks of cancer. Protooncogenes are genetic elements in all normal cells that are capable of causing cancer if they are enhanced through abnormal regulation. The ability of the cancer cell to replicate in an unlimited way may be facilitated by activation or upregulation of an enzyme called *telomerase*. Defects in suppressor oncogenes or antioncogenes like

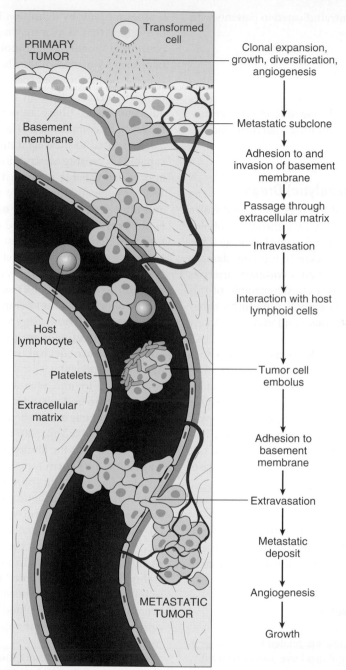

Fig. 16.6 The metastatic cascade. Sequential steps involved in the hematogenous spread of a tumor. Similar events occur during lymphatic spread. (From Zachary, JF. [2012]. *McGavin MD: Pathologic basis of veterinary disease* [5th ed.]. St. Louis: Elsevier.)

the *p53* gene may take away the ability to control the normal cell cycle. Factors that may promote the mechanisms leading to cancer include viruses and chemical, physical, and hormonal influences.

PRINCIPLES OF CHEMOTHERAPY

Proliferating cells, whether they are found in normal tissue or in neoplasms, contain resting and dividing cells that are involved in phases of the cell cycle (Fig. 16.5). These phases of the cell cycle include the S phase (DNA synthesis and replication), the M phase (mitosis), the G1 and G2 phases (RNA synthesis), and the G0 (resting) phase. Chemotherapy can be directed toward a specific phase of the cell cycle or can be cycle nonspecific. Chemotherapy is most effective against rapidly growing tumors because actively dividing cells are more sensitive to DNA damage and cell cycle processes (Withrow & Vail, 2007). All rapidly dividing cells like those found in the bone marrow, gastrointestinal tract, reproductive organs, and hair follicles are affected by antineoplastic drugs. Chemotherapy may be used to treat a tumor with a known sensitivity to a drug or drugs, to make cancer cells more sensitive to radiation or other therapy methods, to reduce or eliminate metastases, to reduce tumor size for the purpose of relieving pain or improving function, and to reduce tumor size to facilitate surgical removal.

The effectiveness of chemotherapy depends on many factors. One of the most important is the length of time that a tumor is exposed to an effective dose of the drug. Another significant factor is the development of specific resistance to a drug by the tumor. A traditional way of using chemotherapy is to give the maximum tolerated dose (MTD) for the shortest time possible. Most of these drugs are dosed on the basis of estimated body surface area (Table 16.2). Many oncologists believe that accuracy of dosing is improved if the dosage is based on body weight rather than surface area for cats and dogs weighing less than 10 kg. Another way of giving chemotherapy drugs is by a frequent low dose over a longer time (metronomic method).

Chemotherapy drugs are often given in combinations to increase their overall effectiveness. Different tumors are treated with specific combinations of drugs at doses, durations, and intervals determined by carefully designed treatment protocols. Chemotherapy agents indiscriminately target rapidly dividing cells and often have a high therapeutic index. Consequently, toxicity is a possibility and side effects are often seen. The side effects can be self-limiting, but constant monitoring of the patient for persistent and/or severe toxic side effects is indicated. Side effects are most often related to the gastrointestinal and hemopoietic systems. Anorexia, nausea, vomiting, and diarrhea may be seen soon after treatment is started because of effects on the chemoreceptor trigger zone (CRTZ), or 3 to 5 days later because of injury to gastrointestinal epithelium. Bone marrow depression (myelosuppression) also may occur, resulting in a moderate to severe reduction in circulating neutrophils and/or platelets. Dogs with continuously growing hair like poodles, terriers, and Old English Sheepdogs may lose their hair as a result of chemotherapy. Cats may lose their whiskers and guard hairs. Other side effects may include cystitis, cardiomyopathy, anaphylactic reactions, and tissue damage due to extravasation of the drug(s). Many chemotherapy drugs are vesicants that cause inflammation and potential sloughing of tissue if leakage outside the vein occurs when the agents are administered. Some protocols call for pretreatment of the patient with drugs like antihistamines, steroids, antiemetics, and analgesics to reduce the severity of side effects.

Great care should be taken to prevent accidental exposure to chemotherapy drugs by technicians, veterinarians, and other employees because of the ability of these drugs to be teratogenic, mutagenic, and carcinogenic at therapeutic doses. Box 16.1 provides a list of recommendations for the safe use of antineoplastic agents.

Antineoplastic drugs have been categorized into the following major classes: alkylating agents, anthracyclines, antimetabolites, antitubulin agents, corticosteroids, and miscellaneous agents. Table 16.3 provides a list of the commonly used antineoplastic agents, as well as their indications, toxicities, and dosages.

Cancer chemotherapy can be a long, emotional, costly, and complicated process. Patients may experience periods of relapse and remission, harmful drug reactions can occur, and treatments can fail. Technicians should be prepared to counsel owners about the potential risks and the high level of commitment they will need to see the process through to completion. They should be able to make the animal owner aware that successful treatment can mean a longer and/or a better quality of life for their pet and a strengthening of the human–companion animal bond.

TABLE 16.2   Body Surface Area Conversion Charts (Body Weight in kg to m².).

kg	m²	kg	m²	kg	m²
Weight to Body Surface Area Conversion Chart—Dogs					
0.5	0.064	17.0	0.668	34.0	1.060
1.0	0.101	10.0	0.004	05.0	1.081
2.0	0.160	19.0	0.719	36.0	1.101
3.0	0.210	20.0	0.744	37.0	1.121
4.0	0.255	21.0	0.769	38.0	1.142
5.0	0.295	22.0	0.785	39.0	1.162
6.0	0.333	23.0	0.817	40.0	1.181
7.0	0.370	24.0	0.840	41.0	1.201
8.0	0.404	25.0	0.864	42.0	1.220
9.0	0.437	26.0	0.886	43.0	1.240
10.0	0.469	27.0	0.909	44.0	1.259
11.0	0.500	28.0	0.931	45.0	1.278
12.0	0.529	29.0	0.953	46.0	1.297
13.0	0.553	30.0	0.975	47.0	1.302
14.0	0.581	31.0	0.997	48.0	1.334
15.0	0.608	32.0	1.018	49.0	1.352
16.0	0.641	33.0	1.029	50.0	1.371
Weight to Body Surface Area Conversion Chart—Cats					
0.1	0.022	3.0	0.208	6.8	0.360
0.2	0.034	3.2	0.217	7.0	0.366
0.3	0.045	3.4	0.226	7.2	0.373
0.4	0.054	3.6	0.235	7.4	0.380
0.5	0.063	3.8	0.244	7.6	0.387
0.6	0.071	4.0	0.252	7.8	0.393
0.7	0.079	4.2	0.260	8.0	0.400
0.8	0.086	4.4	0.269	8.2	0.407
0.9	0.093	4.6	0.277	8.4	0.413
1.0	0.100	4.8	0.285	8.6	0.420
1.2	0.113	5.0	0.292	8.8	0.426
1.4	0.125	5.2	0.300	9.0	0.433
1.6	0.137	5.4	0.307	9.2	0.439
1.8	0.148	5.6	0.315	9.4	0.445
2.0	0.159	5.8	0.323	9.6	0.452
2.2	0.169	6.0	0.330	9.8	0.458
2.4	0.179	6.2	0.337	10.0	0.464
2.6	0.189	6.4	0.345		
2.8	0.199	6.6	0.352		

From Withrow, S. J., & Vail, D. M. (2007). *Withrow & MacEwan's small animal clinical oncology* (4th ed.). St. Louis: Saunders.

℞ Alkylating Agents

Alkylating agents are **cell cycle–nonspecific** drugs that are able to cross-link strands of DNA to change its structure and inhibit its replication. This brings protein synthesis and cell division to a halt; cell death often follows.

Clinical Uses. Clinical uses include treatment of various neoplastic disorders, including lymphoproliferative neoplasms, osteosarcoma, hemangiosarcoma, and squamous cell carcinoma, and treatment of certain immune-mediated diseases (immunosuppression).

Dosage Forms
- **Cyclophosphamide injection** (Cytoxan)
- **Chlorambucil tablets** (Leukeran)
- **Melphalan tablets** (Alkeran)

BOX 16.1 Chemotherapy Safety Recommendations

Safety Issue	Recommendations
To minimize the risk of topical contamination	• Wear approved chemotherapy administration gloves. Latex examination gloves are not impermeable to chemotherapeutic agents. If chemotherapy administration gloves are not available, double-glove with latex examination gloves. • Wear a nonabsorbent chemotherapy administration gown. • Do not push air bubbles out of the syringe. • The use of commercially available closed-system drug transfer devices (e.g., PhaSeal) can decrease the risk of exposure. • Use safety goggles or other protective eyewear.
To avoid the oral route of contamination	• Never eat or drink in the chemotherapy administration room. • Never smoke or apply makeup in the chemotherapy administration room. • Never store chemotherapeutic drugs with food or other drugs. • Caution clients (and veterinary staff) always to wear gloves when administering chemotherapeutic drugs by the oral route.
Chemotherapy waste disposal	• Separate chemotherapy waste from other sharps and biohazards, including needles, syringes, catheters, gloves, and masks. • Contact a local human hospital for aid in disposal of all chemotherapy-associated waste.
Precautions for patient care and cleanup (although the amount of active drug eliminated from the patient is minimal, it is prudent to take precautions)	• Chemotherapeutic drugs are excreted in feces and urine: wear chemotherapy gloves when cleaning up after patients for at least 48 hours after drug administration. • No guidelines have been established for the disposal of pet waste; however, caution clients about cleaning up after their pets. If the patient urinates or defecates inside the home within 48 hours of receiving chemotherapy, owners should wear gloves to clean up waste and should double-bag all waste.

Modified from Withrow, S. J., & Vail, D. M. (2007). *Withrow & MacEwan's small animal clinical oncology* (4th ed.). St. Louis: Saunders.

- **Nitrosoureas, lomustine, and carmustine**
- **Dacarbazine**
- **Ifosfamide** (Ifex)

   Adverse Side Effects. Adverse side effects of the alkylating agents may include neutropenia, nephrotoxicity, thrombocytopenia, vomiting, and hemorrhagic cystitis.

> ### 📋 TECHNICIAN NOTES
>
> Cyclophosphamide is also used as an immunosuppressant.

Anthracyclines

Many of the anthracycline antineoplastic agents are derived from soil fungi of the *Streptomyces* genus. They are cell cycle–nonspecific and exert their effects by binding with DNA and interfering with RNA and protein synthesis. Doxorubicin is the most commonly used drug in this class in veterinary medicine. It is widely used for various neoplastic conditions.

   Clinical Uses. These agents are used for the treatment of lymphoproliferative neoplasms and various carcinomas and sarcomas.

Dosage Forms
- **Doxorubicin hydrochloride for injection** (Adriamycin)
- **Bleomycin** (Blenoxane)
- **Dactinomycin** (Cosmegen)
- **Mitoxantrone** (Novantrone)

   Adverse Side Effects. These include bone marrow suppression, cardiotoxicity (cardiomyopathy), gastroenteritis, and anaphylaxis. Adriamycin may cause the urine to change color (red-brown) for a couple of days.

> ### TECHNICIAN NOTES
>
> - Some clinicians use antihistamines to premedicate animals to be treated with doxorubicin to suppress allergic reactions.
> - Doxorubicin is a strong vesicant. Tissue sloughing can follow extravasation, and skin irritation can result from contact with the drug.
> - Doxorubicin is commonly used in combination with other antineoplastic agents.
> - Dexrazoxane is a drug that may be used to block doxorubicin-induced cardiac toxicity.

Antimetabolites

The antimetabolites are cell cycle–specific drugs that affect the S phase (DNA synthesis) of the cycle. These drugs are analogues of purines and pyrimidines—naturally occurring bases in DNA—that may be incorporated into the DNA molecule to inhibit protein and enzyme synthesis. Cellular functions needed for normal activity are thus blocked.

Clinical Uses. Clinical uses include treatment of lymphoproliferative neoplasms, treatment of gastrointestinal and hepatic neoplasms, and treatment of central nervous system lymphoma.

Dosage Forms
- **Methotrexate** (Mexate), oral tablet or injection
- **Cytosine arabinoside** (Cytarabine) injection
- **5-Fluorouracil** (Adrucil) cream or solution

Adverse Side Effects. These may include anorexia, nausea, vomiting, diarrhea, bone marrow suppression, hepatotoxicity, and neurotoxicity.

> **TECHNICIAN NOTES**
>
> Fluorouracil is contraindicated in cats because of adverse side effects.

Antitubulin Agents

The plant alkaloids are cell cycle–specific for the M phase, inhibiting mitosis and causing cell death. They are thought to bind microtubular proteins and inhibit formation of the mitotic spindle, thus suspending mitosis in metaphase.

The two drugs in this category—vincristine and vinblastine—are natural alkaloids derived from the periwinkle plant (*Vinca rosea*, Linn). Protective clothing should be worn when these drugs are administered so that possible skin contact irritation does not occur.

Clinical Uses. Clinical uses include treatment of lymphoproliferative neoplasms, carcinomas, mast cell tumors, and splenic tumors.

Dosage Forms
- **Vincristine sulfate** (Oncovin, Vincasar) injection
- **Vinblastine sulfate** (Alkaban-AQ, Velban) injection
- **Vinorelbine** (Navelbine)

Adverse Side Effects. These may include gastroenteritis, bone marrow suppression, stomatitis, alopecia, and peripheral neuropathy.

> **TECHNICIAN NOTES**
>
> - Extravasation of plant alkaloids may cause tissue necrosis.
> - Skin contact causes irritation.

Miscellaneous Antineoplastic Drugs
Platinum Drugs

The platinum drugs (carboplatin and cisplatin) are thought to act in a manner similar to the alkylating agents, which interrupt the replication of DNA in tumor cells (Papich, 2016).

Clinical Uses. These products are used for a variety of solid tumors, including osteosarcomas and carcinomas.

Dosage Forms
- **Cisplatin** (Platinol)
- **Carboplatin** (Paraplatin)

Adverse Side Effects. These include renal toxicity, nausea, anorexia, and vomiting (cisplatin). Dyspnea, pulmonary edema, and death may occur in cats. Carboplatin causes less nephrotoxicity, nausea, and vomiting than cisplatin.

> **TECHNICIAN NOTES**
>
> Cisplatin is contraindicated in cats.

Asparaginase

Asparaginase is the most commonly used miscellaneous agent. It is a cell cycle–specific (G1) enzyme extracted from *Escherichia coli* bacteria. Asparaginase acts as a catalyst in the breakdown of asparagine, an amino acid required by cancer cells. Deprived of a needed amino acid, the cancer cells die. Asparaginase has no effect on normal cells, and it is usually used in combination protocols.

Clinical Uses. Asparaginase is used for the treatment of lymphoproliferative neoplasms.

Dosage Form
- **Asparaginase for injection** (Elspar)

Adverse Side Effects. The adverse side effects of this drug include immediate hypersensitivity and gastrointestinal disturbances.

Glucocorticoids

The glucocorticoids prednisone and prednisolone are sometimes used for the treatment of neoplastic disorders. They are cell cycle–nonspecific. Corticosteroids have a

TABLE 16.3 Commonly Used Chemotherapeutic Drugs.

Drug	Main Indications	Toxicities	Dosage
Alkylating Agents			
Cyclophosphamide	Lymphoma, carcinoma, sarcoma	Bone marrow, gastrointestinal (GI) tract, sterile hemorrhagic cystitis	Given orally (PO) or intravenously (IV); many dosing regimens can be used, depending on concurrent anticancer drugs
Chlorambucil	Lymphoma, chronic lymphocytic leukemia, mast cell tumor, IgM myeloma Substitute for cyclophosphamide if hemorrhagic cystitis occurs.	Mild bone marrow toxicity	Given PO only; many dosing regimens can be used, depending on concurrent anticancer drugs
CCNU (lomustine)	Relapsed lymphoma or mast cell tumor, brain tumor	Myelosuppression and idiosyncratic, potentially fatal hepatotoxicity	Dogs: 60–90 mg/m^2 PO every 3 weeks Cats: 50–60 mg/m^2 PO every 3–6 weeks
Dacarbazine	Lymphoma	Myelosuppression, vomiting during administration, perivascular irritation on extravasation Do not use in cats.	Dogs: 200 mg/m^2 IV daily for 5 days every 3 weeks *or* 1000 mg/m^2 IV every 3 weeks
Ifosfamide	Lymphoma	Hemorrhagic cystitis, myelosuppression	Dogs: 275–350 mg/m^2 IV with saline diuresis and mesna, every 3 weeks
Melphalan	Multiple myeloma, anal sac adenocarcinoma	Myelosuppression, potential cumulative thrombocytopenia	Dogs: 0.1 mg/kg every 24 hours for 10 days, then 0.05 mg/kg daily *or* 7 mg/m^2 PO daily for 5 days every 3 weeks Cats: 0.1 mg/kg every 24 hours
Anthracyclines			
Dactinomycin	Lymphoma	Myelosuppression, GI upset, perivascular damage with extravasation	0.75–0.8 mg/m^2 IV every 3 weeks
Doxorubicin	Lymphoma, carcinoma, sarcoma	Myelosuppression, GI upset, hypersensitivity during administration, perivascular damage with extravasation, cumulative (180 mg/m^2) myocardial toxicity, nephrotoxicity (cats)	Dogs: ≥10 kg: 30 mg/m^2 IV every 2–3 weeks Dogs <10 kg: 1 mg/kg IV every 2–3 weeks Cats: 1 mg/kg IV every 3 weeks
Mitoxantrone	Lymphoma, transitional cell carcinoma	Myelosuppression, GI upset, perivascular damage with extravasation	Dogs: 5–5.5 mg/m^2 IV every 3 weeks Cats: 6 mg/m^2 IV every 3 weeks

Continued

TABLE 16.3 Commonly Used Chemotherapeutic Drugs.—cont'd

Drug	Main Indications	Toxicities	Dosage
Antimetabolites			
Methotrexate	Lymphoma	Mild myelosuppression and/or GI upset	Given PO or IV Dogs and cats: 0.8 mg/kg in combination with other chemotherapeutic drugs
Cytosine arabinoside	Lymphoma (myeloproliferative)	Mild myelosuppression and/or GI upset	Given subcutaneously (SC), intramuscularly (IM), or IV; several different regimens can be used, depending on concurrent anticancer drugs.
Antitubulin Agents			
Vinblastine	Mast cell tumor	Myelosuppression, perivascular vesicant	Dogs: 2 mg/m^2 IV every 1–2 weeks
Vincristine	Lymphoma, mast cell tumor, transmissible venereal tumor, immune-mediated thrombocytopenia	Myelosuppression, perivascular vesicant, peripheral neuropathy, constipation in cats	Dogs and cats: 0.5–0.7 mg/m^2 IV weekly or as dictated by concurrent anticancer drugs
Vinorelbine	Primary lung tumor	Myelosuppression, perivascular vesicant	Dogs: 15–18 mg/m^2 IV every 1–2 weeks
Corticosteroids			
Prednisone	Lymphoma, mast cell tumor, myeloma, chronic lymphocytic leukemia Noncytotoxic indications: brain tumor, insulinoma, appetite stimulant	Polyuria, polyphagia, polydipsia, muscle wasting, behavioral changes	Dogs and cats cytotoxic dose: 2 mg/kg/day, taper according to protocol Dogs and cats noncytotoxic dose: 0.5 mg/kg/day
Miscellaneous Drugs			
Asparaginase	Lymphoma	Hypersensitivity reaction after administration	Dogs and cats: 400 IU/kg SQ or IM, maximum dose of 10,000 IU
Carboplatin	Osteosarcoma, carcinoma, sarcoma	Myelosuppression; potentially severe GI effects (small dogs)	Dogs: 300 mg/m^2 IV every 3 weeks Cats: 240–260 mg/m^2 IV every 3 weeks
Cisplatin	Osteosarcoma, carcinoma, sarcoma	Nephrotoxic—must be given with saline-induced diuresis; highly emetogenic; fatal to cats	Dogs: 70 mg/m^2 IV every 3 weeks Cats: Do not use
Hydroxyurea	Polycythemia vera, myeloproliferative diseases	Myelosuppression	Dogs: 50 mg/kg/day, tapering to every other day with remission Cats: 10 mg/kg/day, tapering to every other day with remission
Procarbazine	Lymphoma	GI upset, myelosuppression	Dogs: 50 mg/m^2 daily for 14 days on and 14 days off as part of mechlorethamine, Oncovin (vincristine), procarbazine, and prednisone (MOPP) protocol

Modified from Withrow, S. J., & Vail, D. M. (2007). *Withrow & MacEwan's small animal clinical oncology.* (4th ed.). St. Louis: Saunders.

lympholytic action, which makes them useful for treating lymphoid neoplasms. They are also helpful in the management of secondary complications of neoplastic diseases such as hypercalcemia and immune-mediated (thrombocytopenia) problems. In addition, they can increase appetite and the overall feeling of well-being in patients being treated for neoplasm. They usually are used in combination protocols with other antineoplastic drugs.

Piroxicam

Piroxicam is a nonsteroidal antiinflammatory agent that has been shown to be very effective in the treatment of transitional cell carcinoma of the bladder and squamous cell carcinoma in the dog. Piroxicam's antitumor effects are thought to be due to effects exerted on the immune system rather than on tumor cells.

   Dosage Form
- **Feldene**
- May be obtained from veterinary compounding pharmacy.

   Adverse Side Effects. All nonsteroidal antiinflammatory drugs are capable of causing significant GI effects such as gastrointestinal irritation and ulcerations.

   Hydroxyurea and procarbazine are two other agents in the miscellaneous category. See Table 16.3 for information about these two agents.

Ⓡ Biologic Response Modifiers

Biologic response modifiers (BRMs) are agents that alter the relationship between the tumor and the host animal in a way that improves the host's ability to mount an antitumor response (Grant et al., 1989). BRMs are used as an adjunct to conventional chemotherapy protocols, not as the sole agent of treatment.

Cancer develops in many animals because of an immunosuppressed state, and chemotherapy exacerbates the immunosuppression. BRMs may be used to stimulate or restore the compromised immune response of the host.

Examples of BRMs include bacterial agents, chemical agents, interferons, thymosins, cytokines/lymphokines, and monoclonal antibodies.

Monoclonal Antibodies

Monoclonal antibodies are identical immunoglobulin molecules formed by a single clone of plasma cells. They are produced by a **hybridoma,** a fusion of a specific antibody-producing B cell with **myeloma** cells (Fig. 16.8). Hybridomas secrete large quantities of a very specific (for the tumor) antibody. Monoclonal antibodies may have direct **cytotoxic** effects on tumor cells, or they may be attached (conjugated) to chemotherapeutic agents such as radioisotopes, BRMs, or other agents for direct delivery to the tumor cells. In this way, they become a "magic bullet" directed at cancer cells (Fig. 16.9).

   Clinical Uses. A monoclonal antibody product for the treatment of canine lymphoma that was previously available is no longer being produced. Monoclonal antibody use is a valuable tool in diagnostics and research and has potential value in clinical therapy.

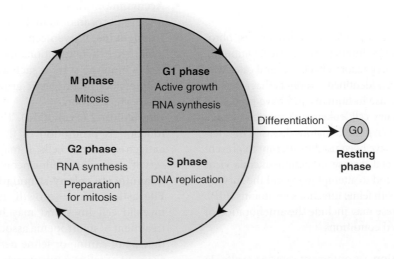

Fig. 16.7 The cell cycle.

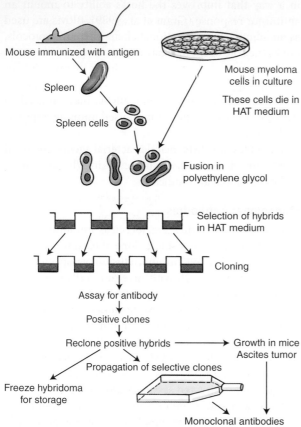

Fig. 16.8 Production of monoclonal antibodies. *HAT,* Hypoxanthine–aminopterin–thymidine. (From Tizard, I. [1987]. *Veterinary immunology: An introduction* [3rd ed.]. Philadelphia: WB Saunders.)

Interferon

Interferons are chemicals produced by leukocytes, fibroblasts, and epithelial cells. Interferons can exert antitumor, antiviral, and immunoregulatory effects. Several categories of interferons have been identified. Products that are available are approved for use in humans and have been used in humans to treat hairy cell leukemia, Kaposi's sarcoma, genital warts, and certain granulomatous diseases. In veterinary medicine, they have been used to attempt to prevent the development of fatal disease in feline leukemia virus (FeLV)–infected cats and to attempt to extend the survival time of cats infected with feline infectious peritonitis (FIP).

   Clinical Uses. These may include the amelioration of FeLV- and FIP-related conditions.

   Dosage Forms
- **Roferon-A injection,** recombinant interferon alfa-2a

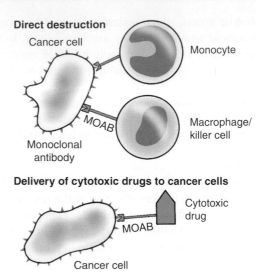

Fig. 16.9 Antitumor mechanisms of monoclonal antibodies. *MOAB,* Monoclonal antibody.

- **Intron A,** recombinant interferon alfa-2b for injection
- **Alferon N injection,** human leukocyte–derived interferon alfa-n3
- **Virbagen Omega,** recombinant interferon of feline origin
- **Actimmune gamma-1b,** recombinant interferon

   Adverse Side Effects. Adverse side effects are uncommon in cats when given orally. Higher dosages given parenterally may cause fever, diarrhea, and loss of appetite.

Other Biologic Response Modifiers

- **Acemannan.** This product is licensed for the treatment of fibrosarcoma in dogs and cats.
- **Interleukins.** Seventeen interleukins have been identified. Their functions include various activities in the immune system such as cell enhancement or suppression, hemopoietic growth, and regulation of leukocyte function.
- **Interleukin-2 (Proleukin).** This substance's primary function is promotion of the clonal expansion of antigen-specific T cells; it may be useful in treating certain canine and feline neoplasias (Kruth, 1998).
- **Granulocyte colony-stimulating factor (G-CSF)— Filgrastim.** These growth factors affect specific myeloid cell lines and may have some use in the treatment of neutropenia associated with the chemotherapy of canine or feline neoplasia or in the management of feline panleukopenia.

- **Bacillus Calmette-Guérin (BCG).** BCG is a live, attenuated strain of *Mycobacterium bovis* that activates B and T cells (Ettinger, 2017).
- *Propionibacterium acnes.* Immunoregulin is a killed suspension of *P. acnes* approved for use in veterinary medicine. It causes nonspecific immunostimulation.
- **Staphylococcal protein A.** This product initiates T- and B-lymphocyte proliferation.
- *Parapox ovis* **virus immunomodulator—Zylexis.** This product is used to treat horses with viral upper respiratory disease caused by equine herpes virus. It is an immunomodulator that may limit the severity of clinical signs.
- **Lymphocyte T-Cell Immunomodulator.** This agent was developed to aid in the treatment of cats with feline leukemia or feline immunodeficiency virus infection.
- **Canine Melanoma Vaccine.** This vaccine carries a conditional U.S. Department of Agriculture approval for the treatment of melanoma in dogs.
- **Oncept.** This product is used for canine malignant melanoma of the oral cavity, stage II and III (Ettinger, 2017).

Immunosuppressive Drugs

Immunosuppressive drugs are used in veterinary medicine to treat various immune-mediated disorders. Some of the diseases related to an overactive or improperly responding immune system include lupus erythematosus, lymphocytic–plasmacytic enteritis, rheumatoid arthritis, immune-mediated skin disease, and hemolytic anemia. Many of the immunosuppressive drugs work by interfering with one of the stages of the cell cycle or by affecting cellular messengers.

Azathioprine

Azathioprine is an antimetabolite that affects cells in the S phase of the cell cycle. It inhibits both T lymphocytes and B lymphocytes to bring about immunosuppression. It has fewer side effects than cyclophosphamide and some of the other immunosuppressants. It is often used in combination with prednisone or prednisolone. This drug should not be used in cats because cats are more likely to be affected by the side effects of this drug.

Clinical Uses. Azathioprine is used primarily for the treatment of immune-mediated disease in dogs.

Dosage Forms
- **Azathioprine (Imuran) tablets, injection**

Adverse Side Effects. Adverse side effects are related to bone marrow suppression. Long-term use may predispose to infection.

Cyclosporine

Cyclosporine is a substance isolated from a fungus that inhibits proliferation of T lymphocytes (Boothe, 2012). It was approved for use in humans for prevention of organ transplant rejection; however, it has also been used to treat several immune-mediated diseases (e.g., uveitis, Graves' disease, psoriasis, pemphigus). It has been used in veterinary medicine for the prevention of organ transplant rejection, for treating immune-mediated skin disorders, and for the management of keratoconjunctivitis sicca (KCS) in dogs.

Clinical Uses. Clinical use of cyclosporine in practice is limited mainly to ophthalmic application for treatment of KCS and atopic dermatitis in dogs.

Dosage Forms
- **Optimmune ophthalmic ointment**
- **Atopica capsules (dogs), atopica oral solution (cats)**
- **Restasis ophthalmic emulsion**
- **Sandimmune, cyclosporine gelatin capsules**
- **Sandimmune, cyclosporine oral solution**
- **Sandimmune, cyclosporine for injection**

Adverse Side Effects. Adverse effects include vomiting, diarrhea, decreased appetite, and weight loss. Nephrotoxicity and hepatotoxicity may occur.

> **TECHNICIAN NOTES**
>
> Monitor the eyes for irritation or infection if cyclosporine is being used for KCS.

Metronidazole

Metronidazole is a substance that has antibacterial, antiprotozoal, and immunosuppressive activities. It may be used in conjunction with corticosteroids to enhance its immunosuppressive effects.

Clinical Uses. Clinical uses include treatment of lymphocytic–plasmacytic enteritis in dogs, treatment of giardiasis, and treatment of anaerobic bacterial infections.

Dosage Forms
- **Flagyl, metronidazole tablets**
- **Flagyl, metronidazole powder for injection**
- **Flagyl IV, injectable**

BOX 16.2 Case Scenario

An 8-year-old spayed female Shih-Tzu, named Lulu, presented to the veterinary hospital with squinting of the right eye, red and irritated conjunctiva, and ocular discharge.

History: Owner noticed that Lulu had been squinting in her right eye for the past week. The eye became red and irritated over the past couple of days and the ocular discharge became thick and appeared yellow in color. Lulu is up-to-date on vaccinations, eating and drinking well, urinating and defecating normally. No history of recurrent eye injuries or ulcers.

Physical examination findings: Lulu was alert and responsive. All vital signs were within normal limits. Reddening of conjunctiva and irritation of the eye tissue in the right eye. She is squinting and blinking excessively indicating a level of discomfort and pain. Right eye appears dull and dry with moderate amount of mucopurulent ocular discharge. The left eye has slight reddening of the conjunctiva and slight mucopurulent discharge. The patient is not squinting or blinking excessively in the left eye.

Diagnostic plan: Schirmer tear test to measure tear production, fluorescein staining test to check for corneal ulcers, ophthalmic exam and intraocular pressure to determine if glaucoma is present.

Diagnostic results: Schirmer tear test: (Normal value is 15 to 20 mm/min) Right eye = 8 mm/min and left eye 15 mm/min.

Fluorescein staining: Right and left eye do not show adherence of stain on the corneal; revealing no corneal ulcers. Passage of fluorescein from the eyes to the external nares is patent. Intraocular pressure: within normal limits.

Diagnosis: Keratoconjunctivitis sicca (KCS) also known as "Dry eye".

Treatment is aimed at restoring tear production and controlling secondary infections. The veterinary techni-

cian cleaned both eyes with warm water and gauze and demonstrated to the owner.

Cyclosporin (Optimmune) was prescribed to help stimulate tear production. The application of the ointment was demonstrated to the client. One quarter-inch strand is to be administered in the right eye every 12 hours. A topical ophthalmic antibiotic ointment (bacitracin-polymixin-neomycin) was prescribed to be given, in both eyes, every 6–8 hours for approximately 2 weeks to control the bacterial overgrowth. Artificial tear ointment was also prescribed to be given, at least 3–4 times daily, in the right eye, to replace tear film.

A recheck visit was scheduled for 4 weeks to re-evaluate the eye, perform another Schirmer tear test, and to evaluate the response to the treatment.

The owner was instructed to keep the eyes clean and free of dried discharge; the eyes should be cleaned multiple times throughout the day with warm water and a washcloth. Discussions about the importance of keeping the eye well lubricated is essential to prevent corneal ulcerations.

The owner was told to contact the hospital if Lulu is experiencing ocular pain or if the mucopurulent discharge persists after 1 week.

KCS causes inflammation of the cornea and surrounding tissues due to inadequate production of the aqueous portion of the tear film by the lacrimal gland. Immune-mediated causes are the most common and the patient's immune system is attacking the lacrimal glands which is affecting tear production.

Prognosis: KCS is usually life-long, chronic disease that is usually controllable but not often curable. Eyes that respond to tear stimulants have a good prognosis. Lulu was diagnosed early and no corneal ulcers or scarring was observed.

Adverse Side Effects. These may include gastrointestinal upset, neurologic disturbances, hepatotoxicity, and lethargy.

TECHNICIAN NOTES

Clients must be warned about the potential side effects of metronidazole, at higher dosages, including neurologic toxicity (Plumb, 2015).

Cyclophosphamide

Cyclophosphamide is an alkylating agent that is used as an antineoplastic agent and an immunosuppressant (see the

earlier section on antineoplastic agents). Cyclophosphamide may produce serious side effects (e.g., hemorrhagic cystitis, bone marrow suppression, and gastroenteritis).

Clinical Uses. Cyclophosphamide is primarily used in combination with other agents both as an antineoplastic (malignant lymphomas, carcinomas, and sarcomas) as an immunosuppressant (autoimmune diseases involving the skin and rheumatoid arthritis) (Plumb, 2015).

Dosage Form

- Cytoxan injection

Adverse Side Effects. These include bone marrow suppression, gastrointestinal signs, alopecia, and hemorrhagic cystitis.

Corticosteroids

Corticosteroids exert antiinflammatory and immuno-suppressive effects through their inhibitory influence on neutrophils, T lymphocytes, blood vessels (decreased permeability), and cellular messengers (e.g., prostaglandin). They are generally considered to be antiinflammatory at lower doses and immunosuppressive at higher doses. Corticosteroids are often used in combination with other immunosuppressant/antineoplastic agents.

Other Immunosuppressive Agents

- **Tacrolimus (Protopic).** This is a topical agent that may be used in the treatment of atopic dermatitis and other dermatologic conditions. It is both an antiinflammatory and an immunosuppressant.
- **Pimecrolimus (Elidel).** This is a topical agent similar to tacrolimus.
- **Oclacitinib (Apoquel).** This agent is a janus kinase inhibitor labeled for the control of pruritus in dogs older than 12 months of age.
- **Mycophenolate mofetil.** This is an immunosuppressive drug that may be used for treating immune-mediated hemolytic anemia, inflammatory bowel disease, or myasthenia gravis in dogs.

REVIEW QUESTIONS

1. Anemia in baby pigs can be treated by the administration of _____.
2. A 10-year-old cocker spaniel is brought to the veterinary clinic with polyuria/polydipsia and mild anemia. What is a potential cause of these signs, and what may be used to treat the anemia?
3. Why are hematinics not indicated for cases of acute blood loss?
4. What is the anticoagulant of choice for collecting blood for hematologic studies?
5. How can you explain the fact that clots may form in the vascular system with no external trauma to blood vessels?
6. You have accidentally cut the quick of a Rottweiler puppy's nail. What would you use to stop the bleeding, and how does this agent work?
7. A 3-month-old Chow is brought to the pet emergency clinic because it has eaten a box of rat poison. What drug would the veterinarian use to treat this condition, and by what route would it be administered?
8. An 8-year-old male Persian cat is brought to the veterinary clinic with an early onset of apparent

rear leg paralysis and tachycardia. The veterinarian determines that there is a thromboembolism occluding the vessel. What agent may be used to treat this condition?
9. Briefly describe the phases of the cell cycle.
10. List the six categories of antineoplastic drugs and give an example of each category.
11. A 12-yr old Labrador retriever has been diagnosed with melanoma, the owner has opted for the use of a BRM vaccine. What agent could be used in this case?
12. List four indications for the use of immunosuppressive agents.
13 Why should you be very careful to avoid extravasation of antineoplastic drugs?
14. List eight precautions that should be taken when antineoplastic drugs are handled.
15. _____ digests fibrin threads and other clotting products to cause clot lysis and the release of fibrin degradation products into the circulation.
16. Which anticoagulant may be used to treat DIC?
17. Why should heparin not be used as an anticoagulant when blood is collected for performance of a differential count?
18. How does EDTA work as an anticoagulant?
19. On what dosage are most antineoplastic agents based?
20. Corticosteroids have a lympholytic action, which makes them useful for treating what type of neoplasia?
21. Cardiomyopathy is a potential side effect of what antineoplastic agent?
22. Vitamin _____ is an antidote for warfarin or dicumarol toxicity.
    a. B_{12}
    b. C
    c. D
    d. K_1
23. A 60-lb dog with a mast cell tumor is being treated with a protocol that includes vincristine at a dosage of 0.5 mg/m². The concentration of the vincristine is 1 mg/mL. How many milliliters would you draw up?
24. A 10-lb cat with rodenticide toxicity needs vitamin K_1 treatment at a dosage of 5 mg/kg. The concentration of the vitamin K_1 is 10 mg/mL. How much would you draw up?
25. How many milliliters of heparin (1000 Units/mL) would you add to a 250-mL bag of saline to prepare a concentration of 5 Units/mL?

REFERENCES

Boothe, D. M. (2012). Immunomodulators or biologic response modifiers. In D. M. Boothe (Ed.), *Small animal clinical pharmacology and therapeutics*. Philadelphia: WB Saunders.

Crow, S. E., & Walshaw, S. O. (1987). Placement and care of intravenous catheters. In S. E. Crow, & S. O. Walshaw (Eds.), *Manual of clinical procedures in the dog and cat*. Philadelphia: JB Lippincott.

Ettinger, S. J., Feldman, E. C., & Cote, E. (2017). *Textbook of veterinary internal medicine expert consult* (8th ed.). St. Louis: Elsevier.

Ganong, W. F. (2003). Endocrine function of the kidneys, heart, and pineal gland. In W. F. Ganong (Ed.), *Review of medical physiology* (21st ed.). New York: McGraw-Hill.

Grant, C. K., & Shelton, G. H. (1989). Biological response modifiers. In R. W. Kirk & J. D. Bonagura (Eds.), *Current veterinary therapy X: Small animal practice*. Philadelphia: WB Saunders.

Kruth, S. A. (1998). Biologic response modifiers: Interferons, interleukins, recombinant products, liposomal products. In D. M. Boothe (Ed.), *The veterinary clinics of North America, small animal practice*. Philadelphia: WB Saunders.

Khan, A. K. (2019). *Merck veterinary manual*. Kenilworth, NJ: Merck & Co., Inc. (Accessed online: October, 2019).

Norsworthy, G. D. (1992). Clinical aspects of feline blood transfusions. *Compendium on Continuing Education for the Practising Veterinarian, 14*, 470.

Papich, M. G. (2016). *Handbook of veterinary drugs* (4th ed.). Philadelphia: WB Saunders.

Plumb, D. C. (2015). *Veterinary drug handbook* (8th ed.). Ames, IA: Wiley-Blackwell.

Pugh, D. M. (1991). Blood formation, coagulation, and volume. In G. C. Brander, D. M. Pugh, R. J. Bywater, et al. (Eds.), *Veterinary applied pharmacology and therapeutics* (5th ed.). London: Bailliere Tindall.

Withrow, S. J., & Vail, D. M. (Eds.), (2007). *Small animal oncology* (4th ed.). St. Louis: Saunders Elsevier.Molenisqui

17

Immunologic Drugs

OBJECTIVES

After studying this chapter, you should be able to

1. Explain the principles associated with vaccination and describe the recommended locations for various feline vaccinations.
2. Describe the differences between infectious and noninfectious vaccines.
3. Discuss the advantages and disadvantages of the many different types of vaccines.
4. Discuss the storage, handling, and reconstitution of vaccines.
5. Describe the different routes of administration of vaccines.
6. Discuss vaccine failure and adverse vaccination responses that may occur.
7. List core and noncore vaccines used in various species, as well as common diseases that have available vaccines.
8. List and discuss drugs used in immunotherapy.

OUTLINE

KEY TERMS

Active immunity
Adjuvant
Anaphylaxis
Antibody
Antigen
Avirulent

Bacterin
Core vaccines
Monovalent
Noncore vaccines
Passive immunity
Polyvalent

PRINCIPLES OF VACCINATION

Keeping animals healthy through the proper use of immunization programs is an important aspect of veterinary medicine. Vaccine protocols (guidelines) recommended by the American Animal Hospital Association (AAHA), American Veterinary Medical Association (AVMA), American Association of Feline Practitioners (AAFP), and American Association of Equine Practitioners (AAEP) should be observed annually. Vaccination guidelines are a source of evidence-based recommendations and expert opinion provided by the AAHA Canine Vaccination Guidelines Task Force (AAHA, 2017) and AAFP feline vaccination guidelines. Veterinary technicians must have knowledge concerning vaccine types and the diseases against which animals are vaccinated. Clients ask many questions regarding this area of their pet's care. As animals enter into their geriatric years, regular laboratory profiles should be done to determine the health of major organ systems. Preventive health care guidelines include a complete history, comprehensive physical examination, assessment, diagnostic plan, therapeutic plan, prevention plan, and a follow-up plan on the animal (JAAHA, 2011). Therefore, immunization programs are only one aspect of the overall health care that should be afforded companion animals. Livestock should be properly immunized to achieve a healthy herd.

Vaccinations are an important part of the preventive health care program for companion animals and food animals alike. Vaccines are given to lessen the chance of a particular disease occurring. A patient's response is determined by (1) health and age, (2) the type of vaccine given, (3) the route of administration, (4) concurrent incubation of infectious disease, (5) exposure to an infectious disease before complete immunity is reached, and (6) drug therapy. The ideal vaccine is safe and effective on challenge and has no undesirable side effects. Immunology is a very complex field of study. This chapter outlines only the basics of common vaccines and immunostimulants. Referencing an immunology textbook may be helpful if further information is desired.

In properly vaccinated females, antibodies are passed to their offspring in the form of maternal antibodies found in colostrum; the colostrum must be ingested within the first

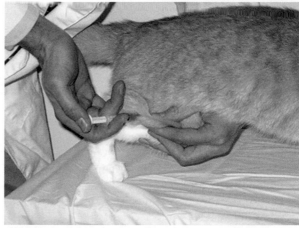

Fig. 17.1 Subcutaneous injection in a cat in the right hind leg, distal to the stifle. (From Bassert, J. M. [2018]. *McCurnin's clinical textbook for veterinary technicians* [9th ed.]. St. Louis: Elsevier.)

24 hours of life. This type of **passive immunity** protects the newborn against disease. It is important not to vaccinate very young animals when maternal antibodies are still present. The neonate's immune system is not capable of producing an active immune response when maternal antibodies are blocking this mechanism. Maternal antibodies will start to wane around 8 weeks of age (8–12 weeks of age); this is the reason we begin vaccinating animals around 8 weeks of age. Repeated boosters are needed due to maternal antibody interference; they are given until maternal antibodies decrease to allow for active immunity, usually at 16–20 weeks of age. (See the tables within this chapter for specific times that various species should be vaccinated.)

It is becoming increasingly important that each vaccine be given at a certain place on a cat's body because of the risk of vaccine-associated sarcomas when inactivated feline vaccines are administered. Although the prevalence of sarcomas after vaccination has been reported at less than one case per 10,000 vaccines administered (AVMA, 2018). The National Vaccine-Associated Sarcoma Task Force studying vaccine site tumors recommends that no vaccine be given in the intrascapular space. Rabies vaccine should be administered in the distal right rear leg (Fig. 17.1), feline leukemia virus (FeLV) vaccine should be administered in the distal left rear leg, and all other vaccines should be administered

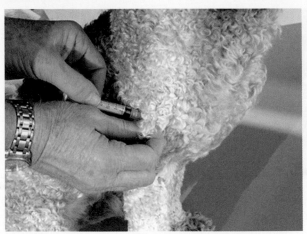

Fig. 17.2 Subcutaneous injection in a dog in the right front limb. (From Bassert, J. M. [2018]. *McCurnin's clinical textbook for veterinary technicians* [9th ed.]. St. Louis: Elsevier.)

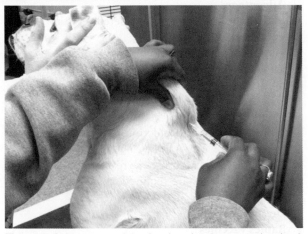

Fig. 17.3 Subcutaneous injection, in a dog, between the shoulder blades. (From Sirois, M. [2011]. *Principles and practice of veterinary technology* [3rd ed.]. St. Louis: Elsevier.)

in the right shoulder area (right front leg, lateral side). It is also recommended that any vaccine lump present 3 months after the time of vaccination be removed, after a biopsy has been performed to reveal the extent of surgery that may have to be performed. The control rate is better for lesions located on the rear limbs because wide surgical margins can be obtained with limb amputation (Morrison & Starr, 2001). Some veterinarians follow the same vaccine site administration for dogs (Fig. 17.2) as is observed in cats. Some veterinarians will administer vaccines subcutaneous between the shoulder blades (Fig. 17.3).

In cattle, the location of vaccine administration is also important. With the advent of the Meat Quality Assurance Program, proper administration of injections and

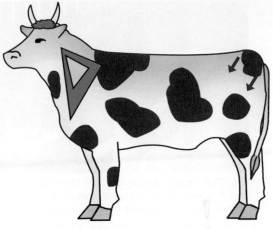

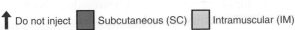
↑ Do not inject ▮ Subcutaneous (SC) ▯ Intramuscular (IM)

Fig. 17.4 All injections in food animals should be given intramuscularly or subcutaneously in the neck region, as outlined in this figure. (From McCurnin, D. M., & Bassert, J. M. [2002]. *Clinical textbook for veterinary technicians* [6th ed.]. St. Louis: WB Saunders.)

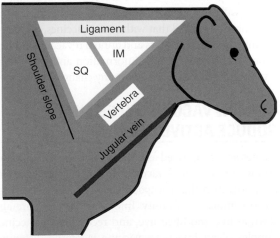

Fig. 17.5 Proper location for intramuscular *(IM)* and subcutaneous *(SQ)* injections in a cow. (Courtesy Dr. Dee Griffin.)

vaccines is critical in all food animal species. All intramuscular and subcutaneous injections in cattle should be given in the neck, if possible. Administration of most vaccines requires observation of a slaughter withdrawal, sometimes up to 60 days postvaccine (Figs. 17.4 and 17.5).

In horses, most vaccines are administered via the subcutaneous and intramuscular route and are administered in the lateral cervical neck or the semitendinosus (Figs. 17.6 and 17.7). In sheep and goats, vaccines are administered in the lateral cervical neck (Fig. 17.8).

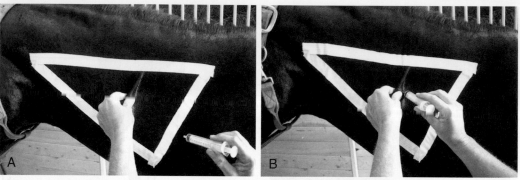

Fig. 17.6 Lateral cervical injection technique in a horse. (A) Pinching the skin before intramuscular injection into the neck. (B) Inserting the needle caudal to the skin pinch. (From Holtgrew-Bohling, K. [2020]. *Large animal clinical procedures for veterinary technicians* [4th ed]. St. Louis: Elsevier.)

The future of vaccination involves development of protocols that individualize vaccine schedules instead of having every animal vaccinated for every disease. Much discussion is ongoing in the veterinary community regarding vaccination of dogs and cats every 3 years rather than yearly. However, some state and county regulations may still mandate the yearly rabies vaccine regimen, and other states may legislate every 3 years. It is hoped that additional research will yield optimal revaccination intervals. Some studies have suggested that with some vaccines, protective immunity may last for years and annual revaccination may not be necessary. With new information and technology, the twenty-first century will see many changes in vaccines.

COMMON VACCINE TYPES THAT PRODUCE ACTIVE IMMUNITY

Vaccines are categorized as either "infectious" or "noninfectious." An infectious vaccine contains a live, but attenuated, organism that is capable of replicating within the host to stimulate immunity. Infectious vaccines are also known as live, modified live, and recombinant vaccines. Examples of an infectious vaccine is canine distemper virus (modified-live) and recombinant canine distemper virus. A noninfectious vaccine contains a whole organism that is killed and not capable of replicating within the host, therefore cannot produce an adequate immune response. In order for the animal to produce an adequate immune response, adjuvants are incorporated into the vaccine. Examples of noninfectious vaccines are rabies, leptospirosis, and *Borrelia burgdorferi* (Lyme).

℞ Inactivated (Killed)

Manufacture of inactivated vaccines involves killing the organisms with heat or chemicals that leave the antigens mostly unchanged. The antigens stimulate protective immunity. Inactivated vaccines are also referred to as *killed* vaccines.

Advantages
- Inactivated vaccines are considered very safe.
- They are stable in storage.
- There is no chance of reversion to virulence.
- Can be used in pregnant or debilitated animals with minimal risk.

Disadvantages
- Inactivated vaccines require repeated doses to achieve adequate protection (shorter duration of immunity).
- Adjuvants may cause adverse reactions.
- If repeated doses are required, costs may be higher for the client.

Dosage Forms
- **Rabies vaccines**
- **Some feline leukemia vaccines**
- **Feline panleukopenia (FPV), rhinotracheitis (herpesvirus), calicivirus vaccines**
- **Feline immunodeficiency virus (FIV) vaccine**
- **Some *B. burgdorferi* (Lyme disease) vaccines**
- ***Bordetella bronchiseptica* vaccines given parenterally**
- **Canine influenza vaccines**

See the vaccine charts within this chapter for a more comprehensive listing of the various vaccine types associated with each disease.

℞ Live

A live vaccine is prepared from live microorganisms or viruses. These organisms may be fully **virulent** (able to cause disease) or avirulent. Few vaccines of this origin are in use, with the exception of several poultry vaccines.

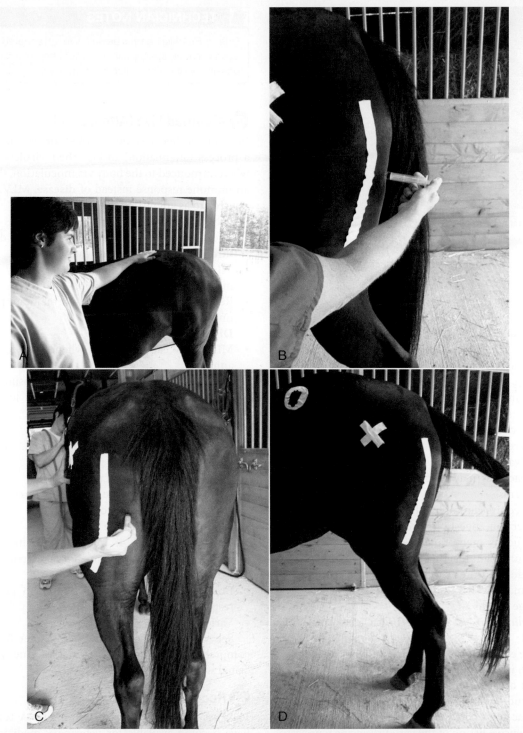

Fig. 17.7 Semitendinosus injection technique in a horse. (A) Location of the most prominent area of the buttocks. (B) Insertion of the needle from cranial to caudal into the semitendinosus muscle. (C) Proper technique for intramuscular semitendinosus injection. (D) Location of the sciatic groove. (From Holtgrew-Bohling, K. [2020]. *Large animal clinical procedures for veterinary technicians* [4th ed.]. St. Louis: Elsevier.)

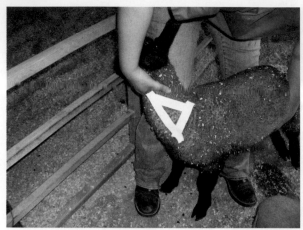

Fig. 17.8 Location of the lateral cervical muscle for intramuscular injections in a sheep and goat. (From Holtgrew-Bohling, K. [2020]. *Large animal clinical procedures for veterinary technicians* [4th ed.]. St. Louis: Elsevier.)

Advantages
- Live vaccines necessitate fewer doses to achieve an immune response.
- Provide longer immunity.
- Adjuvants are unnecessary, but the vaccine may contain preservatives.
- Live vaccines pose less risk of allergic response.
- They are inexpensive.

Disadvantages
- Live vaccines may be contaminated with unwanted organisms.
- They require careful handling. For example, accidental injection, ingestion, or exposure through a cut or the mucous membranes of brucellosis vaccine can cause undulant fever in humans.
- They do not store as well as inactivated vaccines.
- They may possess residual virulence.

Dosage Forms
- *Brucella abortus* **vaccine:** brucella abortus strain RB-51
- **Ovine ecthyma vaccine:** ovine ecthyma virus or sore mouth infection
- **Chick ark bronc:** infectious bronchitis (Massachusetts and Arkansas types)

See vaccine charts within this chapter for a more comprehensive listing of the various vaccine types associated with each disease.

 TECHNICIAN NOTES

Due to *Brucella abortus* being a live, attenuated vaccine used in cattle, special handling must be used due to the possibility of causing disease in humans.

® Modified Live (Attenuated)

In modified live vaccines (MLVs), organisms undergo a process (attenuation) to lose their virulence so that when introduced to the body via inoculation, they cause an immune response instead of disease. MLVs are also referred to as attenuated vaccines.

Advantages
- Effective vaccines for many viruses can be developed through attenuation of the causative virus.
- MLVs stimulate both humoral immunity and cell-mediated immunity.
- Require fewer repeated doses to maintain protective immunity.

Disadvantages
- MLVs may cause abortion when given to pregnant animals.
- Some vaccines can cause mild immunosuppression.
- Residual virulence can cause a mild form of the disease.

Dosage Forms
- **Feline rhinotracheitis (herpesvirus), calicivirus, and panleukopenia**
- **Most canine distemper vaccines**
- **Canine adenovirus type 2 vaccines, parvovirus vaccines, parainfluenza vaccines**
- **Canine measles vaccine**
- **Bovi-Shield Gold 4:** infectious bovine rhinotracheitis (IBR) virus, bovine virus diarrhea (BVD), parainfluenza 3 (PI3) virus
- **Bovi-Shield Gold 5:** IBR, BVD, PI3 and bovine respiratory syncytial virus (BRSV)
- Various others

See vaccine charts within this chapter for a more comprehensive listing of the various vaccine types associated with each disease.

® Recombinant

Vaccines produced by **recombinant DNA technology** have become available for veterinary medicine. These vaccines are recognized as being safe, highly specific, potent, pure, and efficacious. These attributes may be the reason why recombinant vaccines are more desirable than any other vaccine type. Recombinant vaccines are divided into three categories:

Type I recombinant (subunit) vaccines—These vaccines are derived by inserting a foreign gene from a specific pathogen into a recombinant organism (e.g., yeast, bacterium, a virus). The recombinant organism multiplies, and the product of the gene is extracted, purified, and prepared for administration as a vaccine.

Type II recombinant (gene-deleted) vaccines—The manufacturing of these vaccines involves deletion of specific genes from a pathogenic organism. This manipulation produces a vaccine that has a low risk of producing disease but can still stimulate a protective immune response.

Type III recombinant (virus-vectored) vaccines—These vaccines are derived from the insertion of specific pathogenic genetic material into a nonpathogenic or gene-deleted organism (e.g., poxvirus, canarypox). This altered organism then is propagated in vitro and is used to manufacture the vaccine (Van Kampen, 1998).

Advantages
- These vaccines produce fewer adverse effects.
- They provide effective immunity.
- Type I and type III vaccines cannot revert to virulence because of the way they are manufactured.
- Some of these vaccines can also be administered orally.

Disadvantages
- New technology often brings with it a higher cost.

Dosage Forms
- **Lyme:** *B. burgdorferi*, recombinant subunit OspA and polyvalent OspC; recombinant subunit plasmid-expressed OspA
- **Canine distemper;** recombinant canarypox virus-vectored
- **Feline rabies;** recombinant canarypox virus-vectored
- **Feline leukemia;** recombinant canarypox virus-vectored
- **Type III: Raboral V-RG:** oral vaccine for rabies virus (used in baiting devices for wildlife)
- **Type III: Newcastle disease–fowl pox vaccine (recombinant):** Newcastle disease and fowl pox
- **Type III: Trovac-AIV H5:** avian influenza subtype H5 and fowl pox

See vaccine charts within this chapter for a more comprehensive listing of the various vaccine types associated with each disease.

℞ Toxoid

A toxoid is a vaccine that is used to produce an active immune response against a toxin (proteins) rather than a bacterium or a virus. The toxin is treated with heat or chemicals to destroy its damaging properties without eliminating its ability to stimulate antibody production.

Characteristics
- Toxoids provide active immunity.
- Toxoids may require repeated doses to achieve adequate protection, depending on individual patient risk factors.
- Toxoids may contain adjuvants such as aluminium hydroxide.
- Many toxoids contain preservatives such as phenol, thimerosal, and formaldehyde solution.

Dosage Forms
- **Tetanus Toxoid:** *Clostridium tetani*
- **Tetnogen:** *C. tetani*
- **Fermicon CD/T:** *Clostridium perfringens* types C and D, and *C. tetani*
- *Crotalus atrox* toxoid (Western Diamond rattlesnake) vaccine

COMMON VACCINE TYPES THAT PRODUCE PASSIVE IMMUNITY

℞ Antitoxin

An antitoxin is a specific antiserum aimed at a toxin that contains a concentration of antibodies extracted from the blood serum or plasma of a hyperimmunized, healthy animal (usually a horse). For example, tetanus antitoxin is given to animals when there is a risk of developing tetanus secondary to a deep wound.

Characteristics
- An antitoxin neutralizes toxins produced by microorganisms.
- It may contain preservatives such as thimerosal, phenol, or oxytetracycline that may cause adverse reactions.
- Antitoxins produce immediate passive immunity.
- Immunity is short lived (about 7 to 14 days).
- Biologic products of equine origin may be associated with the development of equine serum hepatitis (Theiler's disease). This link has not been proven, but clients should be made aware of the possible risk before these products are administered.

Dosage Forms
- **Clostratox BCD:** *C. perfringens* types C and D
- **Tetanus Antitoxin:** *C. tetani*

Ⓡ Antiserum

An antiserum is a serum that contains specific antibodies extracted from a hyperimmunized animal (usually a horse) or an animal that has been infected with microorganisms that contain antigen.

Characteristics

- An antiserum kills living, infectious antigens.
- It may contain preservatives such as phenol, thimerosal, or oxytetracycline that may cause adverse reactions.
- An antiserum produces immediate passive immunity.
- Immunity is short lived.
- Do not vaccinate within 21 days after antiserum is given. For example, if a calf is treated with a *Corynebacterium–Escherichia coli–Pasteurella–Salmonella* antiserum, then that calf should not be vaccinated with BVD, IBR, PI3, *Haemophilus somnus,* or *Pasteurella haemolytica* within 21 days of receiving the antiserum.

Dosage Forms

- *Erysipelothrix rhusiopathiae* Serum Antibodies: *E. rhusiopathiae*
- *Escherichia-Colicin-B*: *E. coli*
- Septi-Serum: *Salmonella typhimurium*

OTHER TYPES OF VACCINES

Ⓡ Autogenous Vaccine

An autogenous vaccine contains organisms isolated from an infected animal on a farm where a disease outbreak is occurring. This carefully prepared vaccine contains antigens needed for protection at that particular location.

Dosage Forms

- *Streptococcus equi* used for outbreaks of strangles

Ⓡ Mixed Vaccine

A mixed vaccine contains a mixture of different antigens. It is also referred to as a polyvalent vaccine when two or more strains/serotypes of the same antigen are used in a vaccine. Each component of a mixed vaccine is required to achieve an immune response comparable with that of a vaccine containing a single strain of a single antigen (monovalent vaccine).

VACCINE STORAGE, HANDLING, AND RECONSTITUTION

Proper storage and handling of vaccines is vital to their efficacy and safety. All vaccines must be stored according to the manufacturer's product instructions or package inserts.

Most, if not all, vaccines require refrigeration. When vaccines are shipped from the manufacturer, cold packs are put in a styrofoam box to provide refrigeration during shipment. Once a shipment is received, it should be quickly unpacked and placed under refrigeration. Vaccines should never be frozen because cells may rupture when the vaccine thaws, leading to loss of potency. Vaccines should be stored in their original packaging to protect them from sunlight, maintain optimal temperature stability, and manage inventory. Organize vaccines, in the refrigerator, according to their expiration dates, with the earliest expiration dates in front of those with later expiration dates. Many vaccines are sold as a lyophilized (freeze-dried) powder in which a sterile diluent must be added; this will be provided by the manufacturer. It is important to use the sterile diluent that was provided by the manufacturer as diluents vary in volume and have a balanced pH. Diluents are not interchangeable unless specified by the manufacturer. Always double check that you are using the correct vaccine and check the expiration dates of both the vaccine and the diluent prior to reconstitution. Once the vaccine is reconstituted, it should be administered within one hour. Vaccines should only be drawn up at the time of administration.

📋 **TECHNICIAN NOTES**

- All vaccines must be stored according to the manufacturer's product instructions or package inserts, which requires refrigeration.
- Protect vaccines from temperature extremes.
- Diluents are not interchangeable unless specified by the manufacturer; it is important to use the diluent that was provided by the manufacturer.
- Once the vaccine is reconstituted, it should be administered within 1 hour.

Clients purchasing vaccines should be provided with a cold pack if needed and should be warned against leaving such biologics in vehicles or in sunlight, where they may become warm and inactivated.

ADMINISTRATION OF VACCINES

The intramuscular and subcutaneous routes are the most common methods for vaccine administration. These routes are easily accessible and provide systemic immunity, which is important in many diseases. Some diseases also respond well to local immunity. Some vaccines may be administered intranasally such as feline herpes virus-1 (FHV-1), feline calicivirus (FCV), FPV, canine adenovirus type 2, canine parainfluenza, and *B. bronchiseptica*. After administration of these vaccines, the animal may experience occasional sneezing.

All of the previously mentioned routes of vaccine administration necessitate that each animal be handled individually (section on principles of vaccination). When a large number of animals require vaccination, these routes may not be feasible. Some vaccines may be mixed with drinking water or feed. Others can be aerosolized and inhaled by the animal. For example, on mink ranches, vaccine for canine distemper and mink enteritis may be administered in this manner, or poultry houses may vaccinate for Newcastle disease by aerosolization. The margin for incomplete vaccination is greater when aerosolization or mixing with feed or water is used. Some animals may not drink or eat enough to acquire adequate protection, or the aerosolized vaccine may not distribute equally throughout the room. Vaccine failure may be implicated if these animals contract the disease, whereas in reality, the animal did not receive enough vaccine to gain adequate immunity.

When administering vaccinations, it is very important to carefully read the package insert provided, by the manufacturer, with the vaccine. Vaccines should be given only by the route provided by the manufacturer. Some vaccines are administered as an intranasal vaccine providing local immunity and some vaccines are administered intramuscularly or subcutaneously. For example, some rabies vaccines require administration by an intramuscular route to be most effective. Subcutaneous injections should be given according to the manufacturer's instructions.

As stated previously, if a vaccine requires reconstitution, this should be done with the diluent provided by the manufacturer. The vaccine should not be reconstituted until just before it is administered (see Chapter 2 for the proper reconstitution procedure). The full recommended dose should be given. Splitting a vaccine dose may result in an animal's failure to develop an adequate immune response and may lower its protection.

Mixing different vaccines to minimize the number of injections the animal receives is not recommended. This procedure can cause antigen blocking, resulting in one component interfering with the action of another; in this case, the animal does not receive adequate antigen to attain an effective immune response. Mixing of different vaccines may cause an increased chance of an allergic response. When different types of vaccines are administered, each vaccine should be administered at a separate site. It is also advisable to note the locations of administration and vaccine lot numbers on the patient's medical record. If an adverse reaction or a problem develops it should be reported to the manufacturer of the vaccine as well as the USDA Center for Veterinary Biologics.

When food animals are vaccinated, several factors must be considered. Almost all vaccine labels contain information advising not to vaccinate within 21 days of slaughter. Vaccines such as those for *B. abortus* are subject to federal limitations and regulations, and complete records are maintained on administration of these vaccines. Brucellosis vaccines are restricted to use by or under the direction of a licensed veterinarian. Carcass destruction is also a factor that involves food animal producers. Injection site lesions may cause damage to muscle tissue, requiring that area to be trimmed and discarded. If a vaccine may be administered intramuscularly or subcutaneously, the subcutaneous route would produce less tissue reaction and would eliminate muscle damage. This is important when one is dealing with animals used for meat consumption. Most vaccines on the market today can be given subcutaneously.

VACCINE FAILURE

Inappropriate care of vaccines may lead to inactivation of the vaccine and may be perceived as a vaccine failure. Actual vaccine failure is relatively uncommon. If vaccines are purchased from a reputable manufacturer, one can be fairly sure that the vaccine provided will be effective. Failure usually occurs because of improper handling, storage, or administration.

Live vaccines are especially affected by concurrent antibiotic therapy. Live and MLVs can be inactivated by the use of excessive alcohol or other disinfectants to swab the skin before injection. As was mentioned earlier, the route of administration may affect the ability of an animal to achieve an adequate immune response. Immunosuppressed, parasitized, stressed, or malnourished animals and those incubating disease are not able to mount an adequate immune response to prevent disease. Clients should always be advised that such problems can occur. In most cases, an adequate immune response is not achieved before 10 to 14 days. An 8-week-old puppy may not develop a strong immune response to protect against an infectious disease if challenged by maternal antibodies because it is not feasible to check immune titers to determine the presence of maternal antibodies. So, in order for young animals to be protected and mount an immune response, they must receive vaccinations/boosters at certain intervals. Tables 17.1 through 17.7

TABLE 17.1   Recommended Canine Vaccination Protocols.*

Vaccine Type	Initial Vaccination (Dogs ≤16 Weeks of Age)	Initial Vaccination (Dogs >16 Weeks of Age)	Booster Interval Following Last Dose of Initial Vaccination	Subsequent Revaccination	Comments
*Canine Distemper Virus MLV or recombinant (Injection)	1 dose every 2–4 weeks when ≥6 weeks until at least 16 weeks of age Dogs ~16 weeks of age at initial vaccination should receive second booster 2–4 weeks later	1 dose	1 year later	≥ Every 3 years	Combination vaccine including MLV or recombinant Canine Distemper Virus: + MLV Parvovirus + MLV Adenovirus-2 ± MLV Parainfluenza virus **Dogs residing in a HIGH-RISK environment may benefit from receiving a final dose at 18–20 weeks of age.**
*Canine Adenovirus Type 2 (CAV-2) MLV (Injection)	1 dose every 2–4 weeks when ≥6 weeks until at least 16 weeks of age	1 dose	1 year later	≥ Every 3 years	See above: Canine Distemper Virus comment
Canine Adenovirus Type 2 (CAV-2) MLV (Intranasal)	1 dose when ≥3–4 weeks of age	1 dose	1 year later	Every year	Available only as a combination vaccine. The intranasal CAV-2 vaccine is not intended for use in the prevention of canine infectious hepatitis.
*Rabies 1-year killed virus (Injection)	1 dose when ≥12 weeks of age	1 dose	1 year later	Every year	State/local/provincial law applies. For state-specific information on rabies immunization and law, visit aaha.org/CanineVaccineResources
*Rabies 3-year killed virus (Injection)	1 dose when ≥12 weeks of age	1 dose	1 year later	Every 3 years	State/local/provincial law applies. For state-specific information on rabies immunization and law, visit aaha.org/CanineVaccineResources

Vaccine	Initial Vaccination	Dose(s)	Booster	Revaccination	Comments
*Canine Parvovirus MLV (Injection)	1 dose every 2–4 weeks when ≥6 weeks until at least 16 weeks of age	1 dose	1 year later for (≤16 weeks) protocol ≥3 year later for (>16 week) protocol	≥ Every 3 years	See above: Canine Distemper Virus comment
*Canine Parainfluenza Virus MLV (Injection)	1 dose every 2–4 weeks when ≥6 weeks until at least 16 weeks of age	1 dose	1 year later for (≤16 week) protocol ≥3 year later for (>16 week) protocol	≥ Every 3 years	See above: Canine Distemper Virus comment
Canine Parainfluenza Virus MLV (Intranasal)	1 dose when ≥3–4 weeks of age	1 dose	1 year later	Every year	Available in combination with canine *Bordetella bronchiseptica* and/or Canine adenovirus-2. Parenterally administered canine parainfluenza vaccine (CPiV) may not provide a level of protection that is comparable to CPiV vaccine administered by the intranasal route. The duration of immunity for the intranasal CPiV vaccine component is expected to exceed 1 year.
Measles Virus MLV (Injection Intramuscular only)	1 dose when >6 weeks and <12 weeks of age	Not recommended	Not recommended	Not recommended	Do not booster Must be administered intramuscular ONLY
Leptospira interrogans 4-serovar Killed vaccine (Injection)	**2 doses** 2–4 weeks apart when ≥8–9 weeks of age	**2 doses** 2–4 weeks apart regardless of age	1 year later	Every year	Leptospirosis vaccine is available in combination with core vaccines, and as a four-way Leptospirosis only product that is not combined with other vaccines
Leptospira interrogans 2-serovar Killed vaccine (Injection)					The 2-serovar vaccine is not recommended by AAHA

Continued

TABLE 17.1   Recommended Canine Vaccination Protocols.—cont'd

Vaccine Type	Initial Vaccination (Dogs ≤16 Weeks of Age)	Initial Vaccination (Dogs >16 Weeks of Age)	Booster Interval Following Last Dose of Initial Vaccination	Subsequent Revaccination	Comments
Bordetella bronchiseptica Only Monovalent (Injection)	**2 doses** 2–4 weeks apart starting at 8 weeks of age	**2 doses** 2–4 weeks apart regardless of age	1 year following last dose administered	Every year	Available in combination with canine Parainfluenza virus and/or Canine adenovirus-2.
B. bronchiseptica Avirulent Live bacteria (Intraoral – buccal pouch)	1 dose into buccal pouch ≥8 weeks of age	1 dose into buccal pouch	1 year later	Every year	Onset of protective immunity has been shown to be as early as 48–72 hours following a single inoculation.
B. bronchiseptica Avirulent Live bacteria (Intranasal)	1 dose when ≥3–4 weeks of age in puppies at risk of exposure to infected dogs Generally administered between 8–16 weeks of age if at risk of exposure	1 dose if at risk of exposure	1 year later if at risk of exposure	Every year if at risk of exposure	The duration of immunity, based on challenge studies (B. bronchiseptica), is 12–14 months following a single dose of intranasal vaccine.
Borrelia burgdorferi 4 vaccine types: Killed or recombinant subunit OspA, Killed or chimeric-recombinant OspA+C. (Injection)	**2 doses** 2–4 weeks apart when ≥8 or 9 weeks of age (as labeled)	**2 doses** 2–4 weeks apart regardless of age	1 year later	Every year	Dogs traveling into Lyme-disease–endemic areas from nonendemic areas may be at increased risk for exposure and infection. Vaccination may be indicated: administer 2 doses of vaccine, 2–4 weeks apart, so that the last dose is administered approximately 2 to 4 weeks prior to travel.

Canine Influenza H3N8 Killed virus **(Injection)**	**2 doses** 2–4 weeks apart when ≥6–8 weeks of age (see package insert)	**2 doses** 2–4 weeks apart	1 year later	Every year	When vaccination is recommended, dogs intended to be housed in boarding kennels or day-care facilities should BEGIN the initial vaccination series 4 weeks prior to entry (2 weeks between the initial vaccines plus 2 weeks to allow time for a humoral immune response to develop). Dogs at risk of exposure should be vaccinated against both H3N2 and H3N8 strains.
Canine Influenza H3N2 Killed virus **(Injection)**	**2 doses** 2–4 weeks apart when ≥6–8 weeks of age (see package insert)	**2 doses** 2–4 weeks apart	1 year later	Every year	When vaccination is recommended, dogs intended to be housed in boarding kennels or day-care facilities should BEGIN the initial vaccination series 4 weeks prior to entry (2 weeks between the initial vaccines plus 2 weeks to allow time for a humoral immune response to develop). Dogs at risk of exposure should be vaccinated against both H3N2 and H3N8 strains

*Core vaccine.

**Based on recommendations made in the 2017 American Animal Hospital Association Canine Vaccination Guidelines (updated 2018). https://www.aaha.org/aaha-guidelines/vaccination-canine-configuration/vaccination-recommendations-for-general-practice/. Accessed October, 2019.

Note: Canine coronavirus (CCV) vaccination is not recommended on the grounds that infection: (1) causes mild or subclinical disease, (2) generally occurs in dogs 6 weeks of age and younger, and (3) is typically self-limiting.

Note: Administration of multiple doses of parenteral vaccine at the same appointment, particularly among small breed dogs (≤10 kg), may increase the risk of an acute-onset adverse reaction. Alternative vaccination schedules may be indicated, e.g., delaying administration of a noncore vaccine by 2 weeks following administration of core vaccines.

For recommendations on managing dogs who are overdue for this vaccine, visit aaha.org/CanineVaccinesOverdue.

AAHA, American Animal Hospital Association; *MLV,* modified live vaccine.

TABLE 17.2   Recommended Feline Vaccination Protocols.**

Vaccine Type	Initial Vaccination (Cats ≤16 Weeks of Age)	Initial Vaccination (Cats >16 Weeks of Age)	Booster Interval Following Last Dose of Initial Vaccination	Subsequent Revaccination	Comments
*Feline Herpesvirus-1 (FHV-1) and Feline Calicivirus (FCV) Modified live vaccines (MLV) (nonadjuvanted) (Injection)	1 dose starting at 6 weeks of age then every 3–4 weeks until 16–20 weeks of age	**2 doses** 3–4 weeks apart	1 year later	Every 3 years	
*Feline Herpesvirus-1 (FHV-1) and Feline Calicivirus (FCV) Killed (inactivated) adjuvanted (Injection)	1 dose starting at 6 weeks of age then every 3–4 weeks until 16–20 weeks of age	**2 doses** 3–4 weeks apart	1 year later	Every 3 years	
*Feline Herpesvirus-1 (FHV-1) and Feline Calicivirus (FCV) MLV (nonadjuvanted) (Intranasal)	1 dose starting at 6 weeks of age then every 3–4 weeks until 16–20 weeks of age	**2 doses** 3–4 weeks apart	1 year later	Every 3 years	A single dose of intranasal vaccine offers rapid onset of protection (2–6 days), and may be useful for animals entering a high-risk area (boarding facility or shelter).
*Feline Panleukopenia MLV (nonadjuvanted) (Injection)	1 dose starting at 6–8 weeks of age then every 3–4 weeks until 16–20 weeks of age	**2 doses** 3–4 weeks apart	1 year later	Every 3 years	
*Feline Panleukopenia Killed (inactivated) adjuvanted (Injection)	1 dose starting at 6–8 weeks of age then every 3–4 weeks until 16–20 weeks of age	**2 doses** 3–4 weeks apart	1 year later	Every 3 years	
*Feline Panleukopenia MLV (nonadjuvanted) (Intranasal)	1 dose starting at 6–8 weeks of age then every 3–4 weeks until 16–20 weeks of age	**2 doses** 3–4 weeks apart	1 year later	Every 3 years	
Feline leukemia (FeLV) Killed (inactivated) and recombinant (Injection)	Administer two doses, 3–4 weeks apart, beginning as early as 8 weeks of age	Administer two doses, 3–4 weeks apart	Administer a single dose 1 year following administration of the initial two-dose series***	Revaccination every 2 years for cats at low risk of infection and annually for cats at higher risk	AAFP advisory panel recommends administering FeLV vaccines to all kittens up to and including 1 year of age. After the 1-year booster, FeLV vaccine is considered to be noncore unless they are at risk of exposure. At-risk adult cats should continue to be vaccinated against FeLV.

*Rabies Recombinant canarypox virus-vectored vaccine Nonadjuvanted **(Injection)**	1 dose when ≥12 weeks of age	1 dose	1 year later	Every year	State/local/provincial law applies. Where rabies vaccination is required, the frequency of vaccination may differ from these recommendations based on local statutes or requirements
*Rabies 1 year Killed vaccine (Inactivated whole virus) Adjuvanted **(Injection)**	1 dose when ≥12 weeks of age	1 dose	1 year later	Every year	State/local/provincial law applies. Where rabies vaccination is required, the frequency of vaccination may differ from these recommendations based on local statutes or requirements
*Rabies 3 year Killed vaccine (Inactivated whole virus) **Adjuvanted** **(Injection)**	1 dose when ≥12 weeks of age	1 dose	1 year later	Every 3 years	State/local/provincial law applies. Where rabies vaccination is required, the frequency of vaccination may differ from these recommendations based on local statutes or requirements

* Core vaccine.

** Based on recommendations made in the 2013 AAFP (American Association of Feline Practitioners) Feline Vaccination Advisory Panel Report. https://catvets.com/guidelines/practice-guidelines/feline-vaccination-guidelines (Accessed October, 2019).

*** Results of several studies indicate that FeLV vaccine-induced immunity persists for at least 12 months following vaccination.

TABLE 17.3   Vaccinations for Adult Horses.[a]

CORE VACCINATIONS protect against diseases that are endemic to a region, are virulent/highly contagious, pose a risk of severe disease, those having potential public health significance, and/or are required by law. Core vaccines have clearly demonstrable efficacy and safety, with a high enough level of patient benefit and low enough level of risk to justify their use in all equids.

Disease	Broodmares	Other Adult Horses (>1 year of age) *previously vaccinated against the disease indicated*	Other Adult Horses (>1 year of age) *unvaccinated or lacking vaccination history*	Comments
Tetanus	*Previously vaccinated:* Annual, 4–6 weeks pre-partum *Previously unvaccinated or having unknown vaccination history:* **2-dose series:** 2nd dose 4-6 weeks after 1st dose. Revaccinate 4–6 weeks pre-partum	Annual	**2-dose series:** 2nd dose 4–6 weeks after 1st dose. Annual revaccination	Booster at time of penetrating injury or prior to surgery if last dose was administered over 6 months previously.
Eastern / Western Equine Encephalo-myelitis (EEE/ WEE)	*Previously vaccinated:* Annual, 4–6 weeks pre-partum *Previously unvaccinated or having unknown vaccination history:* **2-dose series:** 2nd dose 4 weeks after 1st dose. Revaccinate 4–6 weeks pre-partum.	Annual – spring, prior to onset of vector season.	**2-dose series:** 2nd dose 4–6 weeks after 1st dose. Revaccinate prior to the onset of the next vector season.	Consider 6-month revaccination interval for: In high risk situations such as an early onset of seasonal disease Increase incidence in a geographic area Foals of unvaccinated mares Practitioner in consultation with manufacturer, may consider starting earlier vaccination or using a product more frequently.
West Nile Virus (WNV)	*Previously vaccinated:* Annual, 4–6 weeks pre-partum *Unvaccinated or lacking vaccination history:* It is preferable to vaccinate naïve mares when open. In areas of high risk, initiate primary series as described for unvaccinated, adult horses.	Annual – spring, prior to onset of vector season	**3-dose series:** 1st dose at 4–6 months of age 2nd dose 4–6 weeks after the 1st dose 3rd dose at 10–12 months of age Annual Revaccination	

	Broodmares	Adults	Foals	Comments
Rabies	Annual, 4 - 6 weeks pre-partum OR Prior to breeding*	Annual	Single dose Annual revaccination	*Due to the relatively long duration of immunity, this vaccine may be given post-foaling but prior to breeding and thus reduce the number of vaccines given to a mare pre-partum.

RISK-BASED VACCINES are selected for use based on risk assessment[b] performed by, or in consultation with, a licensed veterinarian. Use of these vaccines may vary between individuals, populations, and/or geographic regions. Note: Vaccines are not listed in order of priority for use.

	Broodmares	Adults	Foals	Comments
Anthrax	Not recommended during gestation	Annual	**2-dose series:** 2nd dose 3–4 weeks after 1st dose. Annual revaccination.	Do not administer concurrently with antibiotics. Use caution during storage, handling and administration. Consult a physician immediately if human exposure to vaccine occurs by accidental injection, ingestion, or otherwise through the conjunctiva or broken skin.
Botulism	*Previously vaccinated:* Annual, 4–6 weeks pre-partum *Previously unvaccinated or having unknown vaccination history:* **3-dose series:** 1st dose at 8 months gestation. 2nd dose 4 weeks after 1st dose 3rd dose 4 weeks after 2nd dose	Annual	**3-dose series:** 2nd dose 4 weeks after 1st dose 3rd dose 4 weeks after 2nd dose Annual revaccination	Horses with history of natural exposure: A vaccination protocol should be initiated once antitoxin immunoglobulins are depleted.
Equine Herpesvirus (EHV)	**3-dose series** with product labeled for protection against EHV **abortion** Give at 5, 7 and 9 months of gestation **It is recommended to also booster broodmares with a product labeled for protection against respiratory disease 4-6 weeks prepartum**	Annual (see comments)	**Inactivated vaccine:** Dependent upon on manufacturer's product recommendation, the vaccine may be a two or three dose series with a 3 to 4-week interval between doses. **Annual revaccination**	Consider 6-month revaccination interval for: 1) Horses less than 5 years of age 2) Horses on breeding farms or in contact with pregnant mares 3) Performance or show horses at high risk

Continued

TABLE 17.3   Vaccinations for Adult Horses.—cont'd

Disease	Broodmares	Other Adult Horses (>1 year of age) *previously vaccinated against the disease indicated*	Other Adult Horses (>1 year of age) *unvaccinated or lacking vaccination history*	Comments
Equine Viral Arteritis (EVA)	Not recommended unless high risk. Mares in foal should not be vaccinated until after foaling and not less than 3 weeks prior to breeding. *The manufacturer does not recommend use of this vaccine in pregnant mares, especially in the last two months of pregnancy.*	Annual • **Breeding stallions previously vaccinated against EVA:** Annual booster every 12 months and not less than 3 to 4 weeks prior to breeding. • **Breeding stallions, unvaccinated or having unknown vaccine history:** All first-time vaccinated stallions should be isolated for 3 weeks following vaccination before being used for breeding. • **Teaser Stallions:** Vaccination against EVA is recommended on an annual basis. *Mares:* Vaccinate when open	**Single dose** (See comments)	**Prior to initial vaccination, intact males and any horses potentially intended for export should undergo serologic testing** and be confirmed negative for antibodies to EAV. Testing should be performed shortly prior to, or preferably at, the time of vaccination.

Influenza	***Pregnant mares, previously vaccinated against influenza:*** Inactivated vaccine: Annually with one dose administered 4–6 weeks pre-partum ***Pregnant mares, unvaccinated or having unknown vaccine history:*** Inactivated vaccine: Dependent upon on manufacturer's product recommendation, the vaccine may be a two or three dose series with a 3 to 4-week interval between doses (IM), with the last dose administered 4–6 weeks pre-partum	Horses with ongoing risk of exposure: Semi-annual Horses at low risk of exposure: Annual revaccination.	**Inactivated vaccine:** Dependent upon on manufacturer's product recommendation, the vaccine may be a two or three dose series with a 3 to 4-week interval between doses **Modified live vaccine:** Administer a single dose (IN application). Annual revaccination	Horses at increased risk of exposure may be revaccinated every 6 months. Some facilities and competitions may require vaccination within the previous 6 months to enter. **USEF Vaccination Rule** https://www.usef.org/forms-pubs/ANcxoLX-1gNs/equine-vaccination-rule-gr845
Leptospirosis	Safe for use in pregnant mares *Previously unvaccinated or having unknown vaccination history:* 2 Initial doses 3–4 weeks apart *Previously vaccinated:* Annual revaccination	Annual	2 initial doses 3–4 weeks apart Annual revaccination	Field safety testing has demonstrated this product is safe for use in pregnant mares
Potomac Horse Fever (PHF)	*Previously vaccinated:* Semi-annual, with one dose given 4–6 weeks pre-partum *Previously unvaccinated or having unknown vaccination history:* **2-dose series:** 1st dose 7–9 weeks pre-partum 2nd dose 4–6 weeks pre-partum	Semi-annual to annual	**2-dose series:** 2nd dose 3–4 weeks after 1st dose Semi-annual or annual booster	A revaccination interval of 3–4 months may be considered in endemic areas when disease risk is high.

Continued

TABLE 17.3   Vaccinations for Adult Horses.—cont'd

Disease	Broodmares	Other Adult Horses (>1 year of age) previously vaccinated against the disease indicated	Other Adult Horses (>1 year of age) unvaccinated or lacking vaccination history	Comments
Rotavirus	**3-dose series** 1st dose at 8 months gestation. 2nd and 3rd doses at 4-week intervals thereafter	Not applicable	Not applicable	
Snake Bite	Please see guidelines for additional information	Please see guidelines for additional information	Please see guidelines for additional information	
Strangles *Streptococcus equi*	*Previously vaccinated:* *Killed vaccine containing M-protein):* Semi-annual with one dose given 4–6 weeks pre-partum *Previously unvaccinated or having unknown vaccination history:* *Killed vaccine containing M- protein):* **3-dose series** 2nd dose 2–4 weeks after 1st dose 3rd dose 4–6 weeks pre-partum	Semi-annual to annual	*Killed vaccine containing M-protein:* **2-3 dose series:** 2nd dose 2–4 weeks after 1st dose 3rd dose (where recommended by manufacturer) 2–4 weeks after 2nd dose Revaccinate semi-annually *Modified live vaccine:* **2-dose series administered intranasally** 2nd dose 3 weeks after 1st dose Revaccinate semi-annually to annually	Vaccination is not recommended as a strategy in outbreak mitigation.

[a] ALL VACCINATION PROGRAMS SHOULD BE DEVELOPED IN CONSULTATION WITH A LICENSED VETERINARIAN

[b] Refer to "Principles of Vaccination" in main document for criteria used in performing risk assessment.

Vaccinations for Adult Horses were developed by the American Association of Equine Practitioners (AAEP) Infectious Disease Committee. These guidelines and charts were reviewed and updated by the committee & Vaccination Guidelines Subcommittee and approved by the Board of Directors in 2020. Please note that updates to these guidelines and charts may occur online at anytime and should always be referenced there for the most current version at www.aaep.org.

TABLE 17.4 Vaccinations for Foals.[a]

The two categories below reflect differences in the foal's susceptibility to disease and ability to mount an appropriate immune response to vaccination based on the presence (or absence) of maternal antibodies derived from colostrum. The phenomenon of maternal antibody interference is discussed in the text portion of these guidelines.

CORE VACCINATIONS protect against diseases that are endemic to a region, those with potential public health significance, required by law, virulent/highly infectious, and/or those posing a risk of severe disease. Core vaccines have clearly demonstrated efficacy and safety, and thus exhibit a high enough level of patient benefit and low enough level of risk to justify their use in all equids.

Disease	Foals and Weanlings (<12 months of age) of mares vaccinated in the prepartum period against the disease indicated	Foals and Weanlings (<12 months of age) of unvaccinated mare or lacking vaccination history	Comments
Tetanus	3-dose series: 1st dose at 4–6 months of age 2nd dose 4–6 weeks after the 1st dose 3rd dose at 10–12 months of age Annual Revaccination	3-dose series: 1st dose at 3–4 months of age 2nd dose 4–6 weeks after the 1st dose 3rd dose 10–12 months of age Annual Revaccination	
Eastern/Western Equine Encephalomyelitis (EEE/WEE)	3-dose series: 1st dose at 4–6 months of age 2nd dose 4–6 weeks after the 1st dose 3rd dose at 10–12 months of age	3-dose series: 1st dose at 4–6 months of age 2nd dose 4–6 weeks after the 1st dose 3rd dose at 10–12 months of age	*Note:* Primary vaccination series scheduling may be amended with vaccinations administered earlier to younger foals that are at increased disease risk due to the presence of vectors. *Foals in the Southeastern USA:* The primary vaccination series can be initiated with an additional dose at 2–3 months of age due to early seasonal vector presence.
West Nile Virus (WNV)	3-dose series: 1st dose at 4–6 months of age 2nd dose 4–6 weeks after the 1st dose 3rd dose at 10–12 months of age Annual revaccination	3-dose series: 1st dose at 4–6 months of age 2nd dose 4–6 weeks after the 1st dose 3rd dose at 10–12 months of age Annual Revaccination	*Note:* Primary vaccination series scheduling may be amended with vaccinations administered earlier to younger foals that are at increased disease risk due to the presence of vectors. *Foals in the Southeastern USA:* The primary vaccination series can be initiated with an additional dose at 2–3 months of age due to early seasonal vector presence.

Continued

TABLE 17.4 Vaccinations for Foals.—cont'd

Disease	Foals and Weanlings (<12 months of age) of mares vaccinated in the prepartum period against the disease indicated	Foals and Weanlings (<12 months of age) of unvaccinated mare or lacking vaccination history	Comments
Rabies	**2-dose series:** 1st dose at 6 months of age 2nd dose 4–6 weeks after 1st dose Annual revaccination	**1 dose** Annual revaccination	The recommendation for a 2-dose initial series in foals from mares vaccinated with rabies within the year prior to foaling is to address the potential for maternal antibody interference. Rabies products are efficacious for at least 12 months (depending on manufacturer) based on efficacy studies with naive foals (no maternal antibodies).

RISK-BASED VACCINATIONS are those having applications which may vary between individuals, populations, and geographic regions. Risk assessment should be performed by, or in consultation with, a licensed veterinarian to identify which vaccines are appropriate for a given horse or population of horses. The listing of a vaccine here is not a recommendation for its inclusion into a vaccination program. Vaccine scheduling is provided for use after it has been determined which, if any, risk-based vaccines are indicated. **Note:** Vaccines are not listed in order of priority for use.

Disease	Foals and Weanlings (<12 months of age) of mares vaccinated in the prepartum period against the disease indicated	Foals and Weanlings (<12 months of age) of unvaccinated mare or lacking vaccination history	Comments
Anthrax	Not applicable. As it is not recommended to vaccinate mares during pregnancy there will be no foals of mares vaccinated prepartum	No age specific guidelines are available for this vaccine. Manufacturer's recommendation is for primary series of 2 doses administered subcutaneously at a 2 to 3-week interval.	Antimicrobial drugs must **not** be given concurrently with this vaccine. Caution should be used during storage, handling and administration of this live bacterial product. Consult a physician immediately should accidental human exposure (via mucus membranes, conjunctiva or broken skin) occur.
Botulism	**3-dose series:** 1st dose 2–3 months of age 2nd dose 4 weeks after 1st dose 3rd dose 4 weeks after 2nd dose	**3-dose series:** 1st dose 1–3 months of age 2nd dose 4 weeks after 1st dose 3rd dose 4 weeks after 2nd dose	Maternal antibody does not interfere with vaccination; foals at high risk may be vaccinated as early as 2 weeks of age.
Equine Herpesvirus (EHV)	*Inactivated or modified live vaccine* **3-dose series:** 1st dose 4–6 months of age 2nd dose 4–6 weeks after 1st dose 3rd dose at 10–12 months of age Revaccinate at 6-month intervals	*Inactivated or modified live vaccine* **3-dose series:** 1st dose at 4–6 months of age 2nd dose 4–6 weeks after 1st dose 3rd dose at 10–12 months of age Revaccinate at 6-month intervals	

			Comments
Equine Viral Arteritis (EVA)	**Colt (male) foals:** Single dose at 6–12 months of age (see comments)	**Colt (male) foals:** Single dose at 6–12 months of age (see comments)	**Prior to initial vaccination, colt (male) foals should undergo serologic testing** and be confirmed negative for antibodies to EAV. Testing should be performed shortly prior to, or preferably at, the time of vaccination. As foals can carry colostral derived antibodies to EAV for up to 6 months, testing and vaccination should **not** be performed prior to 6 months of age.
Equine Influenza	*Inactivated vaccine* **2 or 3-dose series:** Dependent upon the manufacturer's product recommendation, the vaccine is an initial two or three dose series with a 3 to 4-week interval between doses (IM) starting at 4–6 months of age. *Modified live vaccine* Administer a single dose (IN) in foals 11 months of age or older Revaccinate at 6–12month intervals based on risk	*Inactivated vaccine* **2 or 3-dose series:** Dependent upon the manufacturer's product recommendation, the vaccine is an initial two or three dose series with a 3 to 4-week interval between doses (IM) starting at 4–6 months of age. *Modified live vaccine* Administer a single dose (IN) in foals 11 months of age or older Revaccinate at 6-12month intervals based on risk	An increased risk of disease may warrant vaccination of younger foals. Because some maternal anti-influenza antibody is likely to be present, a complete series of primary vaccinations should still be given after 6 months of age.
Leptospirosis	**2 dose series:** 1st dose at 6 months of age 2nd dose 3–4 weeks after 1st dose Annual revaccination	**2 dose series:** 1st dose at 6 months of age 2nd dose 3–4 weeks after 1st dose Annual revaccination	Safety has been demonstrated in foals 3 months of age. The effects of circulating maternal antibody and vaccination have not been determined.
Potomac Horse Fever (PHF)	**2-dose series:** 1st dose at 5 months of age 2nd dose 3–4 weeks after 1st dose	**2-dose series:** 1st dose at 5 months of age 2nd dose 3–4 weeks after 1st dose	If risk warrants, vaccine may be administered to younger foals. Subsequent doses are to be administered at 4-week intervals until 6 months of age.

Continued

TABLE 17.4 Vaccinations for Foals.—cont'd

Disease	Foals and Weanlings (<12 months of age) of mares vaccinated in the prepartum period against the disease indicated	Foals and Weanlings (<12 months of age) of unvaccinated mare or lacking vaccination history	Comments
Snake Bite	Please see guidelines for additional information	Please see guidelines for additional information	
Strangles *Streptococcus equi*	*Killed vaccine* **3-dose series:** **1st** dose at 4–6 months of age **2nd** dose 4–6 weeks after 1st dose **3rd** dose 4–6 weeks after 2nd dose *Modified live vaccine* **3-dose series administered intranasally:** **1st** dose at 6–9 months of age **2nd** dose 3–4 weeks after 1st dose **3rd** dose at 11–12 months of age	*Killed vaccine* **3-dose series:** **1st** dose at 4–6 months of age **2nd** dose 4–6 weeks after 1st dose **3rd** dose 4–6 weeks after 2nd dose *Modified live vaccine* **3-dose series administered intranasally:** **1st** dose at 6–9 months of age **2nd** dose 3–4 weeks after 1st dose **3rd** dose at 11–12 months of age	Vaccination is **not** recommended as a strategy in outbreak mitigation. If risk warrants, the modified live vaccine (MLV) may be safely administered to foals as young as 6 weeks of age. However, vaccine efficacy in this age group has not been adequately studied. If MLV is administered to younger foals, a 3rd dose of vaccine should then be administered 2–4 weeks prior to weaning. The risk of vaccine-associated adverse events is increased when the MLV product is administered to young foals.

[a]ALL VACCINATION PROGRAMS SHOULD BE DEVELOPED IN CONSULTATION WITH A LICENSED VETERINARIAN

Vaccinations for Foals *were developed by the American Association of Equine Practitioners (AAEP) Infectious Disease Committee. These guidelines and charts were reviewed and updated by the committee & Vaccination Guidelines Subcommittee and approved by the Board of Directors in 2020. Please note that updates to these guidelines and charts may occur online at anytime and should always be referenced there for the most current version at www.aaep.org.*

TABLE 17.5 Recommended Bovine Vaccinations.**

Disease or Vaccination	Calves	Replacements	Feedlot Cattle	Adults	Comments
*Bang vaccination (Brucellosis)	Heifer calves 3–12 months old				Depending on local and state laws
*Bovine respiratory syncytial virus	Weaned calves	Heifers and bulls	Feedlot cattle		
*Bovine virus diarrhea type 1 and 2	Calves >2 weeks old, weaned calves	Heifers and bulls		Cows and bulls	Killed bovine virus diarrhea vaccine must be used in pregnant cows and nursing calves
*Clostridial bacteria	Calves >10 days old, weaned calves	Heifers and bulls	Feedlot cattle	Cows and bulls	Known as 5-, 7-, or 8-way vaccines
*Infectious bovine rhinotracheitis	Calves >2 weeks old, weaned calves	Heifers and bulls		Cows	
*Leptospirosis		Heifers and bulls		Cows and bulls	
*Parainfluenza 3 virus	Calves >2 weeks old, weaned calves	Heifers and bulls	On arrival	Cows	
Pasteurella	Weaned calves		Feedlot cattle		
Pinkeye	Calves >30 days old		Feedlot cattle		
Salmonella	Calves >2 weeks old		Feedlot cattle		Entire dairy herd in the presence of an outbreak
Scour vaccine				Cows 30 days before calving	
Somnus		Heifers and bulls	Feedlot cattle		
Trichomonas				Cows and bulls before breeding	
Vibrio		Heifers and bulls		Cows and bulls before breeding	
Anthrax	In the presence of outbreak, by state or federal permission	In the presence of outbreak, by state or federal permission	In the presence of outbreak, by state or federal permission	In the presence of outbreak, by state or federal permission	

*Core vaccines.

**Vaccination protocols should be designed specific to producers by a licensed veterinarian.

Modified from Holtgrew-Bohling, K. J. (2020). *Large animal clinical procedures for veterinary technicians* (4th ed.). St. Louis: Elsevier.

TABLE 17.6   Recommended Vaccinations for Sheep.*

Disease or Vaccination	Ewes	Lambs	Feedlot Lambs	Rams	Comments
*Clostridium perfringens type C	4–6 weeks before parturition. If animals have never been vaccinated, twice 4 weeks apart with last dose 4–6 weeks before parturition	If born to unvaccinated ewe, at birth and booster in 4–6 weeks. Lambs from vaccinated ewes should be vaccinated at 12–16 weeks and booster given in 4–6 weeks	On entering feedlot and booster in 2–4 weeks	Annually	
*Clostridium perfringens type D	4–6 weeks before parturition. If animals have never been vaccinated, twice 4 weeks apart with last dose 4–6 weeks before parturition	If born to unvaccinated ewe, at birth and booster in 4–6 weeks. Lambs from vaccinated ewes should be vaccinated at 12–16 weeks and booster given in 4–6 weeks	On entering feedlot and booster in 2–4 weeks	Annually	
*Clostridium tetani	Can be given during pregnancy with Clostridium types C and D	At time of castration and tail docking	Annually	Annually	Often combined with Clostridium types C and D
Other clostridial diseases (black disease, black-leg, malignant edema, struck, lamb dysentery, botulism)	4–6 weeks before parturition. If animals have never been vaccinated, twice 4 weeks apart with last dose 4–6 weeks before parturition	If born to unvaccinated ewe, at birth and booster in 4–6 weeks. Lambs from vaccinated ewes should be vaccinated at 12–16 weeks and booster given in 4–6 weeks	Annually	Annually	Primarily used only in high-risk herds
Leptospirosis					Primarily used only in high-risk herds
Sore mouth	At least 2 months before parturition and booster every 5–12 months depending on risk	1–2 days of age and booster every 5–12 months depending on risk	4 weeks before risk and booster every 5–12 months depending on risk	4 weeks before risk and booster every 5–12 months depending on risk	Live virus. Vaccinated sheep can spread the disease for up to 8 weeks after vaccination. Use in infected herds only. Performed by scratching skin in area without wool (inner ear or under tail in adults and inner thigh in young animals) and then brushing on the vaccine. Sores will form at application site

Disease					Comments
Foot rot	4 weeks before lambing and booster every 4–6 months	4 weeks of age and booster in 4–8 weeks	4 weeks before wet or rainy season, booster every 4–6 months	4 weeks before wet or rainy season, booster every 4–6 months	Vaccinate behind the ear / Only reduces infection levels / Abscesses not uncommon, discoloration of the wool at the injection site / Booster in 4 weeks from first time of vaccination
Caseous lymphadenitis		Annually	Annually	Annually	Primarily used only in high-risk or infected herds / Booster in 4 weeks after the first dose
Enzootic abortion in ewes (EAE)	4 weeks before breeding / **Do not use in pregnant ewes**				Primarily used only in high-risk or infected herds
Toxoplasma	4 weeks before breeding / **Do not use in pregnant ewes** / Booster every 2 years				Primarily in only high-risk or infected herds / Vaccine not available in the United States
Vibriosis	Annually, 2 weeks before breeding / Booster in mid-pregnancy if first vaccination				Primarily used only in high-risk herds
Brucellosis			Rams test positive if vaccinated		
Rabies					Common in pet sheep and possibly in endemic areas
Escherichia coli	4–6 weeks before parturition / If animals have never been vaccinated, two doses 4 weeks apart	If ewes were unvaccinated, oral antibody can be given at birth			Primarily used only if diarrhea in 1- to 2-day-old lambs is a problem

*Core vaccines.

**Vaccination protocols should be designed specific to producers by a licensed veterinarian.

From Holtgrew-Bohling, K. J. (2020). *Large animal clinical procedures for veterinary technicians* (4th ed.). St. Louis: Elsevier.

TABLE 17.7 **Recommended Vaccinations for Goats.** **

Disease or Vaccination	Comments
Clostridium perfringens types C and D	Use as in sheep
Clostridium tetani	Use as in sheep
Escherichia coli	Use as in sheep, primarily only in high-risk herds
Foot rot	Use as in sheep
Pasteurella	Use as in sheep, primarily only in high-risk herds
Leptospirosis	Primarily used only in high-risk herds
Caseous lymphadenitis	U.S. Food and Drug Administration does not recommend use of the vaccine in goats
Rabies	Use as in sheep, primarily only in high-risk herds
Enzootic abortion in ewes (EAE)	Use as in sheep, primarily only in high-risk herds; goats are more sensitive

*Core vaccine.
** Vaccination protocols should be designed specific to producers by veterinarians.
Most of the vaccines listed above are extra-label use in goats except for *Clostridium perfringens types C and D* and *Clostridium tetani*.
Modified from Holtgrew-Bohling, K. J. (2020). *Large animal clinical procedures for veterinary technicians* (4th ed.). St. Louis: Elsevier.

provide examples of recommended vaccination programs for various species. Therefore, it is recommended that puppies and kittens, starting around 8 weeks of age, receive boosters every few weeks until they are about 4 to 5 months of age. Boosters allow vaccines to produce an optimum immune response. Clients often find it difficult to understand why they need to bring their pet in for boosters. If the reasons are explained and if clients are advised about why they should isolate their pet from animals with questionable vaccination histories, many cases of infectious disease would be prevented among young animals. Clients often perceive one vaccine to be enough or do not understand that their animal is not protected immediately after an injection has been received. Technicians should include this information when educating clients on animal and pet care.

ADVERSE VACCINATION RESPONSES

The most notable risks involving vaccination include residual virulence and toxicity, allergic reactions resulting from hypersensitivity, disease in immunosuppressed animals, possible effects on a fetus, and abortion. The veterinarian assesses these risks before a vaccine is administered. In most cases, the benefits of vaccination far outweigh the risks, but it may occasionally be necessary to omit or delay vaccination because of some of the factors just mentioned.

One of the most common reactions noted with vaccine administration is the sting felt by the animal after injection. This is most often caused by inactivating agents used in manufacturing the vaccine. Manufacturers are constantly researching ways to decrease these undesirable effects while still producing a quality product. This stinging reaction is short lived and does not usually cause a problem unless the animal reacts violently. Other common but not usually serious reactions include a slight fever, lethargy, and soreness at the injection site. These usually subside within 1 day. Hypersensitivity may be caused by several factors, including immunizing antigens, antigens acquired during the manufacture of the vaccine, and reactions to adjuvants used in the vaccine. Adjuvants are substances added to vaccines to enhance a stronger immune response and prolong their effectiveness. Some animals may experience an anaphylactic shock reaction after receiving a vaccine, although this is uncommon. Clinical signs of anaphylaxis include vomiting, salivation, dyspnea, and incoordination. Other possible adverse side effects include vaccine-associated fibrosarcoma in cats and immune-mediated hemolytic anemia in dogs (Ford, 1998). There are various treatment options for vaccine-associated fibrosarcomas that will be determined by the veterinarian which may include surgery, radiation therapy, and chemotherapy. As stated previously, veterinarians should report all adverse reactions to the manufacturer of the vaccine. They may also be reported to the USDA Center for Veterinary Biologics.

CORE VERSUS NONCORE VACCINES

The AAHA and AAFP have established guideline recommendations for vaccines that they consider to be core and noncore. Core vaccines are recommended for most animals to protect them from highly contagious diseases that are widespread in the environment. AAHA suggests vaccines designated as core should be administered to all dogs. However, because exposure risk to vaccine-preventable disease varies, selected noncore vaccines may be recommended as core in individual practices depending on geographic region, patient lifestyle, age, etc. (AAHA, 2017). According to the 2017 AAHA Canine Vaccination Guidelines, core vaccines include canine distemper virus, adenovirus-2 (hepatitis), parvovirus, parainfluenza, and rabies. According to the 2013 AAFP Feline Vaccination advisory panel, core vaccines include FHV-1, FCV, FPV, and rabies.

Noncore vaccines are optional vaccines that should still be considered for animals at risk for developing disease based on geographic location and the lifestyle of the animal.

VACCINATIONS FOR PREVENTIVE HEALTH PROGRAMS

Canine

As was stated earlier, vaccination is an important part of any preventive health program. Many vaccines may be available as a monovalent or polyvalent product. For dogs, a common polyvalent vaccine includes canine distemper (D), respiratory diseases caused by adenovirus type 2 (A_2), canine parainfluenza (P), canine parvovirus (P), and leptospirosis (L). It should be noted that vaccination with the A_2 virus also protects the dog against infectious canine hepatitis (ICH). This vaccine may be referred to as *DA$_2$PPL*. Many different combinations and product names are available. Most veterinarians choose a particular manufacturer from which to buy vaccine products. This helps to lessen the confusion caused by different names used to designate the manufacturers' products. Other available canine vaccines include those given for canine infectious tracheobronchitis *(B. bronchiseptica)*, rabies, and Lyme disease *(B. burgdorferi)*. Manufacturer recommendations should be followed regarding age, route of administration, and follow-up boosters needed for each individual vaccine. Table 17.1 provides an example of a recommended vaccination program for dogs.

An exciting new therapeutic-type vaccine has been developed by Merial. Known as canine (oral) melanoma

vaccine, it is indicated for use in dogs in which local disease has occurred. At present, the vaccine will only be sold to veterinarians who specialize in oncology.

Canine Core Vaccines include:
Canine distemper virus
Canine adenovirus type-2
Canine parainfluenza
Canine parvovirus
Rabies vaccine (1 year or 3 year)
Canine Noncore Vaccines include:
Canine leptospirosis
B. bronchiseptica
Canine influenza
Canine coronavirus
Canine *Giardia*
Canine *B. burgdorferi* (Lyme)

Feline

A common polyvalent vaccine for cats is given for the prevention of feline herpesvirus-1 (FHV-1), feline calicivirus (FCV), and feline panleukopenia (FPV). Other available vaccines include those for feline chlamydiosis, feline leukemia, feline immunodeficiency virus, *B. bronchiseptica*, and rabies. Manufacturer recommendations should be followed regarding age, route of administration, and follow-up boosters needed for each vaccine. Table 17.2 provides an example of a recommended vaccination program for cats.

Feline Core Vaccines
FHV-1
FCV
FPV
Rabies vaccine
Feline Noncore Vaccines
Feline leukemia virus
FIV
Feline *Chlamydia felis*
Feline *B. bronchiseptica*

Equine

Vaccination schedules for horses and foals are based on; individual situations that require an evaluation based on the risk of disease, consequences of the disease, anticipated effectiveness, potential for adverse reactions and cost of immunization versus potential cost of disease (AAEP, 2020). Adult horse and foal vaccines that are available include those for tetanus, equine encephalomyelitis (may include Eastern, Western, and/or Venezuelan strains), West Niles virus, equine herpesvirus, equine influenza, leptospirosis, *Streptococcus* (strangles), equine viral arteritis, equine

BOX 17.1 Case Scenario

A 12-week-old female puppy weighing 14 lb is presented for a new puppy wellness exam and vaccinations.

History: Owner just acquired the puppy 2 weeks ago and brought the paperwork showing that she had her initial vaccination of distemper, adenovirus type 2 (CAV-2), parvovirus, and parainfluenza at another hospital, at 8 weeks of age. The puppy was also dewormed at 8 weeks of age for roundworms and hookworms. The owner stated that she is eating and drinking well, very playful, and normal urination and defecation.

Physical examination findings: Heart rate: 140 bpm, Respiratory rate: 20 bpm and panting, Temperature: 101.5°F, good overall appearance, no fleas observed, all other examination findings unremarkable (within normal limits). A fecal sample was obtained for both direct smear and fecal flotation.

The veterinary technician prepared (reconstituted) the booster vaccine of canine DA2PP (distemper, adenovirus-2, parvovirus, and parainfluenza) and rabies vaccine. She properly identified each vaccine with a label.

Fecal examination findings: No internal parasites observed.

The puppy received its second booster vaccine of DA2PP subcutaneously, between the shoulder blades and a rabies vaccine subcutaneously, in the right hind leg. She also received a second deworming, for roundworms and hookworms, to continue to clear the worms from the intestine.

The veterinary technician discussed the importance of the third booster vaccine in 3–4 weeks (at 16 weeks of age) with the owner as well as another deworming. She explained that the last series of the distemper booster will provide a protective response lasting 1 year. She continued to discuss the importance of revaccinating in 1 year for both the distemper series and the rabies.

The rabies booster vaccine will be administered in 1 year, at which time it will be protective for 3 years. The DA2PP vaccine will be given in 1 year and will also be protective for 3 years.

She discussed the risk of heartworm disease and heartworm preventative was dispensed to the owner and discussed that they also treat for common intestinal parasites. Since this is a new pet owner, the veterinary technician discussed nutritional information, socialization, house breaking, puppy-proofing their home, appropriate crate size, exercise requirements, and the importance of spaying. She explained the ideal age for spaying and will set up an appointment at the next office visit.

Veterinary technicians play an important role during wellness visits, especially initial puppy and kitten visits, educating owners on the importance of vaccinations, preventative products, routine parasite control, spaying or neutering, and nutritional needs. It is also a time to discuss the importance of yearly wellness visits, even when vaccinations are not indicated, to ensure the long-term health of their pet.

monocytic ehrlichiosis (Potomac horse fever), anthrax, botulism, rotavirus, and rabies. Tetanus antitoxin is used in wounded horses with no history of recent tetanus toxoid vaccination. It provides immediate immunity, which lasts for about 2 weeks. Tetanus toxoid may be given to a horse to boost its immunity and provide longer protection. Manufacturer recommendations should be followed regarding age, route of administration, and follow-up boosters needed for each individual vaccine. Tables 17.3 and 17.4 provide a list of vaccination guidelines developed by the American Association of Equine Practitioners (AAEP) Infectious Disease Committee for horses and foals; they are divided into two categories: core and risk-based. Since adverse reactions are not always foreseeable many veterinarians recommend that horses not be vaccinated 2 weeks prior to sales, shipment, or performance events and 3 weeks prior for international travel (AAEP, 2020). Vaccine reactions can be localized or systemic, and clinical signs can vary from loss of appetite, infection at the site of injection, fever, and anaphylaxis.

Equine Core Vaccines

Tetanus

Eastern/Western Equine Encephalomyelitis (EEE/WEE)

West Nile virus

Rabies

Equine Noncore or Risk-Based Vaccines

Anthrax

Botulism

Equine herpesvirus

Equine influenza

Equine viral arteritis

Equine influenza

Leptospirosis

Potomac horse fever

Rotavirus

Strangles (*Streptococcus equi*)

Bovine

Many vaccines are available for cattle in many different combinations. Vaccine schedules for cattle vary depending on the type of cattle-raising operation; a veterinarian can best decide what program an individual operation needs. Examples of commonly used vaccines include those for brucellosis, bovine respiratory syncytial virus (BRSV), bovine viral diarrhea type 1 and 2 (BVD type 1 and 2), clostridial diseases, infectious bovine rhinotracheitis (IBR), parainfluenza 3 (PI3) virus, and leptospirosis. As with all vaccines, manufacturer recommendations should be carefully followed for the best results. Table 17.5 provides examples of preventive health programs for cattle.

TECHNICIAN NOTES

- Many of the vaccines used for food animals have withdrawal times.

Bovine Core Vaccines

IBR
BRSV
BVD type 1 and 2
PI3
Brucellosis (Bang vaccine)
Clostridial diseases
Leptospirosis
Other Bovine Vaccines

Anthrax
Campylobacteriosis (vibriosis)
H. somnus
Mannheimia haemolytica (formerly known as *Pasteurella multocida*)
Moraxella bovis (pinkeye)
Salmonella
Scour vaccine
Trichomonas

Sheep and Goats

Vaccines available for sheep and goats are included in Tables 17.6 and 17.7. These animals may be raised in large numbers on farms, and similar to cattle-raising operations, vaccination schedules may vary according to the type of conditions and location.

TECHNICIAN NOTES

- Rabies vaccinations in sheep and goats are not usually administered unless they are pets, in which case they should be vaccinated.

Core Vaccines for Sheep
Clostridium perfringens **type C**
Clostridium perfringens **type D**
Clostridium tetani
   Other Sheep Vaccines. Other clostridial diseases (black disease, blackleg, malignant edema, struck, lamb dysentery, botulism)
Caseous lymphadenitis
Enzootic abortion in ewes (EAE)
E. coli
Leptospirosis
Sore mouth
Foot rot
Brucellosis
Vibriosis
Rabies
Core Vaccines for Goats
Clostridium perfringens **type C**
Clostridium perfringens **type D**
Clostridium tetani
   ### *Other Goat Vaccines (Use is Extralabel)*
E. coli
Foot rot
Pasteurella
Leptospirosis
Rabies

IMMUNOTHERAPEUTIC DRUGS

It may often be desirable to use drugs to stimulate the body's immunologic response. Immunotherapy involves using drugs to stimulate or suppress the body's immunologic response to diseases or conditions caused by agents such as bacteria, viruses, or cancer cells. Immunostimulants are agents that stimulate the immune response. Immunomodulators are agents used to adjust the immune response to a desired level. Table 17.8 lists some of the drugs commonly used in immunotherapy.

Immunostimulants act by stimulating macrophage activity, producing lymphokines, increasing natural killer cell activity, and enhancing cell-mediated immunity. These drugs may be used in the treatment of chronic pyoderma in dogs, equine sarcoids, and bovine ocular squamous cell carcinoma. They also may be used as adjunctive therapy for some other types of cancers, such as canine malignant lymphoma, fibrosarcoma, and feline retrovirus infection. Some immunostimulants may be used to help reduce the clinical signs and mortality associated with

TABLE 17.8   Immunotherapeutic Drugs and Indications for Their Use.

Product Name and Manufacturer	Product Type	Product Indications
Acemannan Immunostimulant (Carrington)	A complex carbohydrate derived from aloe vera; stimulates macrophage activity	An aid in the treatment of fibrosarcoma in cats and dogs, and feline leukemia; also for stimulating wound healing
Staphage Lysate (SPL) (Delmont)	*Staphylococcus aureus* phage lysate	Treatment for canine pyoderma and related skin infections with a staphylococcal component
Rubeola Virus Immunomodulator (Eudaemonic)	Inactivated rubeola virus with histamine phosphate	Treatment of equine chronic myofascial inflammation
Nomagen (Fort Dodge)	A mycobacterial cell-wall fraction immunostimulant	Treatment of equine sarcoids and bovine ocular squamous cell carcinoma
ImmunoRegulin (Immuno Vet)	*Propionibacterium acnes* immunostimulant	Chronic recurrent pyoderma in dogs
CL/Mab 231 (Synbiotics)	Canine lymphoma monoclonal antibody	Adjunctive therapy for dogs with lymphoma

some infections such as *E. coli* diarrhea in calves. Many other immunostimulants, such as interferons, interleukin-1, and interleukin-2, are being investigated for potential use in veterinary medicine.

Immunosuppressive drugs are used to suppress the body's immunologic response. They are used in veterinary medicine to treat various immune-mediated disorders. Further information on immunosuppressive drugs may be found in Chapter 16.

℞ Immunostimulants
Complex Carbohydrates

Acemannan. This is a complex carbohydrate derived from the gel of the aloe vera leaf.

Clinical Uses. Acemannan is used as an aid in the treatment of fibrosarcoma in cats and dogs. It has also been used for stimulating wound healing and in the treatment of FeLV-infected and FIV-infected cats.

Dosage Form
• **Acemannan immunostimulant**
Adverse Side Effects. There are no known side effects.

Immunomodulatory Bacterins

Staphylococcal Phage Lysate. Staphylococcal phage lysate (SPL) is prepared by lysing *Staphylococcus aureus* with a polyvalent bacteriophage.

Clinical Uses. SPL is used in the treatment of canine pyoderma and related skin infections with a staphylococcal component. It is designed to help control skin infections over time.

Dosage Form
• **Staphage Lysate (SPL)**
Adverse Side Effects. These include malaise, fever, chills, and injection site irritation.

Propionibacterium acnes Bacterin. This is prepared from killed *Propionibacterium acnes*.

Clinical Uses. *P. acnes* is an immunostimulant used as an adjunct to antibiotic therapy in reducing lesions of chronic recurrent pyoderma and as an adjunctive therapy in the treatment of equine respiratory disease complex. It also has been used as an adjunctive therapy in the treatment of feline retrovirus infection.

Dosage Forms
• **ImmunoRegulin**
• **EqStim**
Adverse Side Effects. These include malaise, fever, lethargy, and decreased appetite.

Mycobacterial Cell Wall Fraction. This is an emulsion of cell wall fractions that are modified to reduce their toxicity and allergic effects. It helps stimulate the activation of macrophages and lymphocytes to help kill tumor cells.

Clinical Uses. These include the treatment of equine sarcoids and bovine ocular squamous cell carcinoma. It is also used in the treatment of mixed mammary tumors and mammary adenocarcinoma in dogs (Plumb, 2015).

Dosage Forms

- **Regressin-V**
- **Nomagen**

Adverse Side Effects. These include malaise, fever, and decreased appetite.

 TECHNICIAN NOTES

The effects of immunotherapy may be decreased with the administration of immunosuppressive drugs.

REVIEW QUESTIONS

1. Immunizations should never take the place of regularly scheduled _____.
2. What six factors may determine an animal's response to immunization?
3. What is an inactivated vaccine?
4. What is a live vaccine?
5. What is a modified live vaccine?
6. What is a toxoid?
7. What is an antitoxin?
8. When a shipment of vaccine arrives at a veterinary facility, what should occur immediately?
9. What is the difference between a core and noncore vaccine?
10. What are the recommended sites and routes of administration for feline distemper series, feline leukemia, and rabies vaccines?
11. Explain how vaccines should be stored and handled.
12. List some potential adverse vaccine reactions that may occur in the dog and cat.
13. What type of immunity protects newborn animals against disease?
14. What is immunotherapy?
15. _____ is a complex carbohydrate derived from aloe vera.
16. Vaccines are all that is needed to implement a comprehensive health care plan for animals.
    a. True
    b. False
17. All the following are important factors in a patient's response to vaccine, except _____.
    a. the health and age of the patient
    b. the type of vaccine given
    c. the route of administration

d. administering a medicated bath before vaccination to clean the skin's surface
18. In the manufacture of _____ vaccines, organisms are treated most commonly by chemicals that kill the organisms, but very little change occurs in the antigens that stimulate protective immunity.
    a. live
    b. modified live
    c. inactivated (dead)
    d. recombinant
19. A _____ vaccine is prepared from live microorganisms or viruses. These organisms may be fully virulent or avirulent. Few vaccines of this origin are in use.
    a. live
    b. modified live
    c. inactivated (dead)
    d. recombinant
20. In _____ vaccines, organisms undergo a process (attenuation) to lose their virulence so that, when introduced to the body via inoculation, they cause an immune response instead of disease.
    a. live
    b. modified live
    c. inactivated (dead)
    d. recombinant
21. A(an) _____ vaccine is a specific antiserum aimed at a toxin that contains a concentration of antibodies extracted from the blood serum or plasma of a hyperimmunized animal (usually a horse).
    a. toxoid
    b. antitoxin
    c. recombinant
    d. autogenous
22. Most vaccines for small animals are most commonly administered by what route?
    a. Intramuscular
    b. Subcutaneous
    c. Intravenous
    d. Intranasal
23. All the following may be signs of anaphylaxis, except _____.
    a. vomiting
    b. blepharospasm
    c. salivation
    d. dyspnea

24. *Bordetella bronchiseptica* is a vaccine administered to _____.
   a. equines
   b. dogs
   c. cats
   d. both a and b
   e. both b and c

25. *Borrelia burgdorferi* is an example of a _____ vaccine.
   a. modified live
   b. autogenous
   c. recombinant
   d. toxoid

REFERENCES

AAEP Equine vaccination guidelines, 2020. https://aaep.org/guidelines/vaccination-guidelines. Accessed May 2020.

AAFP Feline vaccination guidelines, 2013. https://catvets.com/guidelines/practice-guidelines/feline-vaccination-guidelines. Accessed October 2019.

AAHA Canine vaccine guidelines, 2017. aaha.org/aaha-guidelines/vaccination-canine-configuration/vaccination-canine. Accessed October 2019.

AVMA. (2018). The continuing conundrum of feline injection-site sarcomas. https://www.avma.org/javma-news/2018-12-01/continuing-conundrum-feline-injection-site-sarcomas. Accessed June 2020.

Ford, R. B. (1998). Vaccines and vaccinations: Issues for the 21st century. *Compendium on Continuing Education for the Practising Veterinarian, 20*(8C), 19–24.

JAAHA (Journal of the American Veterinary Medical Association). (2011). *Development of new canine and feline preventative healthcare guidelines designed to improve pet health, AAHA-AVMA preventative healthcare guidelines task force.* https://www.aaha.org/globalassets/02-guidelines/preventive-healthcare/AAHA-Oncology-Guidelines-for-Dogs-and-Cats. Accessed October 2019.

Morrison, W. B., Starr, R. M., & Vaccine-Associated Feline Sarcoma Task Force (2001). Vaccine-associated feline sarcomas. *JAVMA, 218*(5), 697–702.

Plumb, D. C. (2015). *Veterinary drug handbook* (8th ed.). Ames, IA: Wiley-Blackwell.

Van Kampen, K. R. (1998). Recombinant technology. *Compendium on Continuing Education for the Practising Veterinarian, 20*(8), 28–32.

18

Miscellaneous Therapeutic Agents

OBJECTIVES

After studying this chapter, you should be able to

1. Define *nutraceutical* and *chondroprotectives*, as well as exhibit knowledge of the various types.
2. Discuss and provide a summary of herbal medicine. Also, discuss and evaluate the uses of various herbal products.

3. List and describe three treatment methods used in regenerative medicine.
4. Discuss the use of lubricants.

OUTLINE

KEY TERMS

Autologous
Chondroprotectives
Interleukin-1

Matrix
Nutraceutical
Stem cell

ALTERNATIVE MEDICINES

® Chondroprotectives and Nutraceuticals

The American Veterinary Medical Association (AVMA) defines nutraceutical medicine as "the use of micronutrients, macronutrients, and other nutritional supplements as therapeutic agents." In veterinary medicine, the term is generally used to refer to endogenous substances (not botanicals) that have been prepared or synthesized to support bodily functions. The popularity of these products, which may have characteristics of nutrients and pharmaceuticals, has seen tremendous growth in use by people in recent years. The medical community has acknowledged that some of them may have treatment or preventive effects (Boothe, 1997). Chondroprotectives are substances that are able to decrease the progression of osteoarthritis by providing support to cartilage and promoting its repair; they are available as oral or injectable medications.

As people have become more aware of alternative medical options for themselves, they have come to expect similar options for their pets. Veterinarians and their clients can be expected to use nutraceuticals as treatment options to complement traditional medicine or when traditional treatment options have been exhausted. Veterinary technicians should be familiar with the names of nutraceuticals and chondroprotectants that are commonly used so they can adequately educate the client and answer questions they may have.

The former North American Veterinary Nutraceutical Council proposed that a veterinary nutraceutical be defined as "a nondrug substance that is produced in a purified or extracted form and administered orally to provide agents required for normal body structure and function with the intent of improving the health and well-being of animals." Even though the definitions listed for nutraceutical and veterinary nutraceutical seem straightforward, a great deal of confusion exists over what is actually a nutraceutical. It has been stated that the term *nutraceutical* was developed to refer to a product marketed under the premise of being a dietary supplement but with the real intent of preventing or treating a disease (Warren, 2017).

The question often asked about these products is "Is it a food (nutrient) or a drug?" If it is a food, then it is not subject to U.S. Food and Drug Administration (FDA) approval; if it is a drug, it must go through the FDA approval process at a great deal of expense to the manufacturer. A product is usually determined to be a drug if its label has a claim that indicates a therapeutic or preventive intent. If the product has a label claim of a medical use and does not carry a new animal drug application (NADA) (indicating FDA approval), the product then becomes an unapproved drug and is subject to FDA regulation. Regulatory action may not be taken against these unapproved products because the FDA has limited resources and higher priority issues. If a product is determined to be a food, it is usually determined to be "generally regarded as safe (GRAS)" by the FDA. Any product that is given by injection is considered a drug.

The Dietary Supplement Health and Education Act (DSHEA) of 1994 listed dietary supplements as vitamins, minerals, amino acids, herbal products, and substances that supplement the diet by increasing total dietary intake. This action made these products "food" and excluded them from FDA regulation. The Act does require, however, that the manufacturer show a disclaimer on the label after the product claim that says, "This statement has not been evaluated by the Food and Drug Administration. This product is not intended to diagnose, treat, cure, or prevent any disease." The Center for Veterinary Medicine (CVM) of the FDA has stated that the DSHEA does not apply to animals or animal feeds because of concerns about potential residues and the potential differences in response across species.

Because nutraceuticals have not been through an extensive evaluation process to validate their purity, safety, and efficacy, it is up to the veterinarian to evaluate the suitability of particular products for use in companion animals and to promote their use in the context of a valid veterinarian–client–patient relationship. Veterinary technicians should consult with their veterinarians to formulate sound advice to give to clients regarding use of these products. Some questions that should be answered when a nutraceutical product is evaluated include the following:

- What controlled studies have been done to determine whether the product does what it claims to do, and who performed the studies? Are these studies published in reputable veterinary journals?
- Does the product contain what it says it does, and is that product bioavailable? Bioavailability may be influenced by the source and form of the product (e.g., glucosamine hydrogen chloride [HCl] vs. glucosamine sulfate).
- Is the label easily understandable and are all ingredients listed in the same units? Ingredients should be listed by the order of magnitude by weight.
- Is the dosage listed on the label, along with clear instructions for use?
- Is the product free of contaminants? Were good manufacturing practices (GMPs) followed?
- Does the label carry a United States Pharmacopeia (USP)–verified label for the product or ingredient/s?

(Courtesy United States Pharmacopeia [USP].)

- Is the manufacturer a member of the National Animal Supplement Council (NASC)? NASC provides animal supplement manufacturers with guidelines for product quality assurance, adverse event reporting, and labeling standards. Successful completion of this program allows the member company to display the

NASC Quality Seal on their products, website, product literature, and advertisements (Ettinger, 2017) .

(Courtesy National Animal Supplement Council [NASC].)

- Does the product have a lot number and expiration date on the label?
- Does the product rely on testimonials rather than scientific evidence for validation?

Clients should be urged to make use of information regarding nutraceutical quality by making use of the ConsumerLab (www.consumerlab.com) and USP (www.usp.org) websites.

The following is a partial list of the substances marketed as nutraceuticals and chondroprotectives. Some of these products may not be "endogenous substances" as defined earlier.

Polysulfated Glycosaminoglycans

Polysulfated glycosaminoglycan (PSGAG) consists of a repeating chain of hexosamine and hexuronic acid (Boothe, 2012). The complex nature of the molecule allows water to be trapped in hyaline cartilage to provide resistance to compression and resiliency to the proteoglycan and collagen matrix. PSGAGs are extracted for commercial use from the tracheal tissue of the bovine. After intramuscular injection, PSGAG is deposited in articular cartilage and is preferentially taken up by osteoarthritic cartilage (Plumb, 2015). When used to treat degenerative joint conditions, these PSGAGs increase synovial fluid viscosity and inhibit enzymes that damage cartilage matrix within joints. PSGAGs also reduce inflammation by inhibiting prostaglandin released in joint injury.

Clinical Uses. PSGAG is used in the treatment of noninfectious degenerative or traumatic joint dysfunction and associated lameness of the carpal and hock joints in horses. It also has been used to treat degenerative joint disorders in dogs. It is FDA approved for dogs and horses.

Dosage Forms
- **Adequan I.M.** for intramuscular injection
- **Adequan Canine**

Adverse Side Effects. Adverse side effects are minimal with use of this product. It should be used with caution in dogs with renal or hepatic dysfunction.

TECHNICIAN NOTES

- PSGAG should not be used in horses intended for food.
- Safety in breeding, pregnant or lactating animals has not been evaluated.

Glucosamine and Chondroitin Sulfate

Glucosamine is an amino sugar manufactured by animal cells from glucose and used by the body in the synthesis of glycoproteins and PSGAGs. Chondroitin sulfate is a glycosaminoglycan that combines with hyaluronic acid, proteins, and other glycosaminoglycans to form the basic cartilage matrix. Glucosamine and chondroitin sulfate are believed to act synergistically (Davidson, 2000) to exert a positive effect on cartilage metabolism and inhibition of cartilage breakdown. They have been used extensively in the treatment of osteoarthritis in dogs and horses and are referred to as nutraceuticals. Administration for 4 to 6 weeks may be necessary for a therapeutic effect to be seen. A common veterinary product that contains these substances is called Cosequin; it is composed of glycosaminoglycan derived from the chitin of crab shell and chondroitin sulfate from bovine trachea. Dasuquin and Dasuquin advanced for cats are products that contain glucosamine and chondroitin sulfate with avocado/soybean unsaponifiables, green tea extract, and other ingredients with claims of enhanced chondroprotection. GlycoFlex derive its glycosaminoglycan from the *Perna canaliculus,* an edible green-lipped mussel. Synoflex contains glucosamine and chondroitin sulphate with *N*-acetyl-D-glucosamine, zinc, and vitamin C. Synoquin EFA contains glucosamine and chondroitin sulphate with dexahan (highly purified form of krill oil—omega-3), zinc, and vitamin C.

Dosage Forms
- **Cosequin canine**—soft chews, chewable tablets, and mini chews
- **Cosequin feline**—soft chews and sprinkle capsules
- **Cosequin equine**—powder or easy pack
- **Dasuquin for dogs**—soft chews and chewable tablets
- **Dasuquin for cats**—sprinkle capsules
- **Dasuquin advanced**—soft chews for dogs and cats and sprinkle capsules for cats
- **Glycoflex Everyday, Classic, Sport, and Stage 1, Stage 2, Stage 3 for dogs**

- **Glycoflex Classic** for dogs
- **Glycoflex Plus** for dogs and cats
- **Synoflex**—chewable tablets for dogs
- **Synoquin Growth and EFA for dogs**

Hyaluronic Acid

Hyaluronic acid is a major constituent of synovial (joint) fluid. It has an increased viscosity (thickness) and therefore encourages joint lubrication. Acute injury to the joint can cause inflammation, allowing excess fluid to form, which can lead to swelling and pain. Hyaluronic acid decreases inflammation to the tissue surrounding the joint and repairs the joint cartilage. It is widely used to treat osteoarthritis in horses. Hyaluronic acid can be administered by intravenous or intraarticular injections. Intraarticular injections must be administered under strict aseptic conditions.

Dosage Forms
- **Legend multi dose and Legend 4 mL**—intravenous injection only
- **Legend 2 mL**—intravenous or intraarticular injection
- **Hyalovet**—intraarticular injection
- **Hylartin**—intraarticular injection

Fatty Acids

The omega-6 and omega-3 fatty acids are the ones most often found in commercial veterinary fatty acid supplements. Omega-6 fatty acids have a double bond six carbons from the methyl end, whereas omega-3 fatty acids have a double bond three carbons from the methyl end. Fatty acid supplementation has been shown to be useful in treating certain dermatologic conditions in dogs, such as flea allergy dermatitis and atopic dermatitis, because of their antiinflammatory effects. Omega-3 fatty acids are normally found in low concentrations in the cellular plasma membrane compared with omega-6 fatty acids, but the omega-3 level can be increased by a food or supplement that is enriched in this substance (Roudebush & Freeman, 2000). The breakdown products of the omega-3 acids are apparently less powerful mediators of the inflammatory response than those derived from the omega-6 fatty acids. The omega-3 and omega-6 fatty acids also may be helpful in treating heart disease, cancer, autoimmune disease, and rheumatoid arthritis. The proper ratio of omega-6 to omega-3 fatty acids in a product has apparently not been determined and is often debated. Fish oil and plant oils are common sources of these fatty acids. Many pet foods are rich in essential fatty acids and therefore supplementation is not necessary. Side effects may include increased bleeding times and possible decreased immune function when very high doses of fatty acids are used.

S-Adenosylmethionine

S-Adenosylmethionine (SAMe) SD4 is a molecule produced in the body from methionine and adenosine triphosphate (ATP) by the enzyme SAMe synthetase (Davidson, 2002). It is recommended for veterinary use as a dietary supplement to support normal structure and function of the liver. Some studies have shown that this substance increases levels of glutathione in the liver. Glutathione is an antioxidant that may protect liver cells from injury.

Dosage Forms
- **Denosyl tablets**—for dogs and cats
- **Denamarin** tablets for dogs and cats, chewable tablets for dogs
- **Vetri SAMe tablets**—for dogs and cats
- **Novifit** tablets for dogs and cats
- **Zentonil** tablets for dogs and cats

Superoxide Dismutase

Superoxide dismutase (antioxidant) from protein sources is an oxygen radical scavenger that has been used as an antiinflammatory agent for musculoskeletal problems. Antioxidants play a role in neutralizing the effects of inflammation therefore supplementation may be beneficial.

Coenzyme Q

This substance is an enzyme cofactor of mitochondrial membranes (parts of the cell that produces energy from oxygen), which is important in electron transport and ATP formation. It is a supplement used to support the cardiovascular system. It may be used as an adjunct therapy along with conventional medications for pets with heart disease.

Ⓡ Herbal Medicines

The use of plants to treat veterinary patients is classified by the AVMA as a modality in the category of complementary and alternative veterinary medicine (CAVM). The AVMA in its policy guidelines states that "the theoretical bases and techniques for CAVM may diverge from veterinary medicine routinely taught in North

American veterinary schools or may differ from current scientific knowledge or both." Even though it can be a controversial topic, the demand for herbal medicine by veterinary clients appears to have grown as an extension of the trend toward the increased use of "natural" dietary supplements and the "holistic" approach to good health in people. People may conclude that if herbal supplements make them feel better, the supplements will also make their pets feel better. The two main branches of herbal medicine are traditional and modern.

Traditional use of plant materials to treat ailments in people and animals can be traced to many ancient cultures, including highly refined traditions in China and India. The basis of Traditional Chinese Medicine (TCM), still practiced by some CAVM advocates, is the alteration of energetic systems in the body such as yin, yang, heat, cold, warm, dry, and moist through botanical interventions.

Modern herbal medicine makes use of the fact that plants or plant material contain chemicals (drugs) that may be used in a manner similar to drugs supplied by the pharmaceutical industry. Proponents of herbal medicine argue that whole plants (as opposed to a purified product) provide the advantages of synergy and safety. Synergy, they state, occurs when the primary therapeutic chemical in a plant/plants interacts with other chemicals in the plant/plants to provide a magnified or more efficacious effect. Safety, they believe, occurs because multiple chemicals in a plant may dilute any singly toxic ingredient. Some herbal practitioners report that plants "may contain antimicrobial, anticancer, and immune modulating factors" (Wynn, 2002) not presently known in currently used drugs. Herbal medicine, when used in conjunction with conventional medicine, can provide another dimension of service to the veterinary client and patient.

Very few controlled studies have been performed to document the safety and efficacy of herbal products. Veterinarians must rely on empiric data, anecdotal information, and personal experience to guide their use of botanicals. The Cochrane Collaboration provides a library of papers from studies conducted with the use of botanical medicine. Botanicals are classified as supplements by the FDA according to the DSHEA and fall into a regulatory gray zone where few monitoring programs are in place to ensure the potency and purity of these products. Plants may vary in their makeup according to climate conditions, soil type, fertilizer used, and other factors. Manufacturing practices, packaging procedures,

and storage conditions also may influence the quality of the product. Quality control practices regarding the actual content of the product as well as its strength and purity may vary widely from manufacturer to manufacturer and from country to country. A coalition of animal supplement manufacturers formed the NASC, www.nasc.cc, a voluntary membership group, to address issues of quality control in the industry in the United States. Some veterinarians have advised against using herbal products manufactured in China because of reported contamination with heavy metals, herbs found in the product not listed on the label, or the presence of "spiked" (added) substances like anabolic steroids, glucocorticoids, thyroxine, and other substances (Rishniw, 2006). A useful resource for checking the quality of herbal products is the ConsumerLab website.

When choosing a product, veterinarians also must consider potential interactions of botanicals with conventional drugs that are being simultaneously administered and possible breed or species differences in drug responses. Certain herbs like ginkgo biloba, red clover, and feverfew may decrease platelet aggregation and should not be given before surgery or with conventional drugs that inhibit clotting. St. John's Wort should not be given with some drugs that modify behavior (monoamine oxidase inhibitors [MAOIs]). Potential herb–drug interactions are listed in Table 18.1. Other potential interactions can be found at the PubMed and ConsumerLab websites.

Botanicals are usually available from suppliers in three primary forms. These forms include the following:

Dried bulk herb: The plant has been harvested, dried, and often powdered. If powdered, it may be sold in loose powder form or placed in capsules.

Dried extracts: The plant is simmered in water, strained of residue, and sprayed into a vacuum chamber, which produces a powder or granules. A common extract is a 5:1 ratio that allows the use of less product because of the concentrated form. Water extracts may exclude plant substances that are alcohol soluble.

Liquid extracts: The ingredients are extracted in alcohol and the residue discarded. Advantages of alcohol extraction are thought to include concentration of the ingredient and improved absorption from the intestinal tract. Alcohol extractions usually taste bad to pets and must be added to another ingredient to improve palatability. Many botanical products can be administered in capsule, tablet, liquid, powder, and ointment preparations.

TABLE 18.1 Potential Herb–Drug Interactions.

Herb	Interacting Drugs	Result
St. John's Wort	Cyclosporine	Decreased plasma drug concentrations
	Fexofenadine	
	Midazolam	
	Digoxin	
	Tacrolimus	
	Amitriptyline	
	Warfarin	
	Theophylline	
	Sertraline	Serotonin syndrome
	Buspirone	
Gingko	Warfarin	Bleeding
	Heparin	
	NSAIDs	
	Omeprazole	Decreased plasma concentrations
Ginseng	Warfarin	Bleeding
	Heparin	Falsely elevated serum digoxin levels (laboratory test interaction with ginseng)
	NSAIDs	
	Opioids	Decreased analgesic effect
		Falsely elevated serum digoxin levels (laboratory test interaction with ginseng)
Garlic	Warfarin	Bleeding
Chamomile	Heparin	
Ginger	NSAIDs	

NSAIDs, Nonsteroidal antiinflammatory drugs.

Most of the current dosing of botanicals for animals is extrapolated from human dosage information because few herbal products are produced specifically for animals. Dosage recommendations vary between forms and between extract dilutions (e.g., a 1:1 extract will be dosed differently than a 5:1 extract).

Summary of Herbal Medicines

Herbal medicine has added another dimension outside of conventional therapy to the treatment of veterinary patients. Its practice provides a holistic approach to veterinary health care for those veterinarians and clients who wish to use it as an ancillary method or when conventional

BOX 18.1 Useful Herbal References

National Animal Supplement Council	www.nasc.cc
Veterinary Botanical Medicine Association	www.vbma.org
Drug Digest	www.drugdigest.org
PubMed	www.pubmed.gov
ConsumerLab	www.consumerlab.com
Cochrane Collaboration	www.cochrane.org
HerbMed	www.herbmed.org
American Association of Feed Control Officials	www.aafco.org
American Herbal Products Association	www.ahpa.org

methods have been exhausted. Until strict regulation of the botanical industry is achieved, however, veterinary technicians should counsel clients with judicious information about their use. The following factors may be helpful when one is advising clients about herbal use:

- The use of herbal medicine should not be started without discussion of the process with the attending veterinarian.
- Clients should purchase products from reputable manufacturers approved by the NASC.
- Clients can find product evaluation information at the ConsumerLab website.
- The recommended dosage should be followed closely.
- Herbs may cause harmful interactions with conventional drugs.
- Herb use may cause bleeding tendencies during surgical procedures.
- Adverse side effects of herbs should be reported to the Veterinary Botanical Medicine Association and to the manufacturer.

Box 18.1 includes a list of useful herbal references.

TECHNICIAN NOTES

The American Society of Anesthesiology recommends that patients should discontinue all herbal medicines 2 to 3 weeks before elective surgical procedures are performed.

Aloe. *Aloe vera* is a plant native to Africa that was used as early as 1500 BC for the treatment of various conditions and as a cathartic (Wynn & Fougere, 2007). Today, it is used primarily for the treatment of burns and skin inflammation. Some herbalists believe that aloe stimulates wound healing.

Bloodroot. The rhizome of *Sanguinaria canadensis* has traditionally been used as an expectorant and to treat respiratory conditions like bronchitis, asthma, and laryngitis. It is also reported to have antiinflammatory and antimicrobial effects.

Boswellia. Boswellia *(Boswellia serrata)* may reduce pain, inflammation, and arthritis and is commonly combined with curcumin in Ayurvedic arthritis remedies (Wynn, 2003).

Echinacea. *Echinacea purpurea* is a commonly used remedy for colds and flu in people in the United States and Europe, where research has been done to show that it is an immunostimulant. It is derived primarily from the American coneflower. No major side effects have been reported other than the occasional allergic reaction.

Garlic. Garlic is a perennial bulb in the lily family *(Allium sativum)* that is related to the onion. This plant has been used for centuries for its reported medicinal value. People have claimed that it produces disinfectant, diuretic, and/or expectorant effects. Evidence suggests that it does lower cholesterol values in people. No evidence, however, shows that garlic has any value in the treatment of parasites in animals. Garlic can produce Heinz body anemia in cats and possibly in dogs at high dosages.

Ginger. Ginger root *(Zingiber officinale)*, along with turmeric and other food-based herbs, has been found to have significant antiinflammatory and antioxidant actions; ginger has been used for its antiinflammatory effect, as an antiemetic for cancer, renal disease, and it may also be helpful in cases of asthma and other inflammatory lung conditions (August, 2019).

Ginkgo. *Ginkgo biloba* is thought to increase circulation to the brain and extremities and has been reported to improve memory and symptoms of senile dementia in people.

Ginseng. Ginseng is made from the dried roots of several species of plants from the Panax family. Several varieties of ginseng, including American *(Panax quinquefolius)*, Asian, Korean *(Panax ginseng)*, and Siberian *(Eleutherococcus senticosus)*, have been identified. The Korean and American ginseng have shown promise in managing diabetes; shown to reduce hyperglycemia in humans (Wynn, 2003). The Chinese believe that ginseng increases vitality and overall strength, possibly by improving aerobic metabolism. Side effects may include hypertension, nervousness, and excitement.

Goldenseal. The goldenseal plant *(Hydrastis canadensis)* produces an alkaloid ingredient called *berberine* that may have antimicrobial and vasoactive properties. Its potential veterinary indications include stomatitis, gastritis, enteritis, giardiasis, and focal bacterial skin infections (Wynn & Fougere, 2007). Goldenseal should not be used in pregnant animals because of its potential to cause uterine contractions (Romich, 2005). Goldenseal is becoming very scarce in the wild.

Hawthorn. Hawthorn *(Crataegus oxyacantha)* may increase myocardial contractility and reduce peripheral vascular resistance (Wynn, 2003). The main active ingredient of hawthorn is thought to be an antioxidant bioflavonoid.

Licorice. Licorice *(Glycyrrhiza glabra)* contains multiple flavonoids and other constituents. It has shown potential hepatoprotective benefits through its antiinflammatory and antioxidant actions and topically, it has been used as an antiinflammatory and antimicrobial treatment (August, 2019).

Marshmallow. Marshmallow *(Althaea officinalis)* is a mucilaginous plant, high in flavonoids and polysaccharides; its primary role is soothing membranes of the gastrointestinal and respiratory tracts. It has been used with other herbs for urinary tract infection and inflammation, and as a topical wound treatment (August, 2019).

Milk Thistle. The milk thistle plant *(Silybum marianum)* contains an ingredient called *silymarin* that comprises biologically active flavonoids. This plant has been used as a hepatoprotectant and to enhance liver regeneration (Goodman & Trepanier, 2005). Milk thistle is thought to provide antioxidants that improve hepatocyte regeneration.

St. John's Wort. St. John's Wort is a plant that has reported (anecdotal) antianxiety and antidepression effects in people.

Saw Palmetto. Saw palmetto *(Serenoa repens)* plant extract may be of value in treating benign prostatic hyperplasia because of its possible ability to reduce testosterone formation.

Yunnan Bai Yao. Yunnan Bai Yao is used as a hemostatic (blood clotting) granular/powder formula to offer relief of bleeding in inoperable abdominal hemangiosarcoma. It contains San Qi, an herb that is able to stop bleeding in the body and has been shown to decrease clotting times and initiate platelet release (Wynn, 2003).

BOX 18.2   Case Scenario

A 9-year-old neutered male Golden Retriever, named Cooper, was presented for weakness and a distended abdomen.

History: Cooper has been slowing down over the past several weeks; he has been eating and drinking, no vomiting or diarrhea, and is still playful. He ate this morning and went for his normal morning walk. In the afternoon, he was not interested in eating and seemed lethargic. While Cooper was laying down, the owner felt that his stomach appeared bloated or distended and he had a hard time rising. He is up-to-date on vaccines. No travel history. He has seasonal allergies but is not on any medications.

Physical examination findings: The patient was quiet, alert, and responsive, and wagging his tail. Temperature: 101.5°F, Pulses: 140 bpm and bounding, Respiration: panting but normal effort, MM/CRT: mucous membranes pale pink, CRT (capillary refill time) was 2 seconds. Auscultation of the thorax did not reveal a heart murmur or abnormal lung sounds.

Diagnostic tests: Obtain ECG and blood pressure to further assess hemodynamics and determine if IV fluids are needed, attempt to gain IV access and obtain PCV/TP and blood glucose given the pale mucous membranes. Abdominal radiographs to assess free fluid and to rule out gastric dilatation volvulus. Depending on results from abdominal radiographs, an abdominal ultrasound may be performed.

Diagnostic results: ECG revealed accelerated idioventricular rhythm (AIVR); an ectopic rhythm with three or more consecutive ventricular premature beats and an abnormally fast ventricular escape rate, wide QRS complexes and P waves popping in and out. Blood pressure: 70 mm Hg, Blood glucose: 120 mg/dL, PCV: 24%, TP: 5 g/dL. Abdominal radiographs revealed an empty stomach in normal position, decreased abdominal detail, increased soft tissue opacity in the region of the spleen. Abdominal ultrasound revealed moderate peritoneal effusion.

Further diagnostic tests: Perform an abdominocentesis for fluid analysis. A PT/PTT to rule out coagulopathy if hemorrhagic peritoneal effusion. CBC/Chemistry to assess anemia, platelet counts, albumin levels, and concurrent organ dysfunction. Thoracic radiographs to assess heart and metastasis check.

Second set of diagnostic results: The CBC revealed regenerative anemia, mild inflammatory leukogram, and a platelet count of 120,000/uL. The chemistry was within normal limits. Thoracic radiographs were unremarkable. PT/PTT were normal. Abdominal ultrasound confirmed a cavitated mass at the tail of the spleen but otherwise normal. Abdominocentesis: 3 mL of nonclotting hemorrhagic effusion with a PCV of 36% and TP of 4.6 g/dL.

Diagnosis: Hemoabdomen from bleeding splenic mass with suspicion of hemangiosarcoma.

Treatment: Cooper was given packed red blood cell (pRBC) transfusion and over a period of time hemodynamically stabilized. He began eating and drinking. The veterinarian discussed the need to perform a splenectomy and histopathology to determine malignancy. The owner did not wish to pursue a splenectomy and elected palliative care only.

Cooper was discharged the following day with Yunnan Bai Yao and instructions to monitor for signs of recurrent hemoabdomen was discussed.

Two months post-diagnosis, Cooper is doing well and continues to be stable.

Courtesy Tara J. Fetzer, DVM, DACVECC.

℞ Regenerative Medicine

Regenerative medicine refers to the use of cells, cytokines, scaffolds, and growth factors to improve the repair of damaged or poorly functioning tissues or organs (Fitzwater, 2013). This therapy involves collecting tissue (generally fat, bone marrow, or blood) from the patient, isolating the desired cells or products, and administering the products back to the patient. These autologous products function to replace damaged tissue or stimulate the body's own repair mechanisms to bring about healing. Much of the focus of regenerative medicine is on the use of stem cells but also includes the use of interleukin antagonists, platelet-rich plasma (PRP), and other products. Regenerative medicine is used most often in the treatment of orthopedic disorders in horses and dogs. Other potential uses include chronic kidney disease and asthma in cats, as well as immune-mediated disorders like inflammatory bowel disease and autoimmune hemolytic anemia in companion animals. The efficacy of regenerative medicine is somewhat controversial at this time because of questions related to the lack of extensive data from controlled studies. Some uncertainty remains whether positive results are due to tissue repair, an antiinflammatory effect, or postprocedure rest and restrictions.

Stem Cell Therapy

Stem cells are cells that reside in most native tissues of both the adult and the embryo and are essential for the maintenance of homeostasis. All organisms continuously renew various tissues and organs. This renewal process can occur because of a source of cells that are able to differentiate into the appropriate tissue or organ. These reserve cells are called stem cells.

The two types of stem cells are embryonic and adult. Embryonic stem cells are derived from the early embryo and are called totipotent or pluripotent because they can give rise to multiple tissue types and complete organs needed for the entire organism. These embryonic stem cells can be grown in vitro and form immortal cell lines. They are very useful in research but have two characteristics that limit their clinical use: (1) they form tumors called teratomas when implanted into a patient, and (2) they are foreign tissue that may be rejected by the host. Adult stem cells have a reduced capability for differentiation when compared with embryonic stem cells and are thus called *multipotent*. They are the cells that are used to make the daily renewals to tissues and organs. When used clinically, they do not form teratomas and because they are autologous they are not rejected as foreign. The use of adult stem cells also avoids the controversy of collecting from embryonic tissue. Stem cells derived from bone marrow or fat are called mesenchymal cells or stromal cells. Mesenchymal stem cells can differentiate into fat, cartilage, or bone and are the stem cells used clinically in veterinary medicine. The beneficial effect of stem cell therapy is a result of several mechanisms that include (1) production of growth factors and cytokines that foster growth and regeneration of tissue, (2) production and secretion of antiinflammatory mediators and other immune modulators, (3), differentiation into target tissues like cartilage and/or bone, and (4) the ability to "home" to an inflamed site through the vascular system. Stem cells are harvested from either bone marrow or fat. Fat yields a significantly larger number of cells than bone marrow but a definitive number of cells for therapy has not been established. In dogs and cats, fat tissue is usually harvested from the falciform ligament, the caudal scapular space, or the inguinal fold. The harvest site in the horse is usually the tail head area. Dogs and cats require general anesthesia for collection while collection can usually be performed with the use of sedation in the horse. After harvest, stem cells are sent to a commercial laboratory for isolation and culture or prepared in-hospital with the use of a bench-top technique. After preparation, the mesenchymal stem cells are injected with the use of aseptic technique either into the injury site or intravenously.

Companies providing stem cell products or services include the following:
- Vet Stem
- MediVet
- Animal Cell Therapies

Platelet-Rich Plasma

PRP is the platelet-concentrated plasma obtained from anticoagulated whole blood by a centrifugation process. The platelets are concentrated around the buffy coat near the top of the red cells at the distal end of the plasma. PRP provides several growth factors that signal local mesenchymal, epithelial, and endothelial cells to migrate, divide, and increase collagen and matrix formation. The body's healing response is enhanced by distributing increased concentrations of growth factors to the injured tissue. PRP therapy is used primarily by equine veterinarians for tendon and ligament injuries and to promote granulation of tissue defects. It has also been used for canine orthopedic diseases and injuries. Blood is collected from the injured patient and centrifuged with a specialized tube. Plasma containing the autologous platelets is then separated from the red blood cells and injected into the injured tissue by intraarticular or peritendinous injection. It may also be applied topically.

Companies supplying PRP products include:
- Vet Stem
- Medivet Biologics

Interleukin-1 Antagonist Protein

Interleukin-1 (IL-1) is a proinflammatory cytokine that acts as a major mediator of joint disease. It is produced by synoviocytes, chondrocytes, and white blood cells and stimulates neutral proteinase production. Neutral proteinases promote synovial membrane thickening, cartilage breakdown, and general tissue destruction. The healthy joint has a balance of IL-1 and IL-1 antagonist (IL-1Ra). The theory of IL-1a therapy says that the injured or diseased joint has increased IL-1 that can be offset with IL-1Ra treatment. In this therapy blood is drawn from the equine patient with the use of a special syringe. This syringe contains glass beads that stimulate the production of IL-1Ra from white blood cells. The syringe containing the patient's blood and the glass beads is incubated and spun in a centrifuge to separate the plasma containing the IL-1Ra. The specially prepared plasma is then injected into the injured or diseased joint. This modality is mainly used to treat synovitis, capsulitis, arthritis, and, potentially, bursitis and tenosynovitis. Treatment with IL-1Ra is often called IRAP therapy.

Companies providing IRAP products include the following:

- Arthrex Vet Systems
- Dechra

Lubricants

Lubricants are used to lubricate hands, arms, or instruments before gynecologic and rectal examinations are performed.

Dosage Forms

- **K-Y Jelly**
- **Lube Jelly**
- **Lubrivet**

Adverse Side Effects. Adverse side effects are uncommon.

> ### TECHNICIAN NOTES
>
> Petroleum jelly (Vaseline) is not recommended for use as a lubricant because it is not water soluble and is not easily rinsed from instruments.

REVIEW QUESTIONS

1. Glycosaminoglycans occur naturally in what part(s) of the body?
2. What role do glycosaminoglycans (GAGs) provide in the treatment of degenerative joint conditions?
3. Define *nutraceutical*. Give an example.
4. A product usually is determined to be a drug if its label has a claim that indicates a therapeutic or preventive intent.
   a. True
   b. False
5. What Act defined dietary supplements, such as vitamins, minerals, amino acids, herbal products, and substances that supplement the diet by increasing total dietary intake, as "food" and excluded them from FDA regulation?

6. What is the purpose of the NASC and what do they provide to animal supplement manufacturers?
7. Cosequin and Glycoflex are tradenames for what type of supplement?
8. What is the tradename for polysulfated glycosaminoglycans?
9. Which supplement is used to support the cardiovascular system in domestic animals?
   a. Superoxide dismutase
   b. S-adenosylmethionine
   c. Fatty acids
   d. Coenzyme Q
10. _____ supplementation has been shown to be useful in treating certain dermatology conditions in dogs and cats.
11. What are two possible side effects of using fatty acids as a dietary supplement?
12. Petroleum jelly is not recommended as a lubricant because it is not _____.
13. A dietary supplement for support of normal structure and function of the liver is _____.
14. Botanicals are available from suppliers in what three forms?
15. _____ is a plant native to Africa and is used primarily to treat burns and skin inflammation.
16. What factors should be discussed with clients about the use of herbal products?
17. _____ is used as a hemostatic to relieve bleeding in inoperable abdominal hemangiosarcoma.
18. Echinacea may be used concurrently via the intraarticular route to prevent infections resulting from possible contamination.
    a. True
    b. False
19. Petroleum jelly (Vaseline) is an excellent choice for use in veterinary medicine because it is not easily rinsed from instruments and thereby prolongs the life of those instruments.
    a. True
    b. False
20. The order for a 65-lb arthritic dog is 5 mg/kg of Adequan (100 mg/mL). What quantity would you draw up for IM injection?

REFERENCES

August, K. (2019). Herbs for animal end-of-life and palliative care. *American Holistic Veterinary Medical Association Journal, 56*. ahvma.org. Accessed October 2019.

Boothe, D. M. (2012). Antiinflammatory drugs. In D. M. Boothe (Ed.), *Small animal clinical pharmacology and therapeutics*. Philadelphia: WB Saunders.

Boothe, D. M. (1997). Nutraceuticals in veterinary medicine: part I definitions and regulations. *Compendium on Continuing Education for the Practising Veterinarian, 19*(11), 1248–1255.

Davidson, G. (2000). Glucosamine and chondroitin sulfate. *Compendium on Continuing Education for the Practising Veterinarian, 22*(5), 454–458.

Davidson, G. (2002). S-adenosylmethionine. *Compendium on Continuing Education for the Practising Veterinarian, 24*(8), 600–603.

Ettinger, S. J., Feldman, E. C., & Cote, E. (2017). *Textbook of veterinary internal medicine expert consult* (8th ed.). St. Louis: Elsevier.

Fitzwater, K. Regenerative stem cell, module 1: principles of stem cells—what is regenerative medicine? Veterinary Information Network (website). http://www.vin.com/members/proceedings/proceedings.plx?CID=ABVP2012&PID=83732. Accessed March 5, 2013.

Goodman, L., & Trepanier, L. (2005). Potential drug interactions with dietary supplements. *Compendium on Continuing Education for the Practising Veterinarian, 27*(10), 780–790.

Plumb, D. C. (2015). *Veterinary drug handbook* (8th ed.). Ames, IA: Wiley-Blackwell.

Rishniw, M. (2006). *Evaluating herbal medicines*. Davis, CA: Veterinary Information Network.

Romich, J. A. (2005). *Fundamentals of pharmacology for veterinary technicians*. Clifton Park, NY: Thompson Delmar Learning.

Roudebush, P., & Freeman, L. M. (2000). Nutritional management of heart disease. In J. D. Bonagura (Ed.), *Kirk's current veterinary therapy small animal practice. XIII*. Philadelphia: WB Saunders.

Warren, E. Nutraceuticals. Veterinary Information Network (website). http://www.vin.com/doc/?id=2994084. Accessed June 4, 2019.

Wynn, S. G., & Marsden, S. (2003). *Manual of natural veterinary medicine science and tradition*. St. Louis: Elsevier.

Wynn, S. G. (2002). An introduction to herbal medicine. In *Proceedings. West veterinary conference*. Las Vegas, NV.

Wynn, S. G., & Fourgere, B. J. (2007). *Veterinary herbal medicine*. St. Louis: Mosby Elsevier.

19

Pharmacy Management and Inventory Control

OBJECTIVES

After studying this chapter, you should be able to

1. Explain why having an inventory control system is important.
2. Describe ways in which inventory control benefits a business.
3. Explain why inventory turnover is important and perform calculations related to inventory turnover.
4. Discuss ways of becoming an efficient inventory control manager.
5. Describe various inventory record-keeping systems and discuss ways to organize inventory.
6. Describe the differences in vendor types.
7. Describe good communication techniques that can be used with sales representatives and discuss drug enforcement administration forms, special orders, and human pharmacy.
8. Discuss ways that veterinary management computer software aids in tracking pharmaceutical inventory.

OUTLINE

KEY TERMS

Average cost of inventory on hand
DEA form
Delayed billing
FIFO
Fob
FOB destination
FOB shipping point

Full-service companies
Inventory
Inventory control manager (ICM)
Invoice
Mail order discount house
Margin
Markup

Packing slip
Statement
Total cost

Turnover
Veterinary supply distributor

INTRODUCTION

Control of inventory is an important concern for companies both large and small, and veterinary businesses are no exception. Proactively maintaining pharmaceutical inventory is an ongoing endeavor for veterinary hospitals (Fig. 19.1). Deciding how much trade or generic name product to buy, keeping expired items off the shelves, and performing a physical inventory are all integral parts of keeping a veterinary facility functioning as a healthy business. When a product is depleted before the next order arrives, it is frustrating for both veterinary staff and the clientele. When a product is not available, it cannot be sold and no profit can be made. Deciding which employee to entrust with this responsibility is an important decision for veterinary practice owners that should be made with careful consideration. Therefore, the employee chosen for this job should treat the position with respect and make every effort to be frugal with the employer's money.

The veterinary technician often is the employee chosen to perform this job. Therefore, knowledge of pharmaceutics and the ability to observe quantities of product used within a month are important skills that the veterinary technician must possess.

 TECHNICIAN NOTES

Along with knowledge of nursing skills, accepting the role of inventory control manager (ICM) boosts the veterinary technician's value as an employee.

In our technologically advanced society, pharmaceutics change rapidly because new products are constantly being developed. The veterinary technician who is charged with being the ICM must be willing to learn about new products and to pass this information on to the entire veterinary staff. Communication and good people skills are useful when one is dealing with pharmaceutical sales representatives. Sales representatives are invaluable to veterinary practices because they are armed with all available information about drugs, both old and new.

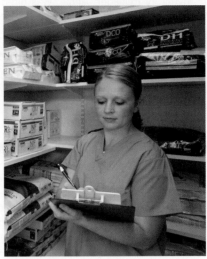

Fig. 19.1 A veterinary technician taking inventory. (From Prendergast, H. [2011]. *Front office management for the veterinary team*. St. Louis: Saunders, Elsevier.)

The ICM has many responsibilities. These responsibilities include keeping the staff informed regarding discontinued items, knowing the dates on which backordered items will be released from the vendor, packing up goods awaiting return to the vendor (e.g., expired items), rotating stock correctly, maintaining current prices on all products, organizing inventory for ease of location and counting, receiving and inspecting orders on arrival at the veterinary facility, and learning about new products. These are only a few of the responsibilities the ICM will meet daily. Inventory should be handled as an ongoing process. Each day, inventory must be visually counted, and physical inventory must be done at least once a month for good results.

INVENTORY

 TECHNICIAN NOTES

The value of all assets owned by the veterinary facility has important tax and insurance implications.

BOX 19.1   Case Scenario

A veterinary hospital decided to hire a veterinary inventory manager to be responsible for inventory control at their practice to increase profitability, improve cash flow, and client fulfilment by having the products available to them. An inventory manager, Angie, was hired and has been employed for 3 months. She is detail oriented, committed to making sure inventory costs are in line with the budget, computer savvy, and communicates very well with the hospital manager and veterinarians.

She developed standard operating procedures for inventory policies which decreased frustration, fewer mistakes were made, and adequate supplies were on the shelves. She trained another staff member, who is a licensed veterinary technician, on the policies and procedures for inventory control. She established protocols for ordering appropriate quantities of items to have on hand, established reorder points, and reorder quantities for all inventory items, protocols for receiving items, restocking items, and processing invoices. A regular schedule for ordering was implemented to improve efficiency. Angie also created inventory codes for all products in the management software system. She audited and reconciled controlled substance logs.

Angie developed professional relationships with a few vendors, discussed a specific day to meet each month to discuss discounted items, new products, and offerings. Discussed the company's payment policy and if delayed billing (option for paying within a 60- to 90-day period) is offered, free shipping, and discounts for early payment. Also discussed their return policy for expired drugs.

Price markups were established using the practice management software system for all inventory items. Inventory items were entered into the computer every week to ensure the correct fees are updated in the system.

She developed a protocol for receiving inventory; the purchase order and packing list must be compared to see if they match; and note if any items are backordered. Pricing information and quantities are then entered into the management software system. As inventory is used up the management system will trigger purchasing needs.

On a daily and sometimes weekly basis, Angie purchases inventory (what is needed and reorder points),

reviews vendor prices, and updates client costs to reflect price changes, if necessary.

Angie developed a method to accurately inventory products using both an inventory management system and manual inventory counts (monthly). Weekly inspections of expiration dates were enforced so that products could be returned to the vendor, if necessary. A rotation system FIFO for products on the shelves was implemented.

Having the ability to use the veterinary management software system allowed for tracking quantities being ordered, dispensed (both prescription and medical supplies), and allowed for printing of daily, monthly, and annual reports. These reports are valuable especially when expiration reports are printed to let you know when inventory is about to expire so items can be returned for reimbursement.

Angie just started planning for an online pharmacy and supply web page for the veterinary hospital so that items can be sold online. This will offer a valuable service to the clients but also provide convenience.

Hiring an inventory manager provided the practice with an individual who:

Manages and orders all retail, over the counter products, and pharmaceuticals.

Maintains good working relationships with vendors and meets with vendors regularly, on a monthly basis.

Ensures that a central area is being utilized for medications.

Controls pricing and markups.

Generates the reorder list.

Purchases inventory to maintain a 1-month supply with balanced turnover.

Ensures rotation of stock items on shelves.

Having a dedicated inventory manager responsible for all product inventory and training of other hospital staff is essential so that the standard operating procedures for inventory control are understood. Also having other staff members trained as a backup is essential for when the inventory manager goes on vacation or is sick. Training hospital staff has eliminated confusion and errors such as double-ordering, inappropriate rotation of stock on shelves, and unchecked expiration dates. Inventory control is crucial to both patient care and the success of the veterinary hospital.

Accounting of inventory items is very important when one is filing income taxes or in the event of a fire or natural disaster. Veterinary practices providing an accurate inventory of their business assets are assured that their insurance companies will reimburse the

business accurately should a disaster occur. The primary goal of inventory is to have sufficient quantities of inventory available to serve clients' needs, while at the same time minimizing the cost of carrying that inventory. Purchasing too many units of a slow-selling item can cost the practice money, and not purchasing enough of a high-selling item can result in the item being out of stock, which can cause frustration for the veterinary team (Libby et al., 2004).

An accounting system plays three roles in the inventory management process:

1. The system must provide accurate information for preparation of periodic financial statements and tax returns.
2. The system must provide up-to-date information on inventory quantities and costs, to facilitate ordering decisions.
3. The system also must provide the information needed to protect assets because inventories are subject to theft and other forms of misuse.

Thus, what exactly is the definition of inventory? It is tangible property that is sold in the normal course of a business day. In veterinary medicine, this would include such items as antibiotics, anthelmintics, shampoos, topical medications, prescription feeds, and even the dispensing bottles used to dispense liquid medication, as well as the syringes sold to clients that they must use to orally medicate their pets at home. Dispensing bottles, syringes, needles, ointment tins, and so forth could be classified as raw materials because they are carriers for the actual medicine that is being prescribed and dispensed. However, raw materials cost the practice money, just as pharmaceutics do. It is just as frustrating to run out of these items as it is to run out of a broad-spectrum antibiotic.

Most veterinary practices use the first in, first out (**FIFO**) method of inventory. This is not necessarily done by choice but rather because of the expiration dates on merchandise that the practice sells. Generally speaking, the expiration date that is the earliest should be sold first. A perpetual inventory control system, which is a detailed record for each type of merchandise stocked, shows the following:

- Units and costs of the beginning inventory
- Units and costs of each purchase
- Units and costs of the goods for each sale
- Units and costs of the goods on hand at any point in time

Luckily, most veterinary computer management software programs do the above listed items automatically. In today's business world, inventory is much easier to keep up with than it was in the days of periodic inventory, when businesses did not have computers (Libby,

Libby, & Short, 2004). However, it is better to use a balance between a perpetual inventory control system and a periodic inventory because sometimes the amount of each item listed within the computer system may not be a true reflection of what is actually on hand. Nothing can ever take the place of a periodic inventory and physically counting the amount of each item on hand. The primary disadvantage of a periodic inventory system is the lack of inventory information that is available to the practice owner; that is, veterinary management software makes inventory easier because it shows up-to-date amounts of each item sold, along with trends during the summer or winter months that can help staff to decide how much inventory needs to be purchased in the coming years.

Inventory is an ongoing process, and trends within the practice must be observed daily. The ICM must be able to recognize the products that each veterinarian in the practice uses and dispenses, to ensure that items are on hand when needed. Nothing is more frustrating than needing a drug or other inventory item to treat a patient with, only to find it is not in stock. Computer software designed for the veterinary business can help tremendously with tracking trends within the practice. Most software has the ability to provide printouts of day-by-day, week-by-week, month-by-month, and yearly sales trends (Fig. 19.2).

Through the establishment of a workable inventory control system within a realistic budget, expenses can be kept at a minimum.

 TECHNICIAN NOTES

For many veterinary practices, inventory represents the second-highest expense. Payroll is usually the highest overhead item.

After determination and implementation of a realistic budget that might be based on the mission statement of the facility and practice needs, followed by implementation of that budget, there should be no danger of running out of inventory items because there always should be sufficient quantities of product on hand. An annual inventory evaluation is beneficial when a vision for the practice and its potential growth has been developed.

℞ The Time Equation

When one is dealing with inventory, no equation is more important than the following:

$$\text{Time} = \text{Money}$$

Date: 05-21-20

Inventory report

Page: 4
Anthelmintics

Code	Description	U/M	Price	On hand	Avg cost	Stock value	Unit cost	Pkg. cost	cost	Codes Cls	Last sold	Document
May	Jun	Jul	Aug	Sep	Oct	Nov	Dec	Jan	Feb	Mar	Apr	May
		Anthelmintics					**0.00**					
Canine vaccines												
1008	Bordetalla (Injection)	Ds	0.00	14	0.000	0.00	0.000	0.000		1		
Qty sold, last 12 months												
May	Jun	Jul	Aug	Sep	Oct	Nov	Dec	Jan	Feb	Mar	Apr	May
1009	Bordetalla (Intra-nasal)	Ds	0.00	1	0.000	0.00	0.000	0.000		0		
Qty sold, last 12 months												
May	Jun	Jul	Aug	Sep	Oct	Nov	Dec	Jan	Feb	Mar	Apr	May
9010	DA2PP/CV	Ds	0.00	15	0.000	0.00	0.000	0.000		0		
Qty sold, last 12 months												
May	Jun	Jul	Aug	Sep	Oct	Nov	Dec	Jan	Feb	Mar	Apr	May
9052	Rabies vaccine	Ds	0.00	21	0.000	0.00	0.000	0.000		1		
Qty sold, last 12 months												
May	Jun	Jul	Aug	Sep	Oct	Nov	Dec	Jan	Feb	Mar	Apr	May
		Canine vaccines					**0.00**					
Miscellaneous items												
1007	Large garbage sacks	Box	0.00	0	0.000	0.00	0.000	0.000		1		May
Qty sold, last 12 months												
May	Jun	Jul	Aug	Sep	Oct	Nov	Dec	Jan	Feb	Mar	Apr	
7022	Small garbage sacks	Box	0.00	0	0.000	0.00	0.000	0.000		1		May
Qty sold, last 12 months												
May	Jun	Jul	Aug	Sep	Oct	Nov	Dec	Jan	Feb	Mar	Apr	
7023	Computer printer paper	Pack	0.00	0	0.000	0.00	0.000	0.000		1		May
Qty sold, last 12 months												
May	Jun	Jul	Aug	Sep	Oct	Nov	Dec	Jan	Feb	Mar	Apr	

Fig. 19.2 AVI-Mark Veterinary Software Management System (McAllister Software Systems, Piedmont, MO).

Although it is important to have merchandise on hand for retail sale, a fine balance is needed to keep products from sitting too long on pharmacy shelves. Products that stay on the shelf for too long will not make money for the veterinary practice. Instead, this is similar to placing money in a jar and burying it in the backyard; the money is there, but it is not earning interest and it is not working for you. It is the same with inventory products. A fine inventory balance is crucial to the financial health of a business. In addition, clients do not like to buy products that have been sitting on pharmacy shelves for a long time because the labels begin to show signs of age or the products are dusty.

A periodic evaluation of inventory is crucial for keeping the balance in fine adjustment. Items that are not selling well or are used infrequently within the practice should be deleted from the inventory master list and should not be ordered in the future. Turnover, then, becomes an important issue.

Turnover

Inventory turnover is the number of times inventory is sold and replenished each year. This indicates how frequently the practice sells its physical products. The more frequently the inventory is turned, the greater the profit to the practice. Storing inventory costs money; inventory is not generating money when it sits on the shelf.

TECHNICIAN NOTES

- Turnover is the number of times a product is sold or used in-house on an annual basis.
- The ideal situation is to use all inventory each month and reorder in time to begin the next month because there are 12 months in a year. However, in the real world, this simply does not happen.
- Four turnovers are a workable goal, and 12 turnovers may be set as the ideal goal. A mean turnover rate of eight turns per year is acceptable for most veterinary practices.

Calculating Average Cost of Inventory on Hand

The average cost of inventory on hand is determined by the year's beginning inventory plus the year's ending inventory divided by 2.

The following equation determines the **average cost of inventory on hand**:

Average cost of inventory on hand =
$$\frac{\text{Year's beginning inventory} + \text{Year's ending inventory}}{2}$$

Example:

$$\frac{\$150,000 + \$35,000}{2} = \$92,500$$

Calculating Turnover Rate

Inventory turnover rate is calculated by dividing the yearly inventory expense by the average cost of inventory on hand.

The following equation is used to determine **turnover rate**:

$$\text{Turnover rate} = \frac{\text{Yearly inventory expense}}{\text{Average cost of inventory on hand}}$$

Example:

$$\frac{\$100,000}{\$20,000} = 5$$

CONTROLLING INVENTORY

Establishing effective inventory control in a veterinary practice necessitates placing a person in charge of ordering and stocking supplies. An additional person trained as a backup is a must because when the ICM goes on vacation or is sick, someone else must be knowledgeable about the system. These two people can work effectively as a team to keep product supplies on hand.

The duties of the ICM are intense. This person is responsible for keeping an adequate supply of all products used, dispensed, and sold; organizing inventory items for easy location; identifying when products should be reordered; keeping accurate inventory records; ordering, receiving, and inspecting shipments; and maintaining price and price updates for all items. The ICM also is responsible for rotating stock, keeping expired items off the shelves, learning about new products, and keeping the practice owner apprised of the specials that suppliers may offer. This responsibility must be acted on every day. The veterinary technician who accepts the role of ICM must be able to perform clinical and nursing duties as well as manage inventory levels.

TECHNICIAN NOTES

The objectives of an inventory control system are two-fold:
1. To make certain that items are on hand when needed
2. To be able to purchase needed items while staying within a budget

Proactive Inventory Control System

For an inventory control system to be workable, it must be easy to use and have a turnover rate of at least four turns per year. It is the ICM's job to make sure that all supplies are on hand when needed. Expenses can be reduced when inventory amounts are ordered properly.

Proper handling of Drug Enforcement Administration (DEA) substances is an important concern.

TECHNICIAN NOTES

Controlled substances (e.g., Sleepaway, diazepam) must be kept in a locked cabinet and all amounts used must be correctly recorded in the controlled substance log.

Each pharmaceutical company has their own policy regarding ordering controlled substances. Therefore, it is best to check with the company prior to placing an order so that proper policy can be followed.

Each invoice (Fig. 19.3) that arrives at the veterinary hospital should be checked to verify amounts ordered

---

The Pharmaceutical Warehouse
1546 Warehouse Road
Plains, Georgia 36945

INVOICE

Ship to:
All Pets Veterinary Hospital
1785 Lawrenceville Road
Lawrenceville, Georgia 37965

Bill to:
All Pets Veterinary Hospital
1785 Lawrenceville Road
Lawrenceville, Georgia 37965

Bill to	Invoice total
A7796	$335.10
Invoice number	**Invoice date**
953146-000	10-20-19
Customer account number	**Ship to**
198531	Lawrenceville, Georgia

Item code	Unit/Size	Description/ Strength	Quantity Ordered	Quantity Shipped	Item Status	Unit price	Extension	Box No.	REM
15637	18/box	Vetrap	3	3	Sent	$54.95	$164.85	1	
15937	9/pack	Gauze bandage rolls	5	5	Sent	$25.65	$128.25	1	
13465	Each	Roll cotton	12	12	Sent	$3.50	$42.00	1	

• *Please note that late payments are subject to a 1.5% monthly finance charge*

Merchandise total
$335.10

Invoice total
$335.10

* Please pay within thirty days of receipt of this invoice.

Fig. 19.3 A sample invoice.

The Pharmaceutical Warehouse

PACKING LIST

Ship to:
All Pets Veterinary Hospital
1785 Lawrenceville Road
Lawrenceville, Georgia 37965

Bill to:
All Pets Veterinary Hospital
1785 Lawrenceville Road
Lawrenceville, Georgia 37965

Customer account number	Ship to
198531	Lawrenceville, Georgia

Item code	Unit/Size	Description/ Strength	Quantity Ordered	Quantity Shipped	Item Status	Unit price	Extension	Box No.	REM
15637	18/box	Vetrap	3	3	Sent	$54.95	$164.85	1	
15937	9/pack	Gauze bandage rolls	5	5	Sent	$25.65	$128.25	1	
13465	Each	Roll cotton	12	12	Sent	$3.50	$42.00	1	

Fig. 19.4 A sample packing slip. (Some vendors do not record prices on their packing slips.)

and prices the practice is charged. A packing slip (Fig. 19.4), an invoice, and a statement (Fig. 19.5) are three different forms. Mistakes can be made on these forms unintentionally by the product vendor, but it may fall to the ICM to audit these mistakes and notify the vendor so the account can be adjusted to receive proper credit.

Backordered items can present problems. Backordered items are those items not on hand at the vendor for any number of reasons. Sometimes, the product may be on backorder for manufacturing reasons; or it may be that the manufacturer is redesigning the product's label. Buyouts of large pharmaceutical corporations also can cause product to be on backorder until all minor details are worked out concerning the merger.

Identification of expired items may be one of the most frustrating experiences an ICM may face.

 TECHNICIAN NOTES

Most products have an expiration date on the label, and these must be checked frequently so they can be removed from the pharmacy when they are out-of-date.

Veterinary practice management systems software can be an invaluable aid in tracking expired items. When products are received, the *earliest* expiration date should

be the one that is recorded in the computer system. Therefore, at the beginning of each month, the computer will reflect those products that expire first, and the ICM can print a list of the old drugs and quickly remove them from the pharmacy. As soon as the old products have been removed from the pharmacy shelves, the next earliest expiration date is recorded in the computer. Some pharmaceutical companies have policies that entitle the practice to free replacement of expired items. However, other vendors do not concur with this arrangement; therefore, the ICM must be able to distinguish which expired product will produce a free product refund and which will not. Some pharmaceutical companies prefer to credit the facility's account instead of sending replacement merchandise; others offer no reimbursement whatsoever for expired items.

It is hoped that pilferage will not occur in the veterinary facility. However, an effective inventory control system will deter employees who may elect to steal because they know that inventory is counted on a regular basis. Likewise, merchandise displayed (e.g., leashes, collars, shampoo, grooming brushes) in the reception area of a veterinary facility can be enticing to some clients who may decide to "pick up" an item instead of paying for it. This is another reason why proper inventory control plays an important role.

The Pharmaceutical Warehouse
1546 Warehouse Road
Plains, Georgia 36945

STATEMENT

0100000034569786221321313213213213245656654

Statement Date	Account Number	Due Date
10-20-19	198531	10-20-19
New Balance	Indicate Amount Enclosed	
$335.10		

The Pharmaceutical Warehouse
1546 Warehouse Road
Plains, Georgia 36945

Please detach here and return the above portion with yhour payment

Questions? Call 1-800-897-3679

Account Name	Account Number	Statement Date	Statement Number	Page
All Pets Veterinary Hospital	198531	10-20-19	3596342	1 of 1

BALANCE SUMMARY

Previous Balance	Add Purchases	Payments	Credits	Late Charge	Adjustments	Balance Due
$120.00	$335.10	$120.00	0.00	0.00	0.00	$335.10

ACCOUNT AGING

1-30 Days Past Due	31-60 Days Past Due	61-90 Days Past Due	91-120 Days Past Due	>120 Days Past Due	Current Balance
0.00	0.00	0.00	0.00	0.00	$335.10

Fig. 19.5 A sample statement.

℞ Keeping Accurate Records

An orderly way of keeping track of data regarding inventory should be employed. Most veterinary facilities in this age of computer technology use software designed especially for the veterinary business. Remember, when dealing with computers, the old adage—"garbage in, garbage out" ("GIGO")—can detract from the quality of information that a computer contains.

℞ Inventory Records

Many types of inventory records may be used in a veterinary facility. At least some of the following should be used, although some practices may elect to use them all.

A reorder log, sometimes called a "want book" (Fig. 19.6), is an effective way to track products to be ordered. Each member of the veterinary staff can use this log to record items that should be ordered.

Reorder Log

Date of Order	Amount	Item Description	Catalog Number	Cost		Extended Cost	
10-17-19	6	Sharps' containers	796029	$ 3	79	$ 22	74
10-17-19	3 boxes	Tuberculin slyringes	194356	$ 9	59	$ 28	77
10-18-19	6 boxes	Needles 22ga. x 3/4"	355796	$ 7	50	$ 45	00

Fig. 19.6 An example of a reorder log.

TECHNICIAN NOTES

All veterinary personnel should know the importance of maintaining inventory and should make every effort to record in the reorder log any product that has been depleted.

In a busy practice, this habit is of utmost importance because once supplies have been exhausted, obtaining interim product from the neighboring veterinary facility becomes an "emergency." Afterward, the amounts borrowed must be replaced or paid for.

TECHNICIAN NOTES

The reorder point is the level reached that necessitates a product reorder.

It is the responsibility of the ICM to set the reorder point. If orders are placed each week, then a minimum of a 3-week supply should be kept in stock. Larger veterinary hospitals, emergency clinics, and colleges of veterinary medicine may require that inventory be ordered via a purchase order. A purchase order is a written form accompanied by a purchase order number. Generally, the form is mailed, although it may be faxed to the vendor, who then will send the merchandise.

TECHNICIAN NOTES

In keeping basic order records, it is imperative to keep a copy of each order.

Regardless of whether a purchase order form is mailed to the vendor or an order is given over the phone, all of the following items should be recorded: order date, order amount, order size, name of the product, vendor(s), product catalogue number, unit cost, total cost, receive date, amount received, and discount or special cost (if applicable). When these items are kept in a written form, an inaccurate order can be corrected easily by contacting the company involved.

An inventory master list provides endless quantities of information. Each veterinary practice should strive to keep a current list of all products in stock. An inventory master list provides information such as name of the product, item number code, usage, order status, and price. Some veterinary management software includes information regarding the seasonal use of products. One category in which this may be important is the area of flea and tick products. Today's computer software designed for veterinary businesses has the ability to reflect the months during which the greatest amount of product was sold. For instance, it may be that flea and tick shampoo is purchased more frequently during the months of March through September compared with other times of the year. By using this information, the ICM can better predict how much merchandise should be ordered. The master list also reflects trade names, generic names, unit size, strength, name of the product's manufacturer, phone numbers, addresses, practice account numbers, order information, unit price, and a formula for calculating markup. (Some of these items are optional.)

TECHNICIAN NOTES

Markup is the difference between the actual cost of the item and the selling price (usually as a percentage). Margin is how much actual profit the practice is making on each sale.

There is a difference between cost and retail value. Cost is what the practice pays for an item. *Total cost* is the amount the item costs plus tax. The retail price is the amount the practice charges a client for an item. Retail price usually includes a profit margin. Each practice has a way of figuring markup, and the percentages used may vary. A common way to figure total cost is to multiply the product's cost by the appropriate tax. When the total cost of an item is obtained and is multiplied by 2, a 100% markup (i.e., retail price) is the result. This is illustrated below.

The following is an equation to figure **total cost**:

$$Cost + Tax = Total\ cost$$

Example:

Amoxicillin(100 mg,100 tablets in bottle) cost = $26.75

$$Tax\ (@\ 10\%) = 0.100$$
$$\$26.75 \times 0.100 = \$2.675$$
$$\$26.75 + \$2.675 = \$29.425$$

The following shows how to find retail price @ 100% markup:

$$Total\ cost\ of\ the\ item \times 2$$
$$= Retail\ Price\ @\ 100\%\ markup$$

$$\$29.43 \times 2 = \$58.86$$

Then : $58.86 divided by 100 tablets in the bottle
= 0.5886 or $0.59 each

Thus, each tablet can be retailed for $0.59 (or $0.60 to make accounting easier).

Reorder Quantity

When the reorder quantity is determined, a good idea is to set the amount equal to a 1-month supply. By ordering a 1-month supply of product, the ICM will not have to micromanage inventory. The reorder quantity can be posted on the computer's master inventory list.

Rabies Vaccine

Records regarding rabies vaccine are very important. Each rabies certificate reflects the vaccine's expiration date and serial number (Fig. 19.7). Therefore, the ICM must ensure that the certificates reflect those numbers by checking that the serial number and expiration date are posted correctly in the computer. This is not optional; it *must* be done.

Organizing Inventory
Pharmacy and Inventory Control Manager Office

> **TECHNICIAN NOTES**
>
> A room in the veterinary facility that is set up to serve as the pharmacy office and the ICM office provides a place to organize catalogs, journals, magazines, and sales lists.

Other items, such as DEA order records, Occupational Safety and Health Administration (OSHA) manuals, material safety data sheets (MSDSs), and suppliers' catalogues, also can be stored in the pharmacy office.

Organizing Inventory in the Veterinary Hospital

The ideal situation for organizing inventory in the veterinary hospital is to establish a centrally located pharmacy area. In this manner, all pharmaceutics can be counted easily. Inventory can be arranged alphabetically, by drug class (i.e., antibiotics, antiparasitics, gastrointestinal), etc.

> **TECHNICIAN NOTES**
>
> Inventory within the pharmacy area can be arranged in a variety of ways. The most common ways to arrange products are alphabetically, by therapeutic use, or by classification of the drug.

An easy way to organize inventory is to print the master inventory list and then stock products on the shelf in the same way that they are listed on the master list. In this way, when it is time to perform inventory, products are arranged on the pharmacy shelves in the same order they appear on the master inventory list, thereby enabling inventory to be performed in a timely fashion.

Staff Memos

> **TECHNICIAN NOTES**
>
> The ICM should designate a bulletin board for memos to the veterinary staff.

Memos attached to a bulletin board can alert all hospital staff of company buyouts, discontinued items, and backordered items. The use of a bulletin board provides the ICM with freedom from frustrating interruptions by office staff concerning inventory questions. Additionally, this bulletin board is a good location for the reorder log (i.e., "want book").

Special Conditions

Some special conditions must be recognized when one is arranging inventory. Products that require refrigeration have only a limited amount of storage space in the refrigerator. Care should be taken to avoid ordering too large a quantity of these items because the available amount of refrigeration may not be able to contain the order amount. DEA substances must be kept in a locked cabinet. The space within the cabinet should be considered before increased amounts of merchandise are ordered. Some bulky items and large volume purchases may need to be placed in other storage areas. It is important that other staff members know where the bulk items are stored.

Physical Inventory
Monthly Inventory Versus Rotating Inventory

When and how often to perform this necessary function needs to be decided. One effective method is to perform a rotating inventory. A rotating inventory necessitates the division of like products into categories. These categories are given a number of one through four. For example, each category designated as one is counted during the month of January. Each category designated as two is counted during the month of February; three is

CERTIFICATE OF VACCINATION

Date of rabies vaccination	16 MAY 19
Next rabies vaccination on	16 MAY 20
Certificate number	N/A
Previous rabies vaccination	N/A
Best Veterinary Hospital	
Taylor Lane, DVM	
621 Banner Street	
Camden, Arkansas 71701	
501-536-8390	
Owner's name	**Best Veterinary Client**
Owner's address	**1313 Schnauzer Lane** **Camden, Arkansas 71701**
County of owner's residence	Ouachita

This is to certify...
That I have vaccinated against rabies the animal described below:

Patient Information and Signalment	
Patient's name	Tangent
Species	Canine
Breed	Mix
Gender	Male/Neutered
Color and markings	Brindle/White on chest
Tag number	N/A
Weight	101.4 lbs.
Age	2 years

Signed: _Taylor Lane, DVM_

Vaccinations administered:

Vaccines administered
RV/DA2PP/CV/Bordetella

Rabies Vaccine Information	
Manufactured by	Zoetis Animal Health
Serial number	A232705A
Lot expiration date	26 NOV 20
Administration of vaccine	SC right hind

Fig. 19.7 A sample rabies certificate.

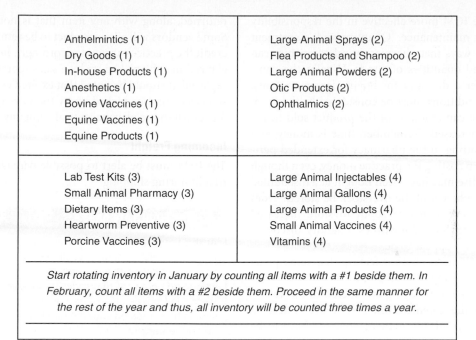

Anthelmintics (1)	Large Animal Sprays (2)
Dry Goods (1)	Flea Products and Shampoo (2)
In-house Products (1)	Large Animal Powders (2)
Anesthetics (1)	Otic Products (2)
Bovine Vaccines (1)	Ophthalmics (2)
Equine Vaccines (1)	
Equine Products (1)	
Lab Test Kits (3)	Large Animal Injectables (4)
Small Animal Pharmacy (3)	Large Animal Gallons (4)
Dietary Items (3)	Large Animal Products (4)
Heartworm Preventive (3)	Small Animal Vaccines (4)
Porcine Vaccines (3)	Vitamins (4)

Start rotating inventory in January by counting all items with a #1 beside them. In February, count all items with a #2 beside them. Proceed in the same manner for the rest of the year and thus, all inventory will be counted three times a year.

Fig. 19.8 An example of how to divide inventory.

counted in March, and four in April. During the month of May, the inventory begins again, starting with those categories designated with number one. Thus, each category is counted three times a year (Fig. 19.8). Although this may not be acceptable to all veterinary practice owners, it certainly can be an efficient way to perform a physical inventory. This process allows for monitoring overstock items, accurate inventory of what is available on hand (in stock on the shelves), and identify expired or soon to expire items. Often, only one person is responsible for inventory control within the veterinary facility, and counting every item stocked in a practice may take a single person 1 to 2 days to complete. If inventory is done on a monthly basis (i.e., all items counted each month), the ICM cannot perform other nursing or technical duties on the day inventory is taken. When a rotating method is used, a smaller amount of inventory is counted each month, thus enabling the ICM to have time available to perform other job duties.

Some practice owners may require a monthly inventory count. However, performing inventory on a rotational 3- to 4-month cycle makes the ICM's job easier. A veterinary technician may perform many functions in a veterinary practice; use of a rotating inventory ensures an accurate count and good use of the veterinary technician's nursing skills.

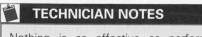 Purchasing Information

In a busy veterinary facility, an ideal situation is to deal with as few suppliers as possible. The ICM will constantly be involved in an appointment with sales representatives if various vendors are used. Dealing with as few suppliers as possible releases the ICM to perform regular nursing and technical duties required by the facility. If sales representatives are asked to make an appointment, the ICM will know when to expect a visit and can better prepare the normal work schedule around this visit. The ICM should ensure that sales representatives are aware of lunch breaks and quitting time; otherwise, they may just "pop in" to make a sale without considering the ICM's schedule.

In dealing with pharmaceutical and supplier sales representatives, it is advantageous to be aware of several things. Knowledge of the following information

---

TECHNICIAN NOTES

Nothing is as effective as performing a physical inventory.

will make the ICM more effective in the responsibility of inventory maintenance. Quantity and assortment discounts are ways that pharmaceutical companies can offer increased quantities of goods. Usually, the company will offer a discount for buying larger amounts, but several conditions must be considered by the ICM. First, how fast can amounts of the product sold in the practice be increased? Remember, time is money, and product left sitting in the pharmacy for extended periods will end up costing the practice money, even though the merchandise may have been bought at a discounted rate. Second, where will the overstock be stored? Does the practice have sufficient room to store increased quantities of product? Sometimes, quantity discounts are not what they appear to be.

Delayed billing is another feature that some pharmaceutical and supplier companies may offer. When discounts for quantity buying are offered to the veterinary practice, the statement often will reflect a delayed billing option (i.e., the statement does not have to be paid within the usual 30-day span). Instead, the option of paying within a 60- to 90-day period will extend the discount. Usually, no interest is charged to the buyer, and the practice owner may be able to purchase increased amounts of stock at a reduced rate without the trial of coming up with funds to pay for it all within a 30-day limit. Consideration must still be given to whether sufficient room exists for storage of overstock and how soon the product can be sold.

When an order is placed, many companies waive the shipping fee if the veterinary practice orders a minimum amount of product. For example, if the minimum order amount is $250 per order, the ICM can save the practice shipping fees by ordering the minimum amount. Keep in mind that a shipping fee of $10 when multiplied over 10 orders adds up to $100. Shipping costs multiplied by 12 months could be used to buy other products instead of being spent on shipping fees.

Some pharmaceutical and supplier companies offer discounts for early payment. Veterinary practices can save money by paying the statement early. This too is a way to save the practice money. On the other hand, penalties may be imposed for statements paid after the 30-day time limit. The amount paid in penalties can also buy product instead of being spent on late fees. Every practice should endeavor to pay within 30 days.

The ICM should be familiar with each vendor's return policy. Items that are expired may have to be returned, along with any item that is not selling well. Some vendors will allow product to be returned and will credit the practice's account accordingly. Items that have expired may be picked up by a sales representative and replaced. It should be noted that expired controlled substances cannot be picked up by the sales representative for return to the pharmaceutical company.

Incoming Freight

The ICM must be alert to possible damage incurred to freight during shipping.

 TECHNICIAN NOTES

> At the time freight is being unloaded at the veterinary facility, the ICM should visually check for damage by noting any boxes that are not intact. Wetness to the cardboard container may indicate breakage of the contents, and boxes should be counted and the number should be compared with the number of containers listed on the packing slip.

As soon as freight arrives, it should be opened and any damage should be noted. Evidence of damage should be reported to the vendor as soon as possible so that credit can be received and/or damaged items replaced. Some companies have a 24-hour reporting period (i.e., all damaged items must be reported within 24 hours of arrival time). Damaged goods should be returned to the vendor from which they were ordered, in the original shipping carton with the damaged goods inside. In this way, the vendor can assess the damage and correctly apply credit to the veterinary facility's account.

Free on Board Rules and Shipment Contracts

A vendor delivers freight to the purchaser. The veterinary facility may make an order with a telephone representative, email or fax a purchase order, or make an order with the sales representative during his or her appointment at the veterinary facility. A shipment contract is one in which the seller turns the goods over to a carrier for delivery to the buyer. The seller has no responsibility for seeing that the goods reach their destination. In a shipment contract, both title and risk of loss pass to the buyer when the goods are given to the carrier. Shipment contracts are often designated by the term *FOB Place of Shipment* (such as FOB Camden, Arkansas). When goods are sent **FOB** (free on board) followed by place of shipment, they will be delivered free to the place of shipment. The buyer must pay all shipping charges from there to the place of destination. The terms indicate that title to the goods and risk of loss pass at the point of origin. Delivery to the carrier by the seller and acceptance by the carrier completes the transfer of both title and risk of loss. Therefore, the buyer accepts full responsibility during the transit of goods (Brown & Sukys, 2006).

A vendor uses a form of transportation to send required items to the veterinary hospital (e.g., UPS [United Parcel Service], Averitt Express, Federal Express, or U.S. Postal Service). Once the vendor releases freight to the carrier, the freight becomes subject to two FOB rules: FOB destination and FOB shipping point.

TECHNICIAN NOTES

Vendors place different terms of delivery on freight that is leaving a pharmaceutical facility. Basically, FOB rules state which business (vendor or buyer) has the title to freight and who will be responsible in cases of loss of freight when the vendor uses outside transportation companies to deliver goods. **FOB destination** means that the title of ownership (freight) is being passed from the vendor to the purchaser, and said freight becomes the property of the purchaser when the shipment is delivered to the veterinary hospital. **FOB shipping point** means that the title of ownership (freight) passes from the vendor to the purchaser when the vendor places the goods in possession of a carrier. FOB shipping point requires the purchaser to determine what responsibility the carrier will take if damage or loss occurs to freight. The ICM should realize that shipments can be refused (not signed for) on delivery. In such cases, if the ICM deems that damage has or may have occurred because of the condition of the shipping container, the shipment may be refused, in which case the carrier will send the goods back to the vendor.

Receiving Freight

TECHNICIAN NOTES

It is best to allow the person who placed the order to unpack the freight once the order has been received.

If the order is incorrect, the person who placed the order will know it immediately, whereas a person unpacking freight who did not place the order will not know what is correct. Several important questions should be asked when one is unpacking an order, such as "Did I get exactly what I ordered?"; "Did I get the right drug form (i.e., capsules, tablets, or powder)?"; "Did I receive the correct size and/or strength?"; "Is the product's expiration date far enough into the future?"; "Does the invoice list the price I was quoted by the phone representative or sales representative?"; "Does this order cost more than the last order of the same items?"; "Is anything backordered, and if so, when will that item be shipped?"; "Is any freight damaged or missing?"; and "Is the order correct, and if so, can the bill be paid?" (Lukens & Landon, 1993). By asking all these questions, the ICM is assured that the veterinary facility will be treated fairly by the vendor.

Stocking Shelves

TECHNICIAN NOTES

It should be remembered when shelves are stocked that newly received items should be placed behind older items, so that the old is used and/or sold first.

When stock is rotated in this manner, the facility is assured that the product is sold or used by the hospital before the expiration date. When stocking shelves, the ICM should record expiration dates. The earliest date should be the one recorded in the computer, so the software will present an accurate list of expired items when the command is given to print an expired items list. Stocking shelves also presents a convenient time to dust and wipe off labels and lids on products that have been sitting on the shelf for extended periods. It should be noted that after cleaning, products should be replaced in specific locations to facilitate accurate inventory.

Vendors

Several different types of vendors may be used. The ICM must have adequate knowledge of these types to correctly place an order. Some vendors allow ordering by phone; others require that the order be given to a sales representative. Still others require a faxed order or an order sent through the mail.

Full-service companies are those that send a sales representative to visit the veterinary facility and offer full service. A technical staff, usually made up of veterinarians, is employed. Full-service companies usually carry a limited product line. Some products may be newly developed products that still retain a patent with the federal government and cannot be ordered through a distributorship. A full-service company has sales representatives who call on the veterinary hospital and take orders. Most full-service companies will replace outdated product with new or will credit the hospital's account accordingly.

 TECHNICIAN NOTES

The sales representative may not pick up expired controlled substances; these must be mailed back to the company.

A full-service company may have several "deals" that the ICM must decide to accept or decline. Examples of full-service companies include Pfizer Animal Health, Pharmacia-Upjohn, Schering-Plough Animal Health, and Fort Dodge Animal Health. These companies employ veterinarians as technical support staff, and their product lines are often limited compared with distributorships. However, full-service companies are forerunners in the development of new drugs protected under U.S. patent laws, in which case they may not be sold under a generic name until the patent expires.

Mail order discount houses provide a good source for ordering items such as gauze, syringes, needles, paper towels, paper drapes, and even isopropyl alcohol. Ordering from this type of vendor occurs over the telephone because most do not employ sales representatives to visit the hospital, although catalogues may be supplied and mailed to the buyer.

Veterinary supply distributors provide the most common way of acquiring supplies for the veterinary facility. A distributor is an intermediate between a full-service company and the mail order discount house. If a full-service company gives its approval and a contract is signed between two companies, some products normally sold only through a full-service company may be obtained from a distributor. Many times, products sold by the full-service company to the distributor are those with a patent about to expire or those with an already expired patent. The distributor may elect to sell under a generic name instead of the full-service company's trade name. A distributorship usually maintains a huge inventory and employs sales representatives who call on veterinary facilities. Products ordered from a

distributorship should be documented carefully. Should expired product need to be returned, the ICM may have to provide invoice numbers to prove which distributorship the product was purchased from before credit is applied to the facility's account.

Communicating With Sales Representatives

It is important for the ICM to be certain that sales representatives that visit the facility are aware of certain things. Sales representatives should know the ICM's scheduled lunch and quitting times. Additionally, the ICM should make sure that the sales representative is aware that all emergencies take priority over scheduled sales appointments. It is usually best to schedule an appointment with a visiting sales representative because this is much easier than having to drop other responsibilities in order to talk to the representative.

Drug Enforcement Administration Forms

Dealing with U.S. DEA forms can be a frustrating experience if they are not handled correctly. However, if certain rules are kept in mind, ordering controlled substances need not be stressful.

 TECHNICIAN NOTES

All veterinarians have a DEA number assigned to them and their veterinary license. This number is private and should never be given out for any reason.

Forms must be ordered from the DEA and kept in a secure location once mailed to the veterinarian. **DEA forms** are multicopy forms (i.e., carbon copies are made). The veterinarian keeps a copy of the order for his or her records. All information contained on these forms must be correct. Important considerations to keep in mind when one is filling out these forms include no markouts, no use of correction fluid or tape, no misspellings or incorrect drug strength, and inclusion of the veterinarian's signature on the form. These forms must be filled out with an ink pen or typewriter.

Special Orders

Often, clients may require "special orders." Clients must be made aware that once a "special order" is made, it must be purchased. If this is not understood, the veterinary facility may have to hold on to a slow-moving item or one that is never sold at all. Once this "special order" has been received by the hospital, the ICM should let the client know that the item has arrived. It is best to place these "special orders" near the receptionist's desk because the ICM may be busy with other duties when the client arrives to pick up the order.

Human Pharmacy

At various times, the veterinary practitioner may have to use a human pharmacy to supply drugs for clients' pets. A veterinarian may call the order into the pharmacy or provide the order on a written prescription. Keeping a good working relationship between pharmacist and veterinarian is important because a pharmacist may have additional knowledge about pharmaceutical products.

℞ Computers and Inventory

The advent of computer software technology has made inventory easier for all businesses. Many types of veterinary management software programs are available. Most programs offer features such as provisions for entering client information, inventory control, print-out of common forms (e.g., rabies certificates), medical history, and accounting information. It is important to enter all inventory products used for each patient because the software has the ability to automatically subtract inventory amounts used. This is where "GIGO" is very important. Although each employee has good intentions, the ICM may find discrepancies in the total amount of product on hand. Staff meetings represent a good time to remind employees of the importance of "GIGO." All newly received inventory items must be added to amounts already posted in the computer. Bar coding is available on most pharmaceutical products. Using a device capable of reading bar codes greatly enhances the counting and maintaining of inventory.

Additionally, most software can be used to produce automatic expiration lists from computer files each month. Utilizing the management software program to track expiration dates is important; the system allows for entry of expiration dates for each product. The total amount of money spent on inventory in a day, week, month, or year can be obtained when computer software systems are used.

℞ The Job of Inventory Control Manager

It cannot be overemphasized how important inventory control is to the veterinary facility. Veterinary technician who are willing to take on this added responsibility will find themselves to be invaluable members of the staff. Keeping in mind that inventory is the second highest expense for the veterinary hospital will enable the ICM to use care when considering sales offers. Understanding the practice's mission is crucial in inventory control. Remember, time is money, and product left sitting on the shelf for extended periods does not benefit the facility. Keeping a turnover of at least four turns per year is a minimum goal. Training a backup person to monitor inventory during times of vacation or sickness experienced by the ICM is crucial. Reminding employees during staff meetings of the importance of "GIGO" and documenting items in low supply on the reorder log will allow the facility to keep a continuous supply of needed product on hand. DEA products must be controlled by effective documentation of their use in a log book kept solely for this purpose (e.g., controlled substance log book).

Many other factors are also important. Establishing a formula for markup is critical. The way inventory is arranged within the pharmacy has a great deal to do with the ease of counting it. No better method of counting inventory can replace doing a physical inventory. Keep sales representatives abreast of lunch breaks and leaving times. Carefully observe all freight for damage, and report claims as soon as possible after receiving the product. Always rotate product on shelves so that the oldest product is sold first. Be knowledgeable about the different types of vendors. Decide which method of inventory counting is most advantageous to your particular situation by deciding whether to count all inventory monthly or on a rotating basis. Keep a good relationship with a local pharmacy because these businesses serve as a valuable source of knowledge and enable the veterinarian to order human products not normally sold through veterinary vendors. Decide whether a manual or a computerized system is best for your facility. However, keep in mind that, in this age of technology, a computer system facilitates efficient work flow.

REVIEW QUESTIONS

1. What is inventory?
2. Name the five principles used to control expenses:
   a. _____
   b. _____
   c. _____
   d. _____
   e. _____

3. When dealing with inventory, it is crucial to remember that time is _____.

4. Define the term "turnover."

5. Calculate the turnover rate by using the following information: Yearly inventory expense = $125,000; average cost of inventory on hand = $31,250.

6. Calculate the average cost of inventory on hand by using the following information: Year's beginning inventory = $75,000; year's ending inventory = $130,000.

7. Name two objectives of an inventory control system.

8. What is a packing slip?

9. What is an invoice?

10. What is a statement?

11. What is the reorder point?

12. Why is recording the expiration date and serial number for rabies vaccine so important?

13. Once the reorder point is reached, a basic rule of thumb is to order a _____ month supply.

14. List some rules for filling out a DEA form.

15. Time = Money.
    a. True
    b. False

16. A mean turnover rate of _____ is acceptable for most veterinary practices.
    a. 12
    b. 4
    c. 2
    d. 8

17. Inventory should be placed on pharmacy shelves in such a way so as to ensure _____.
    a. LILO
    b. FIFO

c. FOB
d. ICM

18. DEA forms are issued by _____.
    a. state governments
    b. county governments
    c. city governments
    d. the federal government

19. The expiration date and the serial number of rabies vaccine administered must be recorded on each pet's rabies certificate.
    a. True
    b. False

20. When a DEA form is used to order a controlled substance, it is acceptable to draw a line through a misspelled word and then write it correctly beside the mistake.
    a. True
    b. False

21. The percent difference between the actual cost of an item and the price the item sold for is called:
    a. Reorder point
    b. Markup
    c. Average cost
    d. Statement

22. Why is it important to perform an actual physical inventory of items?

23. Why is it important to have the person who placed the order also unpack the freight order?

24. What process should be used when stocking shelves with newly received items?

25. Inventory reports printed off from the practice management software system can be used for what purpose?

REFERENCES

Brown, G. W., & Sukys, P. A. (2006). *Business law with UCC applications* (11th ed.). New York: McGraw-Hill Irwin.

Libby, R., Libby, P., & Short, D. G. (2004). *Financial accounting* (4th ed.). New York: McGraw-Hill Irwin.

Lukens, R. L., & Landon, R. M. (1993). *A guide to inventory management for veterinary practices: Effective inventory control.* Westchester, PA: SmithKline Beecham Animal Health.

http://veterinarybusiness.dvm360.com/5-problems-with-inventory-and-how-solve-them.

https://www.aaha.org.

https://www.vhma.org.

https://www.cliniciansbrief.com.

20

Emergency Drugs

OBJECTIVES

After studying this chapter, you should be able to

1. Define terms related to emergencies and list common veterinary emergencies.
2. Determine the purpose of having a crash cart routinely maintained and list the appropriate items contained in a crash cart.
3. List and discuss drugs used as bronchodilators in respiratory and cardiac conditions.
4. Discuss corticosteroids and respiratory stimulants.
5. List the indications and potential side effects of antiarrhythmic drugs.
6. Describe the use of diuretics to treat cardiovascular conditions, as well as their potential side effects.
7. List drugs that are used as inotropes in the treatment of cardiac conditions.
8. Describe the actions and potential side effects of vasodilators.
9. List examples of drugs used to control seizures, as well as describe their potential side effects.
10. Describe the difference between antiemetics and emetics, their clinical uses, and their potential side effects.
11. Describe the uses and potential side effects of common antidotes.
12. Describe the use of reversal agents.

OUTLINE

KEY TERMS

Arrhythmias

Anticholinergic

Antihistamine

Bronchodilation

Chelating agent

Crash cart

Diuretic

Emetic

Inotrope

Methemoglobinemia

Triage

INTRODUCTION

One of the most important roles of veterinary technicians in emergencies is the ability to communicate, problem solve, anticipate needs, and triage patients. Triage can be applied to multiple animals entering a hospital or multiple traumas occurring in one animal. The goal is to quickly and systematically evaluate an animal for their function/injuries and determine which body system or which animal needs attention first (Fig. 20.1). Fig. 20.2 is an example of a triage questionnaire. Veterinary technicians must have a thorough knowledge of emergency drugs, their dosage forms, adverse reactions, and how to properly handle controlled substances. Proper documentation, in the medical record, of administered treatments is also important so that treatments are not repeated. Veterinary technicians must be able to accurately calculate the amount of drug to be given, know the appropriate syringe size and know the appropriate administration route. An important task that veterinary technicians perform is the administration of drugs, by all available routes, to patients on the order of a veterinarian. So, having knowledge of pharmacological drugs and therapeutics is vital. Their role in emergencies is critical to the outcome of the patient (Box 20.1).

Emergency Preparedness

Most veterinary hospitals have a designated area for emergency patients (Fig. 20.3). This area should have supplies, medications, and equipment that are organized and easily accessible and should be compiled in a crash cart (stationary or mobile). Written protocols, quick reference guidelines and an emergency drug chart (Fig. 20.4) should be posted in this area as well. All veterinary team personnel must be familiar with the location of the crash cart, supplies, equipment, and medication.

BOX 20.1   List of Common Emergencies

Allergic reactions	Hemorrhage
Anemia	Lacerations
Burns	Pneumothorax
Cardio pulmonary arrest	Respiratory distress
Congestive heart failure	Seizures
Dystocia	Shock
Foreign body	Toxins
Gastric dilatation volvulus	Tracheal collapse
Gastroenteritis	Trauma
HBC (Hit By Car)	Urethral Obstruction
Heat Stroke	

TECHNICIAN NOTES

Monthly, and after each use, check the crash cart to be sure it is fully stocked and confirm that all equipment is in working order and that no medications are expired; this will ensure preparedness during an emergency.

The Emergency Crash Cart

The emergency crash cart (Fig. 20.5) should be located in a centralized area. It must be routinely inventoried, checked for expiration and sterilization dates, and equipment function verified at least monthly and after every use. The crash cart should be organized and supplies clearly labeled. After restocking the crash cart, two pieces of tape can be placed in an "X" pattern so if the tape is broken you would know that the cart must be restocked. Maintaining the crash cart will ensure preparedness in an emergency situation (Boxes 20.3 and 20.4; Fig. 20.6).

There are many different life-threatening conditions that are emergencies. Many of these conditions involve delivery of supplemental oxygen. It is important to have oxygen concentrations as high as possible in these patients. Different methods of delivering high concentrations of

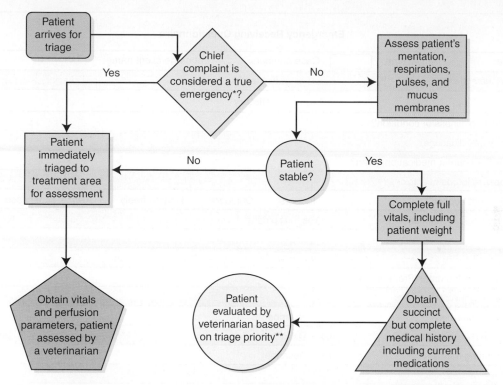

*True Emergencies include but not limited to an unresponsive patient, respiratory distress, active seizure, active bleeding/hemorrhage, inability to urinate, inability to stand/walk, toxin ingestion, collapse
**Triage priority is a means of sorting patients need for treatment based on the severity of their condition with the goal to increase the number of overall survivors

Fig. 20.1 Triage flow chart. (Courtesy Tara J. Fetzer, DVM, DACVECC.)

supplemental oxygen include nasal catheters, nasal cannulas, oxygen cages, and oxygen masks (Figs. 20.7 and 20.8).

 TECHNICIAN NOTES

- Oxygen is a drug that can save lives and has no side effects in a short-term situation.

Commonly Used Emergency Drugs

Drugs that cause bronchodilation include antihistamines, cholinergic blockers, beta-2- adrenergics, and methylxanthines (discussed in Chapter 5).

Antihistamines

Clinical Uses. Antihistamines work by blocking the effects of histamine. They are used to treat acute inflammation such as allergic reactions (anaphylactic shock) and upper respiratory conditions. They may also be used for their antiemetic properties because of the effects on the brain and nervous system.

Dosage Forms
- **Diphenhydramine tablets and injectable**
- **Hydroxyzine injectable, tablets, oral syrup**

Adverse Side Effects. These include sedation (central nervous system [CNS] depression), urinary retention, dry mucous membranes, and occasionally gastrointestinal effects such as diarrhea.

Anticholinergics

Clinical Uses. Cholinergic blockers (Anticholinergics) combine with acetylcholine receptors on smooth muscle fibers and prevent bronchoconstrictive effects of acetylcholine to produce bronchodilation. Anticholinergics are also used to prevent and treat bradycardia and decrease respiratory and gastrointestinal secretions. Atropine is also an antidote for organophosphate poisoning.

Emergency Receiving Questionnaire

Date:	Arrival time:		Case number:	Pet name/client name:
Sex/age/species:			Presenting complaint:	

History

Duration of illness or condition?				
Current medications?				
Over-the-counter medication given?				
Exposure to potential toxins?				
How is pet housed?	Indoors	Outdoors	Roams freely	Always supervised
Environmental changes?	Yes	Describe:		No
Diet?				
Appetite?	Normal	Decreased	Absent	
Rabies vaccine date: (Proof needed)				
Other vaccine date:				
Vomiting/diarrhea?	Yes	Describe:		No
Urinating without difficulty?	No	Describe:		Yes
Ambulating normally?	No	Describe:		Yes
Other changes?				

Initial Exam

Respiratory rate/ventilatory nature
Lung sounds
Heart rate/sounds
Pulse rate/quality
CRT/MM color
Temperature
Pain scale rating*
If painful, location
Ambulatory?
Activity level (BAR-bright alert reactive, QAR Quiet alert reactive, Lethargic)
Behavior (Blue-friendly, interactive, Yellow-reserved, Red-caution)

Overall Assessment

Non-urgent	Urgent	Emergent	Life threatening
Time assessment completed:			

*http://www.vasg.org/pdfs/CSU_Acute_Pain_Scale_Canine.pdf

*http://www.csuanimalcancercenter.org/assets/files/csu_acute_pain_scale_feline.pdf

Fig. 20.2 Triage questionnaire. (From Battaglia, A. M., & Steele, A. M. [2016]. *Small animal emergency and critical care for veterinary technicians* [3rd ed.]. St. Louis: Elsevier.)

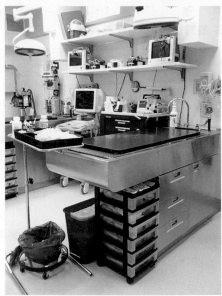

Fig. 20.3 Emergency area. (From Battaglia, A. M., & Steele, A. M. [2016]. *Small animal emergency and critical care for veterinary technicians* [3rd ed.]. St. Louis: Elsevier.)

Dosage Forms
- **Atropine Sulfate injectable**

Adverse Side Effects. These are generally dose related; an overdose can cause tachycardia, disorientation, slow gastrointestinal motility (constipation), anxiety, and burning at the injection site.

 TECHNICIAN NOTES

- Atropine can slow gastrointestinal motility and cause retention of toxic agents.

Beta-2-Adrenergic Agonists

Clinical Uses. Beta-2-adrenergic agonists cause relaxation of smooth muscle fibers and dilation of the airway when they act on the beta-2-adrenergic receptors. They also stabilize mast cells, preventing lysis and reducing the amount of histamine released (Bill, 2017). Epinephrine is a potent bronchodilator that is primarily used in life-threatening situations, like anaphylactic shock and cardiac resuscitation (asystole), because it also produces significant tachycardia. Epinephrine is also a potent sympathetic nervous system stimulant that increases the heart rate and increases the strength of heart contractions (Plumb, 2015), thereby increasing cardiac output.

Albuterol is used in airway diseases for bronchodilation to relieve bronchospasms and bronchoconstriction (Papich, 2016).

Dosage Forms
- **Epinephrine injectable**
- **Albuterol tablets, syrup, and inhalation**
- **Terbutaline injectable**

Adverse Side Effects. These include tachycardia, and hypertension.

Epinephrine can cause anxiety, vomiting, cardiac arrhythmias, and tremors (Plumb, 2015).

 TECHNICIAN NOTES

- Monitoring the heart rate and rhythm is essential when epinephrine is administered as it predisposes the heart to arrhythmias. Arrhythmias are variations from the normal rhythm of the heart.

Methylxanthines

Clinical Uses. Methylxanthines are used for bronchodilation in respiratory and cardiac conditions and for mild heart stimulation (positive inotropic effect). They are used for treating inflammatory airway diseases such as asthma, collapsing trachea, and bronchitis (Papich, 2016). The drug acts to relax smooth muscles in the bronchi and pulmonary vasculature and also has mild diuretic activity.

Dosage Forms
- **Aminophylline injectable**
- **Theophylline oral solution/elixir, tablets and injectable (in 5% dextrose)**

Adverse Side Effects. These drugs should be administered with caution in patients with severe cardiac disease (may cause tachycardia and arrhythmias), seizures, gastric ulcers, renal and hepatic disease, and severe hypertension. They can produce CNS stimulation (excitement, muscle tremors, and seizures), vomiting, diarrhea, gastrointestinal irritation, polyuria, polydipsia, and polyphagia (Plumb, 2015).

 TECHNICIAN NOTES

- Appropriate precautions should be taken before using this drug on a patient as theophylline may adversely react with many other drugs. Examples are furosemide, phenobarbital, propranolol, enrofloxacin, ketamine, and corticosteroids (Plumb, 2015).

CPR Emergency Drugs and Doses

Weight (kg)		2.5	5	10	15	20	25	30	35	40	45	50
Weight (lb)		8	10	20	30	40	50	60	70	80	90	100
DRUG	**DOSE**	ml	ml	ml	ml	ml	ml	ml	ml	ml	ml	ml
Epi Low (1:1000; 1mg/ml) every other BLS cycle x3	0.01 mg/kg	0.03	0.05	0.1	0.15	0.2	0.25	0.3	0.35	0.4	0.45	0.5
Epi High (1:1000; 1 mg/ml) for prolonged CPR	0.1 mg/kg	0.25	0.5	1	1.5	2	2.5	3	3.5	4	4.5	5
Vasopressin (20 U/ml)	0.8 U/kg	0.1	0.2	0.4	0.6	0.8	1	1.2	1.4	1.6	1.8	2
Atropine (0.54 mg/ml)	0.04 mg/kg	0.2	0.4	0.8	1.1	1.5	1.9	2.2	2.6	3	3.3	3.7
Amiodarone (50 mg/ml)	5 mg/kg	0.25	0.5	1	1.5	2	2.5	3	3.5	4	4.5	5
Lidocaine (20 mg/ml)	2 mg/kg	0.25	0.5	1	1.5	2	2.5	3	3.5	4	4.5	5
Naloxone (0.4 mg/ml)	0.04 mg/kg	0.25	0.5	1	1.5	2	2.5	3	3.5	4	4.5	5
Flumazenil (0.1 mg/ml)	0.01 mg/kg	0.25	0.5	1	1.5	2	2.5	3	3.5	4	4.5	5
Atipamezole (5 mg/ml)	100 µg/kg	0.06	0.1	0.2	0.3	0.4	0.5	0.6	0.7	0.8	0.9	1
External Defib (J)	4-6 J/kg	10	20	40	60	80	100	120	140	160	180	200
Internal Defib (J)	0.5-1 J/kg	2	3	5	8	10	15	15	20	20	20	25
External Defib (J)	2-4 J/kg	5	10	20	30	40	50	60	70	80	90	100
Internal Defib (J)	0.2-0.4 J/kg	1	2	2	3	4	5	6	7	8	9	10

Row groups (left margin labels): Arrest (Epi Low–Atropine), Anti-Arrhythmic (Amiodarone–Lidocaine), Reversal (Naloxone–Atipamezole), Defib Monophasic (External/Internal Defib 4-6/0.5-1), Defib Biphasic (External/Internal Defib 2-4/0.2-0.4).

Fig. 20.4 CPR Emergency Drug and Dose Chart. (From RECOVER evidence and knowledge gap analysis on veterinary CPR. Part 7: Clinical guidelines. *Journal of Veterinary Emergency and Critical Care.* 2012;22[S1]:S102–S131 and Thomas. J., & Lerche, P. [2017]. *Anesthesia and analgesia for veterinary technicians* [5th ed.]. St. Louis: Elsevier.)

Corticosteroids

Clinical Uses. Glucocorticoids are used to treat many emergency conditions such as inflammation, anaphylaxis, spinal cord injury, and immune mediated diseases. Their effects on the cardiovascular system are to reduce capillary permeability and enhance vasoconstriction (Plumb, 2015). Corticosteroids are used for their antiinflammatory (low-dose) and immunosuppressive (high-dose or long-term use) effects.

Dosage Forms
- Prednisolone injectable, tablets and syrup
- Prednisolone sodium succinate (Solu-Delta-Cortef) injectable
- Dexamethasone (Azium) injectable, powder, tablets and oral solution
- Dexamethasone sodium phosphate injectable

Adverse Side Effects. There are many side effects associated with the use of corticosteroids which include

BOX 20.2   Case Scenario

Sophie, a 7-year-old, spayed female, toy poodle was presented to the emergency clinic with an intermittent cough that the owner stated "seems to worsen when excited or exercised." The owner also explained that the cough seemed to be dry and she appeared to be retching or gagging. Sophie's appetite, drinking, urination, and defecation seemed normal.

On physical examination, Sophie appeared comfortable and not stressed. The mucous membranes were pink and moist, CRT (capillary refill time) was 1 second. No wheezes or crackles were heard on auscultation of the chest. Her heart rate and rhythm were within normal limits. She was mildly dehydrated. Upon palpation of the trachea, Sophie coughed. The cough was nonproductive. Wheezes were heard when the trachea was ausculted. An oral exam revealed no obstruction in the laryngeal area. The soft palate was normal and not elongated.

A presumptive diagnosis of tracheal collapse was made and thoracic radiographs were performed. The radiographs revealed a narrowing of the trachea at the thoracic inlet: the lungs were clear and there were no signs of pulmonary edema. The technician drew blood for a CBC (Complete Blood Count) and Chemistry profile.

The blood work was unremarkable except for slight elevations in the PCV/TP which were caused by the mild dehydration. No oxygen therapy was indicated. Mild dehydration was treated with 0.9% NaCl fluids subcutaneously. An antitussive, butorphanol was given to help reduce irritation in the trachea and prednisone was given to decrease laryngeal and tracheal inflammation. Albuterol was given for bronchodilation and to relieve coughing. No surgical consideration was given at this time.

The owner was given information on tracheal collapse and was told that it is a common congenital disorder in middle-aged to older toy breeds. They were advised to use a harness rather than a collar when walking her to decrease pressure exerted on the trachea. They were advised to continue monitoring the cough and to call if clinical signs persist after 5 days. The owner reported that Sophie was doing much better.

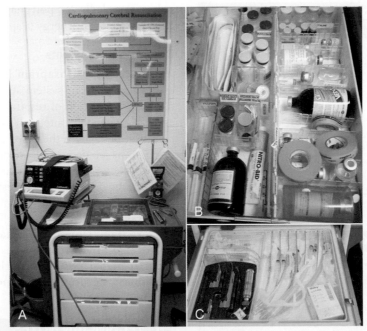

Fig. 20.5 Emergency Crash Cart. **A.** Rolling crash cart with defibrillator, **B.** Crash cart drawer containing emergency medications, syringes, and other supplies, **C.** A laryngoscope and various endotracheal tubes. (From Bassert, J. M., & Thomas, J. A. [2014]. *McCurnin's clinical textbook for veterinary technicians* [8th ed.]. St Louis: Elsevier.)

BOX 20.3   Emergency Crash Cart Items

Various sizes of endotracheal tubes (ET) with ties connected	Micro and Macro IV drip administration sets
12 mL syringe to inflate the ET cuff	Porous tape
Gauze rolls for tying in endotracheal tube	Sterile gauze sponges
Sterile Lubricant	Bandage material
Tracheostomy tube	Fluids (LRS and 0.9 % NaCl)
Scalpel blades and handles	Tourniquet
Suture material	Clippers
Bandage scissors	Tissue glue
Hemostats	Pulse oximeter/capnograph
Laryngoscope with small and large blade	Blood gas machine
Sterile gloves	Respiratory monitor
Stethoscope	Thermometer
Ambu-bag (room air or connected to an oxygen source)	Emergency Drug dose chart
Various sizes of mouth gags	Urinary catheters
Nasal catheters	Lab supplies (blood collection tubes, capillary tubes, clay)
Chest tubes	**Equipment nearby:**
Three-way stop cocks	ECG machine/monitor
Various size butterfly catheters	Suction with suction tips
Various size syringes (1, 3, and 10 mL)	Defibrillator
Various size needles (25, 22, and 20 gauge)	
Various size IV catheters	
Male adapters	

BOX 20.4   Emergency Drugs Stocked in a Crash Cart

Atropine	Furosemide, Mannitol
Aminophylline, Theophylline	Hydralazine, Nitroglycerin
	Lidocaine, Procainamide, Propanolol, Atenolol
Diphenhydramine	
Dobutamine, Digoxin, Dopamine	Vasopressin
	Prednisolone, Dexamethasone
Doxapram	Sodium bicarbonate
Dextrose	**Reversal agents**—naloxone,
Epinephrine, Albuterol	flumazenil, atipamezole, yohimbine

 TECHNICIAN NOTES

- Short-term administration of low doses of corticosteroids can reduce the amount of inflammation with upper airway conditions.
- Corticosteroids control the clinical signs of disease and not the underlying problem.
- Corticosteroids should not be given along with nonsteroidal antiinflammatory drugs (NSAIDs) as this can increase the risk of gastrointestinal ulcers (Papich, 2016).

polyuria, polydipsia, polyphagia, vomiting, diarrhea, and general loss of energy (Papich, 2016).

Respiratory Stimulants

Clinical Uses. Doxapram Hydrochloride is a general central nervous system stimulant that is primarily used for stimulation of respirations during or after anesthesia, in neonates after a dystocia or cesarean section or conditions where the respiratory rate and depth of respirations are decreased. Doxapram is not be used as a substitute for artificial respiratory support in animals with cardiac or respiratory arrest and may be contraindicated in states of apnea.

Dosage Forms
- **Doxapram (Dopram) injectable**

Adverse Side Effects. These effects are likely to occur at higher doses and include hypertension, arrhythmias, seizures, and hyperventilation (Plumb, 2015).

TECHNICIAN NOTES

- Doxapram is used to increase tidal volume and respiratory rate.

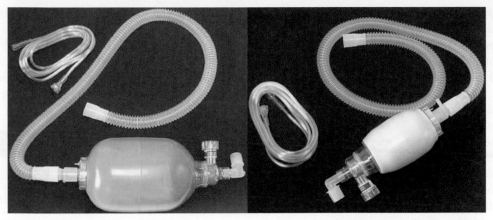

Large Ambu bag | Small Ambu bag

Fig. 20.6 Ambu (Artificial Manual Breathing Unit) bags. Ambu Inc., Columbia, MD. (From Sonsthagen, T. [2014]. *Veterinary instruments and equipment a pocket guide* [3rd ed.]. St. Louis: Elsevier.)

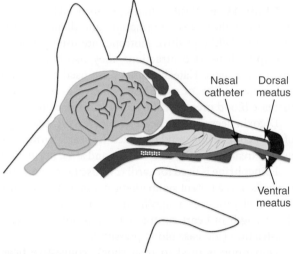

Fig. 20.7 Illustration of the nasal passages of the dog and correct placement of a nasal catheter in the ventral meatus. (From Battaglia, A. M., & Steele, A. M. [2016]. *Small animal emergency and critical care for veterinary technicians* [3rd ed.]. St. Louis: Elsevier.)

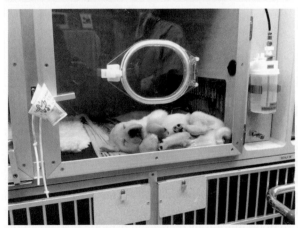

Fig. 20.8 An oxygen cage with heating, cooling, and humidifying and dehumidifying functions. (From Battaglia, A. M., & Steele, A. M. [2016]. *Small animal emergency and critical care for veterinary technicians* [3rd ed.]. St. Louis: Elsevier.)

Antiarrhythmics

Clinical Uses. Antiarrhythmic drugs are used to treat abnormal heart rhythms such as tachyarrhythmias (atrial fibrillation and ventricular tachycardia) and bradyarrhythmias (discussed in Chapter 7). Procainamide is used to treat atrial and ventricular tachycardia by depressing cardiac muscle excitability and is also used to treat ventricular premature complexes.

Lidocaine is a local anesthetic that has antiarrhythmic properties; it is used to treat ventricular tachycardia and ventricular premature complexes.

Propanolol reduces the heart rate, blood pressure, and cardiac output. It is used to treat atrial and ventricular premature complexes, atrial fibrillation, and hypertrophic cardiomyopathy.

Atenolol is a beta-blocker that is primarily used as an antiarrhythmic to reduce the heart rate and blood pressure. It is used to treat tachyarrhythmias, cardiomyopathy, hypertension, and ventricular premature complexes (Papich, 2016).

Dosage Forms
- **Procainamide injectable and tablets**
- **Lidocaine injectable**
- **Propanolol injectable, tablets, and oral solution**
- **Atenolol injectable, tablets, and oral suspension**

Adverse Side Effects. Procainamide adverse effects are dose related and include vomiting, diarrhea, and hypotension.

Lidocaine adverse effects may include depression, ataxia, and muscle tremors.

Propanolol adverse effects include bradycardia, worsening of heart failure, hypotension, hypoglycemia, and bronchoconstriction.

Atenolol adverse effects include lethargy, hypotension, bradycardia, and hypoglycemia (Plumb, 2015).

TECHNICIAN NOTES

- Lidocaine should be used with caution in cats; they are more sensitive to the CNS and cardiovascular depressant effects (Plumb, 2015).
- Propanolol should not be discontinued abruptly as tachycardia or hypertension may occur.

Diuretics

Diuretics promote the loss of body water through decreased reabsorption by the kidney tubules. Furosemide, a loop diuretic, is most commonly used in the treatment of heart failure due to its ability to decrease preload (amount of blood in the ventricles after diastole) through diuresis. Mannitol is an osmotic diuretic that promotes diuresis by increasing osmotic pressure in the renal tubules and reducing water reabsorption thereby increasing urine production and diuresis.

Clinical Uses. Furosemide is commonly used to treat pulmonary edema, congestive heart failure, uremia, and as an adjunct in the treatment of hyperkalemia (Plumb, 2015). Loop diuretics increase renal excretion of water and electrolytes.

Mannitol is used for oliguric renal failure, reduction of intraocular pressure and cerebral edema associated with head trauma, and enhance urinary excretion of toxins (Plumb, 2015).

Dosage Forms
- **Furosemide injectable, tablets, and oral solution**
- **Mannitol injectable**

Adverse Side Effects. Caution should be taken when using diuretics in patients with hypovolemia or hypotension

as diuretics will further decrease blood fluid volume and blood pressure (Bill, 2017).

Prolonged use of diuretics may cause hypotension, dehydration, hypokalemia, and hyponatremia. It is contraindicated in patients with anuria secondary to renal disease, preexisting electrolyte abnormalities, and in patients that are dehydrated (Plumb, 2015).

TECHNICIAN NOTES

- It is important to continually monitor patients on diuretics as the patient can become dehydrated and hypotensive, and electrolyte imbalances can occur.

Inotropes

Inotropes are a group of drugs that affect the contractility of the heart muscle by increasing the strength of contractions.

Clinical Uses. Positive inotropes are used for congestive heart failure, atrial fibrillation, and dilated cardiomyopathy. While positive inotropes are used primarily to help with heart contractions, they also have antiarrhythmic effects. Catecholamines are used to increase the contractility of the heart, increase heart rate, increase blood pressure, and increase cardiac output.

Digoxin decreases the heart rate, increases the strength of heart contractions, and regulates the heart rhythm. It is used to treat congestive heart failure and atrial fibrillation.

Epinephrine is used for cardiac resuscitation and anaphylaxis. It is a potent sympathetic nervous system stimulant that produces a significant tachycardia, increases the strength of heart contractions, and produces vasoconstriction (increase blood pressure).

Dopamine is used to treat shock, congestive heart failure, and to increase renal perfusion. Dopamine increases the force of cardiac muscle contractions and increases the heart rate.

Dobutamine is used for short-term treatment of heart failure. It increases the force of cardiac muscle contractions with little or no increase in the heart rate.

Dosage Forms
- **Digoxin tablets and elixer**
- **Epinephrine injectable**
- **Dopamine injectable**
- **Dobutamine injectable**

Adverse Side Effects. Cardiac glycosides (digoxin) can cause vomiting, diarrhea, anorexia, and arrhythmias if they achieve toxic levels in the blood.

Digoxin is contraindicated in cats with hypertrophic cardiomyopathy as they can increase cardiac muscle oxygen demand and lead to outflow obstruction (Plumb, 2015).

Epinephrine adverse effects include hypertension, arrhythmias, anxiety, and excitability.

Dopamine can cause adverse effects that include tachycardia, hypotension or hypertension, dyspnea, and vasoconstriction (Plumb, 2015).

Dobutamine adverse effects include tachycardia, muscle tremors, and seizures (Plumb, 2015).

> **TECHNICIAN NOTES**
>
> • Heart rate and ECG monitoring is extremely important when patients are being treated with inotropes.

Vasodilators

Clinical Uses. Vasodilators are used to decrease preload (amount of blood in the ventricles after diastole) and decrease afterload (resistance) to improve cardiac output. Giving vasodilators will dilate (open) the vessels and decrease resistance, therefore reducing the workload of the heart.

Hydralazine is an arterial vasodilator that reduces peripheral resistance, reduces arterial blood pressure, and improves cardiac output in patients with congestive heart failure by opening up blood vessels and reducing the stress on the heart.

Nitroglycerin is a venodilator that is used primarily in heart failure to improve cardiac output and decrease pulmonary edema. Nitroglycerin comes as an ointment and a transdermal patch and is applied to hairless areas; gloves must be worn when applying nitroglycerin.

Nitroprusside is a peripheral vasodilator that is used in acute heart failure when blood pressure must be reduced rapidly. It must be further diluted before giving as an intravenous (IV) infusion (Plumb, 2015).

Dosage Forms
• **Hydralazine injectable and tablets**
• **Nitroglycerin injectable, ointment, and transdermal patch**
• **Nitroprusside injectable—must be further diluted and given by IV only**

Adverse Side Effects. Hydralazine can cause excess vasodilation and hypotension resulting in tachycardia. Other effects include lethargy, sodium/water retention, vomiting, and diarrhea (Papich, 2016).

Nitroglycerin ointment/patch can cause irritation at the application site and hypotension.

> **TECHNICIAN NOTES**
>
> • The blood pressure must be constantly monitored during therapy.
> • When applying nitroglycerin to a patient, gloves must be worn.

Anticonvulsants

Anticonvulsants are drugs used to control seizures.

Clinical Uses. Anticonvulsants such as diazepam and phenobarbital are commonly used in emergencies. Diazepam is a central acting CNS depressant used for sedation, as an anesthetic adjunct and the drug of choice for status epilepticus (Papich, 2016). Diazepam is not used for long-term seizure control because of its short duration.

Phenobarbital is used as an adjunct to diazepam for intractable seizures and has sedative properties.

Dosage Forms
• **Diazepam (Valium) injectable**
• **Phenobarbital injectable**

Adverse Side Effects. In general, these include drowsiness, CNS depression, anxiety, polyuria, and polydipsia.

Antiemetics

Antiemetics are drugs used to prevent and control vomiting.

Clinical Uses. Maropitant is used for treating acute vomiting and vomiting due to motion sickness.

Chlorpromazine is a phenothiazine tranquilizer that is used to control vomiting associated with gastrointestinal inflammation, parvo virus, and vomiting from chemotherapy (Bill, 2017).

Metoclopramide hydrochloride is used to control vomiting and to treat gastric motility disorders.

Ondansetron is used to treat severe vomiting and is effective for controlling chemotherapy-associated vomiting.

Dosage Forms
• **Maropitant (Cerenia) injectable and tablets**
• **Chlorpromazine injectable**
• **Metoclopramide** Hydrochloride **(Reglan) injectable, tablet, and oral solution**
• **Ondansetron (Zofran) injectable**

Adverse Side Effects. Maropitant may cause excess salivation and muscle tremors.

Chlorpromazine causes sedation and may cause hypotension.

Metoclopramide may cause behavioral changes, seizures, and constipation (Bill, 2017).

Ondansetron is well tolerated; constipation, sedation, and hypotension are possible.

> **TECHNICIAN NOTES**
>
> • Metoclopramide should not be used in animals if there is a gastrointestinal obstruction.

Emetics

Clinical Uses. Emetics are drugs that induce vomiting in animals that have ingested toxins and must be administered within 2 to 6 hours of toxic ingestion to be effective. Apomorphine is an opioid that depresses the CNS (Fig. 20.9).

Dosage Forms
- **Apomorphine injectable and tablets (dissolve in saline for use in conjunctival sac)**
- **Hydrogen peroxide (3%) solution for oral administration**
- **Xylazine or dexmedetomidine injectable (not classified as emetics, but used to produce vomiting in cats)**

Adverse Side Effects. Emetics are contraindicated in animals that are comatose, seizing, are in shock, have dyspnea, have depressed pharyngeal reflexes, or have ingested strong acid, alkali, or other caustic substances (Plumb, 2015).

Apomorphine can produce respiratory depression. It may cause irritation to the ocular conjunctival membrane if given topically in the conjunctival sac.

Hydrogen peroxide (3%) can cause esophageal irritation and aspiration is possible. It is contraindicated in cats.

Xylazine and dexmedetomidine may cause excessive sedation.

> **TECHNICIAN NOTES**
>
> • Respiratory depressant effects of apomorphine can be reversed with naloxone, an opioid antagonist.
> • Apomorphine is the drug of choice to induce vomiting in dogs. If using dissolved tablets in the conjunctival sac, the eye should be flushed copiously once vomiting occurs.
> • Xylazine (not classified as an emetic) is the preferred drug to induce vomiting in cats. The CRTZ is stimulated by alpha-2 adrenergic drugs (xylazine, dexmedetomidine) and therefore induce emesis in the cat.
> • The emetic effect of xylazine can be reversed with yohimbine or atipamezole (alpha-2-antagonists).
> • After the patient vomits, other systemic antidotes and/or activated charcoal should be used to prevent further absorption of the toxin.

® Miscellaneous Antidotes (Box 20.5)
Activated Charcoal

Activated charcoal is a fine, black, odorless, tasteless powder that is used to adsorb certain drugs or toxins to prevent or reduce their systemic absorption from the upper gastrointestinal tract.

Clinical Uses. These include oral administration to prevent or reduce the systemic absorption of certain drugs or toxins (Fig. 20.10).

Dosage Forms
- **Toxiban** Suspension ± sorbitol
- **Toxiban Granules**
- **UAA Gel ± sorbitol**
- **Activated charcoal powder (generic) (for reconstitution with water)**

Adverse Side Effects. These include vomiting after very rapid administration of activated charcoal. Activated charcoal can also cause constipation or diarrhea, and the stool is black in color.

> **TECHNICIAN NOTES**
>
> • Activated charcoal is not considered effective against heavy metals (e.g., lead, mercury, or inorganic arsenic), mineral acids, caustic alkalis, nitrates, sodium, chloride/chlorate, ferrous sulfate, or petroleum distillates.
> • Other oral therapeutic agents should not be administered within 3 hours after administration of activated charcoal therapy.
> • Dairy products and mineral oil reduce the adsorptive properties of activated charcoal.
> • Only give products with sorbitol for the first dose. Subsequent activated charcoal doses must not contain sorbitol, or severe diarrhea could develop.

Calcium Ethylenediaminetetraacetic Acid

Calcium ethylenediaminetetraacetic acid (Ca-EDTA) is a heavy metal **chelating agent** that is available commercially (human label) as an injection. It also may be referred to as edetate calcium disodium, calcium disodium edetate, calcium edetate, calcium disodium ethylenediaminetetraacetate, and sodium calcium edetate.

Clinical Uses. In veterinary medicine, calcium EDTA is used for the treatment of lead poisoning.

Dosage Forms
- **Calcium Disodium Versenate injection** (human label)
- **Calcium Disodium Edetate**
- **Calcium Edetate-Hey**

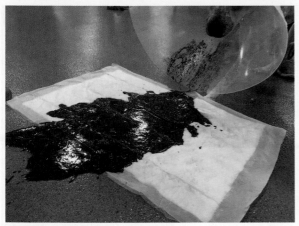

Fig. 20.9 Patient given apomorphine for chocolate toxicity. (Courtesy Tara J. Fetzer, DVM, DACVECC.)

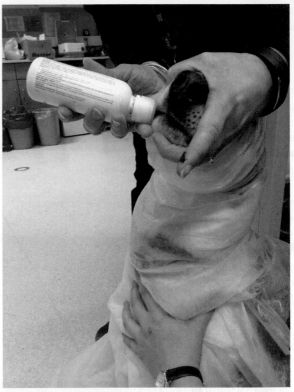

Fig. 20.10 Administration of activated charcoal; a sleeve from a disposable gown is placed over the animal to keep the patient clean. (From Battaglia, A. M., & Steele, A. M. [2016]. *Small animal emergency and critical care for veterinary technicians* [3rd ed.]. St. Louis: Elsevier.)

BOX 20.5 List of Common Antidotes

Antidote	Indication
Activated charcoal	Reduces systemic absorption of certain toxic substances
Calcium-EDTA	Lead, copper, zinc, and other heavy metal toxicity
Methylene blue	Methemoglobinemia
acetylcysteine (*N*-Acetylcysteine)	Acetaminophen overdose
Dimercaprol (BAL—British anti-Lewisite)	Lead, arsenic, mercury, copper, zinc, gold
Pralidoxime chloride	Nicotinic signs of organo-phosphate toxicity
Penicillamine	Lead, iron, zinc, mercury, copper
Sodium Thiosulfate	Cyanide poisoning
Ethanol	Ethylene glycol (antifreeze) toxicity
Fomepizole	Ethylene glycol (antifreeze) toxicity
Antivenin *Crotalidae*	Neutralizes poisonous snake venom from rattlesnakes, copper heads, and water moccasins
Antivenin *Micrurus*	Neutralizes poisonous snake venom from coral snakes
Vitamin K_1	Anticoagulant; used in rodenticide and plant poisoning
Thiamine	Thiamine deficiency and lead poisoning

Adverse Side Effects. These include renal toxicity, depression (dogs), and vomiting/diarrhea (dogs). Zinc deficiency may occur from long-term therapy.

TECHNICIAN NOTES

- Calcium EDTA should not be used in anuric patients, and caution should be exercised when it is used in patients with renal insufficiency.
- Calcium EDTA should not be administered orally.
- Do not confuse with edetate disodium, which may cause severe hypocalcemia.
- Magnesium sulfate (Epsom salt) or sodium sulfate may be used orally to prevent further intestinal absorption of lead.

Methylene Blue

Methylene blue is a thiazine dye that appears as dark green crystals or crystalline powder with a bronze-like luster. It is an oxidating agent that helps to convert methemoglobin (a compound formed from hemoglobin by oxidation of the iron atom) from the ferrous (Fe^{2+}) to the ferric (Fe^{3+}) state. It does not function as an oxygen carrier to hemoglobin.

Clinical Uses. Methylene blue is used for the treatment of methemoglobinemia caused by oxidative agents (e.g., nitrites, nitrates, and chlorates) in ruminants. It may be used for cyanide toxicity in ruminants and for the treatment of acetaminophen poisoning in the dog. It can also be used in dogs to preferentially stain pancreatic islet cell tumors intraoperatively.

Dosage Forms
- **Methylene blue injection** (generic) (human label)
- **Methylene blue tablets** (generic)
- **Methylene blue powder** (generic)

Adverse Side Effects. These include the development of Heinz body anemia or other morphologic changes in red blood cells, and decreased red blood cell life span. Methemoglobinemia may occur but is usually dose and species dependent. Tissue necrosis may occur with subcutaneous administration or extravasation during IV injection.

 TECHNICIAN NOTES

- Methylene blue usually is contraindicated in cats.
- Dogs and horses may show a greater occurrence of side effects than ruminants.
- Methylene blue should not be used in patients with renal insufficiency.
- Safety during pregnancy is unknown.

Acetylcysteine

Acetylcysteine is a white crystalline powder that is soluble in water or alcohol. It also may be referred to as *N*-acetylcysteine or *N*-acetyl-L-cysteine.

Clinical Uses. These include oral therapy for acetaminophen poisoning in dogs and cats. It also may be used as a mucolytic agent for pulmonary (via nebulization) or ophthalmic (via topical application) conditions.

Dosage Forms
- **Mucomyst** (human label)
- **Mucosil** (human label)
- **Acetylcysteine** (human label)

Adverse Side Effects. These include nausea, vomiting, and, occasionally, urticaria (hives) when admin-

 TECHNICIAN NOTES

- Acetylcysteine is incompatible with amphotericin B, chlortetracycline hydrochloride, erythromycin lactobionate, oxytetracycline hydrochloride, ampicillin sodium, tetracycline hydrochloride, iodized oil, hydrogen peroxide, chymotrypsin, and trypsin.
- Activated charcoal may adsorb acetylcysteine, reducing its effectiveness in treating acetaminophen toxicity.
- Carefully monitor patients that have bronchospastic diseases and that receive pulmonary treatment.
- The oral solution has a bad taste, and a masking agent (e.g., colas or juices) may be used.
- Open vials should be refrigerated and discarded after 96 hours.

istered orally. Chest tightness, bronchoconstriction, bronchial or tracheal irritation, and acetylcysteine hypersensitivity are rare but possible side effects when administered into the pulmonary tract. Acetylcysteine may cause bronchospasm in some patients receiving treatment via the pulmonary tract. Subcutaneous injections can cause abscess formation.

Dimercaprol

Dimercaprol is a dithiol chelating agent that occurs as a colorless or nearly colorless viscous liquid with a disagreeable odor. The commercial solution may be cloudy or may contain small amounts of flaky material or sediment. This is normal and does not indicate deterioration of the product. It also may be referred to as British anti-Lewisite (BAL), dimercaptopropanol, or thioglycerol.

Clinical Uses. Dimercaprol is used primarily for the treatment of toxicity resulting from arsenic compounds but may be used for lead, mercury, copper, zinc, or gold toxicity.

Dosage Forms
- **Dimercaprol injection 100 mg/mL** (human label)
- **BAL in oil** (human label)

Adverse Side Effects. Intramuscular injections are painful. Vomiting and seizures may occur with high doses. It is potentially nephrotoxic (Plumb, 2015). Most side effects subside quickly because of rapid elimination of the drug.

Pralidoxime Chloride

Pralidoxime chloride is a quaternary ammonium oxime cholinesterase reactivator. It reverses the action of cholinesterase inhibitors such as certain organophosphates. It also may be referred to as a 2-PAM chloride or 2-pyridine aldoxime methyl chloride.

Clinical Uses. Pralidoxime chloride is used for oral treatment of organophosphate poisoning. It must be given within 24 to 48 hours, or it is ineffective in treating the toxicity. It may be used in conjunction with atropine and supportive therapy.

Dosage Form
- **Protopam injection** (human label)

Adverse Side Effects. These are uncommon, but rapid IV injection may cause tachycardia, muscle rigidity, transient neuromuscular blockade, and laryngospasm.

> **TECHNICIAN NOTES**
>
> - Pralidoxime, similar to other anticholinesterases, may potentiate the action of barbiturates.
> - Patients with impaired renal function require a lower dose and careful monitoring.

Penicillamine

Penicillamine is a chelating agent of metals such as copper, lead, iron, zinc, and mercury. It is a degradation product of penicillins but does not have antimicrobial activity. It also may be referred to as D-penicillamine, β,β-dimethylcysteine, or D,3-mercaptovaline.

Clinical Uses. Penicillamine is used for copper-associated hepatopathy, and for long-term oral treatment of lead poisoning and cystine urolithiasis.

Dosage Forms
- **Depen Titratabs, tablets** (human label)
- **Cuprimine capsules** (human label)

Adverse Side Effects. These include nausea and vomiting. Other rare side effects include fever, lymphadenopathy, skin hypersensitivity reactions, and immune complex glomerulonephropathy.

> **TECHNICIAN NOTES**
>
> Absorption of penicillamine may be reduced by concurrent administration of food, antacids, or iron salts.

Sodium Thiosulfate

Sodium thiosulfate uses the enzyme rhodanese to convert cyanide to a nontoxic thiocyanate ion, which is excreted in urine.

Clinical Uses. Sodium thiosulfate is used in the treatment of cyanide poisoning in horses and ruminants. It may be used in combination with sodium molybdate for the treatment of copper poisoning in ruminants. It also has been used for the treatment of arsenic poisoning. When applied topically, sodium thiosulfate may be useful for treating some fungal infections (Plumb, 2015).

Dosage Forms
- **Cya Dote Injection**
- **Sodium Thiosulfate for Injection 25%** (human label)

Adverse Side Effects. These are uncommon.

> **TECHNICIAN NOTES**
>
> When sodium thiosulfate is administered intravenously, it should be given slowly.

Ethanol

Ethanol is an alcohol that is a competitive inhibitor of ethylene glycol metabolism. It also may be referred to as pure grain alcohol, grain alcohol, or ethyl alcohol.

Clinical Uses. Ethanol is used to treat ethylene glycol (antifreeze) poisoning.

Dosage Form
- **Ethanol**

Adverse Side Effects. Ethanol reduces body temperature, CNS depression, and an overdose can be fatal.

> **TECHNICIAN NOTES**
>
> - Recommended ethanol regimen for dogs is 5.5 mL of 20% ethanol/kg IV every 4 hours for five treatments and then every 6 hours for four additional treatments; for cats, 5 mL of 20% ethanol/kg IV every 6 hours for five treatments, then every 8 hours for four additional treatments (Grauer, 2019).
> - Sodium bicarbonate is usually administered to control metabolic acidosis.

Fomepizole

Fomepizole is a competitive inhibitor of alcohol dehydrogenase. Its action prevents the conversion of ethylene glycol into glycoaldehyde and other toxic metabolites. This allows ethylene glycol to be excreted primarily unchanged. It also may be referred to as 4-methylpyrazole (4-MP).

Clinical Uses. Fomepizole is used to treat ethylene glycol (antifreeze) poisoning in dogs. It inactivates alcohol dehydrogenase without the adverse effects of ethanol and is the treatment of choice (Grauer, 2019).

Dosage Form
- **Antizol-Vet**

Adverse Side Effects. Clinical signs of possible anaphylaxis include tachypnea, gagging, excessive salivation, and trembling.

 TECHNICIAN NOTES

- Fomepizole must be diluted with 0.9% NaCl before IV injection.
- Dogs treated within 8 hours of ingestion have a better prognosis than those treated 10 to 12 hours after ingestion. It has been shown to be effective in cats at high dosages if given within 3 hours of ingestion (Plumb, 2015).
- Treatment with fomepizole can cause false positive results on ethylene glycol screening tests.

Antivenin Polyvalent (*Crotalidae*)/Antivenin (*Micrurus fulvius*) Coral Snake

These products are concentrated serum globulins collected from horses or other species vaccinated with different types of snake venoms. When the antivenin contains antibodies against only one species it is called monovalent. If it has antibodies against several species it is called polyvalent. Venom from pit vipers like copperheads, rattlesnakes, and water moccasins has a different molecular structure from elapid snake venom (coral snake, black, brown, tiger, or Taipan snakes). This distinction requires treatment with the appropriate antivenin. Antivenin antibody combines with and inactivates venom at the time of administration but does not reverse damage done before administration. Treatment of snake bite often requires intensive supportive care of the patient with fluids, antibiotics, steroids, and pain medications in addition to antivenin. Antivenin is also called antivenom, venom antiserum, or antivenom immunoglobulin.

Clinical Uses. These products are used in the treatment of snakebite in domestic animals. Because of the high price of antivenin, treatment with these products is potentially cost prohibitive.

Dosage Forms
- **Antivenin (Crotalidae); polyvalent equine origin, labeled for dogs**—Boehringer Ingelheim.
- **Antivenin (Crotalidae); polyvalent equine origin** (human label)—Wyeth

- **Antivenin (Crotalidae); CroFab Polyvalent Ovine Origin** (human label)—Altana
- **Antivenin (Crotalidae and Micrurus) veterinary labels in development**—BioVeteria
- **Antivenin (Crotalidae); polyvalent** (labeled for horses)—Lake Immunogenics
- **Rattler Antivenin (Crotalidae); polyvalent**—MG Biologics

Adverse Side Effects. Anaphylaxis may occur secondary to administration of equine- or ovine-origin products.

Vitamin K₁ (Phytonadione)

Vitamin K_1 is necessary for the synthesis of blood coagulation factors II, VII, IX, and X by the liver.

Clinical Uses. The main use of this product is for the treatment of anticoagulant rodenticide and plant poisoning.

Dosage Forms
- **Phytonadione;** numerous veterinary-approved products are available, including oral capsules and an aqueous colloidal solution for injection. (Vitamin K_1)
- **Phytonadione; Mephyton** oral capsules and Aqua-**Mephyton injectable** (human label).

Adverse Side Effects. Anaphylaxis may occur with IV injection. The intramuscular route is usually recommended.

Thiamine HCl

Thiamine HCl is a water-soluble B vitamin used for the treatment or prevention of thiamine deficiency.

Clinical Uses. Thiamine HCl is used for thiamine deficiency in several species. It is used to treat polioencephalomalacia in cattle, sheep, and goats, as well as thiamine deficiencies associated with dietary lack or thiamine-destroying compounds in the diet.

Dosage Form
- **Thiamine HCl;** numerous veterinary and human label products are available.

Adverse Side Effects. Hypersensitivity or muscle soreness may be seen.

℞ Reversal Agents (Box 20.6)
Atipamezole HCl

Atipamezole acts as a reversal agent for alpha-2–adrenergic agonists by competitively inhibiting alpha-2–adrenergic receptors.

Clinical Uses. Atipamezole HCl is used for the reversal of dexmedetomidine (Dexdomitor), detomidine

BOX 20.6 List of Common Reversal Agents

Atipamezole—reversal of dexmedetomidine, detomidine, medetomidine, amitraz, xylazine

Flumazenil—reversal of benzodiazepines

Naloxone—reversal of opioids (narcotics)

Neostigmine—reversal/ treatment of ivermectin overdose

Tolazoline—reversal of xylazine

Yohimbine—reversal of xylazine, amitraz, medetomidine

(Dormosedan), medetomidine (Domitor). It also works to reverse xylazine. It also has been used in the treatment of amitraz toxicity.

Dosage Form
• **Antisedan**
Adverse Side Effects. These include vomiting, diarrhea, hypersalivation, tremors, and apprehension.

TECHNICIAN NOTES

Pain perception returns after administration of atipamezole.

Flumazenil

Flumazenil acts as a benzodiazepine antagonist by competitively blocking benzodiazepines at benzodiazepine receptors.

Clinical Uses. Flumazenil is used for the reversal of benzodiazepine action.

Dosage Form
• **Romazicon** (human label)
Adverse Side Effects. Seizures may occur.

Naloxone HCl

Naloxone is a narcotic antagonist. It is structurally related to oxymorphone and may be referred to as *N*-allylnoroxymorphone HCl.

Clinical Uses. Naloxone is used for the treatment, prevention, or control of narcotic depression. It is used for the reversal of mu-agonist opioids.

Dosage Forms
• **P/M Naloxone HCl injection**
• **Narcan** (human label)
Adverse Side Effects. These are uncommon.

TECHNICIAN NOTES

• IV injection yields the quickest response.
• A repeated dose may be necessary if the action of the narcotic outlasts the action of naloxone.
• Naloxone also reverses the analgesic effects of butorphanol (Torbugesic), pentazocine (Talwin-V), and nalbuphine (Nubain).

Neostigmine

Neostigmine is a parasympathomimetic agent that competes with acetylcholine for acetylcholinesterase.

Clinical Uses. Neostigmine may be used to treat nondepolarizing neuromuscular blocking agent (curare-type) overdosages. It has also been used to treat ivermectin overdosages in cats.

Dosage Form
• **Prostigmin ICN** (human label)
Adverse Side Effects. Side effects are dose related and include nausea, vomiting, diarrhea, drooling, lacrimation, and others. Neostigmine may interact with atropine, corticosteroids, magnesium, dexpanthenol, and muscle relaxants.

Tolazoline HCl

Tolazoline is a competitive alpha-1–adrenergic and alpha-2–adrenergic receptor blocking agent that reverses the effects of alpha-2–adrenergic agonists.

Clinical Uses. Tolazoline HCl is used in horses for the reversal of xylazine (Rompun).

Dosage Form
• **Tolazine**
Adverse Side Effects. These include transient tachycardia, peripheral vasodilation, licking of lips, piloerection, clear lacrimal and nasal discharge, muscle fasciculations, and apprehension.

TECHNICIAN NOTES

• Tolazoline is not approved for use in food-producing animals.
• Tolazoline has a short duration and may require repeated doses.

Yohimbine HCl

Yohimbine is an alpha-2–adrenergic receptor antagonist that reverses the effects of alpha-2–adrenergic agonists.

Clinical Uses. Yohimbine is used to reverse the effects of xylazine (Rompun). This action usually occurs within 1 to 3 minutes. It is approved for use in dogs and deer, but is also effective in other species. It also reverses medetomidine and other alpha-2-adrenergic agonists.

Dosage Forms

- Yobine
- Antagonil (approved for deer)

TECHNICIAN NOTES

- Normal pain perception remains after administration of yohimbine.
- Caution should be exercised when used in epileptic or seizure-prone patients.
- Yohimbine should not be used in food-producing animals.
- Safety in pregnant or breeding animals is unknown.

REVIEW QUESTIONS

1. What is the goal of triage in an emergency?
2. List emergency drugs that are commonly stocked in a crash cart?
3. How often should a crash cart be checked to be sure it is fully stocked and no medications are expired?
   a. Every 6 months
   b. Monthly
   c. After each use
   d. Both a & b
4. A 2-year-old beagle has clinical signs of lead toxicity and a history to support the diagnosis. Which agent would be the drug of choice for treating this condition?
   a. Yohimbine HCl
   b. 2-PAM
   c. Calcium EDTA
   d. Methylene blue
5. Which of the following is a central nervous system stimulant used in emergency situations during or after anesthesia where respirations are decreased and on apneic neonates?
   a. Doxapram
   b. Aminophylline
   c. Dobutamine
   d. Dopamine
6. Which emergency drug is given to a patient in cardiac arrest?
   a. Dexamethasone
   b. Atropine
   c. Diazepam
   d. Epinephrine
7. What diuretic is administered to an animal with cerebral edema associated with head trauma?
   a. Furosemide
   b. Mannitol
   c. Acetylcysteine
   d. Atropine
8. Which inotropic drug is used to increase the force of cardiac muscle contractions with little or no increase in heart rate?
   a. Dopamine
   b. Digoxin
   c. Dobutamine
   d. Hydralazine
9. Yohimbine HCl is a reversal agent for _____.
   a. Rompun
   b. acepromazine
   c. pentothal
   d. oxymorphone
10. Name four drugs that naloxone effectively reverses.
11. BAL has been administered to a 4-year-old mixed-breed dog for arsenic poisoning. Results of which of the following laboratory tests should be monitored closely?
    a. Packed cell volume (PCV)
    b. Blood urea nitrogen (BUN)
    c. White blood cell count (WBC)
    d. Alanine aminotransferase (ALT)
12. What is activated charcoal used for?
13. In veterinary medicine, calcium EDTA is used primarily for the treatment of _____.
14. _____ is a narcotic antagonist used for the treatment, prevention, or control of narcotic depression.
15. Grain alcohol may be used to treat what poisoning?
16. It is permissible to use calcium EDTA in anuric patients.
    a. True
    b. False
17. Calcium EDTA can be administered orally.
    a. True
    b. False
18. _____ is a central-acting CNS depressant and is the drug of choice for treating status epilepticus.
19. The antidote for organophosphate poisoning is:
    a. diphenhydramine
    b. atropine

c. doxapram

d. lidocaine

20. Methylene blue should not be used in cats.

a. True

b. False

21. Sodium bicarbonate is contraindicated in the treatment of metabolic acidosis.

a. True

b. False

22. Naloxone reverses the effects of butorphanol, pentazocine, and nalbuphine.

a. True

b. False

23. A 48-lb dog needs treatment for postanesthetic respiratory depression with naloxone (0.4 mg/mL). The dosage ordered is 0.02 mg/kg. What quantity (in milliliters) would you give?

24. A 455-kg horse requires reversal of xylazine sedation with yohimbine (2 mg/mL). The reversal dosage for yohimbine in horses is 0.075 mg/kg. How many milliliters would you draw up?

25. Prepare an injection of phytonadione (vitamin K_1) for an 80-lb dog that has ingested rodenticide. The dosage ordered is 2 mg/kg and the concentration of the K_1 solution is 10 mg/mL. What quantity will you draw up?

BIBILIOGRAPHY

Bassert, J. M. (2018). *McCurnin's clinical textbook for veterinary technicians* (9th ed.). St. Louis: Elsevier.

Bill, R. (2017). *Clinical pharmacology and therapeutics for veterinary technicians* (4th ed.). St. Louis: Elsevier.

Grauer, G. F. Overview of ethylene glycol. In *The Merck veterinary manual* (online edition). http:merckveterinary-manual.com/. Accessed May 2019.

Papich, M. G. (2016). *Saunders handbook of veterinary drugs* (4th ed.). St. Louis: Elsevier.

Plumb, D. C. (2015). *Plumb's veterinary drug handbook* (8th ed.). Ames, IA: Wiley-Blackwell.

Common Abbreviations
Used in Veterinary Medicine

AD	right ear (auris dextra)
ad lib	freely, as wanted (ad libitum)
AL	left ear (auris laeva)
AM	morning
AMA	against medical advice
ASAP	as soon as possible
AU	each ear (aures unitas)
bid	twice daily (bis in die)
bol.	large pill, bolus
Bute	Phenylbutazone
c– (cum)	with
caps	capsule
cc	cubic centimeters
d	day
DDx	differential diagnosis
DES	diethylstilbestrol
disp	dispense
DMSO	dimethyl sulfoxide
DS	dose or days not acceptable
D$_5$W	5% dextrose with water
Dx	Diagnosis
eod	every other day
g or gm	gram
gal	gallon
GI	gastrointestinal
gr	grain
gtt	drops (guttae)
GU	genitourinary
h or hr	hour
IC	intracardiac
IM	intramuscular
IN	intranasal
IP	intraperitoneal
IV	intravenous
IVP	intravenous pyelogram
K	potassium
l or L	liter
LA	long-acting
lb	pound
LRS	Lactated Ringer's solution
lt	left
mcg or µg	microgram
mEq	milliequivalent
mg	milligram
mL	milliliter
mm	millimeters
Na	sodium
non repetat.	do not repeat (non repetatur)
npo	nothing by mouth (nil per os)
O	pint
OD	right eye (oculus dexter)
OS	left eye (oculus sinister)
OU	both eyes (oculi unitas)
oz	ounce
per os or PO	by mouth, orally
phos	phosphorus
prn	as needed (pro re nata)
PTA	prior to administration
pwd	powder
q	every
q2h	every 2 hours (quaque secunda hora)
q4h	every 4 hours (quaque quarta hora)
qd	every day (quaque die)
qh	every hour (quaque hora)
qid	four times a day (quater in die)
qod	every other day
r or rt	right
Rx	take thou of (prescription)
s–	(sine) without
SC or SQ	subcutaneous
sid	once a day (semel in die)
sig	directions, instructions
SOB	shortness of breath
SR	sustained release
STAT	immediately (statim)
Sx	surgery
tab	tablet
TBL or Tbsp	tablespoon
TD	transdermal
tid	three times a day
TLC	tender loving care
tsp	teaspoon

Tx	treatment	**Ut dict**	as directed (ut dictum)
U	unit	**V-D or V/D**	vomiting/diarrhea
UG	urogenital	**×**	times, multiply
ung	ointment	**µL, mcl**	microliter

Weights and Measures

WEIGHTS AND MEASURES

The Metric System of Weight
1 microgram (mcg) = 0.000001 gram (g)
1 microgram (mcg) = 0.001 mg
1 milligram (mg) = 0.001 g
1 milligram (mg) = 1000 mcg
1 gram (g) = 1000 mg
1 gram (g) = 0.001 kilogram (kg)
1 kilogram (kg) = 1000 g

The Metric System of Liquid Measure
1 milliliter (mL) = 1000 microliters (µL or mcL)
1 milliliter (mL) = 1 cubic centimeter (cc)
1 milliliter (mL) = 0.001 L

1 liter (L) = 1000 mL
1 liter (L) = 10 deciliters (dL)
1 teaspoon (tsp) = 5 mL
1 tablespoon (Tbsp) = 15 mL
1 tablespoon (Tbsp) = 3 teaspoons

The Avoirdupois Weights
1 grain (gr) = 65 milligrams (mg)
1 ounce (oz) = 437.5 grains (gr)
16 oz = 1 pound (lb)
1 pound (lb) = 0.454 kilograms (kg)
1 kilogram (kg) = 2.2 pounds (lb)

EQUIVALENTS

1 grain (gr)	65 milligrams (mg) (64.8 mg)
1 ounce (oz)	28.35 gram (g)
1 pound (lb)	454 g (453.6 g)
1 dram	1.772 g
1 minim	0.06 milliliter (mL)
1 fluid dram	3.7 mL
1 fluid ounce	30 mL (29.57 mL)
1 pint	473 mL
1 gallon	3786 mL
1 mg	0.0154 gr
1 g	15.432 gr
1 kilogram (kg)	2.2 pounds (lb)
1 gallon (water)	8.35 pounds (lb)
1 mL	1 cubic centimeter (cc)
1 liquid pint	473 mL (473.18 mL)
1 liquid quart	946 mL (946.35 mL)
1 drop	0.05 mL
1 teaspoonful (tsp)	5 mL
3 teaspoons (tsp)	1 tablespoon (Tbsp)
1 tablespoonful (Tbsp)	15 mL

CONVERSIONS FOR CALCULATING DOSAGE

w/v%*(%)	mg/mL	µg/mL (mcg/mL)	Dilution g to mL
10	100	100,000	1:10
5	50	50,000	1:20
2	20	20,000	1:50
1	10	10,000	1:100
0.1	1	1,000	1:1000
0.2	0.2	200	1:5000
0.01	0.1	100	1:25,000
0.004	0.04	40	1:25,000
0.002	0.02	20	1:50,000
0.001	0.01	10	1:100,000
0.0001	0.001	1	1:1,000,000

*The definition of w/v is grams/dL.
From Boothe, D. M. (2012). *Small animal clinical pharmacology and therapeutics* (2nd ed.). St. Louis: Elsevier.

DRY WEIGHT AND VOLUME CONVERSIONS

Dry Weight	Volume Conversions
1 pound (lb)	454 grams (g)
1 gram (g)	0.0022 pound (lb)
1 gram (g)	1000 milligrams (mg)
1 gram (g)	1,000,000 micrograms (μg) or mcg
1 kilogram (kg)	1000 grams
1 kilogram (kg)	2.2 pounds (lb)
1 milligram (mg)	0.001 gram (g)
1 microgram (μg)	0.001 milligrams (mg)
1 microgram per gram (μg/g)	1 part per million (ppm)
1 liter (L)	1000 milliliter (mL)
1 milliliter (mL)	1000 microliter (μL) or mcL

Modified, 2019, from Boothe, D. M. (2012). *Small animal clinical pharmacology and therapeutics* (2nd ed.). St. Louis: Elsevier.

COMMON UNITS AND CONVERSION FACTORS

Unit	Abbreviation
Concentration of Solutions	
grams per deciliter	g/dL
grams per liter	g/L
international units per liter	IU/L
micrograms per deciliter	μg/dL
micromoles per liter	μmol/L
microunits per milliliter	μU/mL
milliequivalents per liter	mEq/L
milligrams per deciliter	mg/dL
millimoles per kilogram	mmol/kg
millimoles per liter	mmol/L
milliosmoles per kilogram	mOsm/kg
parts per million	ppm
units per liter	U/L
Distance	
centimeter	cm
meter squared	m^2
millimeter	mm
Fluids	
deciliter (10^2 mL)	dL
liter (10^3 mL)	L
microliter (10^{-6})	μL (mcL)
milliliter (1 mL or 10^{-3} L)	mL
Pressure	
centimeters of water	cm H_2O
millimeters of mercury	mm Hg
Time	
every	q
hour	h
minute	min
month	mo

Unit	Abbreviation
second	sec
week	wk
year	yr
Weights	
grain (1 gr = 65 mg)	gr
gram (1 g or 10^{-3} kg)	g
kilogram (10^3 g)	kg
microgram (10^{-6} g)	μg (mcg)
milligram (10^{-3} g)	mg
nanogram (10^{-9} g)	ng
pictogram (10^{-12} g)	pg

Common Conversions	
Volume or Weight	Equivalent
1 dram	1.772 grams (g)
1 drop (gt)	0.05 milliliter (mL)
20 drops	1 milliliter (1 cc)
1 glass (8 ounces)	240 milliliters
1 grain	0.065 gram or 65 milligrams
1 gram	15.43 grains
1 kilogram	2.2 pounds
1 liter	1.06 quarts
1 liter	33.81 fluid ounces
1 measuring cup	236.59 milliliters
1 milligram	0.015432 grain
1 milliliter	16.23 minims
1 ounce	28.35 grams
1 ounce	29.574 milliliters
1 pint	473 milliliters
1 quart	946 milliliters
1 tablespoon	15 milliliters
2 tablespoons	30 milliliters
1 teaspoon	5 milliliters

TEMPERATURE EQUIVALENTS

Fahrenheit (°F)	Celsius (°C)
Temperature Conversions	
°Fahrenheit to °Celsius:	°Celsius to °Fahrenheit:
$(°F - 32°)(5/9)$	$(°C)(9/5) + 32°$
98.6	37.0
99.0	37.2
100.0	37.7
101.0	38.3
102.0	38.8
103.0	39.4
104.0	40.0
105.0	40.5
106.0	41.1

Antidotes

Toxic Agent	Systemic Antidote	Dosage and Method for Treatment
Acetaminophen	N-Acetylcysteine (Mucomyst)	140 mg/kg loading dose, IV (dilute to 5% and give slow IV over 15–20 minutes) or PO (dilute in 5% dextrose or sterile water), then 70 mg/kg PO or IV every 6 hours for seven treatments. Larger overdoses may require up to 17 doses[*]
	Cimetidine	5 mg/kg, orally, every 6–8 hours for 2–3 days; prevents biotransformation of acetaminophen in dogs only
Amphetamines	Chlorpromazine	1 mg/kg IM, IV; administer only half dose if barbiturates have been given: blocks excitation. Titrate to effect. Treatment of increased intracranial pressure may be indicated (mannitol, furosemide)
	Urinary alkalinization: Ammonium chloride	100–200 mg/kg/day divided every 8–12 hours (contraindicated with myoglobinuria, renal failure, or acidosis)
Amitraz	Atipamezole	50 mcg/kg IM. Signs should reverse in 10 minutes. Repeat every 4–6 hours as needed.[*] Can follow with 0.1 mg/kg yohimbine IM every 6 hours
	Yohimbine	**Dogs:** 0.11 mg/kg IV slowly **Cats:** 0.5 mg/kg IV slowly
Antitussives	Naloxone	If narcotic (e.g., hydrocodone, codeine)
Arsenic, mercury, lead, copper, and other heavy metals except cadmium, silver, iron, selenium, and thallium	Dimercaprol (BAL)	10% solution in oil; give small animals 2.5–5 mg/kg IM every 4 hours for 2 days, bid for the next 10 days or until recovery. Note: In severe acute poisoning, 5-mg/kg dosage should be given only for the first day
	D-Penicillamine (Cuprimine)	For lead poisoning: 110 mg/kg/day divided q6–8h PO 30 minutes. Before feeding for 1–2 weeks[*]
Aspirin	No specific antidote (See also Nonsteroidal antiinflammatory drugs)	Acute toxicosis: urinary alkalinization, other supportive therapy; doses of 50 mg/kg/day (**dog**) and 25 mg/kg/day (**cat**); 7 mL/kg/day of bismuth subsalicylate (dogs and cats) may be toxic
Atropine, belladonna alkaloids	Physostigmine salicylate	0.02 mg/kg q12h IV (do not use neostigmine)

Continued

Toxic Agent	Systemic Antidote	Dosage and Method for Treatment
Barbiturates	Doxapram (Dopram)	2% solution: give small animals 3–5 mg/kg IV only (0.14–0.25 mL/kg); repeat as necessary
Barium, bismuth salts	Sodium sulfate/magnesium sulfate	20% solution given orally, 2–25 g
Bleach	Treat as alkali	Use of emetics is controversial; treat as an alkali poisoning. Therapies have included milk or water (large volumes), milk of magnesia (2–3 mg/kg), egg whites, or powdered milk slurry. Sodium bicarbonate is *not* recommended
Borates (roach killers, fleas products, fertilizers, herbicides, antiseptics, disinfectants, contact lens solutions)	No specific antidote	Supportive therapy includes emetics and gastric lavage, fluid therapy and diuresis; treatment of seizures and hyperthermia as indicated
Botulism	Antitoxin	Use is controversial. Supportive care may be sufficient. Supportive therapy may include penicillin, physostigmine or neostigmine, and atropine
Bromethalin	No specific antidote	Supportive care may include treatment of cerebral edema
Bromides	Chlorides (sodium or ammonium salts)	0.5–1 g daily for several days; hasten excretion
Caffeine/chocolate	No specific antidote	General treatment, diazepam (2–5 mg/kg) for tremors; treat arrhythmias as indicated
Carbon monoxide	Oxygen	Pure oxygen at normal or high pressure; artificial respiration; blood transfusion
Cholinergic agents	Atropine sulfate	0.02–0.04 mg/kg, as needed
Cholinesterase inhibitors	Atropine sulfate	Dosage is 0.2–0.4 mg/kg, repeated as needed for atropinization. Treat cyanosis (if present) first. Blocks only muscarinic effects. Atropine in oil may be injected for prolonged effect during the night. *Avoid atropine intoxication!*
	Pralidoxime chloride (2-PAM) (organophosphates, some carbamates; but not carbaryl, dimethan, or carbam piloxime)	5% solution;20 mg/kg IM or IV (diluted in IV fluids) injection (maximum dose is 500 mg/min), repeat as needed; discontinue after 3 - 4 treatments.* 2-PAM alleviates nicotinic effect and regenerates cholinesterase. Morphine, succinylcholine, and phenothiazine tranquilizers are contraindicated
	Diphenhydramine	1–4 mg/kg IM, PO every 8 hours to block nicotinic effects
Cocaine	No specific antidote	Chlorpromazine may lower seizure threshold, use cautiously; butylcholinesterase may convert cocaine to inactive metabolites (currently under investigation); fluids, metoprolol, or isopropanol to treat cardiac arrhythmias; phentolamine or sodium nitroprusside if beta blockers cause hypertension; lidocaine (instead of beta blockers) to control cardiac arrhythmias

Toxic Agent	Systemic Antidote	Dosage and Method for Treatment
Crayons (aniline dyes)	Ascorbic acid	20–30 mg/kg PO or 20 mg/kg IV slowly
	Methylene blue (if ascorbic acid fails)	**Dogs:** 3–4 mg/kg IV **Cats:** 1.5 mg/kg. (Methylene blue may cause Heinz body formation in the absence of methemoglobinemia, and sometimes in the presence of methemoglobinemia)
Copper	D-Penicillamine (Cuprimine)	52 mg/kg for 6 days (*See also* Arsenic)
	Ammonium molybdate	50–500 mg, PO, once a day
	Sodium thiosulfate	300–1000 mg, PO, once a day
	Ammonium tetrathiomolybdate	100–500 mg, PO on alternate days for three treatments
Coumarin-derivative anticoagulants	Vitamin K_1 (Aqua-mephyton, 5-mg caps) (Vita K_1, Eschar, 25-mg caps)	Give 3–5 mg/kg/day with canned food. Treat 7 days for warfarin-type, treat 21–30 days for second-generation anticoagulant rodenticides. Oral therapy is more efficacious than IV
	Whole blood or plasma	Blood transfusion, 25 mL/kg
Curare	Neostigmine methylsulfate	Solution: (1 mL = 0.25, 0.5, or 1 mg/mL) Dose is 0.04 mg/kg, SC. Follow with IV injection of atropine (0.04 mg/kg)
	Edrophonium chloride (Tensilon) Artificial respiration	1% solution; give 0.05–1 mg/kg IV
Cyanide	Methemoglobin (sodium nitrite is used to form methemoglobin) Sodium thiosulfate	1% solution of sodium nitrite, dosage is 16 mg/kg IV (1.6 mL/kg). Follow with sodium thiosulfate 20% solution at dosage of 150 - 500 mg/kg (0.6-2 mL/kg) IV. If treatment is repeated, use only sodium thiosulfate Note: These may be given simultaneously as follows: 0.5 mL/kg of combination consisting of 10 g sodium nitrite, 15 g sodium thiosulfate, distilled water quantity sufficient 250 mL. Dosage may be repeated once. If further treatment is required, give only 20% solution of sodium thiosulfate at level of 0.2 mL/kg
Decongestants	No specific antidote	Treat symptomatically
Detergents: anionic (Na, K, NH_4^+)		Milk or water followed by demulcent (e.g., oils, acacia, gelatin, starch, egg white)
Detergents: cationic (chlorides, iodides)		Castile soap dissolved in four times bulk of hot water. Albumin
Diatomaceous earth		No treatment indicated unless pulmonary, then supportive
Digitalis glycosides, oleander, and *Bufo* toads	Potassium chloride	**Dog:** 0.5–2.0 g, orally in divided doses or, in serious cases, as diluted solution given IV by slow drip (ECG control is essential)
	Diphenylhydantoin (Phenytoin)	25 mg/min IV control is established
	Propranolol (beta-blocker)	0.02 - 0.06 mg/kg IV slowly as needed to control cardiac arrhythmias (ECG control is essential)
	Atropine sulfate	0.02–0.04 mg/kg as needed for cholinergic control
	Diazepam (Valium)	0.2 - 0.5 mg/kg IV; in the case of *Bufo* toads, must treat convulsions first

Continued

Toxic Agent	Systemic Antidote	Dosage and Method for Treatment
Ethylene glycol	Ethanol	*See* Methanol and Ethylene glycol. Minimal lethal dose of ethylene glycol is 4.2–6.6 mL/kg (4.5 ounces in 20-lb dog) and 1.5 mL for cats. **Dogs:** as a 20% solution, give 5.5 mL/kg IV every 4 hours for five treatments, then every 6 hours for four additional treatments; dosed as a CRI over 1 hour. **Cats:** as a 20% solution, give 5 mL/kg IV every 6 hours for five treatments, then every 8 hours for four additional treatments; dosed as a CRI over 1 hour.* To prevent or correct acidosis, use sodium bicarbonate IV, 0.4 g/kg. Activated charcoal: 5 g/kg orally if within 4 hours of ingestion
	4-Methylpyrazole (fomepizole) Treatment of choice	**Dogs:** loading dose at 20 mg/kg IV, then 15 mg/kg at 12 hours, 15 mg/kg at 24 hours, and 5 mg/kg at 36 hours **Cats:** Initially, 125 mg/kg slow IV, 31.25 mg/kg IV at 12, 24, and 36 hours; treat supportively with fluids. Cats must be treated within 3 hours of ingestion.* It should not be given with ethanol due to fatal alcohol toxicosis
	Sodium bicarbonate 5%	8 mL/kg (**dog**) or 6 mL/kg (**cat**) IP every 4 hours for five treatments, then every 6 hours for four more treatments
Fertilizer	No specific antidote	Supportive therapy may include treatment for electrolyte disorders, vomiting, H_2 receptor blockers for gastritis, (sucralfate and analgesics as needed)
Fluoride	Calcium borogluconate	3–10 mL of 5%–10% solution
Fluoroacetate (Compound 1080)	Glyceryl monoacetin	0.1–0.5 mg/kg IM hourly for several hours (total 2–4 mg/kg), or diluted (0.5%–1%) IV (danger of hemolysis). Monoacetin is available only from chemical supply houses
	Acetamide	Animal may be protected if acetamide is given before or simultaneously with Compound 1080 (experimental)
	Pentobarbital Note: All treatments are generally unrewarding.	May protect against lethal dose (experimental)
Formaldehyde		Ammonia water (0.2% orally) or ammonium acetate (1% for lavage). Starch: 1 part to 15 parts hot water, added gradually. Gelatin soaked in water for 30 minutes. Albumin (four to six egg whites to 1 quart warm water); sodium thiosulfate (10% solution given orally). 0.5–3 g for small animals, followed by lavage or emesis
Garbage	No specific therapy	Supportive therapy may include antiemetics (metoclopramide or phenothiazines) and treatment of endotoxemia
Hallucinogens (LSD, PCP)	Diazepam (Valium)	As needed; avoid respiratory depression 0.2 - 0.5 mg/kg IV
Heparin	Protamine sulfate	1% solution; give 1–1.5 mg to antagonize 100 units of heparin; slow IV injection. Reduce dose as time increases between heparin injection and start of treatment (after 30 minutes give only 0.5 mg/kg)

Toxic Agent	Systemic Antidote	Dosage and Method for Treatment
Iron salts	Deferoxamine (Desferal)	Dose for animals not yet established. Dose for humans is 5 g of 5% solution given orally, then 20 mg/kg IM every 4–6 hours. In case of shock, dose is 40 mg/kg by IV drip over 4-hour period; may be repeated in 6 hours, then 15 mg/kg by drip every 8 hours
Ivermectin	Physostigmine	0.06 mg/kg IV very slowly; actions should last 30–90 minutes
	Picrotoxin (GABA antagonist)	Use is controversial. May cause severe seizures. Other treatment may include epinephrine and, if the product causing toxicosis is Eqvalan, an antihistamine to counteract polysorbate 80 (releases histamine in dogs) and atropine
Lead	Calcium disodium edetate (CaNa$_2$ EDTA)	Dosage: maximum safe dose is 75 mg/kg per 24 hours (only for severe cases). EDTA is available in 20% solution; for IV drip, dilute in 5% glucose to 0.5%; for IM, add procaine to 20% solution to give 0.5% concentration of procaine
	EDTA and BAL	BAL is given as 10% solution in oil. Treatment: (1) In severe case (CNS involvement with >100 µg Pb/100 g whole blood) give 4 mg/kg. BAL only as initial dose; follow after 4 hours, and every 4 hours for 3–4 days, with BAL and EDTA (12.5 mg/kg) at separate IM sites; skip 2 or 3 days, and then treat again for 3–4 days (2) In subacute case with <100 µg Pb/100 g whole blood, give only 50 mg EDTA/kg per 24 hours for 3–5 days
	Penicillamine (Cuprimine)	(3) May use after treatments either *1* or *2*; 100 mg/kg/day orally for 1–4 weeks
	Thiamine HCl	Experimental for nervous signs; 5 mg/kg, IV, bid, for 1–2 weeks; give slowly and watch for untoward reactions
	Succimer (Chemet)	Oral human dose: 10 mg/kg every 8 hours for 5 days, then 10 mg/kg bid for 2 weeks (total of 19 days of therapy). Animal dosages have not been established. (Used if blood lead levels >45 ppm)
Local anesthetics	See treatment for methemoglobinemia	Particularly cats
Marijuana	No effective antidotes	Protein: milk, egg whites (four to six egg whites to 1-quart warm water). Magnesium oxide (1:25 dilution with warm water). Sodium formaldehyde sulfoxylate: 5% solution for lavage. Starch (1 part to 15 parts hot water, added gradually). Activated charcoal: 5–50 g.
Metaldehyde	Diazepam (Valium)	0.2 - 0.5 mg/kg IV to control tremors
	Triflupromazine	0.2–2 mg/kg IV
	Pentobarbital	To effect; Note: should monitor liver function and treat accordingly

Continued

Toxic Agent	Systemic Antidote	Dosage and Method for Treatment
Methanol and ethylene glycol	Ethanol	**Dogs:** as a 20% solution, give 5.5 mL/kg IV every 4 hours for five treatments, then every 6 hours for four additional treatments, dosed as a CRI over 1 hour **Cats:** as a 20% solution, give 5 mL/kg IV every 6 hours for five treatments, then every 8 hours for four additional treatments; dosed as a CRI over 1 hour.* To prevent or correct acidosis, use sodium bicarbonate IV, 0.4 g/kg. Activated charcoal: 5 g/kg orally if within 4 hours of ingestion
	4-Methylpyrazole (fomepizole) Treatment of choice	**Dogs:** loading dose at 20 mg/kg IV, then 15 mg/kg at 12, 15 mg/kg at 24 hours, and 5 mg/kg at 36 hours. **Cats:** Initially, 125 mg/kg slow IV, 31.25 mg/kg IV at 12, 24, and 36 hours; treat supportively with fluids. Cats must be treated within 3 hours of ingestion.* It should not be given with ethanol due to fatal alcohol toxicosis
Methemoglobinemia-producing agents (nitrites, chlorates)	Methylene blue	1% solution (maximum concentration), given by *slow* IV injection, 1.5 - 4 mg/kg IV over several minutes*; lower doses can be repeated if needed. To prevent fall in blood pressure in case of nitrite poisoning, use a sympathomimetic drug (ephedrine or epinephrine). (Not recommended for cats)
	Ascorbic acid	30–33 mg/kg PO every 6 hours* or 20 mg/kg IV slowly; methylene blue; **dogs:** 3–4 mg/kg IV slowly if ascorbic acid not effective; **cats:** 1.5 mg/kg
Morphine and related drugs	Naloxone chloride (Narcan)	0.01 mg/kg IV Do not repeat if respiration is not satisfactory. See Note
	Levallorphan tartrate (Lorfan)	Give IV, 0.1–0.5 mL of solution containing 1 mg/mL. **Note:** Use either of these antidotes only in acute poisoning. Artificial respiration may be indicated. Activated charcoal is also indicated
Mothballs (naphthalene, paradichlorobenzene)	No specific antidote	Supportive care includes fluid therapy and maintenance of renal and hepatic function
Narcotics	Naloxone	Emesis: indicated only if patient is sufficiently alert. **Dog:** 0.01–0.04 mg/kg IV; repeat as needed. **Cat:** 0.01–0.04 mg/kg IV; repeat as needed. Supportive therapy may include anticonvulsants (especially for meperidine), fluid therapy
Nicotine	No specific antidote	Emesis: indicated only within 60 minutes and in absence of clinical signs. Atropine indicated to control parasympathetic signs
Nonsteroidal antiinflammatory drugs	Sucralfate	500–1000 mg PO every 8 hours
	Misoprostol	3–5 µg/kg PO every 8–12 hours
	Omeprazole	0.7 mg/kg every 24 hours (**dog**); alternative, ranitidine or famotidine (**dog and cat**)

Toxic Agent	Systemic Antidote	Dosage and Method for Treatment
Oxalates	Calcium	Treatment: 23% solution of calcium gluconate IV. Give 3–20 mL (to control hypocalcemia). Or calcium hydroxide as 0.15% solution or chalk or other calcium salts. Magnesium sulfate as cathartic. Other alkalines are contraindicated because their salts are more soluble. Maintain diuresis to prevent calcium oxalate deposition in kidney
Onion/garlic	No specific antidote	Supportive therapy should address methemoglobinemia and hemoglobinuria. Avoid acidic urine
Organic solvents: acetone, benzene, benzol, methanol, methylene chloride, naphtha, trichloroethane, acetonitrile, chloroform, trichloroethylene, toluene, xylene, xylol	No specific antidote	Emesis contraindicated. Supportive therapy includes treatment of cardiac arrhythmias, methemoglobinemia, renal failure, chemical pneumonia
Petroleum distillates (aliphatic hydrocarbons)		Olive oil, other vegetable oils, or mineral oil given orally. After 30 minutes, sodium sulfate as cathartic. Emesis and lavage are contraindicated for ingested volatile solvents, but petroleum distillates are used as carrier agents for more toxic agents
Phenols and cresols		Soap and water or alcohol lavage of skin Sodium bicarbonate (0.5%) dressings Activated charcoal and/or mineral oil given orally
Phenothiazine	Methylamphetamine (Desoxyn)	0.1–0.2 mg/kg IV; also transfusion. Only available in tablet form
	Diphenhydramine HCl	For CNS depression, 2–5 mg/kg IV for extrapyramidal signs
Phytotoxins and botulin	Antitoxins not available commercially, except for botulism	As indicated for specific antitoxins; examples of phytotoxins: ricin, abrin, robin, crotin
Plants		Treat signs as necessary
Red squill	Atropine sulfate, propranolol, potassium chloride	*See* Digitalis and oleander
Scorpion sting	Antivenin (may not be recommended)	Supportive therapy includes analgesia to control pain (morphine and meperidine, but not butorphanol, are contraindicated because of potential synergy with scorpion venom); methocarbamol (if muscle spasms evident) and fluid therapy
Smoke inhalation	Supportive therapy	Supportive therapy should target the respiratory system and treatment of carbon monoxide intoxication. Oxygen therapy; intermittent positive pressure ventilation with positive end-expiratory pressure with positive inotropic support, bronchodilators, treatment for cyanide poisoning if indicated, and treatment for cerebral edema

Continued

Toxic Agent	Systemic Antidote	Dosage and Method for Treatment
Snake bite Rattlesnake Copperhead Water moccasin	Antivenin; Trivalent Crotalidae	Caution: equine origin. Administer one to two vials, IV, slowly, diluted in 250–500 mL of saline or lactated Ringer's. Also administer antihistamines. *Corticosteroids are contraindicated*
Coral snake	Antivenin	Caution: equine origin. May be used as with pit viper antivenin
Spider bite Black widow	Antivenin	Caution: equine origin. Administer one to two vials reconstituted and diluted in 100 mL of normal saline and administered slowly IV over 30 minutes. Pretreatment with 2–4 mg/kg of diphenhydramine SQ to protect against allergic reaction.* Supportive therapy should include muscle relaxants (dantrolene or methocarbamol) analgesics, calcium gluconate for severe muscle cramping
	Dantrolene sodium (Dantrium)	1 mg/kg IV, followed by 1 mg/kg PO every 4 hours
Brown recluse	Dapsone	1 mg/kg, PO, tid for 10 days*
Strontium	Calcium salts	Usual dose of calcium borogluconate
	Ammonium chloride	0.2–0.5 g orally three to four times daily
	Potassium chloride	Give simultaneously with thiocarbazone or Prussian blue, 2–6 g orally daily in divided doses
Strychnine and brucine	Pentobarbital	Give IV to effect; higher dose is usually required than that required for anesthesia. Place animal in warm, quiet room
	Amobarbital	Give by slow IV infusion; inject to effect. Duration of sedation is usually 4–6 hours
	Methocarbamol (Robaxin)	10% solution; average first dose is 149 mg/kg IV (range: 40–300 mg). Repeat half dose as needed
	Glyceryl guaiacolate (Guaifenison)	110 mg/kg IV, 5% solution. Repeat as necessary
	Diazepam (Valium)	0.2 - 0.5 mg/kg IV, control convulsions, induce emesis, then use other agents
Thallium	Prussian blue	0.2 gm/kg orally in three divided doses daily
	Potassium chloride	Give simultaneously with Prussian blue, 2–6 g orally, daily in divided doses
Theobromine	*See* Caffeine/chocolate	
Toad poisoning (*Bufo alvarius, Bufo marinus*)	Propranolol (*Bufo* poisoning only)	0.02 - 0.06 mg/kg IV; repeat in 20 minutes if ECG does not normalize; supportive therapy includes fluid therapy
	Atropine	0.04 mg/kg IV to control hypersalivation or asystole
	Lidocaine	**Dogs:** 1–2 mg/kg IV followed by continuous infusion of 25–75 µg/kg/min; **cats:** 0.25–1 mg/kg IV bolus followed by 5–40 µg/kg/min continuous IV infusion
	Diazepam (Valium)	0.2 - 0.5 mg/kg IV in the case of *Bufo* toads; must treat convulsions first

Toxic Agent	Systemic Antidote	Dosage and Method for Treatment
Tricyclic antidepressants	No specific antidote	Supportive therapy should target seizures (diazepam, phenobarbital, or general anesthesia with pentobarbital or short-acting thiobarbiturates; or, if unsuccessful, neuromuscular blockade with pancuronium [0.03–0.06 mg/kg IV] or vecuronium [10–20 µg/kg IV in dogs or 20–40 µg/kg in cats]; cardiotoxicity [*see* Toad poisoning]: propranolol, lidocaine [quinidine, procainamide, disopyramide are contraindicated]; sodium bicarbonate [1–3 mEq/kg])
Unknown (e.g., toxic plants or other materials)	No specific antidote	Activated charcoal 2–5 g/kg (replaces universal antidote). For small animals: through stomach tube, as a slurry in water. Follow with emetic or cathartic, and repeat procedure
Vitamin D_3 rodenticides	Treatment of hypercalcemia	Supportive therapy should target treatment of hypercalcemia (0.9% saline solution); control of seizures and treatment of hyperthermia. Calciuria can be promoted with furosemide (1–5 mg/kg every 6–12 hours for 2–4 weeks); prednisolone; calcitonin (4–6 IU/kg every 6–12 hours if calcium >18 mg/dL); sodium bicarbonate if severe metabolic acidosis
	Amphojel, Basagel	As phosphate binders (aluminum hydroxide 30–90 mg/kg PO every 8–24 hours for 2 weeks)
Xylitol		Hypoglycemia: 1–2 mL of 25% dextrose followed by 2.5%–5% dextrose infusion as needed to maintain normoglycemia. Add potassium to fluids to maintain serum potassium (treat for 12–24 hours). Hepatic necrosis: 140–280 mg/kg *N*-acetylcysteine IV followed by 70 mg/kg qid IV or PO; *S*-adenosylmethionine 17–20 mg/kg/day PO, silymarin 20–50 mg/kg/day PO
Zinc	Chelation therapy (*see* Lead)	CaEDTA, Succimer. Other supportive therapy includes fluid therapy and antisecretory drugs such as ranitidine, famotidine, or omeprazole to decrease oral absorption of zinc

*Plumb, D. C. (2015). *Veterinary drug handbook* (8th ed.). Ames, IA: Wiley-Blackwell.
BAL, British anti-Lewisite; bid, twice a day; *CNS*, central nervous system; *ECG*, electrocardiogram; *EDTA*, ethylenediaminetetraacetic acid; *GABA*, gamma-aminobutyric acid; *IM*, intramuscular; *IP*, intraperitoneal; *IV*, intravenous; *LSD*, lysergic acid diethylamide; *PCP*, phencyclidine; *PO*, by mouth; *qid*, four times a day; *SC*, subcutaneous.
Modified, 2019, from Boothe, D. M. (2012). *Small animal clinical pharmacology and therapeutics* (2nd ed.). St. Louis: Elsevier.

Drug Dosages

Drug Name	Other Names	Formulations Available	Dosage
Acepromazine	Acepromazine maleate, PromAce	10- and 25-mg tablets, 10 mg/mL injection	0.025–0.1 mg/kg SC, IM, IV 0.5–2.2 mg/kg PO
Acetaminophen	Tylenol and many generic brands	120-, 160-, 325-, and 500-mg tablets	Dog: 15 mg/kg PO q8h Cat: Not recommended
Acetaminophen with codeine	Tylenol with codeine and many generic brands	Oral solution and tablets Many forms (e.g., 300 mg acetaminophen plus either 15-, 30-, or 60-mg codeine)	Follow dosing recommendations for codeine
Acetazolamide	Diamox	125- and 250-mg tablets	5–10 mg/kg PO q8–12h (glaucoma) 4–8 mg/kg PO q8–12h (other diuretic uses)
Acetylcysteine	Mucomyst	20% solution	Antidote: 140 mg/kg (loading dose) then 70 mg/kg IV or PO q4h for five doses. Eye: 2% solution topically q2h
Acetylsalicylic acid	*See* Aspirin		
ACTH	*See* Corticotropin		
Activated charcoal	*See* Charcoal, activated		
Adequan	*See* Polysulfated glycos-aminoglycan (PSGAG)		
Albendazole	Valbazen	113.6-mg/mL suspension and 300-mg/mL paste	25–50 mg/kg PO q12h for 3 days For *Giardia* use 25 mg/kg q12h for 2 days
Albuterol	Proventil or Ventolin	2-, 4-, and 8-mg tablets; 2 mg/5 mL syrup	20–50 mcg/kg q6–8h; up to maximum of 100 mcg/kg q6–8h PO
Allopurinol	Lopurin, Zyloprim	100- and 300-mg tablets	10 mg/kg q8h, then reduce to 10 mg/kg q24h
Altrenogest	Regu-Mate		
Aluminum carbonate gel	Basaljel	Capsule (equivalent to 500 mg aluminum hydroxide)	10–30 mg/kg PO q8h (with meals)
Aluminum hydroxide gel	Amphojel	64-mg/mL oral suspension; 600-mg tablet	10–30 mg/kg PO q8h (with meals)
Amikacin	Amiglyde-V (veterinary) and Amikin (human)	250-mg/mL injection	Dog: 15–30 mg/kg IV, SC, IM q24h Cat: 10–14 mg/kg IV, SC, IM q24h

Drug Name	Other Names	Formulations Available	Dosage
6-Aminosalicylic acid	*See* Mesalamine, Olsalazine		
Amiodarone	Cordarone	200-mg tablets; 50-mg/mL injection	Dog: Start with 15-mg/kg loading dose, then 10 mg/kg/day thereafter
Aminophylline	Many (generic) (Theophylline is preferred for oral therapy)	100-, 200-, 300-, 400-mg tablets; 25-mg/mL injection	Dog: 10 mg/kg PO, IM, IV q8h Cat: 6.6 mg/kg PO q12h
Amitraz	Mitaban	10.6-mL concentrated dip (19.9%). 10.6 mL per 7.5 L water (0.025% solution)	Apply three to six topical treatments q2wk. For refractory cases, this dose has been exceeded to produce increased efficacy. Doses that have been used include 0.025%, 0.05%, and 0.1% concentration applied twice per week and 0.125% solution applied to one-half body every day for 4 weeks to 5 months
Amitriptyline	Elavil	10-, 25-, 50-, 75-, 100-, and 150-mg tablets	Dog: 1–2 mg/kg PO q12–24h (range: 0.25–4 mg/kg q12–24h) Cat: 2–4 mg/cat/day PO; for cystitis: 2 mg/kg/day (2.5–7.5 mg/cat/day)
Amlodipine besylate	Norvasc	2.5-, 5-, and 10-mg tablets	Dog: 2.5 mg/dog or 0.1 mg/kg PO once daily Cat: 0.625 mg/cat/day PO initially and increase if needed to 1.25 mg/cat/day (average is 0.18 mg/kg)
Ammonium chloride	Generic	Available as crystals	Dog: 100 mg/kg PO q12h Cat: 800 mg/cat (approx. ⅓ to ¼ tsp) mixed with food daily
Amoxicillin trihydrate	Amoxi-Tabs, Amoxidrops, Amoxil, and others	50-, 100-, 200-, and 400-mg tablets; 50-mg/mL oral suspension	6.6–20 mg/kg PO q8–12h
Amoxicillin/ clavulanic acid	Clavamox	62.5-, 125-, 250-, and 375-mg tablets; 62.5-mg/mL suspension	Dog: 12.5–25 mg/kg PO q12h Cat: 62.5 mg/cat PO q12h; consider administering these doses q8h for gram-negative infections
Amphotericin B	Fungizone	50-mg injectable vial	0.5 mg/kg IV (slow infusion) q48h, to a cumulative dose of 4–8 mg/kg
Amphotericin B (liposomal)	Amphotec, Abelcet, AmBisome	50-, 100-mg vials	Dog: 2–3 mg/kg IV three times/wk for 9–12 treatments for a cumulative dose of 24–27 mg/kg Cat: 1 mg/kg IV 3 times/wk for 12 treatments
Ampicillin	Omnipen, Principen, others	250- and 500-mg capsules; 125-, 250-, and 500-mg vials of ampicillin sodium; also 1- and 2- gram vials	10–20 mg/kg IV, IM, SC q6–8h (ampicillin sodium); 20–40 mg/kg PO q8h
Ampicillin + sulbactam	Unasyn	1.5- and 3- g vials in 2:1 combination for injection	22–30 mg/kg IV every 6–8 hours (as combined ampicillin+sulbactam)
Ampicillin trihydrate	Polyflex	10- and 25-mg vials for injection	Dog: 10–50 mg/kg SC, IM q24h Cat: 10–20 mg/kg SC, IM q24h

Continued

Drug Name	Other Names	Formulations Available	Dosage
Amprolium	Amprol, Corid	9.6% (9.6 g/dL) oral solution; soluble powder	1.25 g of 20% amprolium powder to daily feed, or 30 mL of 9.6% amprolium solution to 3.8 L of drinking water for 7 days
Antacid drugs	*See* Aluminum hydroxide gel, Magnesium hydroxide, and Calcium carbonate		
Apomorphine hydrochloride	Generic	6-mg tablet; also compounded into injection, various strengths	0.44 mg/kg IM; 0.05 mg/kg IV; 0.1 mg/kg SC, or instill 0.25 mg in conjunctiva of eye (dissolve 6-mg tablet in 1–2 mL of saline)
Ascorbic acid	Vitamin C	Various forms	100–500 mg/animal/day (diet supplement) or 100 mg/animal q8h (urine acidification)
L-Asparaginase	Elspar	10,000 U per vial for injection	400 Units/kg IV, IP, IM weekly; or 10,000 Units/m^2 weekly for 3 weeks
Aspirin	Many generic and brand names (Bufferin, Ascriptin)	81-mg and 325-mg tablets	Dog: Mild analgesia: 10 mg/kg q12h Antiinflammatory: 20–25 mg/kg q12h Antiplatelet: 5–10 mg/kg q24–48h Cat: 81 mg q48h PO
Atenolol	Tenormin	25-, 50-, and 100-mg tablets; 25-mg/mL oral suspension	Dog: 6.25–12.5 mg/dog q12h (or 0.25–1.0 mg/kg q12–24h) PO Cat: 6.25–12.5 mg/cat q12h (approx. 3 mg/kg) PO
Atipamezole	Antisedan	5-mg/mL injection	Inject same volume as used for medetomidine
Atracurium	Tracrium	10-mg/mL injection	0.2 mg/kg IV initially, then 0.15 mg/kg q30min (or IV infusion at 4–9 mcg/kg/min)
Atropine	Many generic brands	400-, 500-, and 540- mcg/mL injection; 15-mg/mL injection	0.02–0.04 mg/kg IV, IM, SC q6–8h; 0.2–0.5 mg/kg (as needed) for organophosphate and carbamate toxicosis
Auranofin (triethylphosphine gold)	Ridaura	3-mg capsule	0.1–0.2 mg/kg PO q12h
Azathioprine	Imuran	50-mg tablet; 100 mg vial for injection	Dog: 2 mg/kg PO q24h initially then 0.5–1 mg/kg q48h Cat (use cautiously): 0.3 mg/kg PO q48h
Azithromycin	Zithromax	250-mg capsule; and 250- 500- and 600-mg tablets; 20- and 40-mg/mL oral suspension	Dog: 10 mg/kg PO q48h or 3.3 mg/kg once daily Cat: 5–10 mg/kg PO every other day
AZT (azidothymidine)	*See* Zidovudine		
Bactrim (sulfamethoxazole + trimethoprim)	*See* Trimethoprimsulfonamide combinations		
BAL	*See* Dimercaprol		

Drug Name	Other Names	Formulations Available	Dosage
Benazepril	Lotensin	5-, 10-, 20-, and 40-mg tablets	Dog: 0.25–0.5 mg/kg PO q24h Cat: 0.5–1 mg/kg q24h PO or 2.5 mg/cat/day up to a maximum of 5 mg/cat/day
Betamethasone	Celestone	600-mcg (0.6-mg) tablet; 3-mg/mL sodium phosphate injection	0.1–0.2 mg/kg PO q12–24h
Bethanechol	Urecholine	5-, 10-, 25-, and 50-mg tablets; 5-mg/mL injection	Dog: 5–15 mg/dog PO q8h Cat: 1.25–5 mg/cat PO q8h
Bisacodyl	Dulcolax	5-mg tablet	5 mg/animal PO q8–24h
Bismuth subsalicylate	Pepto-Bismol	Oral suspension: 262 mg/15 mL or 525 mg/mL in extra-strength formulation; 262-mg tablet	1–3 mL/kg/day (in divided doses) PO
Bleomycin	Blenoxane	15-Unit vials for injection	10 Units/m^2 IV or SC for 3 days, then 10 Units/m^2 weekly (maximum cumulative dose 200 Units/m^2)
Bromide	*See* Potassium bromide		
BSP (Bromsulphalein)	*See* Sulfobromophthalein (BSP)		
Budesonide	Entocort	3-mg capsule	Dog, cat: 0.125 mg/kg q8–12h PO; dose interval may be increased to q24h when condition improves
Bupivacaine	Marcaine and generic	2.5-, 5-, 7.5-mg/mL solution injection	0.2 mL/kg of 0.5% solution for an epidural
Buprenorphine	Buprenex (human label) Simbadol (Veterinary label)	Buprenex: 0.3-mg/mL solution Simbadol: 0.24 mg/kg SC once daily for up to 3 days	Dog: 0.006–0.02 mg/kg IV, IM, SC q4–8h Cat: 0.005–0.01 mg/kg IV, IM q4–8h Buccal administration in cats: 0.01–0.02 mg/kg q12h
Buspirone	BuSpar	5- and 10-mg tablets	Dog: 2.5–10 mg/dog PO q12–24h; or 1 mg/kg q12h PO Cat: 2.5–5 mg/cat PO q24h (may be increased to 5–7.5 mg/cat twice daily for some cats)
Busulfan	Myleran	2-mg tablet	3–4 mg/m^2 PO q24h
Butorphanol	Torbutrol, Torbugesic	1-, 5-, and 10-mg tablets; 0.5-, 1-, 2-, or 10-mg/mL injection	Dog: Antitussive: 0.055 mg/kg SC q6–12h or 0.55 mg/kg PO Preanesthetic: 0.2–0.4 mg/kg IV, IM, SC (with acepromazine) Analgesic: 0.2–0.4 mg/kg IV, IM, SC q2–4h or 0.55–1.1 mg/kg PO q6–12h Cat: Analgesic: 0.2–0.8 mg/kg IV, SC q2–6h, or 1.5 mg/kg PO q4–8h
Calcitriol	Rocaltrol, Calcijex	Available as injection (Calcijex) and capsules (Rocaltrol): 0.25- and 0.5-mcg capsules; 1- or 2-mcg/mL injection; 1 mcg/mL oral solution	Dog: 2.5–5 nanograms/kg (0.0025–0.005 microgams/kg) PO once daily Cat: 0.25 mcg/cat every other day; or 0.01–0.04 mcg/kg/day

Continued

Drug Name	Other Names	Formulations Available	Dosage
Calcium carbonate	Many brands available: Titralac, Tums, generic	Many tablets or oral suspension (e.g., 650-mg tablet contains 260 mg calcium ion)	For phosphate binder: 60–100 mg/kg/day in divided doses PO For calcium supplementation: 70–180 mg/kg/day added to food
Calcium chloride	Generic	10% (100 mg/mL) solution	0.1–0.3 mL/kg IV (slowly)
Calcium citrate	Citracal (OTC)	950-mg tablet (contains 200 mg calcium ion)	Dog: 20 mg/kg/day added to food Cat: 10–30 mg/kg PO q8h (with meals)
Calcium disodium EDTA	*See* Edetate calcium disodium		
Calcium gluconate	Kalcinate and generic	10% (100 mg/mL) injection	0.5–1.5 mL/kg IV (slowly)
Calcium lactate	Generic	OTC tablet	Dog: 0.5–2 (no trailing zero) g/dog/day PO (in divided doses) Cat: 0.2–0.5 g/cat/day PO (in divided doses)
Captopril	Capoten	25-mg tablet	Dog: 0.5–2 mg/kg PO q8–12h Cat: 3.12–6.25 mg/cat PO q8h
Carbimazole	Neomercazole	Available in Europe	Cat: 5 mg/cat PO q8h (induction), followed by 5 mg/cat PO q12h
Carboplatin	Paraplatin	50- and 150-mg vial for injection	Dog: 300 mg/m^2 IV q3–4wk Cat: 200 mg/m^2 IV q4wk
Carprofen	Rimadyl (Zenecarp in the UK), Novox, generic	25-, 75-, and 100-mg tablets; 50 mg/mL solution	Dog: 2.2 mg/kg PO q12h; or 4.4 mg/kg once daily PO; 2.2 mg/kg q12h or 4.4 mg/kg once daily SC Cat: 4 mg/kg SC once prior to surgery
Carvedilol	Coreg	3.125-, 6.25-, 12.5-, and 25-mg tablets	Dog: 0.2–0.4 mg/kg q12h PO; titrate dose up to 1.5 mg/kg q12h PO if needed
Cascara sagrada	Many brands (e.g., Nature's Remedy)	100- and 325-mg tablets	Dog: 1–5 mg/kg day PO Cat: 1–2 mg/cat/day
Castor oil	Generic	Oral liquid (100%)	Dog: 8–30 mL/day PO Cat: 4–10 mL/day PO
Cefadroxil	Cefa-Tabs, Cefa-Drops	50-mg/mL oral suspension; 50-, 100-, 200-, and 1000-mg tablets	Dog: 22–30 mg/kg PO q12h Cat: 22 mg/kg PO q24h
Cefazolin sodium	Ancef, Kefzol, and generic	50 and 100 mg/50 mL for injection	20–35 mg/kg IV, IM q8h For perisurgical use: 22 mg/kg q2h during surgery
Cefdinir	Omnicef	300-mg capsules; 25-mg/mL oral suspension	Dose not established (human dose is 7 mg/kg PO q12h)
Cefixime	Suprax	20-mg/mL and 40-mg/mL oral suspension and 100-, 200- and 400-mg tablets	10 mg/kg PO q12h For cystitis: 5 mg/kg PO q12–24h
Cefotaxime	Claforan	500-mg and 1-, 2-, and 10-g vials for injection	Dog: 50 mg/kg IV, IM, SC q12h Cat: 20–80 mg/kg IV, IM q6h
Cefotetan	Cefotan	1-, 2-, and 10-g vials for injection	30 mg/kg IV, SC q8h
Cefovecin	Convenia	80 mg/mL injection	Dog, cat: 8 mg/kg SC once q7–14d
Cefoxitin sodium	Mefoxin	1-, 2-, and 10-g vials for injection	30 mg/kg IV q6–8h

Drug Name	Other Names	Formulations Available	Dosage
Cefpodoxime proxetil	Simplicef	100- and 200-mg tablets; 10- or 20-mg/mL human label suspension	Dog: 5–10 mg/kg PO once daily Cat: Dose not established
Ceftazidime	Fortaz, Ceptaz, Tazicef	0.5-, 1-, 2-, and 6-g vials reconstituted to 280 mg/mL	30 mg/kg IV, IM q6h
Ceftiofur	Naxcel (ceftiofur sodium); Excenel (ceftiofur HCl)	50-mg/mL injection; 1- and 4-gram vials	2.2–4.4 mg/kg SC q24h (for urinary tract infections)
Cephalexin	Keflex and generic forms Rilexine	250- and 500-mg capsules; 250- and 500-mg tablets; 100-mg/mL or 125- and 250-mg/5-mL oral suspension Rilexine: 150, 300, and 600 mg	10–30 mg/kg PO q6–12h; for pyoderma, 22–35 mg/kg PO q12h Rilexine: 22 mg/kg PO q12 h
Cetirizine	Zyrtec	1-mg/mL oral syrup; 5- and 10-mg tablets	Dog: 5–10 mg/dog q12h, PO, up to a dose of 2 mg/kg q12h, PO Cat: 5 mg/cat, PO, q24h
Charcoal, activated	Acta-Char, Charcodote, Toxiban, generic	Oral suspension	1–4 g/kg PO (granules); 6–12 mL/kg (suspension)
Chlorambucil	Leukeran	2-mg tablet	Dog: 2–6 mg/m² or 0.1–0.2 mg/kg PO q24h initially, then q48h Cat: 0.1–0.2 mg/kg q24h initially, then q48h PO
Chloramphenicol and chloramphenicol palmitate	Chloromycetin, generic forms	30-mg/mL oral suspension (palmitate); 250-mg capsule; and 100-, 250-, 500-, and 1000-mg tablets	Dog: 40–50 mg/kg PO q8h Cat: 12.5–20 mg/kg PO q12h
Chlorothiazide	Diuril	250- and 500-mg tablets; 50-mg/mL oral suspension and injection	20–40 mg/kg PO q12h or IV
Chlorpheniramine maleate	Chlor-Trimeton, Phenetron, and others	4- and 8-mg tablets	Dog: 4–8 mg/dog PO q12h (up to a maximum of 0.5 mg/kg q12h) Cat: 2 mg/cat PO q12h
Chlorpromazine	Thorazine	25-mg/mL injection solution	Dog: 0.5 mg/kg IM, SC q6–8h (before cancer chemotherapy administer 2 mg/kg SC q3h) Cat: 0.2–0.4 mg/kg q6–8h IM, SC
Chorionic gonadotropin	See Gonadotropin		
Cimetidine	Tagamet (OTC and prescription)	100-, 150-, 200-, and 300-mg tablets and 60-mg/mL injection	10 mg/kg IV, IM, PO q6–8h (in renal failure administer 2.5–5 mg/kg IV, PO q12h)
Ciprofloxacin	Cipro and generic	250-, 500-, and 750-mg tablets; 2-mg/mL injection	Dog: 10–20 mg/kg IV q24h; 25 mg/kg PO q24h Cat: 15 mg/kg PO q24h
Cisapride		Must be compounded	Dog: 0.1–0.5 mg/kg PO q8–12h (doses as high as 0.5–1.0 mg/kg have been used in some dogs) Cat: 2.5–5 mg/cat PO q8–12h (as high as 1 mg/kg q8h has been administered to cats)

Continued

Drug Name	Other Names	Formulations Available	Dosage
Cisplatin	Platinol	1-mg/mL injection; 50-mg vials	Dog: 60–70 mg/m² q3–4wk (administer fluid for diuresis with therapy) Cat: Not recommended
Clavamox	*See* Amoxicillin–clavulanic acid combination		
Clavulanic acid	*See* Amoxicillin–clavulanic acid combination		
Clindamycin	Antirobe, Cleocin, and generic	Oral liquid 25-mg/mL; 25-, 75-, 150-, and 300-mg capsule; and 150-mg/mL injection (Cleocin)	Dog: 11–33 mg/kg q12h PO; for oral and soft tissue infection: 5.5–33 mg/kg q12h PO Cat: 11–33 mg/kg q24h PO for skin and anaerobic infections Toxoplasmosis: 12.5–25 mg/kg PO q12h for 4 weeks
Clomipramine	Anafranil (human label); Clomicalm (veterinary label)	10-, 25-, 50-, 75-mg capsules (human); 5-, 20-, 40- and 80-mg tablets (veterinary)	Dog: 1–2 mg/kg PO q12h up to a maximum of 3 mg/kg PO q12h Cat: 1–5 mg/cat PO q12–24h
Clonazepam	Klonopin	0.5-, 1-, and 2-mg tablets	Dog: 0.5 mg/kg PO q8–12h Cat: 0.1–0.2 mg/kg q12–24h PO
Clopidogrel	Plavix	75-mg tablets	Dog: 2–4 mg/kg q24h PO; give oral loading dose of 10 mg/kg Cat: 19 mg per cat (¼ tablet) q24h PO
Clorazepate	Tranxene	3.75-, 7.5-, 11.25-, 15-, and 22.5-mg tablets	Dog: 2 mg/kg PO q12h Cat: 0.2–0.4 mg/kg q12–24h PO (up to 0.5–2 mg/kg)
Cloxacillin	Cloxapen, Orbenin, Tegopen	250- and 500-mg capsules; 25-mg/mL oral solution	20–40 mg/kg PO q8h
Codeine	Generic	15-, 30-, and 60-mg tablets; 5-mg/mL syrup; 3-mg/mL oral solution	Analgesia: 0.5–1 mg/kg PO q4–6h Antitussive: 0.1–0.3 mg/kg PO q4–6h
Colchicine	Generic	500- and 600-mcg tablets	0.01–0.03 mg/kg PO q24h
Colony-stimulating factor	Sargramostim (Leukine) and filgrastim (Neupogen)	300 mcg/mL (Neupogen) and 250 or 500 mcg/mL (Leukine)	Leukine: 0.25 mg/m² q12h SC or IV infusion. Neupogen: 0.005 mg/kg (5 mcg/kg) q24h SC for 2 wk
Corticotropin (ACTH)	AcatharGel 80 U/mL	Response test: collect pre-ACTH sample and inject	2.2 IU/kg IM; collect post-ACTH sample in 2 hours in dogs and at 1 and 2 hours in cats
Cosequin	*See* Glucosamine chondroitin sulfate		
Cosyntropin	Cortrosyn	250 mcg per vial (can be stored in freezer for 6 months)	Response test: Dog: Collect pre-ACTH sample and inject 5 mcg/kg IV or IM and collect sample at 30 and 60 minutes Cat: 0.125 mg IV or IM and collect sample at 30 and 60 min after IV administration and 30 and 60 min after IM administration
Cyanocobalamin (vitamin B₁₂)	Many	1000-mcg/mL injection	Dog: 200–500 mcg/day IM, SC Cat: 250 mcg/day IM, SC

Drug Name	Other Names	Formulations Available	Dosage
Cyclophospha-mide	Cytoxan, Neosar	25-mg/mL injection; 25- and 50-mg capsules	Dog: Anticancer: 50 mg/m² PO once daily 4 days/wk or 150–300 mg/m² IV or PO and repeat in 21 days Immunosuppressive therapy: 50 mg/m² (approx. 2.2 mg/kg) PO q48h or 2.2 mg/kg once daily for 4 days/wk Cat: 6.25–12.5 mg/cat once daily 4 days/wk
Cyclosporine (cyclosporin A)	Atopica, Neoral, Optim-mune (ophthalmic)	Atopica: 10-, 25-, 50-, and 100-mg capsule, 100 mg/mL oral solution. Neoral: 25-mg and 100-mg microemulsion capsules; 100-mg/mL oral solution (for microemulsion). Optim-mune: 0.2% ointment	Dog: 3–7 mg/kg/day; for atopic derma-titis some dogs are controlled with q48h dosing Cat: 7 mg/kg PO q24h
Cyproheptadine	Periactin	4-mg tablet; 2-mg/5-mL syrup	Antihistamine: 1.1 mg/kg PO q8–12h Appetite stimulant: 2 mg/cat PO
Cytarabine (cytosine arabi-noside)	Cytosar-U	20 mg/mL and 100-mg/mL solution for injection	Dog (lymphoma): 100 mg/m² IV, SC once daily or 50 mg/m² twice daily for 4 days Cat: 100 mg/m² once daily for 2 days
Dacarbazine	DTIC	100- and 200-mg vial for injection	200 mg/m² IV for 5 days q3wk; or 800–1000 mg/m² IV q3wk
Dalteparin	Fragmin	2500 units/0.2 mL or 5000 units/0.2 mL, 7500 units/0.3 mL, 10,000 units/mL, 12,500 units/0.5 mL, 15,000 units/0.6 mL, 18,000 units/0.72 mL pre-filled syringes, or 25,000 units/mL multidose vials for injection	Dog: 100–150 units/kg q8h SC Cat: 180 units/kg q6h SC
Danazol	Danocrine	50-, 100-, and 200-mg capsules	5–10 mg/kg PO q12h
Dantrolene	Dantrium	25-, 50-, and 100-mg capsule; 20 mg and 250 mg vials for injection	For prevention of malignant hyperther-mia: 2–3 mg/kg IV For muscle relaxation: Dog: 1–5 mg/kg PO q8h Cat: 0.5–2 mg/kg PO q12h
Dapsone	Generic	25- and 100-mg tablets	Dog: 1.1 mg/kg PO q8–12h Cat: Do not use
Deferoxamine	Desferal	500-mg and 2 gram vials for injection	10 mg/kg IV, IM q2h for two doses; then 10 mg/kg q8h for 24 hours
Dembrexine	Sputolysin		
Deprenyl (ʟ-deprenyl)	*See* Selegiline (Anipryl)		
Deracoxib	Deramaxx	25-, 100-mg tablets	Dog: 3–4 mg/kg q24h PO for 7 days; or 1–2 mg/kg q24h PO for long-term use Cat: Dose not established

Continued

Drug Name	Other Names	Formulations Available	Dosage
Desmopressin acetate	DDAVP	4-mcg/mL injection; 100 mcg/mL desmopressin acetate nasal spray/solution for injection; 27.7 mcg, 55.3 mcg, 1010 mcg and 200 mcg tablets	Diabetes insipidus: 2–4 drops (2 mcg) q12–24h intranasally or in eye Animal oral dose: 0.05–0.1 mg/dog q12h PO initially, then increase to 0.1–0.2 mg/dog q12h as needed von Willebrand disease treatment: 1 mcg/kg SC, IV, diluted in 20 mL saline administered over 10 min
Desoxycorticosterone pivalate	Percorten-V, DOCP, or DOCA pivalate	25 mg/mL injection	1.5–2.2 mg/kg IM q25days
Dexamethasone (dexamethasone solution and dexamethasone sodium phosphate)	Azium solution in polyethylene glycol. Sodium phosphate forms include DexaJect SP, Dexavet, and Dexasone. Tablets include Decadron and generic	Azium solution, 2 mg/mL; sodium phosphate forms are 3.33 mg/mL; 0.25-, 0.5-, 0.75-, 1-, 1.5-, 2-, 4-, and 6-mg tablets	Antiinflammatory: 0.07–0.15 mg/kg IV, IM, PO q12–24h Dexamethasone suppression test: Dog: 0.01 mg/kg IV Cat: 0.1 mg/kg IV Collect sample at 0, 4, and 8 hours
Detomidine Hydrochloride	Dormosedan	10 mg/mL injection	Dogs: 5 mcg/kg IV or 10-20 mcg/kg IM Cats: 0.5 mg/kg transmucosal
Dexmedetomidine	Dexdomitor	0.5-mg/mL and 100 mcg/mL injectable solution	Dog: Sedative and analgesic: 375 mg/m² IV or 500 mg/m² IM Dog: Preanesthetic: 125 mg/m² IM Cat: Sedative and analgesic: 40 mcg/kg IM
Dexmedetomidine oromucosal gel	Sileo	0.09 mg/mL oral transmucosal gel	125 mcg/m² oral transmucosal; may repeat after 2 hours, but no more than 5 doses per single noise event
Dexpanthenol	D-Panthenol	250 mg/mL injection	11 mg/kg IM; may repeat after 2 hours, then every 6-8 hours thereafter
Dextran	Dextran 70, Gentran-70	Injectable solution: 250, 500, and 1000 mL	10–20 mL/kg IV to effect
Dextromethorphan	Benylin and others	Available in syrup, capsule, and tablet; many OTC products	0.5–2 mg/kg PO q6–8h has been reported, but effective dose not established
Dextrose solution 5%	D5W	Fluid solution for IV administration	40–50 mL/kg IV q24h
Diazepam	Valium and generic	2- and 5-mg tablets; 5-mg/mL solution for injection	Preanesthetic: 0.5 mg/kg IV Status epilepticus: 0.5 mg/kg IV, 1 mg/kg rectal; repeat if necessary Appetite stimulant (cat): 0.2 mg/kg IV
Dichlorophen	Vermiplex (*See* Toluene)		
Dichlorphenamide	Daranide	50-mg tablet	3–5 mg/kg PO q8–12h
Dichlorvos	Task	10- and 25-mg tablets	Dog: 26.4–33 mg/kg PO Cat: 11 mg/kg PO
Dicloxacillin	Dynapen	125-, 250-, and 500-mg capsules; 12.5-mg/mL oral suspension	25 mg/kg IM q6h Oral doses not absorbed
Diethylcarbamazine (DEC)	Caricide, Filaribits	Chewable tablets; 50-, 60-, 180-, 200-, and 400-mg tablets	Heartworm prophylaxis: 6.6 mg/kg PO q24h

Drug Name	Other Names	Formulations Available	Dosage
Diethylstilbes-trol (DES)	DES, generic (no longer manufactured in the United States)	1- and 5-mg tablet; 50-mg/mL injection; compounded	Dog: 0.1–1 mg/dog PO q24h Cat: 0.05–0.1 mg/cat PO q24h
Difloxacin	Dicural	11.4-, 45.4-, and 136-mg tablets	Dog: 5–10 mg/kg/day PO Cat: Safe dose not established
Digoxin	Lanoxin, Cardoxin	0.0625-, 0.125-, 0.25-mg tablets; 0.05- and 0.15-mg/mL elixir; 0.1-, 0.25-, 0.5-mg/mL Injection	Dog: (rapid digitalization): 0.0055–0.011 mg/kg IV q1h to effect Cat: 0.008–0.01 mg/kg PO q48h (approx. of a 0.125-mg tablet/cat) Dog: <20 kg body weight: 0.01 mg/kg q12h; >20 kg use 0.22 mg/m^2 PO q12h (subtract 10% for elixir)
Dihydrotachys-terol (vitamin D)	Hytakerol, DHT	0.125-mg tablet; 0.5-mg/mL oral liquid	0.01 mg/kg/day PO; for acute treatment administer 0.02 mg/kg initially, then 0.01–0.02 mg/kg PO q24–48h thereafter
Diltiazem	Cardizem, Dilacor	30-, 60-, 90-, 120-, 180-, and 240-mg tablets; 5 mg/mL injection Ext release/long-acting capsules: 120-, 180-, 240-, 300-, 360-, 420-mg	Dog: 0.5–1.5 mg/kg PO q8h, 0.25 mg/kg over 2 min IV (repeat if necessary) Cat: 1.75–2.4 mg/kg PO q8h For Dilacor XR or Cardizem CD: dose is 10 mg/kg PO once daily
Dimenhydrinate	Dramamine (Gravol in Canada)	25- and 50-mg tablets; 50-mg/mL injection	Dog: 4–8 mg/kg PO, IM, IV q8h Cat: 12.5 mg/cat IV, IM, PO q8h
Dimercaprol (BAL)	BAL in oil	Injection	4 mg/kg IM q4h
Dinoprost tro-methamine	*See* Prostaglandin F$_2\alpha$ 5-mg/mL injection		
Dioctyl calcium sulfosuccinate	*See* Docusate calcium		
Dioctyl sodium sulfosuccinate	*See* Docusate sodium		
Diphenhydramine	Diphenhydramine	Available OTC: 2.5-mg/mL elixir; 25- and 50-mg capsules and tablets; 50-mg/mL injection	Dog: 25–50 mg/dog IV, IM, PO q8h Cat: 2–4 mg/kg q6–8h PO or 1 mg/kg IM, IV q6–8h
Diphenoxylate	Lomotil	2.5 mg	Dog: 0.1–0.2 mg/kg PO q8–12h Cat: 0.05–0.1 mg/kg PO q12h
Diphenyl-hydantoin	*See* Phenytoin		
Diphosphonate disodium etidronate	*See* Etidronate disodium		
Dipyridamole	Persantine	25-, 50-, 75-mg tablets; 5-mg/mL injection	4–10 mg/kg PO q24h
Disopyramide	Norpace (Rythmodan in Canada)	100- and 150-mg capsules (10-mg/mL injection in Canada only)	6–15 mg/kg PO q8h

Continued

Drug Name	Other Names	Formulations Available	Dosage
Divalproex sodium	*See* Valproic acid		
Dobutamine	Dobutrex	250-mg/20 mL vial for injection (12.5 mg/mL)	Dog: 5–20 mcg/kg/min IV infusion Cat: 2 mcg/kg/min IV infusion
Docusate calcium	Surfak, Doxidan	60-mg tablet (and many others)	Dog: 50–100 mg/dog PO q12–24h Cat: 50 mg/cat PO q12–24h
Docusate sodium	Colace, Doxan, Doss, many OTC brands	50-, and 100-mg capsules; 10-mg/mL liquid	Dog: 50–200 mg/dog PO q8–12h Cat: 50 mg/cat PO q12–24h
Dolasetron mesylate	Anzemet	50-, 100-mg tablets; 20-mg/mL injection	Dog, cat: Prevention of nausea and vomiting: 0.6 mg/kg IV or PO q24h Treating vomiting and nausea: 1.0 mg/kg PO or IV once daily
Domperidone	Motilium	Not available in the United States	2–5 mg/animal PO
Dopamine	Intropin	40-, 80-, or 160-mg/mL	Dog, cat: 2–10 mcg/kg/min IV infusion
Doxapram	Dopram, Respiram	20-mg/mL injection	5–10 mg/kg IV Neonate: 1–5 mg (total dose) SC, sublingual, or via umbilical vein
Doxorubicin	Adriamycin	2-mg/mL injection	30 mg/m^2 IV q21 days, or >20 kg use 30 mg/m^2 and <20 kg use 1 mg/kg Cat: 20 mg/m^2 or approx. 1–1.25 mg/kg IV q3wk
Doxycycline	Vibramycin and generic forms	10-mg/mL oral suspension; 100-mg injection vial; 20-, 50- or 100-mg tablets or capsules	3–5 mg/kg PO, IV q12h or 10 mg/kg PO q24h For *Rickettsia* in dogs: 5 mg/kg q12h
Edetate calcium disodium (CaNa$_2$EDTA)	Calcium disodium verse-nate	20-mg/mL injection	25 mg/kg SC, IM, IV q6h for 2–5 days
Edrophonium	Tensilon and others	10-mg/mL injection	Dog: 0.11–0.22 mg/kg IV Cat: 0.25–0.5 mg/cat (total dose) IV
Enalapril	Enacard, Vasotec	2.5-, 5-, 10-, and 20-mg tablets	Dog: 0.5 mg/kg PO q12–24h Cat: 0.25–0.5 mg/kg PO q12–24h
Enflurane	Ethrane	Available as solution for inhalation	Induction: 2%–3% Maintenance: 1.5%–3%
Enilconazole	Imaverol, Clinafarm-EC	10% or 13.8% emulsion	Nasal aspergillosis: 10 mg/kg q12h instilled into nasal sinus for 14 days (10% solution diluted 50/50 with water) Dermatophytes: Dilute 10% solution to 0.2% and wash lesion with solution four times at 3- to 4-day intervals
Enoxaparin	Lovenox	30 mg/0.3 mL, 40 mg/0.4 mL, 60 mg/0.6 mL, 80 mg/0.8 mL, 100 mg/mL, 120 mg/0.8 mL, and 150 mg/mL in prefilled syringes for injection as well as 100 mg/mL multi-dose vials	Dog: 0.8 mg/kg SC q6h Cat: 1.25 mg/kg SC q6h

Drug Name	Other Names	Formulations Available	Dosage
Enrofloxacin	Baytril	22.7mg, 68 mg, and 136 mg in tablets and chewtabs; 22.7 mg/mL injection	Dog: 5–20 mg/kg/day PO, IM Cat: 5 mg/kg/day PO (do not exceed dose)
Ephedrine	Many, generic	25- and 50-mg/mL injection	Vasopressor: 0.75 mg/kg, IM, SC; repeat as needed
Epinephrine	Adrenaline and generic forms	1-mg/mL injection solution	Cardiac arrest: 10–20 mcg/kg IV or 200 mcg/kg intratracheal (may be diluted in saline before administration) Anaphylactic shock: 2.5–5 mcg/kg IV or 50 mcg/kg intratracheal (may be diluted in saline)
Epoetin alpha (Erythropoietin) (r-HuEPO)	Epogen, epoetin alfa (r-HuEPO)	2000-, 3000-, 4000-, 10,000-, 20,000-Units/mL injection	Doses range from 35 or 50 U/kg three times/wk to 400 U/kg/wk IV, SC (adjust dose to hematocrit of 0.30–0.34) Cat: Start with 100 units/kg three times/wk and adjust dose based on hematocrit
Epsiprantel	Cestex	Coated tablet	Dog: 5.5 mg/kg PO Cat: 2.75 mg/kg PO
Ergocalciferol (vitamin D_2)	Calciferol, Drisdol	400-U tablet (OTC); 50,000-U capsule (1.25 mg); 500,000-U/mL (12.5 mg/mL) injection; 0.2 mg/mL (8,000 units/mL) oral solution	500–2000 Units/kg/day PO
Erythromycin	Many brands and generic	250- or 500-mg capsule or tablet	Antibacterial dose: 10–20 mg/kg PO q8–12h Prokinetic dose: 0.5–1.0 mg/kg PO q8h
Esmolol	Brevibloc	10-mg/mL injection	50 - 100 mcg/kg IV bolus every 5 min. Increase up to 500 mcg/kg max if needed or 50–200 mcg/kg/min IV constant rate infusion
Estradiol cypionate (ECP)	ECP, Depo-Estradiol, generic	5-mg/mL injection	Dog: 22–44 mcg/kg IM (total dose not to exceed 1.0 mg) Cat: 250 mcg/cat IM between 40 hours and 5 days of mating
Etidronate disodium	Didronel	200- and 400-mg tablets; 50-mg/mL injection	Dog: 5 mg/kg/day PO Cat: 10 mg/kg/day PO
Etodolac	EtoGesic, veterinary; Lodine, human	150-, 300-, and 500-mg tablets ; 200-, and 300-mg capsules	Dog: 10–15 mg/kg PO once daily Cat: Dose not established
Famotidine	Pepcid	10-, and 20- mg tablet; 10-mg/mL injection	Dog: 0.1–0.2 mg/kg IM, SC, PO, IV q12h; or 0.5 mg/kg PO q24h, or 0.5 mg/kg IM, SC, PO, IV q24h Cat: 0.2–0.25 mg/kg IM, IV, SC, PO q12–24h

Continued

Drug Name	Other Names	Formulations Available	Dosage
Felbamate	Felbatol	400- and 600-mg tablets; 120-mg/mL oral flavored suspension	Dog: Start with 15 mg/kg PO q8h and increase gradually to maximum of 65 mg/kg q8h
Fenbendazole	Panacur, Safe Guard	Panacur granules 22.2% (222 mg/g); 100-mg/mL liquid	50 mg/kg/day PO for 3 days
Fentanyl	Sublimaze, generic	50-mcg/mL injection	0.02–0.04 mg/kg IV, IM, SC q2h or 0.01 mg/kg IV, IM, SC (with acetylpromazine or diazepam) For analgesia: 0.01 mg/kg IV, IM, SC q2h
Fentanyl transdermal	Duragesic, generic	12-, 25-, 37.5-, 50-, 62.5- 75-, 87.5-, and 100-mcg/h patch	Dog: 10–20 kg, 50-mcg/h patch q72h Cat: 25-mcg patch q120h
Ferrous sulfate	Many OTC brands	Many	Dog: 100–300 mg/dog PO q24h Cat: 50–100 mg/cat PO q24h
Finasteride	Proscar	5-mg tablets	Dog (BPH): 5-mg tablet/dog PO q24h
Firocoxib	Previcox	57- or 227-mg tablets	Dog: 5 mg/kg PO, once daily Cat: 1.5 mg/kg, once; long-term safety in cats has not been determined
Florfenicol	Nuflor	300 mg/mL (cattle)	Dog: 20 mg/kg q6h PO, IM Cat: 22 mg/kg q12h IM, PO
Fluconazole	Diflucan	50-, 100-, 150-, and 200-mg tablets; 10- or 40-mg/mL oral suspension; 2-mg/mL IV injection	Dog: 10–12 mg/kg PO every 24h For *Malassezia*, 5 mg/kg q12h PO Cat: 50 mg/cat PO q12h or 50 mg/cat/day PO
Flucytosine	Ancobon	250-mg capsule; 75-mg/mL oral suspension	25–50 mg/kg PO q6–8h (up to a maximal dose of 100 mg/kg PO q12h)
Fludrocortisone	Florinef	100-mcg (0.1 mg) tablet	Dog: 0.2–0.8 mg/dog or 0.02 mg/kg PO q24h 0.015-0.03 mg/kg/day Cat: 0.1–0.2 mg/cat PO q24h
Flumazenil	Romazicon	100-mcg/mL (0.1 mg/mL) injection	0.01-0.02 mg/kg IV; 0.2 mg (total dose) IV as needed
Flunixin meglumine	Banamine	only 50 mg/mL in US and Canada 50-mg/mL injection	1.1 mg/kg IV, IM, SC once or 1.1 mg/kg/day PO 3 days/wk Ophthalmic: 0.5 mg/kg IV once
5-Fluorouracil	Fluorouracil	50-mg/mL vial	Dog: 150 mg/m^2 IV once/week Cat: Do not use
Fluoxetine	Prozac, Reconcile	8-, 16-, 32-, and 64-mg chewable tablets for dogs. Human formulation is 10- and 20-mg capsules and 4-mg/mL oral solution	Dog: 1–2 mg/kg/day PO q24h Cat: 0.5–4 mg/cat PO q24h
Follicle-stimulating hormone (FSH)	*See* Urofollitropin		
Fomepizole	4-Methylpyrazole, Antizole, and Antizol-vet	5% solution	Dog: 20 mg/kg initially IV, then 15 mg/kg at 12- and 24-hour intervals, then 5 mg/kg at 36 hours; repeat q12h if necessary

Drug Name	Other Names	Formulations Available	Dosage
Furosemide	Lasix, Salix, generic	12.5-, 20-, 40-, 50, and 80-mg tablets; 10-mg/mL oral solution; 50-mg/mL injection	Dog: 2–6 mg/kg IV, IM, SC, PO q8–12h (or as needed) Cat: 1–4 mg/kg IV, IM, SC, PO q8–24h
Gabapentin	Neurontin	100-, 300-, 400-mg capsules; 100-, 300-, 400-, 600-, 800-mg scored tablets; 50-mg/mL oral solution (contains xylitol)	Dog, cat: Anticonvulsant dose: 2.5–10 mg/kg q8–12h PO For analgesia: 10–15 mg/kg q8h PO
Gemfibrozil	Lopid	300-mg capsules; 600-mg tablets	7.5 mg/kg PO q12h
Gentamicin	Gentocin	100-mg/mL solution	Dog: 9–14 mg/kg IV, IM, SC q24h Cat: 5–8 mg/kg IV, IM, SC q24h
Glipizide	Glucotrol	5- and 10-mg tablets	Dog: Not recommended Cat: 2.5–7.5 mg/cat PO q12h. Usual dose is 2.5 mg/cat initially, then increase to 5 mg/cat q12h
Glucosamine chondroitin sulfate	Cosequin and others	Regular (RS) and double-strength (DS) capsules	Dog: 1–2 RS capsules/day (2–4 capsules of DS for large dogs) Cat: 1 RS capsule/day
Glyburide	Diabeta, Micronase, Glynase	1.25-, 2.5-, and 5-mg tablets	0.2 mg/kg/day PO or 0.625 mg/cat
Glycerin	Generic	Oral solution	1–2 mL/kg, up to PO q8h
Glycopyrrolate	Robinul-V	0.2-mg/mL injection	0.005–0.01 mg/kg IV, IM, SC
Gold sodium thiomalate	Myochrysine	10-, 25- and 50-mg/mL injection	1–5 mg IM on first week, then 2–10 mg IM on second week, then 1 mg/kg once/wk IM maintenance
Gold therapy	*See* Aurothioglucose, Gold sodium thiomalate, or Auranofin		
GoLYTELY	*See* Polyethylene glycol electrolyte solution		
Gonadorelin (GnRH, LHRH)	Factrel	50-mcg/mL injection	Dog: 50–100 mcg/dog/day IM q24–48h Cat: 25 mcg/cat IM once
Gonadotropin, chorionic (hCG)	Profasi, Pregnyl, generic, A.P.L.	Injection sizes of 5000, 10,000 and 20,000 Units	Dog: 22 Units/kg IM q24–48h or 44 Units IM once Cat: 250 Units/cat IM once
Gonadotropin-releasing hormone	*See* Gonadorelin		
Granisetron	Kytril	1-mg/mL injection; 1-mg tablet	0.01 mg/kg (10 mcg/kg) IV
Griseofulvin (microsize)	Fulvicin U/F	125-, 250-, and 500-mg tablets; 25-mg/mL oral suspension; 125-mg/mL oral syrup	50 mg/kg PO q24h (up to a maximum dose of 110–132 mg/kg/day in divided treatments)
Griseofulvin (ultramicrosize)	Fulvicin P/G, Gris-PEG	100-, 125-, 165-, 250-, and 330-mg tablets	30 mg/kg/day in divided treatments PO
Growth hormone (hGH, somatrem, somatropin)	Protropin, Humatrope, Nutropin	5- and 10-mg/vial	0.1 Units/kg SC, IM three times/wk for 4–6 weeks (Usual human pediatric dose is 0.18–0.3 mg/kg/wk)

Continued

Drug Name	Other Names	Formulations Available	Dosage
Guaifenesin	Glyceryl guaiacolate, Guaiphenesin, Mucinex	Tablets: 100-, 200-mg; 600-mg extended-release tablets Oral solution: 20 mg/mL or 40 mg/mL	Dog, cat: Expectorant: 3–5 mg/kg q8h PO Dog: Anesthetic adjunct; 2.2 ml / kg/h of a 5% solution IV (must be compounded)
Hemoglobin glutamer	Oxyglobin	13-g/dL in 125-mL single-dose bags	Dog: One-time dose of 10-30 mL/kg IV at a rate not to exceed 10 mL/kg/h Cat: One-time dose of 3–5 mL/kg slowly IV
Heparin sodium	Liquaemin (United States); Hepalean (Canada)	1000- and 10,000-Units/mL injection	100–200 Units/kg IV loading dose; then 100–300 Units/kg SC q6–8h Low-dose prophylaxis (dog and cat): 70 Units/kg SC q8–12h
Hetastarch	Hydroxyethyl starch (HES)	Injectable solution	Dog: 10–20 mL/kg/day IV Cat: 5–10 mL/kg/day IV
Hycodan	*See* Hydrocodone bitartrate		
Hydralazine	Apresoline	10-mg tablet; 20-mg/mL injection	Dog: 0.5 mg/kg (initial dose); titrate to 0.5–2 mg/kg PO q12h Cat: 2.5 mg/cat PO q12–24h
Hydrochlorothiazide	HydroDIURIL and generic	2-4 mg/kg and 25-, 50-, and 12.5-100-mg tablets	24 mg/kg PO q12h
Hydrocodone bitartrate	Hycodan	5-mg tablet; 1-mg/mL syrup	Dog: 0.22 mg/kg PO q4–8h Cat: No dose available
Hydrocortisone	Cortef, and generic	5-, 10-, 20-mg tablets	Replacement therapy: 1–2 mg/kg PO q12h Antiinflammatory: 2.5–5 mg/kg PO q12h
Hydrocortisone sodium succinate	Solu-Cortef	Various size vials for injection	Shock: 50–150 mg/kg IV Antiinflammatory: 5 mg/kg IV q12h
Hydromorphone	Dilaudid, Hydrostat, and generic	1-, 2-, 4-, 10-mg/mL injection	Oral forms are available, but there is no assurance of oral absorption in dogs; 0.22 mg/kg IM or SC Repeat every 4–6 hours, or as needed for pain treatment
Hydroxyethyl starch (HES)	*See* Hetastarch		
Hydroxyurea	Hydrea	200-, 300-, 400-, and 500-mg capsule	Dog: 50 mg/kg PO once daily, 3 days/wk Cat: 25 mg/kg PO once daily, 3 days/wk
Hydroxyzine	Atarax	10-, 25-, and 50-mg tablets; 2-mg/mL oral solution	Dog: 2 mg/kg q12h PO, IV, IM Cat: Safe dose not established
Ibuprofen	Motrin, Advil, Nuprin	200-, 400-, 600-, and 800-mg tablets	Safe dose not established
Imipenem	Primaxin	250- or 500-mg vials for injection	3–10 mg/kg q6–8h IV, SC, or IM; usually 5 mg/kg q6–8h IM, IV, or SC q6–8h

Drug Name	Other Names	Formulations Available	Dosage
Imipramine	Tofranil	10-, 25-, and 50-mg tablets	Dog: 2–4 mg/kg PO q12–24h Cat: 0.5–1.0 mg/kg q12–24h PO
Indomethacin	Indocin		Safe dose not established
Insulin, regular crystalline		100-Units/mL injection	Ketoacidosis: animals <3 kg, 1 Unit/animal initially IM, then 1 Unit/animal q1h; animals 3–10 kg, 2 Unit/animal initially IM, then 1 Unit/animal q1h; animals >10 kg, 0.25 Units/kg initially IM, then 0.1 Unit/kg IM q1h
Insulin	NPH isophane, Ultralente, or PZI	100-Units/mL injection	Dog: Start with 0.75 Units/kg q12h, SC and adjust dose with monitoring Cat: PZI or Ultralente initial dose 0.5–1 Units/kg SC, usually twice/day
Interferon (interferon alpha, HuIFN-alpha)	Roferon	5- and 10-million Units/vial	Dog: 2.5 million Units/kg IV once daily for 3 days Cat: 1 million Units/kg IV once daily for 5 consecutive days at 0, 14, and 60 days
Iodide	*See* Potassium iodide		
Ipecac syrup	Ipecac	Oral solution: 30-mL bottle	Dog: 3–6 mL/dog PO Cat: 2–6 mL/cat PO
Isoflurane	AErrane	100-mL bottle	Induction: 5% Maintenance: 1.5%–2.5%
Isoproterenol	Isuprel	0.2-mg/mL ampules for injection	10 mcg/kg IM, SC q6h; or dilute 1 mg in 500 mL of 5% dextrose or Ringer's solution and infuse IV 0.5–1 mL/min (1–2 mcg/min) or to effect
Isosorbide dinitrate	Isordil, Isorbid, Sorbitrate	2.5-, 5-, 10-, 20-, 30-, and 40-mg tablets; 40-mg capsules	2.5–5 mg/animal PO q12h (or 0.22–1.1 mg/kg PO q12h)
Isosorbide mononitrate	Monoket	10- and 20-mg tablets	5 mg/dog PO two dose/day 7 hours apart
Isotretinoin	Accutane	10-, 20-, and 40-mg capsules	Dog: 1–3 mg/kg/day (up to a maximum recommended dose of 3–4 mg/kg/day PO) Cat: Dose not established
Itraconazole	Sporanox	100-mg capsules; 10-mg/mL oral solution	Dog: 2.5 mg/kg PO q12h or 5 mg/kg PO q24h For dermatophytes: 3 mg/kg/day PO for 15 days For *Malassezia*: 5 mg/kg q24h PO for 2 days, repeated each week for 3 weeks Cat: 5 mg/kg/day on alternating weeks for 3 treatment cycles

Continued

Drug Name	Other Names	Formulations Available	Dosage
Ivermectin	Heartguard, Ivomec, Eqvalan liquid	1% (10 mg/mL) injectable solution; 10-mg/mL oral solution; 18.7-mg/mL oral paste; 68-, 130-, and 272-mcg tablets	Heartworm preventative: Dog: 6 mcg/kg PO q30 days Cat: 24 mcg/kg PO q30 days Microfilaricide: 50 mcg/kg PO 2 weeks after adulticide therapy Ectoparasite therapy (dog and cat): 200–300 mcg/kg IM, SC, PO Endoparasites (dog and cat): 200–400 mcg/kg SC, PO weekly Demodex therapy: Start with 100 mcg/kg, then increase to 600 mcg/kg/day PO for 60–120 days
Kanamycin	Kantrim	200- and 500-mg/mL injection	10 mg/kg IV, IM, SC q6–8h; or 20 mg/kg q24h IV, IM, SC
Kaopectate (kaolin + pectin)	Kaopectate	Oral suspension	1–2 mL/kg PO q2–6h
Ketamine	Ketalar, Ketavet, Vetalar	100-mg/mL injection solution	Dog: 5.5–22 mg/kg IV, IM (recommend adjunctive sedative or tranquilizer treatment) Cat: 2–25 mg/kg IV, IM (recommend adjunctive sedative or tranquilizer treatment)
Ketoconazole	Nizoral	200-mg tablet; 100-mg/mL oral suspension (only available in Canada)	Dog: 10–15 mg/kg PO q8–12h For *Malassezia canis* infection use 5 mg/kg PO q24h Hyperadrenocorticism: 15 mg/kg PO q12h Cat: 5–10 mg/kg PO q8–12h
Ketoprofen	Orudis-KT (human OTC tablet); Ketofen (veterinary injection)	12.5-mg tablet (OTC); 100-mg/mL injection	Dog, cat: 1 mg/kg PO q24h for up to 5 days or 2.0 mg/kg IV, IM, SC for one dose
Ketorolac tromethamine	Toradol	10-mg tablet; 15- and 30-mg/mL injection in 10% alcohol	Dog: 0.5 mg/kg PO, IM, IV q12h for not more than two doses
L-Dopa	*See* Levodopa		
Lactated Ringer's solution	Generic	250-, 500-, and 1000-mL bags	Maintenance: 55–65 mL/kg/day IV For severe dehydration: 50 mL/kg/h IV or for shock 90 mL/kg IV (dogs) and 60–70 mL/kg IV (cats)
Lactulose	Chronulac, generic	10 g/15 mL	Constipation: 1 mL/4.5 kg PO q8h (to effect) Hepatic encephalopathy: Dog: 0.5 mL/kg PO q8h Cat: 2.5–5 mL/cat PO q8h
Leucovorin (folinic acid)	Wellcovorin, generic	5-, 10-, 15-, and 25-mg tablets; 3- and 5- mg/mL injection	With methotrexate administration: 3 mg/m^2 IV, IM, PO Antidote for pyrimethamine toxicosis: 1 mg/kg PO q24h

Drug Name	Other Names	Formulations Available	Dosage
Levamisole	Levasole, Tamisol, Ergamisol	0.184-g bolus; 11.7 g/13-g packet; 50-mg tablet (Ergamisol)	Dog (hookworms): 5–8 mg/kg PO once (up to 10 mg/kg PO for 2 days) Microfilaricide: 10 mg/kg PO q24h for 6–10 days Immunostimulant: 0.5–2 mg/kg PO three times/wk Cat: 4.4 mg/kg once PO For lungworms: 20–40 mg/kg PO q48h for five treatments
Levetiracetam	Keppra	250-, 500-, 750-& 1000 mg tabs, 100 mg/mL oral soln 500 mg vials for injection mg tablets	Dog: Start with 20 mg/kg q8h PO; increase gradually as necessary Cat: 30 mg/kg q12h PO
Levodopa (L-dopa)	Larodopa, L-dopa, in combination with carbidopa	100-, 250-, and 500-mg tablets or capsules	Hepatic encephalopathy: 6.8 mg/kg initially then 1.4 mg/kg q6h
Levothyroxine sodium (T_4)	Soloxine, Thyro-Tabs, Synthroid	0.1- to 0.8-mg tablets (in 0.1-mg increments)	Dog: 18–22 mcg/kg PO q12h (adjust dose via monitoring) Cat: 10–20 mcg/kg/day PO (adjust dose via monitoring)
Lidocaine	Xylocaine, generic	5-, 10-, 15-, and 20-mg/mL injection	Antiarrhythmic: Dog: 2–4 mg/kg IV (to a maximum dose of 8 mg/kg over 10-minute period); 25–75 mcg/kg/min IV infusion; 6 mg/kg IM q1.5h Cat: 0.25–0.75 mg/kg IV slowly; or 10–40 mcg/kg/min infusion For epidural (dog and cat): 4.4 mg/kg of 2% solution
Lincomycin	Lincocin	100-, 200-, and 500-mg tablets; 50 mg/mL oral solution; 100 mg/mL injection	15–25 mg/kg PO q12h or 22 mg/kg q24h IV (diluted and administered as a slow infusion) or IM For canine pyoderma: Doses as low as 10 mg/kg q12h have been used
Linezolid	Zyvox	600-mg tablets; 20-mg/mL oral suspension; 2-mg/mL injection	Dog, cat: 10 mg/kg q8–12h PO, IV
Liothyronine (T_3)	Cytomel	5, 25 and 50-mcg tablet	4.4 mcg/kg PO q8h For T_3 suppression test (cats): Collect presample for T_4 and T_3; administer 25 mcg q8h for seven doses, then collect post samples for T_3 and T_4 after last dose
Lisinopril	Prinivil, Zestril	2.5-, 5-, 10-, 20-, and 40-mg tablets	Dog: 0.5 mg/kg PO q24h Cat: No dose established
Lithium carbonate	Lithotabs	150-, 300-, and 600-mg capsules; 300-mg tablet; 300-mg/5 mL syrup	Dog: 10 mg/kg PO q12h Cat: Not recommended

Continued

Drug Name	Other Names	Formulations Available	Dosage
Lomotil	*See* Diphenoxylate		
Lomustine	CCNU, CeeNU	10-, 40-, 100-mg capsules	Dog: 70–90 mg/m², q4wk PO For brain tumors: Use 60–90 mg/m² q6–8wk PO Cat: 50–60 mg/m² PO q3–6 wk or 10 mg/cat PO q3wk
Loperamide	Imodium, generic	2-mg tablet; 0.2-mg/mL oral liquid	Dog: 0.1 mg/kg PO q8–12h Cat: 0.08–0.16 mg/kg PO q12h
Lufenuron	Program	45-, 90-, 135-, 204.9-, and 409.8-mg tablets; 135- and 270-mg suspension per unit pack	Dog: 10 mg/kg PO q30 days Cat: 30 mg/kg PO q30 days, 10 mg/kg SC q6mo
Lufenuron + milbemycin oxime	Sentinel tablets and Flavor Tabs	Milbemycin/lufenuron ratio is as follows: 2.3/46-mg tablets; 5.75/115–11.5/230-, and 23/460-mg Flavor Tabs	Administer one tablet q30 days; each tablet formulated for size of dog
Luteinizing hormone	*See* Gonadorelin		
L-Lysine	Enisyl-F	250-mg/mL paste	Paste formulation: 1–2 mL/cat, PO, to adult cats (approx. 400 mg/cat) and 1 mL/cat, PO, for kittens
Magnesium citrate	Citroma, Citro-Nesia (Citro-Mag in Canada)	Oral solution	2–4 mL/kg PO
Magnesium hydroxide	Milk of Magnesia	Oral liquid	Antacid: 5–10 mL/kg PO q4–6h Cathartic: Dog: 15–50 PO mL/kg Cat: 2–6 mL/cat PO q24h
Magnesium sulfate	Epsom salts	Crystals, many generic preparations	Dog: 8–25 g/dog PO q24h; for treating arrhythmias: 0.15–0.3 mEq/kg slowly IV over 5–15 minutes followed by 0.75–1.0 mEq/kg/day; fluid supplementation: 0.75–1.0 mEq/kg/day Cat: 2–5 g/cat PO q24h
Mannitol	Osmitrol	5%–25% solution for injection	Diuretic: 1 g/kg of 5%–25% solution IV to maintain urine flow. Glaucoma or central nervous system edema: 0.25–2 g/kg of 15%–25% solution IV over 30–60 minutes (repeat in 6 hours if necessary)
Marbofloxacin	Marbocyl, Zeniquin	25-, 50-, 100-, and 200-mg tablets	Dog, cat: 2.75–5.55 mg/kg PO q24h
Maropitant	Cerenia	10-mg/mL injection; 16-, 24-, 60-, 160-mg tablets	Dog: 1 mg/kg SC, IV once daily for up to 5 days; 2 mg/kg PO once daily for up to 5 days For motion sickness: 8 mg/kg PO once daily for up to 2 days Cat: 1 mg/kg SC, IV once/day for up to 5 days
MCT oil	MCT oil (many sources)	Oral liquid	1–2 mL/kg/day in food
Mebendazole	Telmintic	Each gram of powder contains 40 mg	22 mg/kg (with food) q24h for 3 days

Drug Name	Other Names	Formulations Available	Dosage
Meclizine	Antivert, generic	12.5-, 25-, and 50-mg tablets	Dog: 25 mg PO q24h (for motion sickness, administer 1 hour before traveling) Cat: 12.5 mg PO q24h
Meclofenamic acid (meclo-fenamate sodium)	Arquel, Meclomen	50- and 100-mg capsules	Dog: 1 mg/kg/day PO for up to 5 days Cat: Not recommended
Medium-chain triglycerides	*See* MCT oil		
Medroxyproges-terone acetate	Depo-Provera (injection); Provera (tablets)	150- and 400-mg/mL suspension injection; 2.5-, 5-, and 10-mg tablets	1.1–2.2 mg/kg IM q7 days; for behavioral use, 10–20 mg/kg SC; for prostate, 3–5 mg/kg SC, IM
Megestrol acetate	Ovaban	5-mg tablet	Dog: Proestrus: 2 mg/kg PO q24h for 8 days Anestrus: 0.5 mg/kg PO q24h for 30 days Behavior: 2–4 mg/kg q24h for 8 days (reduce dose for maintenance) Cat: Dermatologic therapy or urine spraying: 2.5–5 mg/cat PO q24h for 1 week, then reduce to 5 mg once or twice/wk Suppress estrus: 5 mg/cat/day for 3 days, then 2.5–5 mg once/wk for 10 weeks
Melarsomine	Immiticide	25-mg/mL injection; after reconstitution retains potency for 24 hours	Administer via deep IM injection. Class 1–2 dogs: 2.5 mg/kg/day for 2 consecutive days Class 3 dogs: 2.5 mg/kg once, then in 1 month two additional doses 24 hours apart
Meloxicam	Metacam (veterinary); Mobic (human)	Veterinary: 0.5- and 1.5-mg/mL oral suspension and 5-mg/mL injection Human: 7.5-mg tablets	Dog: 0.2 mg/kg initially PO, then 0.1 mg/kg q24h PO thereafter; injection 0.1 mg/kg IV or SC Cat: 0.3 mg/kg SC one-time injection; 0.05 mg/kg q24–48h PO for chronic use
Melphalan	Alkeran	2-mg tablet	1.5 mg/m^2 (or 0.1–0.2 mg/kg) PO q24h for 7–10 days (repeat every 3 weeks)
Meperidine	Demerol	50- and 100-mg tablets; 10-mg/mL syrup; 25-, 50-, 75-, and 100-mg/mL injection	Dog: 5–10 mg/kg IV, IM as often as q2–3h (or as needed) Cat: 3–5 mg/kg IV, IM q2–4h (or as needed)
Mepivacaine	Carbocaine-V	2% (20 mg/mL) injection	Variable dose for local infiltration. For epidural: 0.5 mL of 2% solution q30sec until reflexes are absent
6-Mercaptopu-rine	Purinethol	50-mg tablet	Dog: 50 mg/m^2 PO q24h Cat: Do not use

Continued

Drug Name	Other Names	Formulations Available	Dosage
Meropenem	Merrem	500 mg in 20-mL vial, or 1-gm vial in 30-mL vial for injection	Dogs, cats: 8.5 mg/kg SC q12hr up to 12 mg/kg SC q12hr or 24 mg/kg IV q12hr
Mesalamine	Asacol, Mooooal, Pentasa	400-mg tablet; 250-mg capsule	Veterinary dose has not been established, the usual human oral dose is 400–500 mg q6–8h (*also see* Sulfasalazine, Olsalazine)
Metaproterenol	Alupent, Metaprel	10- and 20-mg tablets; 5-mg/mL syrup; inhalers	0.325–0.65 mg/kg PO q4–6h
Methadone	Methadose, generic	2-mg/mL oral solution; 10- and 20-mg/mL solution for injection; 5-, 10-, 40-mg tablets	Dog: 0.5–2.2 mg/kg IV, SC, IM, or 0.5–1 mg/kg IV q3–4h for analgesia Cat: 0.2–0.5 mg/kg SC or IM, or 0.05–0.1 mg/kg up to 0.2 mg/kg IV q3–4h for analgesia
Methazolamide	Neptazane	25- and 50-mg tablets	2–3 mg/kg PO q8–12h
Methenamine hippurate	Hiprex, Urex	1-g tablet	Dog: 500 mg/dog PO q12h Cat: 250 mg/cat PO q12h
Methenamine mandelate	Mandelamine, generic	1-g tablet; granules for oral solution; 50- and 100-mg/mL oral suspension	10–20 mg/kg PO q8–12h
Methimazole	Tapazole	2.5-, 5- and 10-mg tablets	Cat: 2.5 mg/cat q12h PO for 7–14 days then 5–10 mg/cat PO q12h and adjust by monitoring T_4
DL-Methionine	*See* Racemethionine		
Methocarbamol	Robaxin-V	500- and 750-mg tablets; 100-mg/mL injection	44 mg/kg PO q8h on the first day then 22–44 mg/kg PO q8h
Methohexital	Brevital	0.5-, 2.5-, and 5-g vials for injection	3–6 mg/kg IV (give slowly to effect)
Methotrexate	MTX, Mexate, Folex, Rheumatrex, generic	2.5-mg tablet; 2.5- or 25-mg/mL injection	2.5–5 mg/m² PO q48h (dose depends on specific protocol) Dog: 0.3–0.5 mg/kg IV once/wk Cat: 0.8 mg/kg IV q2–3wk
Methoxamine	Vasoxyl	20-mg/mL injection	200–250 mcg/kg IM or 40–80 mcg/kg IV
Methoxyflurane	Metofane	4-oz bottle for inhalation	Induction: 3% Maintenance: 0.5%–1.5%
Methylene Blue	Generic, also called New Methylene Blue	1% solution (10 mg/mL)	1.5 mg/kg IV, once slowly
Methylprednisolone	Medrol	1-, 2-, 4-, 8-, 18-, and 32-mg tablets	0.22–0.44 mg/kg PO q12–24h
Methylprednisolone acetate	Depo-Medrol	20-, 40-, and 80-mg/mL suspension for injection	Dog: 1 mg/kg (or 20–40 mg/dog) IM q1–3wk Cat: 10–20 mg/cat IM q1–3wk
Methylprednisolone sodium succinate	Solu-Medrol	1- and 2-g and 125- and 500-mg vials for injection	For emergency use: 30 mg/kg IV and repeat at 15 mg/kg IV in 2–6 hours
4-Methylpyrazole (fomepizole)	Antizole, Antizol-Vet (Fomepizole)	5% solution	*See* Fomepizol for dose
Methyltestosterone	Android, generic	10- and 25-mg tablets	Dog: 5–25 mg/dog PO q24–48h Cat: 2.5–5 mg/cat PO q24–48h

Drug Name	Other Names	Formulations Available	Dosage
Metoclopramide	Reglan, Clopra, and others	5- and 10-mg tablets; 1-mg/mL oral solution; 5-mg/mL injection	0.2–0.5 mg/kg IV, IM, PO q6–8h or IV loading dose at 0.4 mg/kg followed by 0.3 mg/kg/h IV
Metoprolol tartrate	Lopressor	25-, 50-, and 100-mg tablets; 1-mg/mL injection	Dog: 5–50 mg/dog (0.5–1 mg/kg) PO q8h Cat: 2–15 mg/cat PO q8h
Metronidazole and metronidazole benzoate	Flagyl, generic	250- and 500-mg tablets; 50-mg/mL suspension; 5-mg/mL injection; the benzoate form is not available commercially and must be obtained from a compounding pharmacist	For anaerobes: Dog: 15 mg/kg PO q12h or 12 mg/kg q8h Cat: 10–25 mg/kg PO q24h For *Giardia:* Dog: 12–15 mg/kg PO q12h for 8 days Cat: 17 mg/kg (⅓ tablet/cat) q24h for 8 days
Mexiletine	Mexitil	150-, 200-, and 250-mg capsules	Dog: 5–8 mg/kg PO q8–12h (use cautiously) Cat: Do not use
Midazolam	Versed	1 mg/mL and 5 mg/mL injection	Dogs and Cats: 0.1-0.3 mg/kg SC, IM, IV
Milbemycin oxime	Interceptor Flavor Tabs	2.3-, 5.75-, 11.5-, and 23-mg tablets tablets	Dog: Microfilaricide; 0.5 mg/kg; Demodex: 2 mg/kg PO q24h for 60–120 days Heartworm prevention: 0.5 mg/kg PO q30 days Cat: 2 mg/kg q30 days PO
Milk of Magnesia	*See* Magnesium hydroxide		
Mineral oil	Generic	Oral liquid	Dog: 10–50 mL/dog PO q12h Cat: 10–25 mL/cat PO q12h
Minocycline	Minocin	50-, 75-, and 100-mg tablets or capsules; 10-mg/mL oral suspension	5–12.5 mg/kg PO q12h
Mirtazapine	Remeron	7.5-, 15-, 30-, and 45-mg tablets	Dog: 3.75-30 mg (depending on dogs weight) PO q24h Cat: 1.88 mg per cat PO every other day
Misoprostol	Cytotec	0.1-mg (100 mcg), 0.2-mg (200 mcg) tablets	Dog: 2–5 mcg/kg PO q6–8h; for atopic dermatitis: 5 mcg/kg q8h PO Cat: Dose not established
Mithramycin	*See* Plicamycin (Mithracin)		
Mitotane (o,p'-DDD)	Lysodren	500-mg tablet	Dog: For pituitary-dependent hypercorticism: 50 mg/kg/day (in divided doses) PO for 5–10 days, then 50–70 mg/kg/wk PO For adrenal tumor: 50–75 mg/kg day for 10 days, then 75–100 mg/kg/wk PO
Mitoxantrone	Novantrone	2-mg/mL injection	Dog: 6 mg/m^2 IV q21 days Cat: 6.5 mg/m^2 IV q21 days

Continued

Drug Name	Other Names	Formulations Available	Dosage
Morphine	Generic	1-, 2-, 4-, 5-, 8-, 10-, and 50 mg/mL solution for injection. 10- and 25- mg/mL preservative free (epidural)	Dog: 0.1–1 mg/kg IV, IM, SC (dose is escalated as needed for pain relief) q4–6h Dog: 0.5 mg/kg q2h IV, IM, or CRI 0.2 mg/kg followed by 0.1 mg/kg/h IV Epidural: 0.1 mg/kg Cat: 0.1 mg/kg q3–6h IM, SC (or as needed)
Moxidectin	Proheart 6, Proheart 12, Advantage multi	Injection; Advantage multi (imidacloprid+moxidectin): topical application	Dog: Proheart 6 (dosage = 0.17mg/kg SC every 6 months) Dog: Proheart 12 (dosage = 0.5 mg/kg SC every 12 months) Dogs and Cats: Advantage multi: topical application
Moxifloxacin	Avelox	400-mg tablet	10mg/kg q24h PO
Mycochrysine	*See* Gold sodium thiomalate		
Mycophenolate	Cell Cept	250-mg capsule	Dog: 10mg/kg q12h PO Cat: No dose established
Naloxone	Narcan	20- or 400-mcg/mL injection	0.01–0.04mg/kg IV, IM, SC as needed to reverse opiate
Naltrexone	Trexan	50-mg tablet	For behavior problems: 2.2mg/kg PO q12h
Neomycin	Biosal	500-mg bolus; 200-mg/mL oral liquid	10–20mg/kg PO q6–12h
Neostigmine methylsulfate	Prostigmin	0.5 and 1 mg/mL injection as neostigmine methylsulfate	Injection: Antimyasthenic: 0.04 mg/kg IM, SC q6h Antidote for nondepolarizing neuromuscular block: 40 mcg/kg IV Diagnostic aid for myasthenia gravis: 0.04 mg/kg SC, IM or 0.02 mg/kg IV
Nifedipine	Adalat, Procardia	10- and 20-mg capsules	Dose not established; in humans, the dose is 10mg/human three times/day and increased in 10-mg increments to effect
Nitenpyram	Capstar	11.4- or 57-mg tablet	1 mg/kg PO daily as needed to kill fleas
Nitrates	*See* Nitroglycerin, Isosorbide dinitrate, or Nitroprusside		
Nitrofurantoin	Macrodantin, Furalan, Furantoin, Furadantin, or generic	Macrodantin and generic 25-, 50-, and 100-mg capsules; Furalan, Furantoin, and generic 50- and 100-mg tablets; Furadantin 5-mg/mL oral suspension	10mg/kg/day divided into four daily treatments, then 1mg/kg PO at night
Nitroglycerin ointment	Nitrol, Nitro-Bid, Nitrostat	2% ointment	Dog: 4–12mg (up to 15mg) topically q12 (or 1/2 -1 inch of ointment q6-12h for first 24-48 hours) Cat: 2–4 mg topically q12h (or ¼ inch of ointment per cat)

Drug Name	Other Names	Formulations Available	Dosage
Nitroprusside	Nitropress	50-mg vial for injection	1–5, up to a maximum of 10 mcg/kg/min IV infusion
Nizatidine	Axid	150- and 300-mg capsules	Dog: 5 mg/kg PO q24h
Norfloxacin	Noroxin	400-mg tablet	22 mg/kg PO q12h
Oclacitinib	Apoquel	3.6-, 5.4-, and 16-mg tablets	0.4-0.6 mg/kg PO q12h for 2 weeks, then once daily for maintenance therapy
o,p'-DDD	See Mitotane (Lysodren)		
Olsalazine	Dipentum	500-mg tablet	Dose not established (usual human dose is 500 mg or 5–10 mg/kg PO twice daily)
Omeprazole	Prilosec (formerly Losec), Gastrogard (equine paste)	20-mg capsule	Dog: 20 mg/dog PO once daily (or 0.7 mg/kg q24h) Cat: 0.5–0.7 mg/kg q24h PO
Ondansetron	Zofran	4- and 8-mg tablets; 2-mg/mL injection	0.5–1 mg/kg IV, PO 30 minutes before administration of cancer drugs
Orbifloxacin	Orbax	5.7-, 22.7-, and 68-mg tablets 30 mg/mL oral suspension	2.5–7.5 mg/kg PO once daily
Ormetoprim	See Primor (ormetoprim-sulfadimethoxine)		
Oxacillin	Prostaphlin, generic	250- and 500-mg capsules; 50-mg/mL oral solution	22–40 mg/kg PO q8h
Oxazepam	Serax	10-, 15-, and 30-mg capsules	Cat: Appetite stimulant: 2.5 mg/cat PO; Dog: 0.1 - 1 mg/kg PO q12-24h
Oxybutynin chloride	Ditropan	5-mg tablet	Dog: 5 mg/dog PO q6–8h
Oxymorphone	Numorphan	1-mg/mL injection	Dog, cat: Analgesia: 0.1–0.2 mg/kg IV, SC, IM (as needed), redose with 0.05–0.1 mg/kg q1–2h Preanesthetic: 0.025–0.05 mg/kg IM, SC
Oxytetracycline	Terramycin	250-mg tablets; 100- and 200-mg/mL injection	7.5–10 mg/kg IV q12h; 20 mg/kg PO q12h
Oxytocin	Pitocin and Syntocinon (nasal solution) and generic	10- and 20- Units/mL injection; 40-Units/mL nasal solution	Dog: 5–20 Units/dog SC, IM (repeat q30min for primary inertia) Cat: 2.5–3 Units/cat SC, IM (repeat q30 min)
2-PAM	See Pralidoxime chloride		
Pamidronate	Aredia	30-, 60-, 90-mg vials for injection	Dog: 2 mg/kg IV, SC For treatment of cholecalciferol toxicosis: 1.3–2 mg/kg for two treatments
Pancreatic enzyme	See Pancrelipase		
Pancrelipase	Viokase	Lipase 71,700 units/ teaspoon (2.8g) Protease: 388,000 units/tsp Amylase: 460,000 units/tsp also capsules and tablets	Mix 2 tsp powder with food per 20 kg body weight or 1–3 tsp/0.45 kg of food 20 minutes before feeding

Continued

Drug Name	Other Names	Formulations Available	Dosage
Pancuronium bromide	Pavulon	1- and 2-mg/mL injection	0.1 mg/kg IV or start with 0.01 mg/kg and additional 0.01-mg/kg doses q30 min
Pantoprazole	Protonix	40-mg tablets, 0.4-mg/mL vials for injection	Dog, cat: 0.5 mg/kg q24h IV or 0.5–1 mg/kg IV infusion over 24 hours
Paregoric	Corrective mixture	2 mg morphine per 5 mL of paregoric	0.05–0.06 mg/kg PO q12h
Paroxetine	Paxil	10-, 20-, 30-, and 40-mg tablets	Cat: ⅛ to ¼ of a 10-mg tablet daily PO
D-Penicillamine	Cuprimine, Depen	125- and 250-mg capsules and 250-mg tablets	10–15 mg/kg PO q12h
Penicillin G benzathine	Benzapen and other names	150,000 Units/mL, combined with 150,000 Units/mL of procaine penicillin G	24,000 Units/kg IM q48h
Penicillin G potassium; penicillin G sodium	Many brands	5- to 20-million Units vials	20,000–40,000 Units/kg IV, IM q6–8h
Penicillin G procaine	Generic	300,000 Units/mL suspension	20,000–40,000 Units/kg IM q12–24h
Penicillin V	Pen-Vee	250- and 500-mg tablets	10 mg/kg PO q8h
Pentobarbital	Nembutal and generic	50 mg/mL	25–30 mg/kg IV to effect; or 2–15 mg/kg IV to effect, followed by 0.2–1.0 mg/kg/h IV
Pentoxifylline	Trental	400-mg tablet	Dog: For use in canine dermatology and for vasculitis, 10 mg/kg PO q12h and up to 15 mg/kg q8h Cat: ¼ of 400-mg tab PO, q8–12h
Pepto Bismol	*See* Bismuth subsalicylate		
Phenobarbital	Luminal, generic	15-, 30-, 60-, and 100-mg tablets; 30-, 60-, 65-, and 130-mg/mL injection; 4-mg/mL oral elixir solution	Dog: 2–8 mg/kg PO q12h Cat: 2–4 mg/kg PO q12h Dog and cat: Adjust dose by monitoring plasma concentration Status epilepticus: Administer in increments of 10–20 mg/kg IV (to effect)
Phenoxybenzamine	Dibenzyline	10-mg capsule	Dog: 0.25 mg/kg PO q8–12h or 0.5 mg/kg q24h Cat: 2.5 mg/cat q8–12h or 0.5 mg/cat PO q12h (in cats, doses as high as 0.5 mg/kg IV have been used to relax urethral smooth muscle)
Phentolamine	Regitine (Rogitine in Canada)	5-mg vial for injection	0.02–0.1 mg/kg IV
Phenylbutazone	Butazolidin, generic	100-mg, 200-mg, 400-mg, and 1-g tablets; 200-mg/mL injection	Dog: 15–22 mg/kg PO, IV q8–12h (44 mg/kg/day) (800 mg/dog maximum) Cat: 6–8 mg/kg IV, PO q12h
Phenylephrine	Neo-Synephrine	10-mg/mL injection; 1% nasal solution	0.01 mg/kg IV q15min; 0.1 mg/kg IM, SC q15 min

Drug Name	Other Names	Formulations Available	Dosage
Phenylpropanol-amine	PPA, Propalin, Proin PPA	25-, 50-, and 75-mg chewable tablets and 25-mg/mL liquid	Dog: 1 mg/kg q12h PO and increase to 1.5–2.0 mg/kg as needed q8h PO; Extended release tablets: 2-4 mg/kg PO once daily
Phenytoin	Dilantin	25 mg/mL oral susp (125 mg per 5 mL) oral suspension; 30- and 100-mg capsules; 50-mg/mL injection	Antiepileptic dog: 20–35 mg/kg q8h Antiarrhythmic: 30 mg/kg PO q8h or 10 mg/kg IV over 5 min
Physostigmine	Antilirium	1-mg/mL injection	0.02 mg/kg IV q12h
Phytomenadi-one	*See* Vitamin K$_1$		
Phytonadione	*See* Vitamin K$_1$		
Pimobendan	Vetmedin	2.5- and 5-mg capsules (Europe and Canada); 1.25-, 2.5-, 5-, 10-mg chewable tablets (United States)	Dog: 0.5 mg/kg/day or 0.25 - 0.3 mg/kg PO every 12 hours Cat: 0.1 - 0.3 mg/kg PO q12h
Piperacillin combined with tazobactam	Zosyn	2.25-, 3.375-, 4.5-g vials for injection	50 mg/kg IV q6h
Piperazine	Many	860-mg powder; 140-mg capsule, 170-, 340-, and 800-mg/mL oral solution	44–66 mg/kg PO administered once
Piroxicam	Feldene, generic	10-, and 20-mg capsule	Dog: 0.3 mg/kg PO q48h Cat: 0.3 mg/kg q24h PO
Pitressin (ADH)	*See* Vasopressin, Desmopressin acetate		
Plicamycin (old name is mithramycin)	Mithracin	2.5-mg injection	Dog: Antineoplastic: 25–30 mcg/kg day IV (slow infusion) for 8–10 days Antihypercalcemic: 25 mcg/kg/day IV (slow infusion) over 4 hours Cat: Not recommended
Polyethylene glycol electrolyte solution	GoLYTELY	Oral solution	25 mL/kg PO; repeat in 2–4 hours PO
Polysulfated glycosaminoglycan (PSGAG)	Adequan Canine	100-mg/mL injection in 5-mL vial (for horses vials are 250 mg/mL)	4.4 mg/kg IM twice weekly for up to 4 weeks
Potassium bromide (KBr)	KBroVet	250 and 500 mg chewable tablets; 250 mg/mL oral solution	Dog: 30–40 mg/kg PO q24h; if administered without phenobarbital, higher doses of up to 40–50 mg/kg may be needed. Adjust doses by monitoring plasma concentrations. Loading doses of 600–800 mg/kg divided over 3–4 days have been administered.
Potassium chloride (KCl)	Generic	Various concentrations for injection (usually 2 mEq/mL); oral suspension and oral solution	0.5 mEq potassium/kg/day; or supplement 10–40 mEq/500 mL of fluids, depending on serum potassium

Continued

Drug Name	Other Names	Formulations Available	Dosage
Potassium citrate	Generic, Urocit-K	5-mEq tablet; some forms are in combination with potassium chloride	0.5 mEq/kg/day PO
Potassium gluconate	Kaon, Tumil-K, generic	2-mEq tablet; 500-mg tablet; Kaon elixir is 20-mg/15-mL elixir	Dog: 0.5 mEq/kg PO q12–24h Cat: 2–8 mEq/day PO divided twice daily
Potassium iodide			30–100 mg/cat daily (in single or divided doses) for 10–14 days
Pralidoxime chloride (2-PAM)	2-PAM, Protopam Chloride	50-mg/mL injection	20 mg/kg q8–12h (initial dose) IV slow or IM
Praziquantel	Droncit	23- and 34-mg tablets; 56.8-mg/mL injection	Dog (PO): <6.8 kg, 7.5 mg/kg, once; >6.8 kg, 5 mg/kg, once (IM, SC): <2.3 kg, 7.5 mg/kg, once; 2.7–4.5 kg, 6.3 mg/kg, once; >5 kg, 5 mg/kg, once Cat (PO): <1.8 kg, 6.3 mg/kg, once; >1.8 kg, 5 mg/kg, once (for *Paragonimus* use 25 mg/kg q8h for 2–3 days) (IM, SC): 5 mg/kg
Prazosin	Minipress	1-, 2-, and 5-mg capsules	0.5- and 2-mg/animal (1 mg/15 kg) PO q8–12h
Prednisolone	Delta-Cortef and many others	5- and 20-mg tablets 3 mg/ml oral solution	Dog (cat often requires two times dog dose) Antiinflammatory: 0.5–1 mg/kg IV, IM, PO q12–24h initially, then taper to q48h Immunosuppressive: 2.2–6.6 mg/kg/day IV, IM, PO initially, then taper to 2–4 mg/kg q48h Replacement therapy: 0.2–0.3 mg/kg/day PO
Prednisolone sodium succinate	Solu-Delta-Cortef	100- and 200-mg vials for injection (10 and 50 mg/mL)	Shock: 15–30 mg/kg IV (repeat in 4–6 hours) Central nervous system trauma: 15–30 mg/kg IV, taper to 1–2 mg/kg q12h
Prednisone	Deltasone and generic; Meticorten for injection	1-, 2.5-, 5-, 10-, 20-, 25-, and 50-mg tablets; 1 mg/mL syrup (LiquidPred in 5% alcohol) and 1-mg/mL oral solution (in 5% alcohol); 10- and 40-mg/mL prednisone suspension for injection	Same as prednisolone, except that prednisone is not recommended for cats
Primidone	Mylepsin, Neurosyn (Mysoline in Canada)	50- and 250-mg tablets	8–10 mg/kg PO q8–12h as initial dose, then is adjusted via monitoring to 10–15 mg/kg q8h
Primor (ormetoprim + sulfadimethoxine)	Primor	Combination tablet (ormetoprim + sulfadimethoxine)	55 mg/kg on first day, followed by 27.5 mg/kg PO q24h
Procainamide	generic	100- and 500-mg/mL injection	Dog: 8–20 mg/kg IV IM; 25–50 mcg/kg/min IV infusion (CRI) Cat: 3–8 mg/kg IM, q6–8h

Drug Name	Other Names	Formulations Available	Dosage
Prochlorperazine	Compazine	5-, 10-, and 25-mg tablets (prochlorperazine maleate); 5-mg/mL injection (prochlorperazine edisylate)	0.1–0.5 mg/kg IM, SC q6–8h
Progesterone, repositol	*See* Medroxyprogesterone acetate		
Promethazine	Phenergan	6.25- and 25-mg/5- mL syrup; 12.5-, 25-, 50-mg tablets; 25- and 50-mg/mL injection	0.2–0.4 mg/kg IV, IM PO q6–8h (up to a maximum dose of 1 mg/kg)
Propantheline bromide	Pro-Banthine	7.5- and 15-mg tablet	0.25–0.5 mg/kg PO q8–12h
Propofol	Rapinovet and PropoFlo (veterinary); Diprivan (human)	1% (10 mg/mL) injection in 20-mL ampules	6.6 mg/kg IV slowly over 60 seconds; constant-rate infusions have been used at 5 mg/kg slowly IV, followed by 100–400 mcg/kg/min IV
Propranolol	Inderal	10-, 20-, 40-, 60-, 80-, and 90-mg tablets; 1-mg/mL injection; 4- and 8-mg/mL oral solution	Dog: 20–60 mcg/kg over 5–10 min IV; 0.2–1 mg/kg PO q8h (titrate dose to effect) Cat: 0.4–1.2 mg/kg (2.5–5 mg/cat) PO q8h
Propylthiouracil (PTU)	Generic, Propyl-Thyracil	50- and 100-mg tablets	11 mg/kg PO q12h
Prostaglandin F$_2$ alpha (dinoprost)	Lutalyse	5-mg/mL solution for injection	Pyometra: Dog: 0.1–0.2 mg/kg SC once daily for 5 days Cat: 0.1–0.25 mg/kg SC once daily for 5 days Abortion: Dog: 0.1 - 0.25 mg/kg SC q12h for 4 d Cat: 0.5–1 mg/kg IM for two injections
Pseudoephedrine	Sudafed and many others (some formulations have been discontinued)	30- and 60-mg tablets; 120-mg capsule; 6-mg/mL syrup	0.2–0.4 mg/kg (or 15–60 mg/dog) PO q8–12h
Psyllium	Metamucil and others	Available as powder	1 tsp/5–10 kg (added to each meal)
Pyrantel pamoate	Nemex, Strongid	180-mg/mL paste and 50-mg/mL suspension	Dog: 5 mg/kg PO once and repeat in 7–10 days Cat: 20 mg/kg PO once
Pyridostigmine bromide	Mestinon, Regonol	12-mg/mL oral syrup; 30-, 60-, 180-mg tablet; 5-mg/mL injection	Antimyasthenic: 0.02–0.04 mg/kg IV q2h or 0.5–3 mg/kg PO q8–12h Antidote (nondepolarizing muscle relaxant): 0.15–0.3 mg/kg IM, IV
Pyrimethamine	Daraprim, ReBalance (Equine)	25-mg tablet equine formulation (ReBalance) contains 250 mg sulfadiazine and 12.5 mg pyrimethamine per milliliter	Dog: 1 mg/kg PO q24h for 14–21 days (5 days for *Neospora caninum*) Cat: 0.5–1 mg/kg PO q24h for 14–28 days
Quinidine gluconate	Quinaglute, Duraquin	324-mg tablets; 80-mg/mL injection	Dog: 6–20 mg/kg IM q6h; 6–20 mg/kg PO q6–8h (of base)
Quinidine sulfate	Cin-Quin, Quinora	100-, 200-, and 300-mg tablets; 200- and 300-mg capsules; 20-mg/mL injection	Dog: 6–20 mg/kg PO q6–8h (of base); 5–10 mg/kg IV

Continued

Drug Name	Other Names	Formulations Available	Dosage
Quinidine poly-galacturonate	Cardioquin	275-mg tablet	Dog: 6–20 mg/kg PO q6h (of base) (275 mg quinidine polygalacturonate = 167 mg quinidine base)
Racemethionine (DL-methionine)	Uroeze, MethioForm, generic; human forms include Pedameth, Uracid, and generic	500-mg tablets and powders added to animal's food; 75-mg/5 mL pediatric oral solution; 200-mg capsule	Dog: 150–300 mg/kg/day PO Cat: 1–1.5 g/cat PO (added to food each day)
Ranitidine	Zantac	75-, 150-, and 300-mg tablets; 150- and 300-mg capsules; 25-mg/mL injection 15 mg/mL oral solution	Dog: 2 mg/kg IV, PO q8h Cat: 2.5 mg/kg IV q12h, 3.5 mg/kg PO q12h
Retinoids	*See* Isotretinoin (Accutane), Retinol (Aquasol A), or Etretinate (Tegison)		
Retinol	*See* Vitamin A (Aquasol A)		
Riboflavin (vitamin B$_2$)	*See* Vitamin B$_2$		
Rifampin	Rifadin	150- and 300-mg capsules	5–15 mg/kg PO q24h
Ringer's solution	Generic	250-, 500-, and 1000-mL bags for infusion	55–65 mL/kg/day IV, SC, or IP; 50 mL/kg/h IV for severe dehydration
Robenacoxib	Onsior	5-, 6-, 10-, 20-, 40-mg flavored tablets; 20 mg/mL injection	Dog: 10, 20 & 40 mg tablets (2 mg/kg PO once daily for up to 3 days) Cat: 6 mg tablet (1 mg/kg PO daily for up to 3 days); 20 mg/mL injection (2 mg/kg SC once daily for up to 3 days)
Ronidazole		No commercial formulations are available. However, compounding pharmacies have prepared formulations for cats.	Dog: Dose not established Cat: 30–60 mg/kg/day PO for 2 weeks
Salicylate	*See* Aspirin, acetylsalicylic acid		
Selegiline (deprenyl)	Anipryl (also known as deprenyl, and *l*-deprenyl); human dose form is Eldepryl	2-, 5-, 10-, 15-, and 30-mg tablets	Dog: Begin with 1 mg/kg PO q24h; if no response within 2 months, increase dose to maximum of 2 mg/kg PO q24h Cat: 0.25–0.5 mg/kg q12–24h PO
Senna	Senokot	Granules in concentrate or syrup	Dog: Syrup; 5–10 mL/dog q24h; Granules: ½ to 1 tsp/dog q24h PO with food Cat: Syrup: 5 mL/cat q24h; granules: ½ teaspoon/cat q24h (with food)
Septra (sulfamethoxazole + trimethoprim)	*See* Trimethoprim + sulfonamides		
Sevoflurane	SevoFlo	100 mL and 250 mL liquid	Induction: up to 7% Maintenance: 3-4%
Sildenafil	Viagra	25-, 50-, 100-mg tablets	Dog: 0.5–1 mg/kg q12h PO; higher dose of 2–3 mg/kg q8h may be needed in some cases

Drug Name	Other Names	Formulations Available	Dosage
Silymarin	Silybin, Marin, "milk thistle"	Silymarin tablets are widely available OTC. Commercial veterinary formulations (Marin) also contain zinc and vitamin E in a phosphatidylcholine complex in tablets for dogs and cats	30 mg/kg/day PO
Sodium bicarbonate (NaHCO$_3$)	Generic, Baking Soda, Soda Mint	325-, 520-, and 650-mg tablets; injection of various strengths (4.2%–8.4%), and 1 mEq/mL	Acidosis: 0.5–1 mEq/kg IV Renal failure: 10 mg/kg PO q8–12h Alkalization of urine: 50 mg/kg PO q8–12h (1 tsp is approx. 2 g)
Sodium bromide	No commercial form	Must be compounded	Same as potassium bromide, except dose is 15% lower (30 mg/kg potassium bromide is equivalent to 25 mg/kg sodium bromide)
Sodium chloride	0.9%, Generic	500- and 1000-mL infusion	15–30 mL/kg/h IV
Sodium chloride	7.5%, Generic	Infusion	2–8 mL/kg IV
Sodium thiomalate	See Gold sodium thiomalate		
Somatrem, Somatropin	See Growth hormone		
Sotalol	Betapace	80-, 160-, 240-mg tablets	Dog: 1–2 mg/kg PO q12h (one can start with 40 mg/dog q12h, then increase to 80 mg if no response) Cat: 1–2 mg/kg PO q12h
Stanozolol	Winstrol-V	50-mg/mL injection; 2-mg chew treat; oral suspension	Dog: 2 mg/dog (or range of 1–4 mg/dog) PO q12h; 25–50 mg/dog/wk IM Cat: 1 mg/cat PO q12h; 25 mg/cat/wk IM
Succimer	Chemet	100-mg capsule	Dog: 10 mg/kg PO q8h for 5 days, then 10 mg/kg PO q12h for 2 more weeks Cat: 10 mg/kg q8h for 2 weeks
Sucralfate	Carafate (Sulcrate in Canada)	1-g tablet; 200-mg/mL oral suspension	Dog: 0.5–1 g/dog PO q8–12h Cat: 0.25 g/cat PO q8–12h
Sufentanil citrate	Sufenta	50-mcg/mL injection	2 mcg/kg IV, up to a maximum dose of 5 mcg/kg
Sulfadiazine	Generic, combined with trimethoprim in Tribrissen	500-mg tablet; trimethoprim-sulfadiazine 30-, 120-, 240-, 480-, and 960-mg tablets	100 mg/kg IV, PO (loading dose), followed by 50 mg/kg IV, PO q12h (see also Trimethoprim)
Sulfadimethoxine	Albon, Bactrovet, generic	125-, 250-, and 500-mg tablets; 400-mg/mL injection; 50-mg/mL suspension	55 mg/kg PO (loading dose), followed by 27.5 mg/kg PO q12h (see also Primor)
Sulfamethoxazole combined with trimethoprim	generics	Sulfamethoxazole + Trimethoprim injection (80 mg/16 mg per mL); 400 mg/80 mg tablets and 800 mg/160 mg tablets	100 mg/kg PO (loading dose), followed by 50 mg/kg PO q12h (see also Bactrim, Septra)
Sulfasalazine (sulfapyridine + mesalamine)	Azulfidine (Salazopyrin in Canada)	500-mg tablet	Dog: 10–30 mg/kg PO q8–12h (see also Mesalamine, Olsalazine) Cat: 20 mg/kg q12h PO
Sulfisoxazole	Gantrisin	500-mg tablet; 500-mg/5 mL syrup	50 mg/kg PO q8h (urinary tract infections)

Continued

Drug Name	Other Names	Formulations Available	Dosage
Tamoxifen	Nolvadex	10- and 20-mg tablets (tamoxifen citrate)	Veterinary dose not established; 10 mg PO q12h is human dose
Taurine	Generic	Available in powder	Dog: 500 mg PO q12h Cat: 250 mg/cat PO q12h
Telazol	*See* Tiletamine + zolazepam		
Telmisartan	Semintra	10 mg/mL solution	Dog: 1 mg/kg PO q24h Cat: 1.5 mg/kg PO q12h for 14d, then 2 mg/kg once daily; reduce dose if hypotension develops
Terbinafine	Lamisil	125-, 250-mg tablets	Dog: *Malassezia* dermatitis: 30 mg/kg/day PO Cat: Dermatophytosis: 30–40 mg/kg PO q24h
Terbutaline	Brethine, Bricanyl	2.5- and 5-mg tablets; 1-mg/mL injection (equivalent to 0.82 mg/mL)	Dog: 1.25–5 mg/dog PO q8h Cat: 0.1–0.2 mg/kg PO q12h (or 0.625 mg/cat, ¼ of 2.5-mg tablet) For acute treatment in cats: 5–10 mcg/kg q4h SC or IM
Testosterone cypionate ester	Andro-Cyp, Andronate, Depo-Testosterone	100- and 200-mg/mL injection	1–2 mg/kg IM q2–4wk (*see also* Methyltestosterone)
Testosterone propionate ester	Testex (Malogen in Canada)	100-mg/mL injection	0.5–1 mg/kg two to three times/wk IM
Tetracycline	Panmycin	250- and 500-mg capsules; 100-mg/mL suspension	15–20 mg/kg PO q8h; or 4.4–11 mg/kg IV, IM q8h
Theophylline	Many brands and generic	100-, 125-, 200-, 250-, and 300-mg tablets or capsules; 27-mg/5 mL oral solution or elixir	Dog: 9 mg/kg PO q6–8h Cat: 4 mg/kg PO q8–12h
Theophylline extended-release	Inwood Labs Extended Release	100-, 200-, 300-, and 400-mg tablets or 125-, 200-, 300-mg capsules	Dog: 10 mg/kg q12h PO of extended-release tablet or capsule Cat: 20 mg/kg q24–48h PO extended-release tablet or 25 mg/kg q24–48h PO extended-release capsule
Thiamine (vitamin B$_1$)	Bewon and others	250-mcg/5 mL elixir; tablets of various size from 5 to 500 mg; 100- and 500-mg/mL injection	Dog: 10–100 mg/dog/day PO or 12.5–50 mg/dog IM or SC/day Cat: 5–30 mg/cat/day PO (up to a maximum dose of 50 mg/cat/day) or 12.5–25 mg/cat IM or SC/day
Thiamylal sodium		No longer available	
Thioguanine (6-TG)	Generic	40-mg tablet	40 mg/m^2 PO q24h Cat: 25 mg/m^2 PO q24h for 1–5 days, then repeat every 30 days
Thiomalate sodium	*See* Gold sodium thiomalate		

Drug Name	Other Names	Formulations Available	Dosage
Thiotepa	Generic	15-mg injection (usually in solution of 10 mg/mL)	0.2–0.5 mg/m^2 weekly, or daily for 5–10 days IM, intracavitary, or intra-tumor
Thyroid hormone	*See* Levothyroxine sodium (T$_4$), or Liothyronine		
Thyrotropin, thyroid-stimulating hormone (TSH)	Thytropar, Thyrogen	10-Unit vial; old forms difficult to obtain; 1.1 mg per vial	Dog: Collect baseline sample, followed by 75-150 mcg/dog IV; collect post-TSH sample at 6 hours Cat: Collect baseline sample, followed by 100 mcg/cat IV and collect a post-TSH sample at 6 hours
Tiletamine + zolazepam	Telazol, Zoletil	50 mg of each component per milliliter	Dog: 6.6–10 mg/kg IM (short term) or 10–13 mg/kg IM (longer procedure) Cat: 10–12 mg/kg IM (minor procedure) or 14–16 mg/kg IM (for surgery)
Tobramycin	Nebcin	40-mg/mL injection	Dog: 9–14 mg/kg IM, IV, SC q24h Cat: 5–8 mg/kg IM, SC, IV q24h
Tocainide	Tonocard	400- and 600-mg tablets	Dog: 15–20 mg/kg PO q8h Cat: No dose established
Toceranib	Palladia	10-, 15-, and 50- mg tablets	Dog: 2.5 - 3 mg/kg PO and treat on a schedule of 3 days per week (Monday, Wednesday, and Fridays) Cat: No dose established
Toluene	Vermiplex		267 mg/kg PO (of toluene), repeat in 2–4 weeks
Tramadol hydrochloride	Ultram, generic	Tramadol immediate-release tablets are available in 50-mg tablets	Dog: 5 mg/kg PO q6–8h Cat: 2-4 mg/kg PO every 8-12 hours
Trandolapril	Mavik	1-, 2-, and 4-mg tablets	Not established for dogs; human dose is 1 mg/person/day to start, then increase to 2–4 mg/day
Trazodone	Desyrel	50-, 100-, 150-, and 300-mg tablets	Dog: 5 - 10 mg/kg PO q8-12h Cat: 50 - 100 mg/cat PO prior to transport to vet hosp.
Triamcinolone	Vetalog, Trimtabs, Aristocort, generic	Veterinary (Vetalog) 0.5- and 1.5-mg tablets. Human form: 1-, 2-, 4-, 8-, and 16-mg tablets; 10-mg/mL injection	Antiinflammatory: 0.5–1 mg/kg PO q12–24h, then taper dose to 0.5–1 PO mg/kg q48h; however, manufacturer recommends doses of 0.11–0.22 mg/kg/day
Triamcinolone acetonide	Vetalog	2- or 6-mg/mL suspension injection	0.1–0.2 mg/kg IM, SC, repeat in 7–10 days Intralesional: 1.2–1.8 mg, or 1 mg for every centimeter diameter of tumor
Triamterene	Dyrenium	50- and 100-mg capsules	1–2 mg/kg PO q12h
Tribrissen	*See* Trimethoprim-sulfadimethoxine combination		

Continued

Drug Name	Other Names	Formulations Available	Dosage
Trientine hydro-chloride	Syprine	250-mg capsule	10–15 mg/kg PO q12h
Trifluoperazine	Stelazine	1-, 2-, 5-, and 10-mg tablets	0.03 mg/kg IM q12h
Tri-iodothyronine	See Liothyronine		
Trilostane	Vetoryl	5-, 10-, 30-, 60-, and 120-mg capsules; no formulations approved in the United States; must be imported	Dog: 1.5 - 3 mg/kg PO q12h Cat: 3 - 6 mg/kg PO q12h
Trimeprazine tartrate	Temaril (Panectyl in Canada)	2.5-mg/5 mL syrup; 2.5-mg tablet	0.5 mg/kg PO q12h
Trimethoben-zamide	Tigan and others	100-mg/mL injection; 300-mg capsules	Dog: 3 mg/kg IM, PO q8h Cat: Not recommended
Trimethoprim + sulfonamides (sulfadiazine or sulfamethox-azole)	Tribrissen and others	30-, 120-, 240-, 480-, and 960-mg tablets with trimethoprim to sulfa ratio 1:5	15 mg/kg PO q12h, or 30 mg/kg PO q12–24h For *Toxoplasma*: 30 mg/kg PO q12h
Tripelennamine	Pelamine, PBZ	25- and 50-mg tablets; 20-mg/mL injection	1 mg/kg PO q12h
TSH (thyroid-stimulating hormone)	See Thyrotropin		
Tylosin	Tylocine, Tylan, Tylosin tartrate	Available as soluble powder 2.2 g tylosin per tsp (tablets for dogs in Canada)	Dog, cat: 7–15 mg/kg PO q12–24h Dog: For colitis: 10–20 mg/kg q8h with food initially, then increase interval to q12–24h
Urofollitropin (FSH)	Metrodin	75 Units/vial for injection	75 Units/day IM for 7 days
Ursodiol (ursode-oxycholate)	Actigall	300-mg capsule, 250-mg tablets	10–15 mg/kg PO q24h
Valproic acid, divalproex	Depakene (valproic acid); Depakote (divalproex)	125-, 250-, and 500-mg tablets (Depakote); 250-mg capsule; 50-mg/mL syrup (Depakene)	Dog: 60–200 mg/kg PO q8h; or 25–105 mg/kg/day PO when adminis-tered with phenobarbital
Vancomycin	Vancocin, Vancoled	Vials for injection (0.5–10 g)	Dog: 15 mg/kg q6–8h IV infusion Cat: 12–15 mg/kg q8h IV infusion
Vasopressin (ADH)	Pitressin	20 Units/mL (aqueous)	10 Units IV, IM
Verapamil	Calan, Isoptin	40-, 80-, and 120-mg tablet; 2.5-mg/mL injection	Dog: 0.05 mg/kg IV q10–30 min (maxi-mum cumulative dose is 0.15 mg/kg)
Vinblastine	Velban	1-mg/mL injection	2 mg/m^2 IV (slow infusion) once/week
Vincristine	Oncovin, Vincasar, generic	1-mg/mL injection	Antitumor: 0.5–0.7 mg/m^2 IV (or 0.025–0.05 mg/kg) once/week For thrombocytopenia: 0.02 mg/kg IV once/week
Viokase	See Pancrelipase		
Vitamin A (reti-noids)	Aquasol A	Oral solution: 5000 Units (1500 RE) per 0.1 mL; 10,000-, 25,000-, and 50,000-Units tablets	625–800 Units/kg PO q24h
Vitamin B$_1$	See Thiamine		

Drug Name	Other Names	Formulations Available	Dosage
Vitamin B₂ (riboflavin)	Riboflavin	Various size tablets in increments from 10 to 250 mg	Dog: 10–20 mg/day PO Cat: 5–10 mg/day PO
Vitamin B₁₂ (cyanocobalamin)	Cyanocobalamin	Various size tablets in increments from 25 to 100 mcg and injections	Dog: 100–200 mcg/day PO Cat: 50–100 mcg/day PO
Vitamin C (ascorbic acid)	*See* Ascorbic acid	Tablets of various sizes and injection	100–500 mg/day
Vitamin D	*See* Dihydrotachysterol or Ergocalciferol		
Vitamin E (alpha-tocopherol)	Aquasol E, generic	Wide variety of capsules, tablets, oral solution available (e.g., 1000 units per capsule)	100–400 Units PO q12h (or 400–600 Units PO q12h for immune-mediated skin disease)
Vitamin K₁ (phytonadione, phytomenadione)	Aquamephyton (injection), Mephyton (tablets); Veta-K1 (capsules)	2- or 10-mg/mL injection; 5-mg tablet (Mephyton); 25- and 50-mg tablets or capsules	Short-acting rodenticides: 1 mg/kg/day IM, SC, PO for 10–14 days Long-acting rodenticides: 2.5–5 mg/kg/day IM, SC, PO for 3-4 weeks and up to 6 weeks Birds: 2.5–5 mg/kg q24h
Warfarin	Coumadin, generic	1-, 2-, 2.5-, 4-, 5-, 7.5-, and 10-mg tablets	Dog: 0.1–0.2 mg/kg PO q24h Cat: Thromboembolism: Start with 0.5 mg/cat/day and adjust dose based on clotting time assessment
Xylazine	Rompun and generic	20- and 100-mg/mL injection	Dog: 1.1 mg/kg IV, 2.2 mg/kg IM Cat: 1.1 mg/kg IM (emetic dose is 0.4–0.5 mg/kg IV)
Yohimbine	Yobine	2-mg/mL injection	0.11 mg/kg IV or 0.25–0.5 mg/kg SC, IM
Zidovudine (AZT)	Retrovir	10-mg/mL syrup; 10-mg/mL injection; 100- and 300-mg capsules	Cat: 5-10 mg/kg PO, SC q12h
Zolazepam	*See* Tiletamine + zolazepam combination		
Zonisamide	Zonegran	25-, 50-, and 100-mg capsule	Dog: 5-10 mg/kg PO q12h Cat: Dose not established

Note: Doses listed are for dogs and cats, unless otherwise listed. Many of the doses listed are extralabel or are human drugs used in an off-label or extralabel manner. Doses listed are based on the best available evidence at the time of table preparation; however, the author cannot ensure the efficacy of drugs used according to recommendations in this table. Adverse effects may be possible from drugs listed in this table of which the author was not aware at the time of table preparation. Veterinarians using these tables are encouraged to check current literature, product labels, and the manufacturer's disclosures for information regarding efficacy and any known adverse effects or contraindications not identified at the time of table preparation.
ACTH, Adrenocorticotropic hormone; *ADH*, antidiuretic hormone; *BPH*, benign prostatic hyperplasia; *CRI*, continuous rate infusion; *GnRH*, gonadotropin-releasing hormone; *hCG*, human chorionic gonadotropin; *IM*, intramuscular; *IP*, intraperitoneal; *IV*, intravenous; *LHRH*, luteinizing hormone-releasing hormone; *MCT*, medium-chain triglycerides; *OTC*, over-the-counter (without prescription); *PO*, per os (oral); *PSGAG*, polysulfated glycosaminoglycan; *Rx*, prescription only; *SC*, subcutaneous; *U*, units.
(Modified 2020) From Papich, M. G. (2016. Saunders handbook of veterinary drugs, ed 3, Elsevier, St. Louis, Missouri). Bonagura, J.D., Twedt, D.C. (2014). *Kirk's current veterinary therapy* XV. St. Louis: Saunders Elsevier. Plumb, D.C. (2015). Plumb's veterinary drug handbook, ed 8, Wiley-Blackwell, Ames, Iowa.

Drugs by Therapeutic Class

Drug Classification	Drug Name
Acidifying agent	Ammonium chloride
	Racemethionine
Adrenal suppressant	Trilostane
Adrenergic agonist	Ephedrine hydrochloride
	Epinephrine
	Fenoldopam mesylate
	Phenylpropanolamine hydrochloride
	Pseudoephedrine hydrochloride
Adrenolytic agent	Mitotane
Alkalinizing agent	Potassium citrate
	Sodium bicarbonate
Alpha-2 antagonist	Atipamezole hydrochloride
	Tolazoline
	Yohimbine
Analgesic	Acetaminophen
	Amantadine
	Gabapentin
	Pregabalin
	Tramadol
Analgesic, nonsteroidal antiinflammatory drug	Aspirin
	Carprofen
	Deracoxib
	Etodolac
	Firocoxib
	Flunixin meglumine
	Ibuprofen
	Indomethacin
	Ketoprofen
	Ketorolac tromethamine
	Meclofenamate sodium; Meclofenamic acid
	Meloxicam

Drug Classification	Drug Name
	Naproxen
	Phenylbutazone
	Piroxicam
	Robenacoxib
	Tepoxalin
Analgesic, opioid	Acetaminophen–codeine
	Buprenorphine hydrochloride
	Butorphanol tartrate
	Fentanyl citrate
	Fentanyl transdermal
	Hydrocodone
	Hydromorphone
	Meperidine
	Methadone hydrochloride
	Morphine sulfate
	Oxymorphone hydrochloride
	Pentazocine
	Remifentanil
	Sufentanil citrate
Analgesic, opioid, antitussive	Butorphanol
	Codeine
	Hydrocodone
Anesthetic	Alfaxalone
	Ketamine hydrochloride
	Propofol
	Tiletamine–zolazepam
Anesthetic, alpha-2 agonist	Detomidine hydrochloride
	Dexmedetomidine
	Medetomidine hydrochloride
	Romifidine hydrochloride
	Xylazine hydrochloride

Drug Classification	Drug Name	Drug Classification	Drug Name
Anesthetic, barbiturate	Methohexital sodium	Antibacterial, beta-lactam	Amoxicillin
	Pentobarbital sodium		Amoxicillin–clavulanate potassium
	Thiopental sodium		
Anesthetic, inhalant	Enflurane		Ampicillin
	Halothane		Ampicillin–sulbactam
	Isoflurane		Carbenicillin
	Methoxyflurane		Cefaclor
	Sevoflurane		Cefadroxil
Antacid	Aluminum hydroxide and aluminum carbonate		Cefazolin sodium
			Cefdinir
Antiarrhythmic	Amiodarone		Cefepime
	Carvedilol		Cefixime
	Disopyramide		Cefotaxime sodium
	Lidocaine		Cefotetan disodium
	Mexiletine		Cefovecin
	Procainamide hydrochloride		Cefoxitin sodium
	Quinidine		Cefpodoxime proxetil
	Quinidine gluconate		Cefquinome
	Quinidine polygalacturonate		Ceftazidime
			Ceftiofur crystalline free acid
	Quinidine sulfate		Ceftiofur hydrochloride
	Tocainide hydrochloride		Ceftiofur sodium
Antiarrhythmic, calcium channel blocker	Diltiazem hydrochloride		Cephalexin
	Verapamil hydrochloride		Cloxacillin sodium
Antiarthritic agent	Chondroitin sulfate		Dicloxacillin sodium
	Glucosamine–chondroitin sulfate		Doripenem
			Ertapenem
	Polysulfated glycosaminoglycan		Imipenem–cilastatin
			Meropenem
Antibacterial	Chloramphenicol		Oxacillin sodium
	Dapsone		Penicillin G
	Florfenicol		Piperacillin sodium
	Fosfomycin		Piperacillin-tazobactam
	Isoniazid		Ticarcillin–clavulanate potassium
	Linezolid		
	Methenamine		Ticarcillin disodium
	Nitrofurantoin	Antibacterial, fluoroquinolone	Ciprofloxacin hydrochloride
	Polymyxin B		
	Pyrimethamine		Danofloxacin mesylate
	Rifampin		Difloxacin hydrochloride
Antibacterial, aminoglycoside	Amikacin		Enrofloxacin
	Gentamicin sulfate		Marbofloxacin
	Kanamycin sulfate		Moxifloxacin
	Neomycin		Norfloxacin
	Tobramycin sulfate		Orbifloxacin
Antibacterial, antidiarrheal	Sulfasalazine		Pradofloxacin
Antibacterial, antiparasitic	Metronidazole	Antibacterial, glycopeptide	Vancomycin
	Ronidazole		

Continued

Drug Classification	Drug Name
Antibacterial, lincosamide	Clindamycin hydrochloride
	Clindamycin palmitate
	Clindamycin phosphate
	Lincomycin hydrochloride
	Lincomycin hydrochloride monohydrate
Antibacterial, macrolide	Azithromycin
	Clarithromycin
	Erythromycin
	Tilmicosin phosphate
	Tulathromycin
	Tylosin
Antibacterial, potentiated sulfonamide	Ormetoprim–sulfadimethoxine
	Trimethoprim–sulfadiazine
	Trimethoprim–sulfamethoxazole
Antibacterial, sulfonamide	Sulfachlorpyridazine
	Sulfadiazine
	Sulfadimethoxine
	Sulfamethazine
	Sulfamethoxazole
	Sulfaquinoxaline
Antibacterial, tetracycline	Chlortetracycline
	Doxycycline
	Minocycline hydrochloride
	Oxytetracycline
	Tetracycline
Antibiotic, aminocyclitol	Spectinomycin
Anticancer agent	Asparaginase (L-asparaginase)
	Bleomycin sulfate
	Busulfan
	Carboplatin
	Chlorambucil
	Cisplatin
	Cyclophosphamide
	Cytarabine
	Dacarbazine
	Doxorubicin hydrochloride
	Fluorouracil
	Hydroxyurea
	Lomustine
	Melphalan
	Mercaptopurine
	Methotrexate
	Mitoxantrone hydrochloride

Drug Classification	Drug Name
	Plicamycin
	Streptozocin
	Thioguanine
	Thiotepa
	Toceranib
	Vinblastine sulfate
	Vincristine sulfate
	Vinorelbine
Anticholinergic	Atropine sulfate
	Glycopyrrolate
	Hyoscyamine
	Oxybutynin chloride
Anticholinesterase agent	Neostigmine
	Physostigmine
	Pyridostigmine bromide
Anticoagulant	Dalteparin
	Enoxaparin
	Heparin sodium
	Warfarin sodium
Anticonvulsant	Bromide
	Clonazepam
	Clorazepate dipotassium
	Felbamate
	Levetiracetam
	Lorazepam
	Midazolam hydrochloride
	Oxazepam
	Phenobarbital
	Phenobarbital sodium
	Phenytoin
	Phenytoin sodium
	Primidone
	Valproate sodium
	Valproic acid
	Zonisamide
Anticonvulsant, analgesic	Gabapentin
	Pregabalin
Anticonvulsant, tranquilizer	Diazepam
	Midazolam
Antidiarrheal	Bismuth subsalicylate
	Diphenoxylate
	Kaolin–pectin
	Loperamide
	Mesalamine
	Olsalazine sodium
	Paregoric
	Propantheline bromide
Antidote	Charcoal, activated
	Deferoxamine mesylate
	Dimercaprol

Drug Classification	Drug Name
	Edetate calcium disodium
	Flumazenil
	Fomepizole
	Leucovorin calcium
	Methylene blue 0.1%
	Penicillamine
	Pralidoxime chloride
	Succimer
	Trientine hydrochloride
Antiemetic	Aprepitant
	Dolasetron mesylate
	Dronabinol
	Granisetron hydrochloride
	Maropitant
	Meclizine
	Mirtazapine
	Ondansetron hydrochloride
	Trimethobenzamide
Antiemetic, antidiarrheal	Prochlorperazine edisylate
	Prochlorperazine maleate (with isopropamide iodide)
Antiemetic, phenothiazine	Chlorpromazine
	Prochlorperazine edisylate
	Prochlorperazine maleate
	Trifluoperazine hydrochloride
	Triflupromazine hydrochloride
	Trimeprazine tartrate
Antiemetic, phenothi-azine, antihistamine	Promethazine hydrochloride
	Propiopromazine hydrochloride
Antiemetic, prokinetic agent	Metoclopramide hydrochloride
Antiestrogen	Tamoxifen citrate
Antifungal	Amphotericin B
	Enilconazole
	Fluconazole
	Flucytosine
	Griseofulvin
	Itraconazole
	Ketoconazole
	Posaconazole
	Terbinafine hydrochloride
	Voriconazole
Antifungal, expectorant	Potassium iodide
Antihistamine	Cetirizine hydrochloride

Drug Classification	Drug Name
	Chlorpheniramine maleate
	Cyproheptadine hydrochloride
	Dimenhydrinate
	Diphenhydramine hydrochloride
	Hydroxyzine
	Tripelennamine citrate
Antihypercalcemic agent	Alendronate
	Etidronate disodium
	Pamidronate disodium
	Tiludronate disodium
	Zoledronate
Antihyperglycemic agent	Glipizide
	Glyburide
	Metformin
Antihyperlipidemic	Gemfibrozil
Antiinflammatory	Allopurinol
	Colchicine
	Dimethyl sulfoxide (DMSO)
	Niacinamide
	Pentoxifylline
Antiinflammatory, corticosteroid	Betamethasone
	Budesonide
	Desoxycorticosterone pivalate
	Dexamethasone
	Dexamethasone sodium phosphate
	Flumethasone
	Hydrocortisone
	Isofluoredone acetate
	Methylprednisolone
	Prednisolone
	Prednisolone acetate
	Prednisolone sodium succinate
	Prednisone
	Triamcinolone acetonide
	Triamcinolone diacetate
	Triamcinolone hexace-tonide
Antimyasthenic	Edrophonium chloride
Antiobesity	Dirlotapide
	Mitratapide
Antiparasitic	Afoxolaner
	Albendazole
	Amitraz

Continued

Drug Classification	Drug Name	Drug Classification	Drug Name
	Amprolium		Tinidazole
	Bunamidine hydrochloride		Toltrazuril
	Dichlorvos	Antispasmodic	N-Butylscopolammonium bromide
	Diethylcarbamazine citrate		Butylscopolamine bromide
	Dithiazanine iodide	Antithyroid agent	Carbimazole
	Doramectin		Iopanoic acid
	Epsiprantel		Methimazole
	Febantel		Propylthiouracil
	Fenbendazole	Antitussive, analgesic	Butorphanol
	Fluralaner		Dextromethorphan
	Furazolidone		Hydrocodone bitartrate
	Ivermectin	Antiulcer agent	Misoprostol
	Ivermectin-clorsuon		Sucralfate
	Ivermectin–praziquantel	Antiulcer agent, H_2-blocker	Cimetidine hydrochloride
	Levamisole hydrochloride		Famotidine
	Lotilaner		Nizatidine
	Lufenuron		Ranitidine hydrochloride
	Lufenuron–milbemycin oxime	Antiulcer agent, proton-pump inhibitor	Omeprazole
	Mebendazole		Pantoprazole
	Melarsomine	Antiviral	Acyclovir
	Metaflumizone		Famciclovir
	Milbemycin oxime		Lysine (L-Lysine)
	Moxidectin		Valacyclovir
	Nitenpyram		Zidovudine
	Oxfendazole	Antiviral analgesic	Amantadine
	Oxibendazole	Behavior-modifying drug	Buspirone hydrochloride
	Paromomycin sulfate		Trazodone
	Piperazine	Behavior-modifying drug, SSRI	Fluoxetine hydrochloride
	Praziquantel		Paroxetine
	Pyrantel pamoate	Behavior-modifying drug, tricyclic	Amitriptyline hydrochloride
	Pyrantel tartrate		Clomipramine hydrochloride
	Quinacrine hydrochloride		Doxepin
	Sarolaner		Imipramine hydrochloride
	Selamectin	Beta-agonist	Isoproterenol hydrochloride
	Spinosad	Beta-blocker	Atenolol
	Thenium closylate		Bisoprolol
	Thiabendazole		Esmolol hydrochloride
	Thiacetarsamide sodium		Metoprolol tartrate
Antiplatelet agent	Clopidogrel		Propranolol hydrochloride
	Dipyridamole		Sotalol
Antiprotozoal	Atovaquone	Bronchodilator	Aminophylline
	Diclazuril		Oxtriphylline
	Imidocarb hydrochloride		Theophylline
	Metronidazole	Bronchodilator, beta-agonist	Albuterol sulfate
	Nitazoxanide		Clenbuterol
	Ponazuril		Metaproterenol sulfate
	Pyrimethamine–sulfadiazine		Terbutaline sulfate
	Ronidazole		Zilpaterol

Drug Classification	Drug Name
Calcium supplement	Calcium carbonate
	Calcium chloride
	Calcium citrate
	Calcium gluconate and calcium borogluconate
	Calcium lactate
Cardiac inotropic agent	Digitoxin
	Digoxin
	Dobutamine hydrochloride
	Pimobendan
Cholinergic	Bethanechol chloride
Corticosteroid, hormone	Fludrocortisone acetate
Dermatologic agent	Isotretinoin
Diuretic	Acetazolamide
	Bumetanide
	Chlorothiazide
	Dichlorphenamide
	Furosemide
	Hydrochlorothiazide
	Mannitol
	Methazolamide
	Spironolactone
	Torsemide
	Triamterene
Diuretic, laxative	Glycerin
Dopamine agonist	Bromocriptine mesylate
	Levodopa
	Pergolide
	Pergolide mesylate
	Selegiline hydrochloride
Emetic	Apomorphine hydrochloride
	Ipecac
Expectorant; muscle relaxant	Guaifenesin
Fluid replacement	Dextran
	Dextrose solution
	Hetastarch
	Lactated Ringer's solution
	Pentastarch
	Ringer's solution
	Sodium chloride 0.9%
	Sodium chloride 7.2%
Hepatic protectant	S-adenosylmethionine (SAMe)
	Silymarin
Hormone	Altrenogest
	Colony-stimulating factors
	Corticotropin
	Cosyntropin

Drug Classification	Drug Name
	Danazol
	Darbepoietin
	Desmopressin acetate
	Diethylstilbestrol
	Epoetin alpha (erythropoietin)
	Estradiol cypionate
	Estriol
	Gonadorelin hydrochloride, gonadorelin diacetate tetrahydrate
	Gonadotropin, chorionic
	Growth hormone
	Insulin
	Levothyroxine sodium
	Liothyronine sodium
	Medroxyprogesterone acetate
	Megestrol acetate
	Testosterone
	Urofollitropin
	Vasopressin
Hormone, anabolic agent	Boldenone undecylenate
	Methyltestosterone
	Mibolerone
	Oxymetholone
	Stanozolol
Hormone, antagonist	Finasteride
Hormone, labor induction	Oxytocin
Hormone, thyroid	Thyroid-releasing hormone
	Thyrotropin
Immunostimulant	Interferon
	Lithium carbonate
Immunosuppressive agent	Auranofin
	Aurothioglucose
	Azathioprine
	Cyclophosphamide
	Cyclosporine
	Gold sodium thiomalate
	Leflunomide
	Mycophenolate
	Tacrolimus
Iodine supplement	Iodide
	Potassium iodide
	Sodium iodide (20%)
Laxative	Bisacodyl
	Cascara sagrada
	Castor oil
	Docusate
	Lactulose

Continued

Drug Classification	Drug Name	Drug Classification	Drug Name
	Magnesium citrate	Tranquilizer, benzodiazepine	Alprazolam
	Magnesium hydroxide		
	Mineral oil	Tranquilizer, phenothiazine	Acepromazine maleate
	Polyethylene glycol electrolyte solution	Vasodilator	Hydralazine hydrochloride
	Psyllium		Irbesartan
	Senna		Isosorbide dinitrate
	Ursodeoxycholic acid		Isosorbide mononitrate
	Ursodiol		Isoxsuprine
Laxative, antiarrhythmic	Magnesium sulfate		Nitroglycerin
Local anesthetic	Bupivacaine hydrochloride		Nitroprusside (sodium nitroprusside)
	Mepivacaine		Phenoxybenzamine hydrochloride
Local anesthetic, antiarrhythmic	Lidocaine hydrochloride		Phentolamine mesylate
Mucolytic	Dembrexine		Prazosin
Mucolytic, antidote	Acetylcysteine		Sildenafil
Muscle relaxant	Atracurium besylate	Vasodilator, ACE inhibitor	Benazepril hydrochloride
	Dantrolene sodium		Captopril
	Methocarbamol		Enalapril maleate
	Pancuronium bromide		Irbesartan
Nutritional supplement	Ferrous sulfate		Lisinopril
	Iron dextran		Losartan
	MCT oil		Ramipril
	Taurine		Telmisartan
	Zinc		Trandolapril
Opioid antagonist	Naloxone hydrochloride	Vasodilator, calcium channel blocker	Amlodipine besylate
	Naltrexone		Nifedipine
Pancreatic enzyme	Pancrelipase	Vasopressor	Arginine vasopressin
Phosphate supplement, urine acidifier	Potassium phosphate		Methoxamine
			Phenylephrine hydrochloride
Potassium supplement	Potassium chloride	Vitamin	Ascorbic acid
	Potassium gluconate		Cyanocobalamin
Prokinetic agent	Cisapride		Dihydrotachysterol
	Domperidone		Ergocalciferol
	Methylnaltrexone		Phytonadione
	Metoclopramide		Riboflavin
	Tegaserod		Thiamine hydrochloride
Prostaglandin	Cloprostenol		Vitamin A
	Dinoprost tromethamine		Vitamin E
	Prostaglandin F_2 alpha		Vitamin K
Respiratory stimulant	Doxapram hydrochloride		

ACE, Angiotensin-converting enzyme; *SSRI*, selective serotonin reuptake inhibitors.
From Papich, M. G. (2016). *Handbook of veterinary drugs*. St. Louis: Saunders.

Controlled Substances Information

Drugs that have been determined to have potential for abuse by people are classified as controlled substances. Controlled substances are regulated through the efforts of the U.S. Drug Enforcement Administration (DEA), which enforces the regulations of the Controlled Substances Act (CSA) and the DEA regulations of Title 21, Code of Federal Regulations (CFR), Parts 1300 to 1316. Much valuable information related to the CSA and the CFR is available online at www.deadiversion.usdoj.gov.

Information that may be found at the DEA Diversion website includes but is not limited to the following:

- Applications and online forms, including Form 106, Report of Theft and Loss of Controlled Substances
- A complete list of controlled substances and the schedule of each
- A list of Drugs and Chemicals of Concern that includes both controlled and noncontrolled drugs whose abuse potential concerns the DEA
- Information about proposed or new regulations under the CFR
- Offices and directories, including a list of DEA offices and officials throughout the United States
- A *Practitioner's Manual* that summarizes much of the CSA and CFR

SCHEDULES OF CONTROLLED SUBSTANCES

Drugs that are under the control of the Controlled Substances Act are placed into five schedules, or classes, according to their potential for abuse. Manufacturers of controlled substances must label original containers with the schedule drug classification. This schedule is designated by a *C* with a Roman numeral (I, II, III, IV, or V) inside the C.

Schedule I substances have no accepted medical use and a high potential for abuse. Lysergic acid diethylamide (LSD), heroin, crack cocaine, marijuana, and peyote are substances in this class.

Schedule II drugs have accepted medical uses but have a high potential for abuse. A partial list of schedule II drugs includes morphine, meperidine, codeine, cocaine, fentanyl, Hycodan, oxymorphone, amphetamines, and pentobarbital. Orders for schedule II drugs must be made using the DEA Form 222.

Schedule III substances have less (moderate) potential for abuse than those in schedule II and include ketamine, buprenorphine, and anabolic steroids.

Schedule IV drugs have lower abuse potential than those in schedule III. Included in this class are phenobarbital, diazepam, tramadol, midazolam, pentazocine, and butorphanol.

Schedule V drugs are the lowest on the scale of abuse potential and include mostly antidiarrheal and anticough medications. Lomotil and Robitussin with codeine are in this schedule.

REGISTRATION REQUIREMENTS

Every person or entity that handles controlled substances must be registered with the DEA. DEA registration gives practitioners the authority to handle controlled substances. The DEA-registered practitioner may engage only in those activities that are allowed under state law in the state in which the practice is located. In some cases, state law is more stringent than federal law. In all cases, the most stringent regulation takes precedence.

To obtain DEA registration, a practitioner must apply using DEA Form 224, which can be submitted as a hard copy or online.

A practitioner must be registered with the DEA in each state in which controlled substances are prescribed, administered, or dispensed. Also, a separate registration is required for each place of business or practice where controlled substances are stored or dispensed. An exemption is made that allows affiliated (employee) veterinarians to act on behalf of registered veterinarians to administer or dispense controlled substances. The affiliated practitioner cannot write prescriptions under this exemption and may need state registration.

The person who holds the registration must keep the information on the registration certificate current. A letter of request must be made to alter the name or address or to approve a change in schedule on the certificate. A DEA modification must be issued before applications related to the request may be carried out by the registrant. Registrations must be renewed every 3 years.

SECURITY REQUIREMENTS

CFR regulations require that all registrants provide effective measures and procedures to guard against theft or diversion of controlled substances. The *DEA Practitioner's Manual* lists several factors that may be used to determine the adequacy of security measures. Those factors include the following:

- Location of the premises
- Type of building and its construction
- Type and quantity of controlled substances kept on the premises
- Type of storage container
- Control of public access to the facility
- Adequacy of premise monitoring systems
- Availability of police protection

Regulations require that schedule II through V controlled substances be stored in a securely locked substantially constructed (unmovable) safe or cabinet. If the registrant stores carfentanil, etorphine, and/or diprenorphine, a safe or steel cabinet equivalent to a U.S. Government Class V security container (General Services Administration specifications) must be used.

Regulations state that a registrant should limit access to controlled substances according to the following guidelines. Access should be denied to the following:

- Any person convicted of a felony related to a controlled substance
- Any person denied a DEA registration
- Any person who has had a DEA registration revoked
- Any person who has surrendered a DEA license for cause

Registrants must notify the DEA of any theft or "significant loss" of controlled substances using DEA Form 106 as soon as the theft or loss is discovered.

RECORD-KEEPING REQUIREMENTS

Registrants under the CSA must maintain specific records. The DEA *Practitioner's Manual* states that records, inventories, and records of substances in schedules I and II must be maintained separately from all other records. It further states that records of substances in schedules III, IV, and V must be maintained separately or on a form that is readily retrievable from ordinary business records of the practitioner. Thus, the registrant must have two separate sets of records for controlled substances; logbooks must be bound. The records for schedules III, IV, and V can be kept with records for noncontrolled substances if they can be easily retrieved. Schedule II records are usually kept in a controlled substances log, and schedule III, IV, and V drugs are kept in a controlled substances log and/or in a computer inventory system. The American Animal Hospital Association publishes a controlled substances log for purchase that may avoid pitfalls of hospital/clinic-constructed logs. Entries in the log should be made in ink with great care, and mistakes should be marked through, corrected, and initialed. Each time a controlled drug is administered or dispensed to a patient, this event must be reported in the controlled substance inventory log, as well in the patient's medical record.

Each registrant must maintain a "complete and accurate record of the controlled substances on hand and date the inventory was conducted." This record must be in written, typewritten, or printed form and maintained at the registration location for 2 years. After the first inventory is taken, a new inventory must be carried out, at least, every 2 years. Regulations state that each inventory must contain the following information:

- Whether the inventory was taken at the beginning or the end of the business day
- Names of the controlled substances

- Each form of the controlled substances (e.g., 50-mg tablet)
- Number of dosage units in each container (e.g., 100-tablet bottles)
- Number of commercial containers of each form (e.g., two 100-tablet bottles)
- Disposition of the controlled substances
- Name, address, and DEA registration number of the registrant
- Signature of the person performing the inventory

DISPOSAL OF CONTROLLED SUBSTANCES

A practitioner may dispose of out-of-date, damaged, or otherwise unusable or unwanted controlled substances by transferring them to a registrant who is authorized to receive them. These registrants are referred to as "reverse distributors." The local DEA field office (Appendix E of the DEA *Practitioner's Manual*) should be contacted for a list of authorized reverse distributors. Practitioners are advised to keep copies of the records that document such transfer and disposal of controlled substances for a period of 2 years. Always follow federal and state guidelines. While reverse distributors may be used to dispose of controlled substances held by veterinary clinics, the AVMA recommends that law enforcement agencies be used by clients for the disposal of unwanted controlled substances prescribed for their pets. Never flush unwanted pharmaceuticals down the toilet or drain. Drugs flushed down the toilet or drain may show up in the water supply and may be a cause of potential danger to consumers similar to those caused by drug residues in animal products.

VALID PRESCRIPTION REQUIREMENTS

Controlled substances are also prescription drugs. The dispensing or administering of a prescription drug requires a valid veterinarian–client–patient relationship (VCPR). A prescription for any controlled substance may only be issued by a practitioner (ie. veterinarian), registered with the DEA and authorized by the jurisdiction in which they are licensed. The dispensing or administering of such a drug without a valid VCPR is illegal under federal law. A prescription for a controlled substance must be signed and dated on the date of issue. The prescription must include the patient's (owner's) full name and address, the practitioner's full name and address, and the practitioner's DEA number. It must be written in ink or indelible pencil or printed, and it must be manually signed by the practitioner on the date issued. A designated individual may be assigned to prepare prescriptions for the practitioner's signature. The prescription also must include the following:

- Drug name
- Drug strength
- Dosage form
- Quantity prescribed
- Directions for use
- Number of refills (if any) authorized; refilling of prescriptions for a Schedule II controlled drug is prohibited.

BIBLIOGRAPHY

Ahrens, A. A. (1996). *Pharmacology, the National Veterinary Medical Series for independent study.* Philadelphia: Lippincott Williams & Wilkins.

AAEP equine vaccination guidelines. (2020). https://aaep.org/guidelines/vaccination-guidelines. Accessed May 2020.

AAFP feline vaccination guidelines. (2013). https://catvets.com/guidelines/practice-guidelines/feline-vaccination-guidelines. Accessed October 2019.

American Animal Hospital Association (website). https://www.aaha.org/aaha-guidelines/infection-control-configuration/protocols/intravenous-catheter-placement-and-maintenance2/. Accessed March 26, 2020.

AAHA canine vaccine guidelines. (2017). aaha.org/aaha-guidelines/vaccination-canine-configuration/vaccination-canine. Accessed October 2019.

American Animal Hospital Association and the American Association of Feline Practitioners (AAHA/AAFP). (2013). *Fluid therapy guidelines for dogs and cats, implementation toolkit.* aahanet.org. Accessed September 2019.

American Animal Hospital Association (AAHA). (2015). *AAHA/AAFP pain management guidelines for dogs and cats.* aaha.org/aaha-guidelines/pain-management-config/pain-management-Intro/ Accessed August 2019.

American Animal Hospital Association. (2013). *AAHA/AAFP Fluid therapy guidelines for dogs and cats implementation toolkit (supplemental information).* https://www.aaha.org/globalassets/02-guidelines/fluid-therapy/fluidtherapy_tipsheet.pdf. Accessed August 2019.

American Heartworm Society. (2018). *Current canine guidelines for the prevention, diagnosis, and management of heartworm infections in dogs.* American Heartworm Society. Accessed June, 2019.

American Heartworm Society. (2018). *Current feline guidelines for the prevention, diagnosis, and management of heartworm infections in cats.* American Heartworm Society. Accessed June 2019.

American Veterinary Medical Association: Disposal of controlled substances (website). https://www.avma.org/Advocacy/National/Federal/Pages/Disposal-of-Controlled-Substances.aspx. Accessed January 31, 2012.

American Veterinary Medical Association: Compounding (website). https://www.avma.org/KB/resources/reference/pages/compounding.aspx. Accessed April 6, 2019.

American Veterinary Medical Association: ELDU and AMDUCA (website). https://www.avma.org/KB/Resources/FAQs/Pages/ELDU-and-AMDUCA-FAQs.aspx. Accessed April 4, 2019.

AVMA. (2018). The continuing conundrum of feline injection-site sarcomas. https://www.avma.org/javma-news/2018-12-01/continuing-conundrum-feline-injection-site-sarcomas. Accessed June 2020.

Anderson, K. N., & Anderson, L. (Eds.). (1998). *Mosby's pocket dictionary of medicine, nursing, and allied health.* St. Louis: Mosby.

Anderson, K. N., & Anderson, L. (Eds.). (2002). *Mosby's pocket dictionary of medicine, nursing, and allied health* (4th ed.). St. Louis: Mosby.

Anonymous. (2012). Partnership to promote proper vet drug disposal. *Journal of the American Veterinary Medical Association, 116,* 240.

Anonymous. White paper: Rogue Internet pharmacies (website). http://www.avma.org/noah/members/scientific/prescribing/white_paper.asp. Accessed March 10, 2001.

August, K. (2019). Herbs for animal end-of-life and palliative care. *AHVMA Journal, 56,* Fall. ahvma.org. Accessed October 2019.

Barragry, T. B. (1994). *Cardiac disease: Veterinary drug therapy.* Philadelphia: Lea & Febiger.

Barton, C. L. (2012). Chemotherapy. In D. M. Boothe (Ed.), *Small animal clinical pharmacology and therapeutics.* Philadelphia: WB Saunders.

Bassert, J. M., Samples, O., & Beal, A. (Eds.). (2018). *McCurnin's clinical textbook for veterinary technicians* (9th ed.). St. Louis: Elsevier.

Battaglia, A. M., & Steele, A. M. (2016). *Small animal emergency and critical care for veterinary technicians* (3rd ed.). St. Louis: Elsevier.

Behrend, E., Holford, A., Lathan, P., Rucinsky, R., & Schulman, R. (2018). Diabetes management guidelines for dogs and cats. *Journal of the American Animal Hospital Association, 54,* 1–21.

Bill, R. (2017). Drugs affecting the respiratory system. In R. Bill (Ed.), *Pharmacology for veterinary technicians* (4th ed.). St. Louis: Mosby.

Bill, R. (Ed.). (1993). *Pharmacology for veterinary technicians.* Goleta, CA: American Veterinary Publications.

Birchard, S., & Sherding, R. (Eds.). (1994). *Saunders manual of small animal practice.* Philadelphia. WB Saunders.

Blankenship, J., & Campbell, J. B. (Eds.). (1976). *Laboratory mathematics: Medical and biological applications.* St. Louis: Mosby.

Bonagura, J. D. (Ed.). (2000). *Kirk's current veterinary therapy XIII: Small animal practice.* Philadelphia: WB Saunders.

Bonagura, J. D. (2000). *Kirk's Current veterinary therapy XIII: Small animal practice*. Philadelphia: WB Saunders.

Boothe, D. M. (1997). Nutraceuticals in veterinary medicine: Part I: Definitions and regulations. *Compendium on Continuing Education for the Practising Veterinarian, 19*(11), 1248–1255.

Boothe, D. M. (Ed.). (1998). *The veterinary clinics of North America, small animal practice*. Philadelphia: WB Saunders.

Boothe, D. M. (2012). *Small animal clinical pharmacology and therapeutics*. Philadelphia: WB Saunders.

Brander, G. C., Pugh, D. M., Bywater, R. J., et al. (Eds.). (1991). *Veterinary applied pharmacology and therapeutics* (5th ed.). London: Bailliere Tindall.

Brooks, W. (2019). Grapiprant. Veterinary Information Network. veterinarypartner.vin.com. Accessed April 2020.

Brown, G. W., & Sukys, P. A. (2006). *Business law with UCC applications* (11th ed.). New York: McGraw-Hill Irwin.

Carter, G. R., Chengappa, M. M., & Roberts, A. W. (Eds.). (1995). *Essentials of veterinary microbiology*. Baltimore: Williams & Wilkins.

Christenson, D. E. (2020). *Veterinary medical terminology* (3rd ed.). St. Louis: Elsevier.

Claude, A. (2013). Acute pain management in the small animal practice: Pharmaceutical options. In *Proceedings. Music City Veterinary Conference*, Murfreesboro, TN.

Cowgill, L. D. (1991). *Managing renal disease and hypertension*. Harmon-Smith.

Crow, S. E., & Walshaw, S. O. (Eds.). (1987). *Manual of clinical procedures in the dog and cat*. Philadelphia: JB Lippincott.

Crowe, D. T. (2007). Emergency medicine. In *Proceedings. The Tennessee Veterinary Medical Association annual conference*. Brentwood, TN.

Davidson, G. (1997). Pharmacy update: New FDA policy gives clear guidance for compounding. *Veterinary Technician, 18*(3), 195–201.

Davidson, G. (2000). Glucosamine and chondroitin sulfate. *Compendium on Continuing Education for the Practising Veterinarian, 22*(5), 454–458.

Davidson, G. (2002). S-adenosylmethionine. *Compendium on Continuing Education for the Practising Veterinarian, 24*(8), 600–603. https://www.deadiversion.usdoj.gov/schedules/index.html#define. Accessed April 6, 2019. https://www.fda.gov/animal-veterinary/resources-you/fda-regulation-animal-drugs#dispensing Accessed April 6, 2019.

DeFrancesco, T. (2013). Can we delay progression of heart disease? In *Proceedings. Music City Veterinary Conference*, Murfreesboro, TN.

DeLahunta, A. (Ed.). (1983). *Veterinary neuroanatomy and clinical neurology*. Philadelphia: WB Saunders.

DeNovo, R. C. (2002). Chronic vomiting in the cat and dog. In *Proceedings. American Veterinary Medical Association*, Nashville, TN.

DiBartola, S. P. (Ed.). (2000). *Fluid therapy in small animal practice* (2nd ed.). Philadelphia: WB Saunders.

DiBartola, S. P. (2011). *Fluid therapy in small animal practice* (4th ed.). St. Louis: Elsevier.

Dowling, P. M. (2001). Respiratory drugs. In *Proceedings. Annual meeting of American Veterinary Medical Association*. Boston, MA.

Ettinger, S. J. (Ed.). (1989). *Textbook of veterinary internal medicine* (3rd ed.). Philadelphia: WB Saunders.

Ettinger, S. J. (Ed.). (1993). *Textbook of veterinary internal medicine* (5th ed., Vols. I and II). Philadelphia: WB Saunders.

Ettinger, S. (Ed.). (2000). *Textbook of veterinary internal medicine* (5th ed.). Philadelphia: WB Saunders.

Ettinger, S. J. (Ed.). (2001). *Pocket companion to textbook of veterinary internal medicine*. Philadelphia: WB Saunders.

Ettinger, S. J. (2017). *Textbook of veterinary internal medicine expert consult* (8th ed., Vols. I and II). St. Louis: Elsevier.

Fascetti, A. J. Nutraceuticals and food faddism (website). http://www.avma.org/noah/-default.asp. Accessed January 8, 1998.

FDA. Drugs prohibited from extra-label uses in animals (website). https://www.fda.gov/AnimalVeterinary/ResourcesforYou/ucm380135.htm#. Accessed April 6, 2019.

FDA. Compounding and the FDA (website). https://www.fda.gov/drugs/guidancecomplianceregulatoryinformation/pharmacycompounding/ucm339764.htm. Accessed April 6, 2019.

Fitzwater K. *Regenerative stem cell, module 1: Principles of stem cells—what is regenerative medicine?* Veterinary Information Network (website). http://www.vin.com/members/proceedings/proceedings.plx?CID=ABVP2012&PID=83732. Accessed March 5, 2013.

Ford, R. B. (1998). Vaccines and vaccinations: Issues for the 21st century. *Supplement of Compendium on Continuing Education for the Practising Veterinarian, 20*(8C), 19–24.

Foushee, L. L. (2000). Omeprazole. *Compendium on Continuing Education for the Practising Veterinarian, 22*(8), 746–749.

Ganong, W. F. (2003). *Review of medical physiology* (21st ed.). New York: McGraw-Hill.

Gaynor, J. S., & Muir, W. W. (Eds.). (2015). *Handbook of veterinary pain management* (3rd ed.). St. Louis: Elsevier.

Gelatt, K. N. (1981). *Textbook of veterinary ophthalmology*. Philadelphia: Lea & Febiger.

Giovanoni, R., & Warren, R. C. (1983). Cardiovascular drugs. In R. Giovanoni, & R. C. Warren (Eds.), *Principles of pharmacology*. St. Louis: Mosby.

Goodman, L., & Trepanier, L. (2005). Potential drug interactions with dietary supplements. *Compendium on Continuing Education for the Practising Veterinarian, 27*(10), 780–790.

Gordon S. G., Saunders A. B. P. Inotropes. Antiarrhythmics. In "The Merck Veterinary Manual" (online edition). http://merckveterinarymanual.com/. Accessed June 2019.

Grauer G. F. Overview of Ethylene Glycol. In "The Merck veterinary manual" (online edition). http://merckveterinarymanual.com/ Accessed May 2019.

Hall, J. A., & Washabau, R. J. (1997). Gastrointestinal prokinetic therapy: Dopaminergic antagonist drugs. *Compendium on Continuing Education for the Practising Veterinarian, 19*(2), 214–219.

Hamlin, R. L. (2003). Cardiovascular system, introduction. In *Proceedings. Music City Veterinary Conference*, Nashville, TN.

Hand, M. S., Thatcher, C. D., Remillard, R. L., Roudebush, P. (2000). In *Small animal clinical nutrition* (4th ed.). Topeka, KS: Mark Morris Institute.

Haskins, S. C. (2000). Fluid overload: How to identify and manage. In *Proceedings. International veterinary emergency and critical care symposium*. Orlando, FL.

Hendrix, C. M., & Robinson, E. (Eds.). (2017). *Diagnostic veterinary parasitology* (5th ed.). St. Louis: Mosby.

Hoffman, A. M. (2001). What's new with aerosol medications in the horse. In *Proceedings. Annual meeting of American Veterinary Medical Association*. Boston, MA.

JAAHA (Journal of the American Veterinary Medical Association). (2011). *Development of new canine and feline preventative healthcare guidelines designed to improve pet health, AAHA-AVMA Preventative Healthcare Guidelines Task force*. Available at https://www.aaha.org/globalassets/02-guidelines/preventive-healthcare/AAHA-Oncology-Guidelines-for-Dogs-and-Cats. Accessed October 2019.

Jordan, D. G. (2013). Trends in veterinary therapeutics. In *Proceedings. Music City Veterinary Conference*, Murfreesboro, TN.

Kirk, R. W. (Ed.). (1983). *Current veterinary therapy VIII: Small animal practice*. Philadelphia: WB Saunders.

Kirk, R. W. (1986). *Current veterinary IX: Small animal practice*. Philadelphia: WB Saunders.

Kirk, R. W., & Bonagura, J. D. (Eds.). (1989). *Current veterinary therapy X: Small animal practice*. Philadelphia: WB Saunders.

Kirk, R. W., & Bonagura, J. D. (Eds.). (1995). *Current veterinary therapy XII: Small animal practice*. Philadelphia: WB Saunders.

Kirk, R. W., & Bonagura, J. D. (Eds.). (2014). *Current veterinary therapy XV: Small animal practice*. St. Louis: Elsevier.

Lane, D. R., & Cooper, B. C. (Eds.). (1999). *Veterinary nursing* (2nd ed.). Oxford, England: Butterworth-Heinemann.

Lane, D. R., & Cooper, V. N. (Eds.). (2003). *Veterinary nursing* (3rd ed.). Oxford: Butterworth-Heinemann.

Langston, V. C., & Mercer, H. D. (1988). Nonsteroidal antiinflammatory drugs. In *Proceedings. 17th Seminar for veterinary technicians, the Western Veterinary Conference*, Las Vegas.

Lavoie, J. P. (2001). Inhalation therapy for equine heaves. *Compendium on Continuing Education for the Practising Veterinarian, 23*(5), 475–477.

Libby, R., Libby, P., & Short, D. G. (2004). In *Financial accounting* (4th ed.). New York: McGraw-Hill Irwin.

Locklar, C. F., Jr., & Locklar, M. S. (2003). *Personal interview*.

Loes, N. (2012). Probiotics: Healthy from the inside out. In *Proceedings. Annual meeting of the Tennessee Veterinary Medical Association*, Nashville, TN.

Lukens, R. L., & Landon, R. M. (1993). *A Guide to inventory management for veterinary practices: Effective inventory control*. West Chester, PA: SmithKline Beecham Animal Health.

MacEwen, E. G., & Rosenthal, R. C. (2000). Approach to treatment of cancer Patients. In S. J. Ettinger (Ed.), *Textbook of veterinary internal medicine* (5th ed.). Philadelphia: WB Saunders.

Macintire, D. K., & Tefend, M. (2004). Constant rate infusions: Practical use. In *North American Veterinary Conference clinician's brief*, Orlando, FL.

McCurnin, D. M., & Bassert, J. M. (Eds.). (2002). *Clinical textbook for veterinary technicians* (8th ed.). Philadelphia: WB Saunders.

McCurnin, D. M., Bassert, J. M., & Thomas, J. (Eds.). (2014). *Clinical textbook for veterinary technicians* ((8th ed.). St. Louis: Elsevier.

McKiernan, B. (1988). Respiratory therapeutics. In *Proceedings. 17th Seminar for veterinary technicians, the Western Veterinary Conference*, Las Vegas.

Mealey, K. L. (2002). Clinically significant drug interactions. *Compendium on Continuing Education for the Practising Veterinarian, 24*(1), 10–22.

Morrison, W. B., Starr, R. M., & the Vaccine-Associated Feline Sarcoma Task Force. (2001). Vaccine-associated feline Sarcomas. *Journal of the American Veterinary Medical Association, 218*(5). Available at https://avmajournals.avma.org/doi/pdfplus/10.2460/javma.2001.218.697. Accessed October 2019.

O'Toole, M.T. (2017). (8th ed.). Mosby's pocket dictionary of medicine, nursing and health professionals. (1998). St. Louis, Missouri: Elsevier.

Muir, W. W., & DiBartola, S. P. (1983). Fluid therapy. In R. W. Kirk (Ed.), *Current veterinary therapy VIII: Small animal practice*. Philadelphia: WB Saunders.

Muir, W. W., Hubbell, J. A., Bednarski, R. M., & Lerche, P. (2013). *Handbook of veterinary anesthesia* (5th ed.). St. Louis: Mosby/Elsevier.

Muller, G. H., Kirk, R. W., & Scott, D. W. (1989). *Small animal dermatology* (4th ed.). Philadelphia: WB Saunders.

Sir Alexander Fleming – Biographical. NobelPrize.org. Nobel Media AB 2020. Sat. 23 May 2020. https://www.nobelprize.org/prizes/medicine/1945/fleming/biographical/. From Nobel Lectures, Physiology or Medicine 1942-1962, Elsevier Publishing Company, Amsterdam, 1964.

Norsworthy, G. D. (1992). Clinical aspects of feline blood transfusions. *Compendium on Continuing Education for the Practising Veterinarian, 14,* 470.

Ortel, S. O. (2006). Constant-rate infusions. *Veterinary Technician, 27*(1), 47–50.

Osborne, C. A. (2001). Idiopathic lower urinary tract diseases: Therapeutic rights and wrongs. In *Proceedings. American Veterinary Medicine Association (AVMA) annual meeting,* Boston, MA.

Package insert for Banamine, Merck Animal Health, Madison, New Jersey. (2017).

Package insert for Bravecto, Merck animal Health, United States. (2016).

Package insert for Bravecto, Merck Animal Health. United States. (2019).

Package insert for Bravecto Plus for cats, Merck. Madison, New Jersey. (2020).

Package insert for Credelio, Elanco, Greenfield, Indiana. (2019).

Package insert for Micotil, Elanco, Indianapolis, Indiana, January, 2010.

Package insert for Sentinel, Virbac, United States, 2018.

Package insert for Simbadol, Zoetis, United States, July 2017.

Package insert for Simparica, Zoetis, Kalamazoo, Michigan. (2019).

Package insert for Sileo, Zoetis, United States, November 2017.

Paddleford, R. R. (1999). *Manual of small animal anesthesia.* Philadelphia: WB Saunders.

Papich, M. G. (2016). *Saunders handbook of veterinary drugs* (4th ed.). Philadelphia: Elsevier.

Parker, A. R. (2001). Domperidone. *Compendium on Continuing Education for the Practising Veterinarian, 23*(10), 906–908.

Plumb, D. C. (2015). *Veterinary drug handbook* (8th ed.). Ames, IA: Wiley-Blackwell.

Quinn, P. J., Donnelly, M. E., Carter, B. K., et al. (Eds.). (1997). *Microbial and parasitic diseases of the dog and cat.* London: Saunders.

Rishniw, M. (2006). *Evaluating herbal medicines.* Davis, CA: Veterinary Information Network.

Romich, J. A. (2005). *Fundamentals of pharmacology for veterinary technicians.* Clifton Park, NY: Thompson Delmar Learning.

Rudloff, E. *Fluid therapy series: Colloids in-depth.* http://abbottanimalhealthce.com/. Accessed February 24, 2013.

Scott, D. W., Miller, W. H., & Griffin, C. E. (2001). *Small animal dermatology* (6th ed.). Philadelphia: WB Saunders.

Seibert, L. M. (2013). Behavior drug protocols. In *Proceedings. Music City Veterinary Conference.* Murfreesboro, TN.

Shull, E. A. (1998). Psychopharmacology in veterinary behavioral medicine. In *Proceedings. Annual conference for veterinary technicians.* Knoxville, TN: UT-CVM.

Simpson, B. S., & Simpson, D. M. (1996). Behavioral pharmacotherapy: Part I: Antipsychotics and antidepressants.

Compendium on Continuing Education for the Practising Veterinarian, 18(10), 1067–1081.

Simpson, B. S., & Simpson, D. M. (1996). Behavioral pharmacotherapy: Part II: Anxiolytics and mood stabilizers. *Compendium on Continuing Education for the Practising Veterinarian, 18*(11), 1203–1210.

Smith, P. (1999). New studies, products fuel heartworm debate. *Veterinary Practice News, 11*(4), 34–36.

Snyder, S. (1986). Mood modifiers. In S. Snyder (Ed.), *Drugs and the brain.* New York: Scientific American Library.

Spinelli, J. S., & Enos, L. R. (Eds.). (1978). *Drugs in veterinary practice.* St. Louis: Mosby.

Tams, T. R. (2012). Gastrointestinal medicine—diarrhea. In *Proceedings. Annual meeting of Tennessee Veterinary Medical Association,* Nashville, TN.

Thomas, J. A., & Lerche, P. (2017). *Anesthesia and analgesia for veterinary technicians* (5th ed.). St. Louis: Elsevier.

Tilley, L. P., & Smith, W. K. (2014). *The 5-minute veterinary consult canine and feline* (3rd ed.). Baltimore: Lippincott Williams &Wilkins.

Tizard, I. (1992). *Veterinary immunology: An introduction* (4th ed.). Philadelphia: WB Saunders.

Tizard, I. (2000). *Veterinary immunology: An introduction* (6th ed.). Philadelphia: WB Saunders.

Upson, D. W. (1988). Central nervous system. In D. W. Upson (Ed.), *Handbook of clinical veterinary pharmacology* (3rd ed.). Manhattan, KS: Dan Upson Enterprises.

Van Kampen, K. R. (1998). Recombinant technology. *Supplement of Compendium on Continuing Education for the Practising Veterinarian, 20*(8), 28–32.

Veterinary Information Network. (2010). VIN Proceedings Library (website). In C. N. Reinero, & K. A. Selting (Eds.), *Inhalational therapies in dogs and cats.* http://www.vin.com/members/proceedings.plx?CID=ACVIM2010&PID=559. Accessed March 19, 2013.

Veterinary Information Network. Reuse of intravenous extension tubing or giving sets (website). http://www.vin.com/Members/Boards/DiscussionViewer.aspx?documentid=3995391&ViewFirst=1. Accessed February 9, 2013.

Ware, W. A. (2002). Problems in chronic heart failure management. In *Proceedings. American Veterinary Medical Association annual conference.* TN: Nashville.

Warren E. *Nutraceuticals.* Veterinary Information Network (website). http://www.vin.com/doc/?id=2994084. Accessed June 4, 2019.

Webb, A. I., & Aeschbacher, G. (1993). Animal drug container labels: A guide to the reader. *Journal of the American Veterinary Medical Association, 202,* 1591–1599.

Werth B. J: Cephalosporins. (2018). In "The Merck Veterinary Manual" (online edition). http://merckveterinarymanual.com/. Accessed August 2013.

Whelan N: Treatment of glaucoma. In "The Merck Veterinary Manual" (online edition). http://merckveterinarymanual.com/. Accessed August 2013.

Wickstrom ML. Overview of Antiseptics and Disinfectants. (2015). In "The Merck veterinary manual" (online edition). http://merckveterinarymanual.com/. Accessed April 2020.

Williams, B. R., & Baer, C. (Eds.). (1990). *Essentials of clinical pharmacology in nursing*. Springhouse, PA: Springhouse Corp.

Withrow, S. J., & Vail, D. M. (Eds.). (2007). *Small animal oncology* (4th ed.). St. Louis: Saunders Elsevier.

Wynn, S. G., & Marsden, S. (2003). *Manual of natural veterinary medicine science and tradition*. St. Louis: Elsevier.

Wynn, S. G., & Fourgere, B. J. (2007). *Veterinary herbal medicine*. St. Louis: Mosby Elsevier.

acetylcholine A neurotransmitter that allows a nerve impulse to cross the synaptic junction (gap) between two nerve fibers or between a nerve fiber and an organ (e.g., muscle, gland).

acetylcholinesterase An enzyme that brings about the breakdown of acetylcholine in the synaptic gap.

active immunity Immunity that occurs by an animal's own immune response after exposure to foreign antigen.

Addison's disease A disease or syndrome characterized by inadequate amounts of corticosteroid hormones.

adjuvant A substance given with an antigen to enhance the immune response to the antigen. Adjuvants may form a localized granuloma at the injection site or may produce systemic hypersensitivity. Adjuvants have received much attention as a result of a possible (but not proven) link with the increased incidence of fibrosarcomas in vaccinated cats. Examples of adjuvants are aluminum hydroxide, aluminum phosphate, aluminum potassium sulfate, water in oil, saponin, and diethylaminoethyl (DEAE) dextran.

adrenergic A term used to describe an action or a receptor that is activated by epinephrine or norepinephrine.

adsorbent A drug that inhibits gastrointestinal absorption of drugs, toxins, or chemicals by attracting and holding them to its surface.

adverse drug event Harm to a patient caused by a therapeutic or preventive intervention. It could be due to a medication error or adverse drug reaction.

adverse drug reaction An undesirable response to a drug by a patient. It may vary in severity from mild to fatal.

aerobe Organism that is able to grow in the presence of oxygen.

aerosolization The conversion of a liquid into a fine mist or colloidal suspension in air.

afterload The resistance (pressure) in arteries that must be overcome to empty blood from the ventricle.

agonist A drug that brings about a specific action by binding with the appropriate receptor.

alkylation Formation of a linkage between a substance and DNA that causes irreversible inhibition of the DNA molecule. Alkylating drugs are used in chemotherapy treatment of cancer.

anabolism The constructive phase of metabolism in which body cells repair and replace tissue.

anaerobe Organism that is not able to grow in the presence of oxygen.

analgesia The absence of the sensation of pain.

analogue A chemical compound having a structure similar to another but differing from it in some way.

anaphylaxis A systemic, severe allergic reaction.

anesthesia The loss of all sensation. May be described as local (affecting a small area), regional, or surgical (accompanied by unconsciousness).

angiogenesis The development of blood vessels.

antagonist A drug that inhibits a specific action by binding with a particular receptor.

anthelmintic Drug used to eliminate helminth parasites (e.g., roundworms) from a host.

antibacterial An agent that inhibits bacterial growth, impedes replication of bacteria, or kills bacteria.

antibiotic An agent produced by a microorganism or semisynthetically that has the ability to inhibit the growth of or kill microorganisms.

antibody An immunoglobulin molecule that combines with the specific antigen that induced its formation.

anticholinergic Blocking nerve impulse transmission through the parasympathetic nervous system; also called *parasympatholytic*. Anticholinergic drugs may be used for the treatment of diarrhea or vomiting.

antigen Any substance that can induce a specific immune response, such as toxins, foreign proteins, bacteria, and viruses.

antihistamine A drug that counteracts the action of histamine in the body; are used for treating allergic reactions.

antimicrobial An agent that kills microorganisms or suppresses their multiplication or growth.

antimicrobial residues Presence of an antimicrobial (antibiotic) or its metabolites in food products or animal tissue.

antimicrobial resistance Develops when microorganisms, such as bacteria and fungi, no longer respond to a drug that previously were effective.

antiseptic A substance used on the skin to prevent the growth of bacteria or to provide preoperative cleansing of the skin.

antitussive A drug that inhibits or suppresses the cough reflex.

arrhythmia (dysrhythmia) A variation from the normal rhythm.

astringent An agent that causes contraction after application to tissue.

atony The absence or lack of normal tone or strength.

autologous Belonging to the same organism.

automaticity The ability of cardiac muscle to generate impulses.

autonomic nervous system That portion of the nervous system that controls involuntary activities.

average cost of inventory on hand Average cost of inventory on hand is determined by adding the year's beginning inventory to the year's ending inventory and dividing by two.

avirulent The inability of an infectious agent to produce pathologic effects.

bacteria Single-celled microorganisms that usually have a rigid cell wall and a round, rod-like, or spiral shape.

bactericidal An agent with the capability to kill bacteria.

bacterin A killed bacterial vaccine.

bacteriostatic An agent that inhibits the growth or reproduction of bacteria.

beta-lactamase Enzymes that reduce the effectiveness of certain antibiotics; beta-lactamase I is penicillinase; beta-lactamase II is cephalosporinase.

bioavailability Measure of the degree to which a drug is absorbed and reaches systemic circulation.

blepharospasm   Squinting of the eye.

bots   Larvae of several fly species (e.g., *Gasterophilus* [horse bot]).

bradyarrhythmia   Bradycardia associated with an irregularity of heart rhythm.

bradycardia   A slower-than-normal heart rate.

bronchoconstriction   Narrowing of the bronchi and bronchioles, which results in increased airway resistance and decreased airflow.

bronchodilation   Widening lumen of bronchi and bronchioles, which results from relaxation of smooth muscle in the walls of the bronchi and bronchioles. Airway resistance is decreased, and airflow is increased.

buffer   A substance that decreases the change in pH when an acid or base is added.

callus   Hypertrophy of the horny layer of the epidermis in a localized area as a result of pressure or friction.

cardiac output   Amount of blood pumped by the heart per minute.

cardiac remodeling   Change in the size, shape, structure, and physiology of the heart due to damage to the myocardium.

catalepsy   A state of involuntary muscle rigidity that is accompanied by immobility, amnesia, and variable amounts of analgesia. Some reflexes may be preserved.

catecholamine   The class of neurotransmitters that includes dopamine, epinephrine, and norepinephrine. When given therapeutically, catecholamines mimic the effects of stimulating the sympathetic nervous system.

caval syndrome   A life-threatening condition caused by a large number of heartworms lodged in the vena cava, right atrium, and right ventricle.

ceiling effect   The highest level of a specific drug has been reached; increasing the dose does not provide any additional pain relief but may increase the side effects.

cell cycle–nonspecific   Capable of acting in several or all cell cycle phases.

cell cycle–specific   Capable of acting during a particular cell cycle phase only.

cerumen   A waxy secretion of the glands of the external ear canal.

cestode   A tapeworm.

chelating agent   An agent used in chemotherapy for metal poisoning.

chemoreceptor trigger zone (CRTZ)   An area in the brain that activates the vomiting center when stimulated by toxic substances in the blood.

cholinergic   activated by or transmitted through acetylcholine; also called parasympathomimetic. Cholinergic drugs increase activity in the gastrointestinal tract.

chondroprotectives   Substances that are able to decrease the progression of osteoarthritis by providing support to cartilage and promoting its repair; they are available as oral or injectable medications.

chronotropic   Affecting the heart rate.

closed-angle glaucoma   A type of primary glaucoma of the eye that is characterized by a shallow anterior chamber and a narrow angle that compromises filtration because the iris is blocking the angle and is causing an increase in intraocular pressure.

collagen   A fibrous substance found in skin, tendon, bone, cartilage, and all other connective tissues.

colloid   A chemical system composed of a continuous medium throughout which small particles are distributed and do not settle out under the influence of gravity.

colony forming unit (CFI)   An estimate of viable bacterial or fungal numbers.

comedo (pl. comedones)   A plug of keratin and sebum within a hair follicle of the skin.

compounding   Any manipulation (e.g., diluting, combining) performed to produce a dosage-form drug, other than the manipulations described in the directions for use on the labeling of an approved drug product.

concentration of a drug   The amount of a drug in a given volume of blood plasma.

conjunctivitis   Inflammation of the conjunctiva.

controlled drug or scheduled drug   A drug that is tightly controlled due to its abuse potential or risk.

core vaccines   Recommended vaccines for most animals to protect them from highly contagious diseases that are widespread in the environment.

counterirritant   An agent that produces superficial irritation that is intended to relieve some other irritation.

crash cart   A stationary or mobile cart stocked with supplies, equipment, and drugs for use during an emergency.

cream   A semisolid preparation of oil, water, and a medicinal agent.

Cushing's disease or syndrome   Hyperadrenocorticism; a disease or syndrome characterized by an overabundance of corticosteroid hormones.

cycloplegia   Paralysis of the ciliary muscle.

cytotoxic   Capable of destroying cells.

DEA form   An official federal government DEA changed to non-carbon-copy form in 2020. form from the Drug Enforcement Administration used for ordering controlled substances.

decongestant   A substance that reduces the swelling of mucous membranes.

deep pain   Pain arising from deep receptors in the periosteum, tendons, and joint structures.

delayed billing   A benefit that some companies offer to the buyer who is purchasing increased amounts of merchandise. The date the statement must be paid is usually longer than 30–60 days away.

dentifrice   A preparation for cleansing teeth that is available in a powder, paste, or liquid.

depolarization   Neutralizing of the polarity of a cardiac cell by an inflow of sodium ions. Depolarization results in contraction of the cardiac cell and renders it incapable of further contraction until repolarization occurs.

dermatitis   Inflammation of the skin.

dermatophyte   Fungi parasitic on the skin.

dermatophytosis   A fungal skin infection.

detergent   An agent that cleanses.

detrusor   The smooth muscle of the urinary bladder that is mainly responsible for emptying the bladder during urination.

detrusor areflexia   The absence of detrusor contractions.

diabetes mellitus   A condition that occurs due to insulin deficiency.

diastole   Relaxation phase when the chambers of the heart are filling with blood.

dilution   A process of reducing the concentration of a substance in a solution.

disinfect   To make free of pathogens or make them inactive.

disinfectant   A chemical agent applied to inanimate objects to destroy or inhibit growth of microorganisms.

disseminated intravascular coagulation (DIC)   Widespread formation of clots (thrombi) in the microscopic blood vessels of the circulatory system. DIC occurs as a complication of a wide variety of disorders and consumes clotting factors, with resultant bleeding.

dissociation   The act of separating into ionic components (NaCl → Na and Cl).

distichia (distichiasis)   Eyelashes emerge through the meibomian gland opening at the eyelid margin in a misdirected way, causing the eyelashes to touch and irritate the corneal surface.

diuretic   A drug used to promote urine excretion.

dosage   The amount of a drug dose and the frequency at which the medication must be administered to a patient.

dosage form   A drug's physical appearance; the form in which they are marketed for use.

dosage range   A drug's dosage formula expressed as a set of two numbers; a minimum and a maximum safe dose.

dose   The amount of drug to be administered to a patient (e.g., 100 mg).

downregulation   A decrease in the number of cellular receptors to a molecule resulting in reduced sensitivity to the molecule.

drug   A substance used to diagnose, prevent, or treat disease.

dystocia   Difficult birth.

ectoparasite   A parasite that lives on the outside body surface of its host.

ectropion   A rolling outward (i.e., away from the eye) or sagging of the eyelid. Many times, the conjunctiva is plainly visible.

effector   A gland, organ, or tissue that responds to nerve stimulation with a specific action.

efficacy   The extent to which a drug causes the intended effects in a patient.

electrolyte   A substance that dissociates into ions when placed in solution, becoming capable of conducting electricity.

elixir   A hydroalcoholic liquid that contains sweeteners, flavoring, and a medicinal agent.

emesis   The act of vomiting.

emetic   A substance or drug that induces vomiting.

empirical   Based on observation and personal experience.

emulsion   A medicinal agent that consists of oily substances dispersed in an aqueous medium with an additive to stabilize the dispersion.

endometrium   The mucous membrane lining of the uterus.

endoparasite   A parasite that lives inside the body of its host.

endothelial layer   The smooth layer of epithelial cells that line blood vessels.

enteric coating   Acid resistant coating on a tablet that prevents it from being dissolved in an acid environment such as the stomach and are activated (dissolved) only when they reach an alkaline environment such as the small intestine.

entropion   A rolling inward (i.e., toward the cornea) of the eyelid.

equivalent weight   One gram molecular weight (from periodic chart) divided by the total positive valence of the material.

erythema   Redness of the skin caused by congestion of the capillaries.

erythropoiesis   The formation of erythrocytes.

erythropoietin   A glycoprotein hormone secreted mainly by the kidney; it acts on stem cells of the bone marrow to stimulate red blood cell production.

euthyroid   A normal thyroid gland.

expectorant   A drug that enhances the expulsion of secretions from the respiratory tract.

extralabel use   The use of a drug that is not specifically listed on the U.S. Food and Drug Administration (FDA)-approved label.

exudation   Leakage of fluid, cells, or cellular debris from blood vessels and their deposition in or on the tissue.

fatty acid   Organic compound of carbon, hydrogen, and oxygen that is esterified with glycerol to form fat.

feed efficiency   The rate at which animals convert feed into tissue. It is expressed as the number of pounds or kilograms of feed needed to produce 1 lb or 1 kg of animal.

feedback   The return of some of the output product of a process as input in a way that controls the process.

fibrinolysis   Fibrin (clot) breakdown through the action of the enzyme plasmin.

FIFO   Acronym for "first in, first out."

first-pass effect   Some orally administered drugs are rapidly metabolized in the liver; the concentration of the drug is greatly reduced before it reaches systemic circulation.

FOB   Acronym for "free on board."

FOB destination   Title of possession passes from the pharmaceutic company to the buyer (i.e., the purchaser) when the shipment is delivered to the buyer's business destination (i.e., the veterinary facility).

FOB shipping point   Title passes from the pharmaceutic company to the purchaser when the vendor places the goods in the possession of the carrier (e.g., United Parcel Service, Federal Express, Averitt Express).

full-service company   A pharmaceutic company that offers full service (e.g., the company employs sales representatives [reps] who visit veterinary facilities), usually with a limited number of products.

fungicidal   An agent that kills fungi.

fungistatic   An agent that inhibits the growth of fungi.

furuncle (furunculosis)   A focal suppurative inflammation of the skin and subcutaneous tissue; also known as a *boil*.

ganglionic synapse   The site of the synapse between neuron one and neuron two of the autonomic nervous system.

glaucoma   A group of eye diseases characterized by increased intraocular pressure that results in damage to the retina and the optic nerve.

gonadotropin   A hormone that stimulates the ovaries or testes.

granulation tissue   New tissue formed in the healing of wounds of the soft tissue, consisting of connective tissue cells and ingrown young vessels; it ultimately forms a scar.

Green Book   An on-line resource listing all FDA-approved animal drugs.

half-life   The amount of time (usually expressed in hours) that it takes for the quantity of a drug in the body to be reduced by 50%.

helminths   Parasitic worms, including nematodes, cestodes, and trematodes.

hematemesis   Vomiting of blood (the vomitus often resembles coffee grounds).

hematuria   Blood in the urine.

histamine   A chemical mediator of the inflammatory response released from mast cells. Histamine may cause dilation and increased permeability of small blood vessels, constriction of small airways, increased secretion of mucus in the airways, and pain.

Horner's syndrome   Paralysis of the sympathetic nerve supply to the eye that may cause enophthalmos, ptosis of the upper eyelid, slight elevation of the lower eyelid, constriction of the pupil, and narrowing of the palpebral tissue.

humidification   Addition of moisture to the air.

hybridoma   A cell culture that consists of a clone of a hybrid cell formed by fusing cells of different types, such as stimulated mouse plasma cells and myeloma cells.

hyperalgesia   A heightened sense of pain.

hyperkalemia   An excess of potassium in the blood.

hypernatremia   An excess of sodium in the blood.

hypertension   Persistently high blood pressure.

hypertonic solution   Having an osmolality higher than 300 mOsm/L.

hypertonus   The state characterized by an increased tonicity or tension.

hyphema   A condition in which red blood cells are present in the anterior chamber of the eye(s).

hypokalemia   Abnormally low potassium concentration in the blood.

hyponatremia   A deficiency of sodium in the blood.

hypophyseal portal system   This is the portal system of the pituitary gland in which venules from the hypothalamus connect with capillaries of the anterior pituitary.

hypotonic solution   Having an osmolality less than 300 mOsm/L.

hypovolemia   Decreased volume of circulating blood.

iatrogenic   Caused by the physician (veterinarian).

immunoglobulin A (IgA)   Class of antibody produced on mucous membrane surfaces, such as those of the respiratory tract.

in vitro   Within an artificial environment.

in vivo   Within the living body.

inotrope   A drug that affects the strength or force of cardiac muscle contractions.

inotropic   Affecting the force of cardiac muscle contraction.

inspissated   Thickened or dried out.

integumentary system   Pertaining to, or composed of, skin.

interleukins   A group of polypeptide cytokines that carry signals between cells in the immune system.

intracameral injection   An injection into the anterior chamber of the eye.

intravenous bolus   A single, precise amount of medication or fluids given, one time intravenously.

intravenous infusion   A controlled administration of fluids, including drugs, directly into the vein, over a period of time. The most common method used is an infusion pump.

inventory   The quantity of goods or assets that a veterinary facility possesses, requiring proactive control to keep supplies stable and current.

inventory control manager (ICM)   A person (many times a licensed veterinary medical technician [LVMT]) responsible for monitoring, ordering, and maintaining inventory in a veterinary facility.

invoice   A form generated by a company that documents the quantity and price of each item ordered by the inventory control manager.

involution   The return of a reproductive organ to normal size after delivery.

iodophor   An iodine compound with a longer activity period that results from the combination of iodine and a carrier molecule that releases iodine over time.

isotonic solution   Having an osmolality equal to 300 mOsm/L.

keratitis   Inflammation of the cornea.

keratolytic   An agent that promotes loosening or separation of the horny layer of the epidermis.

keratoplastic   An agent that promotes normalization of the development of keratin.

ketone bodies   Excessive ketones made from fat as an emergency fuel source. Ketone levels increase causing a shift in the acid/base balance.

legend   Legend drugs are required by law to be dispensed on or by the order of a licensed veterinarian or physician.

levo isomer   Left-sided arrangement of a molecule that may exist in a left- or a right-sided configuration. Levo and dextro isomers have the same molecular formula.

liniment   A medicine in an oily, soapy, or alcoholic vehicle to be rubbed on the skin to relieve pain or to act as a counterirritant.

loading dose   It is an initial higher dose of a drug given at the beginning of a treatment to rapidly achieve a therapeutic concentration in the body.

lower motor neurons   Peripheral neurons whose cell bodies lie in the central gray columns of the spinal cord and whose terminations lie in skeletal muscle.

A sufficient number of lesions of lower motor neurons cause muscles supplied by the nerve to atrophy, resulting in weak reflexes and flaccid paralysis.

mail order discount house   A company that accepts orders from the buyer by telephone; a good source for ordering items such as gauze, cotton, isopropyl alcohol, or paper towels.

manufacturing   The bulk production of drugs for resale outside of the veterinarian–client–patient relationship.

margin   The actual profit a practice makes on each sale.

markup   The amount of money over cost for which a product sells. Markup percentages vary from practice to practice, but all markups reflect a retail value over wholesale value.

matrix   The intercellular substance of tissues like cartilage and bone.

melena   Dark or black stools that result from blood staining. Bleeding has occurred in the anterior part of the gastrointestinal tract.

metabolic acidosis   Decreased body pH caused by excess hydrogen ions in the extracellular fluid.

metabolic alkalosis   Increased body pH caused by excess bicarbonate in the extracellular fluid.

metabolism (biotransformation)   The biochemical process that alters a drug from an active form to a form that is inactive or that can be eliminated from the body.

metastasis   Generally refers to the transfer of cancer cells from one site to another.

metered dose inhaler (MDI)   A hand held device that uses a propellant to deliver a specific amount of medication that is inhaled into the lungs by the patient.

methemoglobinemia   The presence of methemoglobin in the blood caused by injury or toxic agents that convert a larger-than-normal proportion of hemoglobin into methemoglobin, which does not function as an oxygen carrier.

microfilaria   A prelarval stage of a filarial worm transmitted to the biting insect from the principal host (e.g., filarial stage of *Dirofilaria immitis*).

microorganism   An organism that is microscopic (e.g., bacterium, protozoan, Rickettsia, virus, and fungus).

milliequivalent A term used to express the concentration of electrolytes in a solution; 1/1000 of an equivalent weight.

minimum alveolar concentration (MAC) A measure of potency and is the alveolar concentration that prevents movement in 50% of patients in response to a painful stimulus. Lower numbers indicate more potent agents.

miosis Contraction of the pupil.

miotic A drug used to constrict the pupil.

modulation The modification of nociceptive transmission.

monovalent A vaccine, antiserum, or antitoxin developed specifically for a single antigen or organism.

motilin A hormone secreted by cells in the duodenal mucosa that causes contraction of intestinal smooth muscle.

MRSA Methicillin-resistant *Staphylococcus aureus.*

mucolytic Having the ability to break down mucus.

multimodal analgesia The use of different drugs with different actions to produce optimal analgesia and minimize individual drug quantities when possible.

muscarinic receptors Receptors activated by acetylcholine and muscarine that are found in glands, the heart, and smooth muscle. An acronym for remembering muscarinic effects is SLUD: S, salivation; L, lacrimation; U, urination; D, defecation.

mydriasis Dilation of the pupil.

myeloma A malignant neoplasm of plasma cells (B lymphocytes).

myelosuppression Inhibition of bone marrow activity that results in decreased production of blood cells and platelets.

myofibril A muscle fibril composed of numerous myofilaments.

nasogastric (intubation) Passing a flexible tube through the nasal passages into the stomach.

nebulization The process of converting liquid medications into a spray that can be carried into the respiratory system by inhaled air.

nematodes Parasitic worms, including intestinal roundworms, filarial worms, lungworms, kidney worms, heartworms, and others.

nephrology The study of the urinary (renal) system.

nephron The basic functional unit of the kidney.

nephrotoxic Toxic to the kidneys.

nerve block A loss of feeling or sensation produced by injecting an anesthetic agent around a nerve to interfere with its ability to conduct impulses.

neuroleptanalgesia A combination of an opioid with a tranquilizer or sedative.

neuropathic pain Pain that originates from injury or involvement of the peripheral or central nervous system.

nicotinic receptors Receptors activated by acetylcholine and nicotine found at the neuromuscular junction of the skeletal muscle and at the ganglionic synapses.

nitrogen balance The condition of the body as it relates to protein intake and use. Positive nitrogen balance implies a net gain in body protein.

nociception The reception, conduction, and central nervous system processing of nerve signals generated by nociceptors.

nociceptor A receptor for pain caused by injury to body tissue. Pain sensation arises in the terminal ends of sensory nerve fibers.

noncore vaccine Optional vaccines that are considered for animals at risk for developing disease based on geographic location and the lifestyle of the animal.

nonproductive cough A cough that does not result in coughing up of mucus, secretions, or debris (a dry cough).

nutraceutical Any nontoxic food component that has scientifically proven health benefits.

ointment A semisolid preparation that contains medicinal agents for application to the skin or eyes.

oncotic pressure The osmotic pressure generated by plasma proteins in the blood.

open-angle glaucoma A type of primary glaucoma of the eye in which the angle of the anterior chamber remains open, but filtration of the aqueous humor is gradually reduced, causing an increase in intraocular pressure.

organophosphate A substance that can interfere with the function of the nervous system by inhibiting the enzyme cholinesterase.

osmotic pressure The ability of solute molecules to attract water.

otoacariasis Infestation of ear mites.

ototoxic Toxic to the ears.

over-the-counter drug A drug that can be purchased without a prescription; these drugs contain ingredients that are safe or have low concentrations of an active ingredient.

packing slip A document supplied by the vendor that accompanies a purchase. A packing slip generally reflects quantities ordered, not prices.

parasitiasis A condition in which an animal harbors an endoparasite or an ectoparasite but no clinical signs of infection or infestation are evident.

parasitosis A condition in which an animal harbors an endoparasite or an ectoparasite and clinical signs of infection or infestation are evident.

parasympathetic nervous system That portion of the autonomic nervous system that arises from the craniosacral portion of the spinal cord, is mediated by the neurotransmitter acetylcholine, and is concerned primarily with conserving and restoring a steady state in the body.

parasympatholytic A drug used to inhibit the activity of the parasympathetic nervous system.

parasympathomimetic A drug that mimics the effects of stimulating the parasympathetic nervous system.

parenteral The route of administration of injectable drugs.

parenteral administration By a route other than the alimentary canal (e.g., intramuscular, subcutaneous, intravenous).

parietal cell A cell located in the gastric mucosa that secretes hydrochloric acid.

partition coefficient The ratio of the solubility of substances (e.g., gas anesthetics) between two states in which they may be found (e.g., blood and gas, gas and rubber goods).

passive immunity Immunity that occurs by administration of antibody produced in another individual.

pathologic pain Pain with an exaggerated response; it is often associated with tissue injury due to trauma or surgery.

percent concentration An expression of the strength of a substance based on the ratio of parts per hundred (e.g., 25%).

perception The processing and recognition of pain in the cerebral hemispheres.

peristalsis   A wave of smooth muscle contraction that passes along a tubular structure (gastrointestinal or other) and moves the contents of that structure forward.

physiologic pain   The protective sensation of pain that allows individuals to move away from potential tissue damage.

polydipsia   Excessive thirst manifested by increased water consumption.

polyuria   Excessive urination.

polyvalent   A vaccine, antiserum, or antitoxin active against multiple antigens or organisms; mixed vaccine.

precision vaporizer   A part of the anesthesia machine, located out of the circuit, used to convert a liquid anesthetic to a gas state and produce a precise concentration of anesthetic vapor in the carrier gas (oxygen) passing through the vaporizer and delivered to the patient. They are designed for use with only one specific anesthetic agent.

preemptive analgesia   Analgesia administered before the painful stimulus to help prevent sensitization and windup.

preload   The volume of blood in the ventricles at the end of diastole.

premature ventricular contraction (PVC)   Contraction of the ventricles without a corresponding contraction of the atria. PVCs arise from an irritable focus or foci in the ventricles.

prescription (legend) drug   A drug that is limited to use under the supervision of a veterinarian because of potential danger, difficulty of administration, or other considerations. The legend that designates a prescription drug states the following: "Caution: Federal law restricts this drug to use by or on the order of a licensed veterinarian."

preservative   A substance, such as an antibiotic, antiinfective, or fungistat, that is added to a product to destroy or inhibit multiplication of microorganisms.

primary hypothyroidism   Hypothyroidism resulting from a pathologic condition in the thyroid.

primary intention healing   Healing of a clean, uninfected, surgical incision that is approximated by sutures.

productive cough   A cough that results in coughing up of mucus, secretions, or debris.

prostaglandin   A substance synthesized by cells from arachidonic acid that serves as a mediator of inflammation and has other physiologic functions.

pruritus   Itching.

pseudomembranous colitis   A severe acute inflammation of the bowel mucosa.

pyoderma   Any skin disease characterized by the presence or formation of pus.

ratio concentration   An expression of the strength of a substance based on the ratio of its parts (e.g., 1:32).

recombinant DNA technology   A process that removes a gene from one organism or pathogen and inserts it into the DNA of another. This also may be referred to as *gene splicing*.

regimen   A program for administration of a drug that includes the route, the dose (how much), the frequency (how often), and the duration (for how long) of administration.

regional anesthesia   Loss of feeling or sensation in a large area (region) of the body after injection of an anesthetic agent into the spinal canal or around peripheral nerves.

regurgitation   Casting up of undigested or semidigested (ruminant) foodstuff from the esophagus or rumen.

releasing factor (releasing hormone)   A hormone produced by the hypothalamus and transported to the anterior pituitary to stimulate the release of trophic hormones.

repolarization   The return of the cell membrane to its resting polarity after depolarization.

residue   An amount of a drug still present in animal tissue or products (e.g., meat, milk, eggs) at a particular point (slaughter or collection).

retroperitoneal   Located behind the peritoneum.

reverse sneeze   Aspiration reflex— short periods of noisy inspiratory effort in dogs.

scheduled drug or controlled drug   Controlled substances are regulated by federal and state laws. They are placed into five categories based on their abuse potential.

seborrhea   An increase in scaling of the skin; sebum production may or may not be increased.

seborrhea oleosa   Condition characterized by scaling and excess lipid production that forms brownish yellow clumps, which adhere to the hair and skin.

seborrhea sicca   Characterized by dry skin and white to gray scales that do not adhere to the hair or skin.

seborrheic dermatitis   An inflammatory type of seborrhea characterized by scaling and greasiness.

secondary intention healing   Healing of a wound by granulation tissue formation, contraction, and epithelization to achieve structural integrity.

sedative   A drug used to suppress brain activity and awareness; reduced excitement by causing sleepiness.

segmentation   Periodic constriction of segments of the intestine without movement backward or forward; a mixing rather than a propulsive movement.

solute   A substance dissolved in a solvent to form a solution.

solution   A mixture of two or more substances that are combined with each other.

solvent   A solution capable of dissolving other substances.

somatic pain   Pain arising from bones, joints, muscle, or skin. Somatic pain is described in humans as localized, sharp, constant, aching, or throbbing.

speculum   An instrument for dilating a body orifice or cavity to allow visual inspection.

sporicidal   An agent capable of killing spores.

statement   A document generated by the vendor that details the quantity and pricing of all goods purchased (usually in 1 month) by the buyer. The total balance is generally expected to be paid in full within 30 days.

stem cell   Cells found in embryonic tissue and the adult animal that have the ability for self-renewal, a lack of cellular specialization, and can give rise to other more specialized cells.

stock solution   A concentrated solution that will be diluted to a weaker solution for use.

stroke volume   The amount of blood ejected by the left ventricle with each beat.

surfactant   A mixture of phospholipids secreted by type II alveolar cells that reduce surface tension in pulmonary fluids.

suspension   A preparation of solid particles dispersed in a liquid but not dissolved in it.

symbiosis   Two living organisms of different species living together.

sympathetic nervous system That portion of the autonomic nervous system that arises from the thoracolumbar spinal cord, is mediated by catecholamines, and is concerned with the fight-or-flight response.

sympatholytic A drug used to inhibit the activity of the sympathetic nervous system; block the effects of the adrenergic neurotransmitters.

sympathomimetic A drug that mimics the effects of stimulating the sympathetic nervous system.

systole Contraction of the heart muscle.

tachyarrhythmia Tachycardia associated with an irregularity in normal heart rhythm.

tachycardia A faster-than-normal heart rate.

tachypnea Rapid breathing.

teratogenic An agent that causes harm to the developing fetus.

therapeutic index Relationship between a drug's ability to achieve the desired effect and its tendency to produce toxic effects.

thrombocytopenia A decreased number of platelets.

thromboembolism The condition that occurs when thrombus material becomes dislodged and is transported by the bloodstream to another site.

thrombophlebitis Inflammation of a vein associated with a thrombus formation.

thrombus A clot in the circulatory system.

total cost A measure that includes the cost of an item plus tax.

total nutrient admixture A solution used for parenteral administration that contains amino acids, lipids, dextrose, vitamins, and minerals.

totipotent (stem cell) A cell existing in the zygote and fertilized oocyte that is capable of creating an entire animal including extra-embryonic membranes.

toxoid Inactivated toxin that has been weakened by a chemical or heat treatment to eliminate the toxic qualities but retain antigenic properties.

tranquilizer A drug used to calm a patient by decreasing anxiety, not necessarily reduce awareness.

transcellular fluid Cerebrospinal fluid, aqueous humor of the eye, synovial fluid, gastrointestinal fluid, lymph, bile, and glandular and respiratory secretions.

transdermal application The use of a patch applied to the skin to deliver a drug through an intact cutaneous surface to the systemic circulation.

transduction The process that involves translation of noxious stimuli into electric activity at sensory nerve endings.

transmission Conduction of pain impulses from peripheral pain receptors to the spinal cord.

triage Process of sorting patients in an emergency based on medical priority. The goal is to quickly and systematically evaluate an animal for their injuries and determine which body system or which animal needs attention first.

trophic hormone A hormone that results in production of a second hormone in a target gland.

turgor Degree of fullness or congestion; describes the degree of elasticity of the skin.

turnover The number of times a product is sold or used up in a veterinary facility. The minimum turnover rate should be established at four times a year.

upper motor neurons Neurons in the cerebral cortex that conduct impulses from the motor cortex to the motor nuclei of the cerebral nerves or to the ventral gray columns of the spinal column. A sufficient number of lesions of upper motor neurons interrupt the inhibitory effect that upper motor neurons have on lower motor neurons, resulting in exaggerated or hyperactive reflexes.

upregulation An increase in the number of cellular receptors to a molecule resulting in an increased sensitivity to the molecule.

uremia Abnormally high concentrations of urea, creatinine, and other nitrogenous end products of protein and amino acid metabolism in the blood.

urinary incontinence Lack of voluntary control over the normal excretion of urine.

urinary tract infection Infection of the urinary tract. Infection may be localized or may affect the entire urinary tract.

uvea The vascular layer of the eye that comprises the iris, ciliary body, and choroid.

uveitis Inflammation of the uvea.

vapor pressure Vapor pressure of an agent indicates how volatile it is and the maximum concentration that can be achieved. Vapor pressure of an inhalant anesthetic is a measure of its tendency to evaporate.

vermicide A drug that kills internal parasites.

vermifuge A drug that paralyzes the internal parasite and gets expelled from the gastrointestinal tract into the feces.

vesicant A substance that causes blister formation.

veterinarian–client–patient relationship The set of circumstances that must exist between the veterinarian, the client, and the patient before the dispensing of prescription drugs is appropriate.

veterinary supply distributor An intermediate company (i.e., not full service, not mail order) that generally stocks a large inventory and employs sales representatives who visit veterinary facilities.

virulence The ability of an infectious agent to produce pathologic effects.

visceral pain Pain arising from stretching, distension, or inflammation of viscera, described in humans as deep, cramping, or aching and difficult to localize.

viscid Sticky.

vomiting center An area in the medulla that may be stimulated by the chemoreceptor trigger zone, the cerebrum, or peripheral receptors to induce vomiting.

withdrawal time The period of time from when the last dose of medication is administered to when the animal can be slaughtered for food or milk and eggs can be consumed safely.

wolbachia A gram-negative intracellular bacteria living in the body of both the immature and adult heartworms; they play an important role in the worm's survival and pathogenesis of the disease.

INDEX

2.5% dextrose solutions
  with half-strength lactated Ringer's
    solution, 311
  with saline 0.45%, 311
2-PAM, 264b, 431t–473t
4-Methylpyrazole, 431t–473t
5-Fluorouracil, 334, 440t–473t
5-HT$_3$ antagonists, 148
6-Aminosalicylic acid, 440t–473t
6-Mercaptopurine, 440t–473t
50% dextrose solutions, 315, 315b

A

Abbreviations, 426
ABCB1 gene, 9
Abdominocentesis, 138
Absorption, 8–10, 8f
ACE inhibitors. *See* Angiotensin-
  converting enzyme (ACE) inhibitors
Acemannan, 338, 374
Acepromazine, 78, 440t–473t
  acepromazine maleate, 79, 79b
  acepromazine/morphine, 86
  acepromazine/oxymorphone, 86
Acepromazine maleate, 79, 79b,
  474t–480t
Acetamide, 431t–439t
Acetaminophen, 280, 431t–480t
  classification of, 474t–480t
Acetaminophen–codeine, 474t–480t
Acetazolamide, 114, 440t–480t
Acetic acid/boric acid, 205
Acetylcholine, 72–73, 75–76, 91
Acetylcholinesterase, 76, 90–91
Acetylcholinesterase inhibitors,
  154–155, 155b
Acetylcysteine, 102, 420, 420b, 440t–480t
  antidotes for, 102
  classification of, 474t–480t
Acetylsalicylic acid, 440t–473t. *See also*
  Aspirin
Acid-base balance, 97, 297
Acid citrate dextrose (ACD) solution,
  327

Acid-fast bacilli, 214
Acidifiers
  classification of, 474t–480t
  urinary, 116–117, 116b
Acidifying agent, 474t–480t
Actimmune gamma-1b, 338
Activated charcoal, 153, 153b, 418–419,
  419f, 440t–473t
Active immunity production, 346–349.
  See also Vaccines
Acute renal failure, 113–114
Acyclovir, 192, 239, 474t–480t
Addison's disease, 287
Additives
  drug, 28
  fluid, 313–315
Adenohypophysis, 161
Adenosine triphosphate (ATP), 9
Adequan, 440t–473t
Adequan Canine, 379
Adequan I.M., 379
ADH. *See* Adrenal-dependent
  hyperadrenocorticism (ADH);
  Antidiuretic hormone (ADH)
Adjuvants, 370–371
Administration routes and techniques,
  6–12
  client education and, 46
  controlled substances and, 43–46,
    45f, 45b. *See also* Controlled
    substances
  dispensed medication labeling and,
    43, 45f
    contents requirements, 43
    examples of, 45f
  dosage forms, 26–28
    capsules, 26–27
    elixirs, 27
    emulsions, 27
    implants, 28
    intravenous (IV) infusions, 27–28
    liniments, 28
    liquid preparations, 27, 27f, 27b
    lotions, 28

Administration routes and techniques
  (Continued)
    microencapsulation, 28
    ointments, 28
    parenteral injections, 27–28, 27f
    preservatives in, 28–32
    reconstitution methods, 29b
    solvents in, 28–32
    suspensions, 27
    syringes and needles for, 28,
      30b–32b
    tablets, 26–27, 27f
    topical, 28
  drug storage and, 46b
  medication orders, 42–43, 44f
  parenteral. *See* Parenteral
    administration
  routes, 6–12, 32–42
    comparisons of, 8
    inhalation, 8, 40, 42f–43f
    intramuscular, 39–40
    oral, 6–8, 32–35, 33f–35f, 33b
    parenteral, 27f, 35–39, 35b, 39b
    subcutaneous, 40
    topical, 8, 42
  veterinary technician roles in, 26,
    32, 46
Adrenal-dependent
  hyperadrenocorticism (ADH),
  173
Adrenal suppressant, 474t–480t
Adrenergic agents, 77–78
Adrenergic agonist, 474t–480t
Adrenergic antagonists, 114–115
Adrenergic receptor
  responses, 76t
  types, 76f
Adrenergic receptor responses, 76t
Adrenocorticotropic hormone, 162,
  163t
  corticosteroids, 285
Adrenolytic agent, 474t–480t
Adsorbents, 152–153, 153b
Adsorbotear, 193

Note: Page number followed by "f" indicate figures, "t" indicate tables, and "b" indicate boxes.